Frontiers in Clinical Drug Research - Anti-Cancer Agents
Volume 3

Edited By

Atta-ur-Rahman, *FRS*

Kings College
University of Cambridge
Cambridge
UK

advertisements or ideas contained in the Work.

Limitation of Liability:

In no event will Bentham Science Publishers, its staff, editors and/or authors, be liable for any damages, including, without limitation, special, incidental and/or consequential damages and/or damages for lost data and/or profits arising out of (whether directly or indirectly) the use or inability to use the Work. The entire liability of Bentham Science Publishers shall be limited to the amount actually paid by you for the Work.

General:

1. Any dispute or claim arising out of or in connection with this License Agreement or the Work (including non-contractual disputes or claims) will be governed by and construed in accordance with the laws of the U.A.E. as applied in the Emirate of Dubai. Each party agrees that the courts of the Emirate of Dubai shall have exclusive jurisdiction to settle any dispute or claim arising out of or in connection with this License Agreement or the Work (including non-contractual disputes or claims).
2. Your rights under this License Agreement will automatically terminate without notice and without the need for a court order if at any point you breach any terms of this License Agreement. In no event will any delay or failure by Bentham Science Publishers in enforcing your compliance with this License Agreement constitute a waiver of any of its rights.
3. You acknowledge that you have read this License Agreement, and agree to be bound by its terms and conditions. To the extent that any other terms and conditions presented on any website of Bentham Science Publishers conflict with, or are inconsistent with, the terms and conditions set out in this License Agreement, you acknowledge that the terms and conditions set out in this License Agreement shall prevail.

Bentham Science Publishers Ltd.
Executive Suite Y - 2
PO Box 7917, Saif Zone
Sharjah, U.A.E.
Email: subscriptions@benthamscience.org

**BENTHAM
SCIENCE**

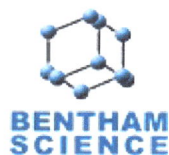

CONTENTS

Saïd C. Azoury, David M. Straughan, Robert D. Bennett and *Vivek Shukla*

PREFACE

The third volume of *Frontiers in Clinical Drug Research - Anti-Cancer Agents* presents seven cutting edge reviews on recent developments in various therapeutic approaches against different types of cancer.

Studies have revealed that the Epidermal Growth Factor Receptor (EGFR) is involved in the pathogenesis and progression of different types of carcinoma. Tumor resistance to agents targeting the Epidermal Growth Factor Receptor (EGFR) is common, and is well recognized as a major challenge. In first two consecutive chapters, Rodney B. Luwor provides an overview of the progress in targeting the EGFR that will lead to overall refractory outcomes to anti-EGFR therapies. In Chapter 1 he discusses on the resistance mechanisms driven by alterations in ligand and receptors of the EGFR family as well as on the cross-talk between EGFR receptors and non-EGFR family members. In Chapter 2 the same author describes the current understanding regarding the resistance mechanisms mediated by alterations in substrates downstream of the EGFR. Luwor has also reviewed the other intracellular mechanisms that mediate both sensitivity and resistance outcomes to anti-EGFR agents in this chapter.

Melanoma is the most dangerous form of skin cancer that develops when unrepaired DNA damage to skin cells triggers mutations, which lead to the formation malignant tumors. In Chapter 3 Shukla *et al.*, present a comprehensive review on the chemotherapeutic, immunologic, and molecularly targeted therapy approaches to the treatment of advanced melanoma.

In various tumor cells, there is increased aerobic glycolysis that represents a major biochemical alteration associated with malignant transformation. This phenomenon is known as the Warburg effect. 18F-deoxyglucose positron emission tomography (18FDG–PET), a metabolic imaging technique, is based on the avidity of cancer cells for glucose; currently, it represents the only successful exploitation of the Warburg effect for medical purposes. In Chapter 4, Abreu and Urbano focus on past and current efforts to target the Warburg effect for selective anti-cancer therapeutics.

Follicular lymphoma (FL) is a B-cell lymphoma and the most common slow-growing form of non-Hodgkin lymphoma (NHL). Studies suggest that immunotherapy, radioimmunotherapy and vaccines result in high response rates and survival in FL patients. Chapter 5 by Panizo *et al.*, briefly describes the biology and conventional treatment of follicular lymphoma with immunochemotherapy. They also discuss novel immunotherapy strategies (active and passive) for the treatment of follicular lymphoma.

The progression of cancer involves epigenetic abnormalities along with genetic alterations. The manipulation of epigenetic alterations holds great promise for the prevention, detection, and therapy of cancer. Evidence indicates that the activities of key epigenetic regulators including DNA methyltransferases and histone modification enzymes are sensitive to cellular metabolism. Wong and Yu in Chapter 6 discuss that the cross-talk between epigenetics and cancer cell metabolism may reveal novel therapeutic opportunities. They also highlight their implications in oncogenesis, and potential therapeutic approaches to target these cancer specific abnormities.

Apoptosis is a programmed cell death, which involves various biochemical events that lead to characteristic cell changes and death. Dysfunctions of apoptosis pathways promote oncogenesis as well as confer resistance of cancer cells to most conventional therapies. In Chapter 7 by Moorthy *et al.* focus their discussion small molecular anticancer drugs, especially target proteins, responsible for apoptosis.

I hope that the current volume of this book series will provide fresh insights into development of new recent approaches to anti-cancer therapy for interested researchers and pharmaceutical scientists. I would like to thank the editorial staff, particularly Mr. Mahmood Alam (Director Publications) and Mr. Shehzad Naqvi (Senior Manager Publications) for their hard work and dedicated efforts.

Atta-ur-Rahman, *FRS*
Kings College
University of Cambridge
Cambridge
UK

List of Contributors

Ana M. Urbano	Unidade de Química-Física Molecular and Departamento de Ciências da Vida, Faculdade de Ciências e Tecnologia, Universidade de Coimbra, Coimbra, Portugal
Ascensión López Díaz de Cerio	Hematology Department, Clínica Universidad de Navarra, Pamplona, Spain
Carlos Panizo	Hematology Department, Clínica Universidad de Navarra, Pamplona, Spain
Chi Chun Wong	Department of Medicine and Therapeutics, State Key Laboratory of Digestive Disease, Li Ka Shing Institute of Health Sciences, Shenzhen Research Institute, The Chinese University of Hong Kong, Hong Kong
C. Karthikeyan	Departamento de Química e Bioquímica, Faculdade de Ciências, Universidade do Porto, s/n, Rua do Campo Alegre, 4169-007 Porto, Portugal
David M. Straughan	Department of Surgery, University of South Florida, Morsani College of Medicine, Tampa, FL, USA
Esther Pena	Hematology Department, Complejo Hospitalario de Navarra, Pamplona, Spain
Jun Yu	Department of Medicine and Therapeutics, State Key Laboratory of Digestive Disease, Li Ka Shing Institute of Health Sciences, Shenzhen Research Institute, The Chinese University of Hong Kong, Hong Kong
N.S. Hari Narayana Moorthy	Departamento de Química e Bioquímica, Faculdade de Ciências, Universidade do Porto, s/n, Rua do Campo Alegre, Porto, Portugal: School of Pharmaceutical Sciences, Rajiv Gandhi Proudyogiki Vishwavidyalaya, Airport Bypass Road, Gandhi Nagar, Bhopal, India
Nicolás Martínez-Calle	Hematology Department, Clínica Universidad de Navarra, Pamplona, Spain
Patrícia L. Abreu	Unidade de Química-Física Molecular and Departamento de Ciências da Vida, Faculdade de Ciências e Tecnologia, Universidade de Coimbra, Coimbra, Portugal
Piyush Trivedi	School of Pharmaceutical Sciences, Rajiv Gandhi Proudyogiki Vishwavidyalaya, Bhopal (MP)-462033, India
Ricardo García-Muñoz	Hematology Department, Hospital San Pedro, Logroño, Spain
Robert D. Bennett	Department of Surgery, University of South Florida, Morsani College of Medicine, Tampa, FL, USA
Rodney B. Luwor	Department of Surgery, The Royal Melbourne Hospital, The University of Melbourne, Parkville, Victoria 3050, Australia
Saïd C. Azoury	Department of Surgery, The Johns Hopkins Hospital, Baltimore, MD, USA

Susana Inogés   Hematology Department, Clínica Universidad de Navarra, Pamplona, Spain

Vivek Shukla   Thoracic and GI Oncology Branch, National Cancer Institute, National Institutes of Health, Bethesda, MD, USA

Frontiers in Clinical Drug Research - Anti-Cancer Agents
Volume 3

2

Frontiers in Clinical Drug Research - Anti-Cancer Agents

[Volume 3]

ISSN (Online): 2215-0803

ISSN (Print): 2451-8905

Frontiers in Clinical Drug Research - Anti-Cancer Agents

Editor: Atta-ur-Rahman, *FRS*

ISBN (eBook): 978-1-68108-289-9

ISBN (Print): 978-1-68108-290-5

©[2016], Bentham eBooks imprint.

Published by Bentham Science Publishers – Sharjah, UAE. All Rights Reserved.

CHAPTER 1

Tumor Resistance Mechanisms to Inhibitors Targeting the Epidermal Growth Factor Receptor– Part I: Extracellular Molecules

Rodney B. Luwor*

Department of Surgery, The Royal Melbourne Hospital, The University of Melbourne, Parkville, Victoria 3050, Australia

Abstract: Since its discovery several decades ago, the Epidermal Growth Factor Receptor (EGFR) has become one of the most extensively studies receptor tyrosine kinases. However, despite continued insight into the cancer promoting properties of the EGFR and its downstream signalling substrates, clinical use of agents targeting the EGFR continue to yield modest outcomes. Clinically, approved anti-EGFR therapeutics can successfully inhibit receptor activation. However major tumour regression is observed in only 10-30% of advanced unselected cancer patients, with most patients showing no therapeutic benefit. Furthermore, those who initially respond commonly relapse presenting with reoccurrence of tumours that are frequently resistant to the original therapy. In addition, the standard course of treatment of such agents is estimated to cost between "US $15,000-80,000/patient" for an improved overall survival of only 1-2 months. Therefore, it is both medically and financially critical to determine the true molecular mechanisms of tumour resistance, and how it can be overcome. In these 2 back-to-back chapters, we will provide an overview of the progress made in targeting the EGFR and discuss the challenges presented by the numerous molecular mechanisms currently identified, leading to overall refractory outcomes to anti-EGFR therapeutics. In this chapter (Part I) we will specifically focus on the resistance mechanisms driven by alterations in ligand and receptors of the EGFR family and cross-talk between EGFR receptors and non-EGFR family members.

Keywords: Afatinib, Cancer, Cetuximab, Epidermal Growth Factor Receptor,

* **Corresponding author Rodney B. Luwor:** Department of Surgery, The Royal Melbourne Hospital, The University of Melbourne, Parkville, Victoria 3050, Australia; Tel: +613 8344 3027 Fax: +613 9347 6488; E-mail: rluwor@unimelb.edu.au

Atta-ur-Rahman (Ed.)

Erlotinib, Gefitinib, Lapatinib, Panitumumab, Resistance, Signaling, Therapeutics, Tumor.

1. INTRODUCTION

Since the discovery of the Epidermal Growth Factor (EGF) in 1962 by Stanley Cohen and colleagues [1] tremendous advances in our understanding of the sophisticated interactions between growth factors and their accompanying cell surface receptors have been made. One of the most intensely studied classes of receptors is the HER or ErbB family [2]. This family consists of four members, the Epidermal Growth Factor Receptor (EGFR) (also referred to as ErbB1 or HER1) [3], HER2 (p185[Neu] or ErbB2) [4], HER3 (ErbB3) [5] and HER4 (ErbB4) [6]. All 4 family members share a similar overall structure consisting of an extracellular domain with 2 cysteine-rich regions, a single membrane-spanning region and a cytoplasmic domain containing multiple tyrosine residues that are phosphorylated upon receptor activation [7, 8].

The *EGFR* gene is located on the short arm of chromosome 7 [9, 10], and encodes an 1186 amino acid long, 140 KDa polypeptide chain [3, 11], which contains approximately 30 – 40 KDa of N-linked oligosaccharides [12, 13]. A single 23 amino acid long hydrophobic sequence transverses the cell membrane. The extracellular N-terminal end (amino acids 1 - 621) can be divided into four domains (I-IV) [14, 15]. The intracellular C-terminal region (amino acids 645 - 1186) is responsible for tyrosine kinase activity and regulatory functions [16].

Currently eight ligands have been identified to bind the EGFR with varying affinity and potentially differential downstream function. They include EGF [1], transforming growth factor alpha (TGF() [17], amphiregulin (AR) [18], heparin-binding EGF-like growth factor (HB-EGF) [19], betacellulin [20], epiregulin [21], neuregulin-2-beta (NRG2β) [22] and the most recently discovered Epigen [23]. These peptide ligands are produced as trans-membrane precursors that are then processed by metalloproteases and released in their soluble form [24] (Fig. **1**).

Ligand induced ATP binding to the EGFR lysine-721 residue is a critical step in tyrosine kinase activation and auto-phosphorylation in the intracellular region of the receptor [11, 25 - 28]. In turn, this auto-phosphorylation results in a more open conformation allowing access to several cellular substrates to the tyrosine kinase domain of the EGFR [25, 29] and subsequent triggering of downstream signaling cascades including the RAS-RAF-MAPK-Erk1/2 pathway, the PTEN regulated phosphatidylinositol 3-kinase (PI3-K)-Akt-mTOR pathway, Src-Signal transducer and activator of transcription (STAT) family members and the Phospholipase C gamma (PLCγ) signaling pathway [30]. These signaling networks and the evidence for alterations or hyper-activity of each of these downstream molecules in providing resistance mechanisms to anti-EGFR therapy will be covered thoroughly in Part II of our series of reviews.

Due to the EGFR's many associations at the cell membrane and the diverse network of signaling, its activation is intimately associated with many cellular activities in both development and in the adult organism including proliferation, survival, differentiation, adhesion, migration and invasion and tumor metastasis. The importance of the EGFR in development is provided from the analysis of genetically altered mice. EGFR knockout mice display impaired epithelial development resulting in either embryonic or perinatal lethality or in mice suffered from abnormalities in multiple organs including the brain, skin, lung and gastrointestinal tract, depending on the genetic background [31 - 34]. Among the functions attributed to the EGFR are the proliferation and development of specific epithelial regions in the embryo, including branch point morphogenesis, maturation of early embryonic lung tissue, skin development and promoting survival of early progenitor cells in the cleft palate [35, 36]. The EGFR is also expressed throughout the brain during development primarily in the early postnatal astrocytes and purkinje cells [37, 38]. The EGFR also plays an important role in the adult organism where it is essential for the differentiation of normal mammary glands and the induction of uterine and vaginal growth [39, 40]. It is also required in the adult neurones of the cerebral cortex where it acts to promote terminal differentiation [41].

In summary these data clearly show the essential role of the EGFR during normal development and homeostasis. Not surprisingly, genetic alterations leading to EGFR over-expression or gain-of-function mutation are frequently observed in cancer [42 - 44]. These findings led to the vigorous pursuit that continues today to develop agents targeting the EGFR (and downstream substrates) in the hope that inhibition of EGFR-driven signal transduction will lead to improved cancer patient outcomes [45, 46]. However, despite the enormous effort and cost, only a very small percentage of tested agents have made it through clinical evaluation to be ultimately approved.

In this review we will particularly highlight the current inhibitors to the EGFR both in clinical application and being examined in translational models. We will also specifically focus on how ligands and receptors of the HER family and alternative non-EGFR family ligand-receptor pairs assist in by-pass therapeutic intervention from anti-EGFR agents and discuss potential strategies to overcome this resistance.

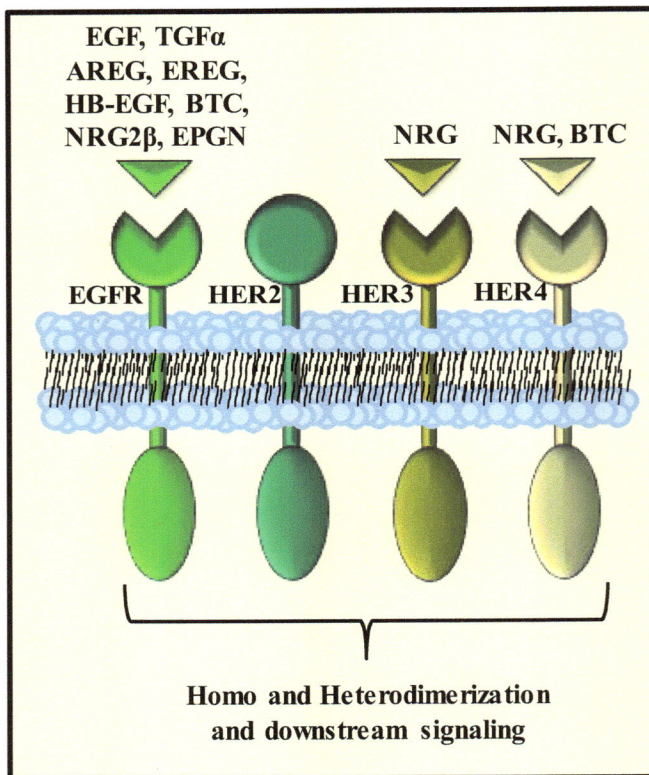

Fig. (1). Schematic of HER family of ligands and receptors. The HER family receptors are made up of 4 family members (EGFR, HER2, HER3 and HER4). These receptors bind a number of ligands. These include EGF, TGFα, AREG, EREG, HB-EGF, NRG2β and EPGN that bind the EGFR; NRG that binds both HER3 and HER4 and BTC that binds both the EGFR and HER4. No known ligand has been identified for HER2.

2. LINKING THE EGFR WITH CANCER THERAPUTICS

One of the major objectives of this 2-part review series is to discuss the most recent advances made in targeting the EGFR in cancer patient management and to thoroughly examine our current understanding of intrinsic and acquired resistance to these therapies. Thus a comprehensive synopsis chronicling all the discoveries made throughout the course of EGFR-based laboratory research is beyond the scope of this review. Nonetheless, it would be remiss of us to not discuss the original pivotal discoveries relating to the EGFR receptor tyrosine kinase system and the original rationale behind focusing on the EGFR as a potential anti-cancer target. Thus we will summarise some of the ground-breaking early findings of EGFR biology and therapeutics that set a strong framework for the body of research and clinical development currently being undertaken.

During the 1970's and 1980's vast knowledge was generated about polypeptide growth factors and growth factor receptors. While Cohen and colleagues were characterizing the tyrosine kinase properties of the EGFR, other researchers were publishing reports showing that growth factors found in serum were essential for cell proliferation in *in vitro* culture experiments [47]. Sporn and Todaro published experiments indicating that cells could secrete ligands such as TGF (to activate their own proliferation by binding the EGFR [48]. Based on these findings, it was postulated that cell proliferation could be inhibited if a monoclonal antibody could block ligand binding to its receptor, thereby preventing receptor activation. In the early 1980's several research groups set out to prove this hypothesis by immunizing mice with crude cellular extracts containing EGFR or partially purified EGFR and subsequently creating hybridomas, a fusion of mouse splenic B cells and immortalized mouse myeloma cells that secreted mature forms of antibodies into their culture supernatant [49 - 52]. Several of these monoclonal antibodies, including mAb 225 the mouse precursor to Cetuximab/Erbitux, could indeed bind the extracellular domain of the EGFR, block ligand binding, prevent receptor tyrosine kinase activation and inhibit cell proliferation [49 - 51, 53].

The first indications that the EGFR could potentially contribute to tumorigenesis came soon after with the discovery that the v-erbB viral oncogene, which caused malignancies in chickens, was very closely related in structure to the EGFR [54,

55]. Thus it, was hypothesised that the over-expression and the subsequent high level of tyrosine kinase activity of the closely related EGFR could also potentially contribute to the development of human malignancies [56]. Investigations of several cultured cell lines supported the fact that the EGFR could cause cell transformation. Velu and colleagues transformed NIH3T3 mouse cells by retroviral transfection of the full-length human EGFR gene. The ability of these cells to grow in agar, or in low levels of serum was dependent on EGFR expression and EGF supplementation [57]. In similar experiments, full length or truncated EGFR transfection into the hematopoietic BaF/3, 32D and IC2 cell lines increased cell proliferation and survival [58 - 61]. Animal studies also support the *in vitro* evidence that expression levels of the EGFR may be correlated to cell transformation. The epidermoid carcinoma cell line, A431, which expresses 2-3 $\times$ 10^6 EGFR/cell was used to examine the relationship between EGFR number and growth *in vivo*. Various clones of the A431 cell line expressing a range of EGFR numbers ($6 \times 10^4 - 1.6 \times 10^6$) were subcutaneously injected into nude mice. Cell lines with higher EGFR levels had shorter latent periods preceding measurable tumor formation, and once established the rate of tumor growth was greater than those with fewer cell surface EGFR [62]. Likewise the *in vivo* tumorigenicity of the MDA-MD-468 breast cell line possessed a significantly greater growth rate in nude mice was compared to MDA-MD-468 cell variants with lower EGFR expression [63].

Thus these studies provided the first lines of evidence that the EGFR was not only responsible for "normal" physiological mitogenic growth factor mediated signalling but also acted as an oncogene responsible for increased malignant phenotypes. As such, the original antibodies generated to study EGFR mitogenic function could also be utilised to target tumor cells expressing the pro-tumorigenic oncogene, EGFR as a therapeutic agent. Importantly, pivotal studies assessing clinical samples taken from patients with a variety of tumors were concurrently being performed. These studies showed conclusively that EGFR expression was significantly enhanced in tumor biopsies compared to normal adjacent tissue. Tumors known to over-express the EGFR include breast, bladder, ovarian, oesophageal, non-small cell and squamous cell lung carcinoma, colon, head and neck cancer and brain [56, 64 - 71]. More importantly EGFR expression was also correlated with OS outcomes in many cancers [64, 69 - 73], although several studies refute this claim that EGFR is of prognostic value for all cancers [74 - 76]. Thus, many lines of evidence were being pieced together to indicate that the EGFR was an important molecule in tumorigenesis in most cancer types and that its activation was indeed critical for tumor development and progression.

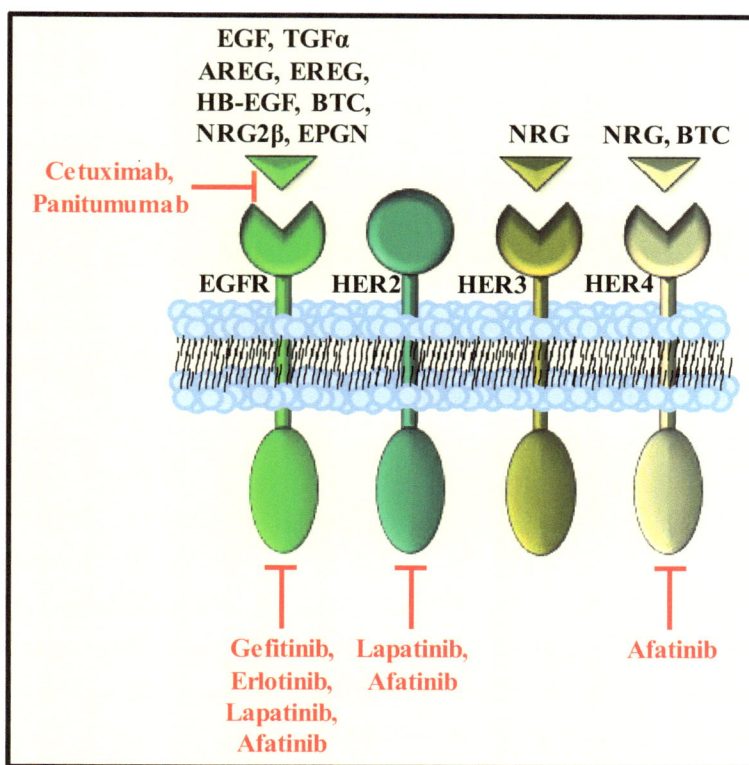

Fig. (2). Schematic of current approved anti-EGFR inhibitors. Current anti-EGFR inhibitors approved for clinical use include mAbs and TKI's. Cetuximab and panitumumab are two mAbs that bind the extracellular region of the EGFR and block ligand binding. Gefitinib and erlotinib are 2 reversible TKI's of the EGFR competing with ATP coupling to the ATP binding region of the EGFR. Lapatinib inhibits both EGFR and HER2, while afatinib can inhibit the EGFR, HER2 and HER4.

These findings in the late 1980 and throughout the 1990's stimulated the ever-growing research effort to isolate anti-EGFR therapeutics. Critical experiments showed that monoclonal antibodies targeting the EGFR, and later another class of inhibitors, the small molecular weight tyrosine kinase inhibitors (TKI's) significantly inhibited the growth of tumor cells in culture and in animal xenograft models [46, 77 - 82]. Pre-clinical evaluation of these anti-EGFR inhibitors in combination with chemotherapy and radiotherapy also produced encouraging tumor inhibition [45, 77, 79, 83 - 86]. These vital pre-clinical studies paved the way for clinical application of many of these inhibitors, ultimately leading to the approved use of a select few (Fig. **2**). In the next section we will discuss the most clinically advanced anti-EGFR therapeutics reviewing the progress each has made from pre-clinical inception to clinical application and approval.

3. THERAPEUTIC AGENTS TARGETING THE EGFR

3.1. Cetuximab/Erbitux (Bristol-Myers Squibb and Eli Lilly and Company)

As mentioned earlier, cetuximab was originally generated through traditional mouse immunization and hybridoma screening in the early 1980's and was named m225 or mAb 225 [49, 50, 53]. Initial studies showed that mAb 225 produced significant inhibitory effects when evaluated against a series of cancer derived cell lines in culture and when grown as xenografts in nude mice [87 - 91]. Subsequent studies showed that mAb 225 inhibit proliferation of cultured cell lines and *in vivo* xenografts by several mechanisms include the blockade of receptor-ligand interactions [53, 87, 92] which often lead to the inhibition of cell-cycle progression [93, 94], the induction of apoptosis [84, 95 - 99], inhibition of pro-angiogenic factors [100 - 102], down-regulation of the EGFR [103, 104] and the recruitment of host immune effector function [105].

A human/mouse chimeric version of mAb 225, (C225, Cetuximab), was produced to alleviate human host immune response, allowing for the continuous mAb delivery that may be required for sustained anti-tumor activity [106, 107]. On the basis of a series of Phase I clinical trials with cetuximab alone or in combination with chemotherapy and radiotherapy [108 - 110] a recommended optimal cetuximab dose was determined; 400 mg/m^2 loading dose, followed by weekly doses of 250 mg/m^2. In 2004, Cunningham and colleagues published the results of a multi-center open-label Phase II study comparing cetuximab plus irinotecan or cetuximab monotherapy in mCRC patients whose disease progressed following irinotecan-based treatment [111]. In this study, the RR of patients treated with both cetuximab and irinotecan was 22.9% (50 out of 218) compared to 10.8% (12 out of 111) of patients treated with cetuximab alone. The median TTP and the median survival time were also enhanced in the combination groups compared to the cetuximab monotherapy group. Based on this landmark trial and earlier trials where cetuximab and irinotecan (17% response rate) or cetuximab monotherapy (8.8% response rate) were assessed independently in mCRC patients who were refractory to fluorouracil and irinotecan [112, 113], cetuximab was approved for the used in EGFR-expressing mCRC patients who are refractory to irinotecan-based chemotherapy in 2004.

Subsequent identification of K-RAS mutations as predictive molecular markers for cetuximab response *(which will be comprehensively reviewed in Part II of this 2 part series)* led to the modified FDA approved of the combination of cetuximab with FOLFIRI (5-fluorouracil, leucovorin and irinotecan) as a first-line treatment for patients with wild-type *K-RAS* and *EGFR*-expressing mCRC in 2012 [114]. The approved use of cetuximab for patients harbouring K-RAS wildtype only was based on the results of the CRYSTAL (Cetuximab Combined with Irinotecan in First-Line Therapy for Metastatic Colorectal Cancer) and OPUS (Oxaliplatin and Cetuximab in First-Line Treatment of mCRC) trials. In the Phase III multi-center CRYSTAL trial, retrospective stratification of patients found that cetuximab in combination with FOLFIRI significantly improved response rate, PFS and OS in the first-line treatment of patients with wild-type K-RAS mCRC compared with FOLFIRI alone [115, 116]. Similarly, the randomised phase II OPUS clinical trial confirmed that wild-type K-RAS expression was significantly more responsive to cetuximab combined with FOLFOX-4 (5-fluorouracil, leucovorin and oxaliplatin) as first-line treatment for mCRC [117, 118].

In addition to mCRC, cetuximab has been approved for the treatment of SCCHN in several settings. In 2006, cetuximab in combination with radiotherapy was FDA approved for patients with locally or regionally advanced SCCHN in first-line therapy [119, 120]. This was based on initial data from a Phase III randomised trial evaluating cetuximab and radiotherapy *versus* radiotherapy alone in patients with loco-regionally advanced SCCHN. In this trial, cetuximab plus radiotherapy significantly increased PFS and OS compared with radiation therapy alone [121, 122]. Cetuximab monotherapy was also approved in 2006 for patients with recurrent or metastatic SCCHN who had previously failed platinum-based therapies [119, 120]. A phase II study by Vermorken and colleagues provided the evidence for the benefit of cetuximab monotherapy in recurrent or metastatic SCCHN patients [123]. In an open-labelled Phase II trial, they showed that single-agent cetuximab was active and well tolerated in the treatment of patients with recurrent and metastatic SCCHN who had disease progression following platinum-based chemotherapy [123]. Most recently, cetuximab (in combination with cisplatin or carboplatin and 5-fluorouracil) was also FDA approved in 2011 for the first-line treatment of patients with recurrent loco-regional or metastatic SCCHN [119]. In addition to several important phase II studies [124 - 126], a pivotal multi-center Phase III trial comparing cetuximab and cisplatin or carboplatin and 5-fluorouracil treatment *versus* chemotherapy alone in recurrent and metastatic SCCHN patients was reported [126 - 128]. The cetuximab and chemotherapy group displayed greater PFS (5.5 *vs.* 3.3 months) and OS (10.1 *vs.* 7.4 months) and higher ORR (36% *vs.* 20%) compared to the chemotherapy treated group.

3.2. Panitumumab/Vectibix (Amgen Inc)

Panitumumab (originally named ABX-EGF clone E7.6.3) was generated from a mouse strain genetically altered to carry human immunoglobulin genes [129]. Thus panitumumab possess the attractive feature of being totally human, reducing the likelihood of eliciting patient immunogenic response. Administration of panitumumab *in vivo* led to significant inhibition of established tumors of breast, ovarian, pancreatic, prostate and colon origin [130]. Panitumumab monotherapy was well tolerated and mediated some response in early trials of chemo-refractory mCRC patients [131, 132]. A pivotal open-labelled Phase III trial was published in 2007 by Van Custem and colleagues reporting the efficacy of Panitumumab and best supporting care *versus* best supportive care alone in 463 EGFR-expressing mCRC patients who failed chemotherapy [133]. Objective response rates of 9.5% (22 out of 231) were seen in the panitumumab treated patients compared to 0% (0 out of 232) in the best supportive care group. Panitumumab also significantly prolonged PFS, but did not enhance OS compared to best supportive care only [133]. Panitumumab was granted accelerated approval as monotherapy in the United States in 2006 and Europe in 2007 prior to the final publication of the Van Custem article [134]. Nonetheless, panitumumab approval remained for the use in EGFR expressing mCRC patients who had originally failed fluoropyrimidine, oxaliplatin and irinotecan based treatment.

3.3. Lapatinib/Tykerb (GlaxoSmithKline)

Lapatinib, originally named GW572016, is an orally-active small molecular inhibitor that competes for binding with ATP for the ATP-binding domain of both the EGFR and HER2 [80, 81]. Lapatinib displays *in vitro* and *in vivo* efficacy against cancer cells with low and high HER2 expression [135 - 137]. Importantly, lapatinib was not cross-resistant with trastuzumab (Herceptin, an anti-HER2 monoclonal antibody) demonstrating significant activity in trastuzumab-resistant breast cancer cell lines [135], and was effective in trastuzumab-refractory breast cancer patients [138, 139]. Lapatinib was also well tolerated when combined with capecitabine in early trials involving breast cancer patients [140]. In a Phase III multi-center trial, HER2-positive advanced or metastatic breast cancer patients progressed after treatment with regimens that included an anthracycline, a taxane, and trastuzumab were randomized to receive either lapatinib and capecitabine in combination or capecitabine monotherapy [141, 142]. Based on a delay in TTP (27.1 *vs.* 18.6 weeks) and improvement in overall RR (23.7% *vs.* 13.9%) comparing lapatinib and capecitabine in combination *versus* capecitabine monotherapy seen in this trial Lapatinib and capecitabine combinational treatment was approved by the FDA in 2007 in patients with advanced breast cancer who had been previously treated with anthracyclines and taxanes and had progressed on trastuzumab-based therapy [143, 144]. Lapatinib and capecitabine has also showed PR in HER2-positive metastatic breast cancer patients with brain metastases [145].

3.4. Gefitinib/Iressa (AstraZeneca)

Gefitinib, originally named ZD1839, is an orally available, first-generation reversible EGFR tyrosine kinase inhibitor that competes with ATP for the ATP-binding region of the EGFR [146]. Initial studies of gefitinib showed that it inhibited the tyrosine kinase activity of EGFR and EGF-dependent proliferation of cancer cells both *in vitro* and showed significant anti-tumor activity against colon, prostate and lung derived human cell lines *in vivo* animal xenograft models [85, 147, 148].

Phase I trials of gefitinib in healthy volunteers and patients with varying tumors including NSCLC found that gefitinib was well tolerated and effective in blocking EGFR phosphorylation, with doses of 250-500mg chosen for larger scale trials [149 - 154]. Two pivotal Phase II trials (The Iressa Dose Evaluation in Advanced Lung Cancer: IDEAL1 and IDEAL 2) were conducted evaluating gefitinib monotherapy in NSCLC patients who had been treated with chemotherapy previously and formed the evidence for original accelerated FDA approval in 2003 [155, 156]. Response rates ranged from 9-19% and approximately 40% of patients showed objective improvement in symptoms. Two subsequent Phase III trials followed where gefitinib was assessed in combination with gemcitabine and cisplatin compared to chemotherapy alone (Iressa NSCLC Trial Assessing Combination Therapy; INTACT 1) [157] or gefitinib in combination with carboplatin and paclitaxel compared to chemotherapy alone (INTACT 2) [158] in chemo naïve NSCLC patients. Disappointingly, no significant difference was seen in RR, median TTP or survival rate between gefitinib plus chemotherapy *versus* chemotherapy alone in either of these trials which enrolled over 1000 patients each. Thus gefitinib in combination with chemotherapy in chemotherapy-naive patients with advanced NSCLC did not have improved efficacy over chemotherapy alone [157, 158]. Furthermore, another Phase III trial (Iressa Survival Evaluation in advanced Lung Cancer - ISEL) evaluating gefitinib and best supportive care *versus* placebo and best supportive care did not show any significant difference in OS between both arms. On the basis of these disappointing trials, gefitinib was restricted for the use in patients that were showing benefit from it prior to the release of the negative data of these trials.

Following the landmark discovery of EGFR mutations in a subset of NSCLC that confer sensitivity to gefitinib [159, 160] (*as discussed in detail in section 5.1.3.1*) selecting patients that harboured these mutations became standard practice and response to gefitinib in this sub-population was significantly better than in overall unselected populations. This was evident in two randomised Phase III trials (West Japan Oncology Group (WJOG) and North-East Japan Study Group (NEJSG)) comparing gefitinib to chemotherapy in the first-line treatment of NSCLC patients containing these sensitizing EGFR mutations [161, 162]. These studies led to the approval of gefitinib for advanced NSCLC patients with activating or sensitizing EGFR mutations in the United States, Europe and many other countries worldwide, however this approval has been withdrawn in the United States due to its failure to demonstrate a survival benefit [163, 164].

3.5. Erlotinib/Tarceva (Genentech)

Erlotinib, earlier named CP-358,774 and OSI-774, is an orally available ATP competitive specific and reversible inhibitor of the EGFR, inhibiting auto-phosphorylation of the EGFR expressed on several tumor cell lines both *in vitro* and in animal xenograft models [165 - 169]. Many Phase I studies evaluating erlotinib as monotherapy or in combination with chemotherapy in patients with a variety of solid tumors showed that erlotinib was well tolerated and produced positive response rates in several patients [170 - 177], although erlotinib plus FOLFIRI (5-fluorouracil, irinotecan and leucovorin) produced increases in toxicities and was terminated early in one study [178]. An important Phase II study showing for the first time erlotinib efficacy as single agent therapy in advanced refractory NSCLC was published by Perez-Soler in 2004 [179]. In this trial, a RR of 12.3% (7 out of 57) was observed and median OS was 8.4 months following Erlotinib monotherapy (150mg/day) in patients with EGFR-expressing Stage IIIB/ IV NSCLC who had failed first-line chemotherapy [179]. Other Phase II studies have also been performed evaluated erlotinib as first-line therapy in advanced NSCLC, with one trial reporting a RR of 22.7% (12 out of 53), median TTP and OS were 84 and 391 days respectively [180]. A pivotal Phase III study (NCIC BR-21 trial) by Shepherd and colleagues randomised patients with stage IIIB or IV NSCLC, who had received one or two prior chemotherapy regimens 2:1 into erlotinib monotherapy or placebo groups [181]. The RR (8.9%; 38 out of 427 *vs.* 0.9%; 2 out of 211), PFS (2.2 *vs.* 1.8 months) and median OS (6.7 *vs.* 4.7 months) were all significantly greater in the erlotinib group *versus* the placebo group. Erlotinib also improved global quality of life [181]. As a result of this trial erlotinib monotherapy was approved and became standard of care in the second or third line setting for patients with NSCLC [182].

As mentioned in section 3.4, the discovery of EGFR sensitizing mutations radically changed the approach to treating NSCLC patients with EGFR inhibitors, with patients selected for these mutations becoming routine practice prior to treatment with either gefitinib or erlotinib. Several pivotal erlotinib based trials aiding in this transition of clinical management have been summarised in Table **1** and discussed in section 5.1.3.1, including both retrospective and prospective analysis of these mutations in both Caucasian and Asian populations [183 - 188]. Currently, both erlotinib and gefitinib are approved in Europe for the treatment of patients with locally advanced and metastatic NSCLC that harbour sensitizing EGFR mutations. Erlotinib approval is for first-line, maintenance, second-line or third line treatment of NSCLC patients harbouring EGFR sensitizing mutations. However, erlotinib is the current EGFR tyrosine kinase Inhibitor of choice in the United States for patients with sensitizing EGFR mutations because of the restricted access of gefitinib [163].

Table 1. EGFR Kinase Domain Mutations and response to EGFR TKI's in NSCLC.

No of Patients[a]	Patient Ethnicity/ Study location	Mutation status	Treatment	Responders (%)	Study
16	Taiwanese	8 w mut[b] 8 w/o[c]	Gefitinib Gefitinib	7 (88) 2 (25)	[650]
18	USA	7 w mut 11 w/o	Gefitinib Gefitinib	7 (100) 3 (33)	[184]
17	USA	5 w mut 12 w/o	Erlotinib Erlotinib	5 (100) 2 (17)	
12	Japan	4 w mut 8 w/o	Gefitinib Gefitinib	4 (100) 0 (0)	[651]
27	South Korea	6 w mut 21 w/o	Gefitinib Gefitinib	6 (100) 2 (10)	[652]
114	USA	15 w mut 99 w/o	Erlotinib Erlotinib	8 (53) 18 (18)	[183]
50	Japan	29 w mut 21 w/o	Gefitinib Gefitinib	24 (83) 2 (10)	[351]
21	Japan	9 w mut 12 w/o	Gefitinib Gefitinib	8 (89) 2 (17)	[653]
90	South Korea	17 w mut 73 w/o	Gefitinib Gefitinib	11 (65) 10 (14)	[654]

(Table 1) contd.....

No of Patients[a]	Patient Ethnicity/ Study location	Mutation status	Treatment	Responders (%)	Study
89	Italy	15 w mut 74 w/o	Gefitinib Gefitinib	8 (54) 4 (5)	[253]
74	USA	13 w mut 61 w/o	Gefitinib Gefitinib	6 (43) 6 (10)	[290]
83	Spain	10 w mut 73 w/o	Gefitinib Gefitinib	6 (60) 6 (8)	[655]
62	Taiwan	29 w mut 33 w/o	Gefitinib Gefitinib	20 (69) 3 (9)	[361]
20	Japan	11 w mut 9 w/o	Gefitinib Gefitinib	11 (100) 3 (33)	[656]
66	Japan	39 w mut 27 w/o	Gefitinib Gefitinib	32 (82) 3 (11)	[657]
34	Japan and Spain	8 w mut 26 w/o	Gefitinib Gefitinib	7 (88) 3 (12)	[658]
54	Taiwan	33 w mut 21 w/o	Gefitinib Gefitinib	17 (52) 4 (19)	[352]
30	China	12 w mut 18 w/o	Gefitinib Gefitinib	8 (67) 1 (6)	[659]
100	Canada	19 w mut 81 w/o	Erlotinib Erlotinib	3 (16) 6 (7)	[186]
68	Asian + Caucasian	17 w mut 51 w/o	Gefitinib Gefitinib	16 (94) 6 (12)	[660]
20	Japan	9 w mut 11 w/o	Gefitinib Gefitinib	7 (78) 0 (0)	[661]
98	Japan	38 w mut 60 w/o	Gefitinib Gefitinib	22 (58) 3 (5)	[292]
82	Taiwan	53 w mut 29 w/o	Gefitinib Gefitinib	38 (72) 7 (24)	[355]
46	Japan	29 w mut 17 w/o	Gefitinib Gefitinib	23 (79) 10 (59)	[207]
223	East Asia	132 w mut 91 w/o	Gefitinib Gefitinib	94 (71) 1 (1)	[350]
69	China	51 w mut 18 w/o	Icotinib Icotinib	28 (55) 2 (11)	[662]
1583[d]	-	618 w mut 965 w/o	-	426 (69) 109 (11)	-

[a]Number of Patients screened for EGFR mutations, treated with EGFR inhibitor and assessed for clinical response.

[b]w mut = with EGFR kinase domain mutation

[c]w/o = without EGFR kinase domain mutation

[d]Totals of all trials (shaded in light blue).

A randomised Phase III trial (NCIC PA.3 trial) has also been conducted evaluating first line treatment of gemcitabine and erlotinib in combination *versus* gemcitabine and placebo in patients with locally advanced, unresectable or metastatic pancreatic cancer [189]. Although it did not significantly increase overall response rates, patients treated with erlotinib and gemcitabine had a significantly enhanced PFS (3.8 *vs.* 3.6 months) and OS (6.2 *vs.* 5.9 months) compared to patients treated with gemcitabine alone [189]. Based on preliminary results of this trail the US FDA approved erlotinib in combination with gemcitabine for patients with locally advanced, unresectable or metastatic pancreatic carcinoma and who have not received previous chemotherapy [190] in 2005.

3.6. Afatinib/Gilotrif (Boehringer Ingelheim Pharmaceuticals)

Afatinib, previously named BIBW2992, is an orally available, selective irreversible inhibitor of EGFR, HER2 and HER4 tyrosine kinase activity. Preclinical studies in cell lines found that afatinib was more potent in blocking the activity of not only the wildtype EGFR, but also EGFR sensitizing mutations and more importantly a point mutation found to provide acquired resistance to gefitinib and erlotinib (EGFR T790M; [191, 192]; which will be discussed in greater detail in section 5.1.3.2 of this review) compared to gefitinib and erlotinib [193, 194]. A series of clinical trials (LUX-Lung) have evaluated afatinib as first-line and following acquired resistance to other EGFR tyrosine kinase inhibitors in patients with EGFR mutation positive NSCLC [195 - 201]. Overall, these trials showed that afatinib increased PFS rates compared to cisplatin and pemetrexed in first-line treatment of NSCLC patient harbouring EGFR mutations but had limited efficacy in EGFR mutation positive patients that had acquired resistance to either gefitinib or erlotinib. Based on these trials, afatinib was approved in the United States in 2013 for the first-line treatment of NSCLC patients whose tumors harbour EGFR mutations and is the only second-generation agents currently approved in the NSCLC setting. Afatinib is also approved in Europe and other countries including Japan, Chile, Mexico, Taiwan and Australia. Interestingly, a combination of afatinib and cetuximab induces tumor regression in a T790M transgenic mouse lung tumor model [202] and produced a 32.4% (23 out of 71 patients) RR in a Phase Ib trial of NSCLC patients who had developed acquired resistance to either gefitinib or erlotinib and were EGFR T790M positive [203]. An overall RR of 29.4% (37 out of 126 patients) was seen in all patients with acquired resistance to gefitinib or erlotinib irrespective of T790M mutation status [203] suggesting that dual inhibition of EGFR may overcome resistance to initial EGFR tyrosine kinase inhibitor monotherapy in some patients.

It is clear that the discovery, pre-clinical and clinical design and production of targeted therapeutics are long and arduous. The 6 anti-EGFR agents reviewed above are the most currently advanced and are clinically prescribed for the treatment of cancer patients of varying origin. However, as highlighted above, the response rates and improvement in patient survival is only modest. The presence of pre-existing intrinsic resistance and the ability of tumors to develop or acquire resistance represents one of the greatest challenges to successful treatment outcome. Resistance to anti-EGFR agents is common and is the main reason for only 10-30% of advanced unselected cancer patients demonstrating major tumor regression [204]. The seemingly never-ending long-term goal to improving patient survival through a greater understanding of tumor resistance has led to a large number of research laboratories searching for the critical mediators of anti-EGFR therapy. Significant progress through both clinical and translational methods has been made, however these advances have not translated linearly into the clinic and thus continued efforts using technological advanced methodology are still required. The remainder of this review will examine the many extracellular (ligand and receptors) mechanisms used by tumor cells to resist anti-EGFR therapeutic intervention particularly discussing molecular markers that predict both increased sensitivity and resistance.

4. BIOMARKERS PREDICTING SENSITIVITY AND RESISTANCE TO ANTI-EGFR THERAPIES - LIGANDS OF THE EGFR AS PREDICTORS OF RESPONSE TO ANTI-EGFR THERAPY

It is not surprising that a common feature predicting response to anti-EGFR is the differential expression of both HER and non-HER ligands intratumorally and in the microenvironment. Discoveries from many research groups have identified a role for ligands of the EGFR as predictive biomarkers for response to EGFR therapy in studies using cell lines and clinical samples. We will examine each ligand in turn.

4.1. Amphiregulin (AREG) and Epiregulin (EREG)

One of the first studies to determine if ligands to the EGFR could act as potential biomarkers of response to anti-EGFR therapy came from Kakiuchi and colleagues in 2004 [205]. In their study they identified 51 differentially expressed genes (from a cDNA microarray set of 27,648 genes tested) in NSCLC tumors from patients that responded *versus* those that did not respond to second – seventh-line gefitinib monotherapy. Although using a small sample size (7 responders *vs.* 10 non-responders), this initial microarray data set was validated by successfully predicting gefitinib response in a subsequent cohort of 16 advanced NSCLC patients [205]. Amphiregulin (AREG) was the only EGFR ligand identified in this microarray screen and was one of the most significantly up-regulated genes that predicted resistance to gefitinib. In addition, validation by RT-PCR and immunohistochemistry confirmed the microarray data, that amphiregulin was up-regulated in non-responders compared to patients that responded to gefitinib. In accordance to these clinical findings, Kakiuchi *et al.* performed laboratory studies and demonstrated that stimulation of NSCLC cell lines with AREG resulted in a desensitisation of the anti-proliferative effects of gefitinib, further supporting the notion that amphiregulin expression provides resistance to gefitinib [205]. Further confirmation of this came from a subsequent report from the same group one year later where they assessed the serum levels of amphiregulin in 50 NSCLC patients who had failed previous chemotherapy and were treated with gefitinib [206]. AREG levels were detected by ELISA in 28% (14 out of 50) of patient serum samples. Of these 14 samples with greater than background levels, 12 were from patients that responded poorly to gefitinib further suggesting that amphiregulin expression correlated to gefitinib response in NSCLC patients [206]. Another report by Masago and colleagues also confirmed that circulating amphiregulin is predictive of an unfavourable response to gefitinib in NSCLC patients [207].

However, others report contradictory findings indicating that AREG may act as a predictor of tumor cell sensitivity to anti-EGFR therapy. Indeed, a study by

Yonesaka *et al.* analysed AREG protein expression in 24 NSCLC patients treated with either gefitinib or erlotinib monotherapy by immunohistochemistry [208]. The AREG staining was significantly greater in patients with SD (more likely responder to anti-EGFR treatment) than that of the tumors from patients who had disease progression. Furthermore, utilising human NSCLC and SCCHN cell lines, Yonesaka and colleagues discovered that cells that expressed and secreted higher levels of AREG were more likely to be inhibited by gefitinib and cetuximab than those that produced minimal or no AREG expression [208]. Another study showed that AREG (and TGFα) gene expression was significantly higher in a series of gefitinib sensitive *versus* refractory SCCHN cell lines [209]. Thus, these reports clearly indicate that AREG expression is a predictive biomarker for better response to EGFR targeted therapy.

Supporting this notion was a report in 2007 from Khambata-Ford and colleagues utilising a much large patient cohort in the mCRC setting [210]. In their study, patients with mCRC were biopsied at the site of metastasis (liver and extrahepatic sites) prior to treatment with cetuximab monotherapy. Large-scale gene expression analysis of the metastatic tumor tissue revealed that AREG and epiregulin (EREG) were 2 of the most significantly differentially expressed genes in patients with disease control *versus* non-responders to cetuximab. Furthermore, patients with high AREG and EREG gene expression had significant longer PFS compared to those with low expression [210]. A series of subsequent articles supporting the findings of Khambata-Ford and colleagues have been more recently reported. However, unlike the study from Khambata-Ford *et al.* these studies further stratified mCRC patients into those with tumors that expressed wild-type K-RAS and those with tumors that harbour a K-RAS mutation (*a validated negative predictor of anti-EGFR response in mCRC that is discussed in greater detail in Part II of our series of reviews*). Similar to the findings in metastatic lesions by Khambata-Ford *et al.* Jacobs and colleagues described comparable results in primary tumor tissue from chemotherapy refractory mCRC patients treated with cetuximab and irinotecan [211]. AREG and EREG gene expression levels correlated with the likelihood of cetuximab response in a subset of wildtype K-RAS mCRC (but not in tumors harbouring K-RAS mutation). Another study evaluating the expression profiles of 110 genes in

226 primary colon tumors (144 wt K-RAS and 82 K-RAS mutated) from mCRC patients treated with cetuximab monotherapy also identified AREG and EREG as predictive markers of response [212]. Both AREG and EREG were 2 of only 9 genes tested that were associated with disease control, objective response to cetuximab and PFS [212]. Likewise, a subsequent study reporting a Phase I clinical trial of mCRC patients treated with first-line cetuximab followed by cetuximab plus fluorouracil, leucovorin and irinotecan disease also supports the above findings [213]. Once more, AREG and EREG gene expression was elevated in tumors from patients that responded to cetuximab compared to low level gene expression in tumors from patients that did not respond. This was evident in tumors in the whole cohort of analysed patients (wt and K-RAS mutated) and in the wt K-RAS subgroup. Other groups found that higher levels of EREG gene expression was significantly associated with an increased likelihood of objective response to first and third line cetuximab therapy [214], TTP and OS in second and third-line cetuximab therapy [215] in independent cohorts of mCRC patients. Another study assessed the predictive value of EREG gene expression and K-RAS status in a Phase III clinical trial of 193 mCRC patients treated with cetuximab and best supportive care *versus* 192 patients treated with best supportive care only [216]. In the wt K-RAS subgroup, 16.7% (11 out of 66) of patients with tumors that had high EREG expression responded to cetuximab compared to a RR of only 6.3% (3 out of 48) in patients with low tumor EREG expression. Lower expression was also associated with worse OS and PFS in the cetuximab treated patients [216]. In addition, Yoshida and colleagues expanded on the above finding to determine if protein expression of ligands to the EGFR family could predict response to not only cetuximab but also panitumumab (albeit using a small sample size) [217]. Immunohistochemical analysis revealed that protein expression of AREG and EREG (along with TGFα and HB-EGF) could act as biomarkers for response to both cetuximab and panitumumab in wt K-RAS mCRC. Likewise, positive staining also correlated to PFS. Finally, a laboratory based study further confirmed the notion of AREG and EREG as positive predictors of cetuximab efficacy [218]. Cetuximab's ability to reduce the colony formation of A431 vulvar squamous carcinoma cells with stable AREG and EREG knockdown was significantly reduced compared to parental A431 cells. In addition, selection of A431 sub-clones that were refractory to cetuximab by long-

term, continuous exposure of the overall population to cetuximab displayed significantly less AREG and EREG mRNA expression compared to parental A431 cells [218, 219]. Similar findings of reduced AREG expression have been shown by the same group when treating breast cancer cells with short term exposure of lapatinib [219]. Likewise, low EREG expression correlated with resistance to *in vitro* efficacy of cetuximab in a series of SCCHN cell lines [220], while high AREG expression levels correlated with cetuximab plus docetaxel treatment benefit in recurrent or initial metastatic SCCHN patients [221].

Taken together, these findings demonstrate the potential of intratumoral AREG and EREG expression to predict anti-EGFR treatment response. However, it should be noted that AREG and EREG serum expression did not correlate to response indicating post-transcriptional modifications or retention of these ligands within the tumor [210]. Meanwhile, another study showed that K-RAS wildtype mCRC patients with high levels of EREG had shorter PFS (4.9 *vs.* 6.6 months) and OS (7.4 *vs.* 13.8 months) compared with those with low levels of EREG [222]. Nonetheless, this large body of evidence also supports the hypothesis that high ligand expression results in tumor cell addiction or dependence on EGFR signaling for tumor progression, and thus renders these sub-populations of tumors more sensitive to the shutting down of this pathway with anti-EGFR inhibitors.

4.2. Transforming Growth Factor Alpha (TGFα)

Studies evaluating expression of other EGFR ligands, most notably TGFα promote contradictory theories. Several studies have shown that the presence of TGFα in patient serum predicts a poor response. The study by Ishikawa and co-workers determined that TGFα levels were detectable in the serum of 86.7% (13 out of 15) of advanced NSCLC patients that responded poorly to gefitinib [206]. In contrast, TGFα was detected in only 51.4% (18 out of 35) patients that responded better to gefitinib [206]. Likewise another study examining a cohort of Japanese patients showed a similar trend despite a far less number of patients with detectable TGFα in their serum [207]. In this study, TGFα was detected in the serum of 32.4% (11 out of 34) of NSCLC patients treated with gefitinib who had progressive disease compared to only 8.5% (5 out of 59) in patients with PR and SD [207]. Similarly, high serum TGFα levels predicted reduced response to lapatinib and capecitabine in breast cancer patients with high HER2 expression [223]. High TGFα serum levels were observed in 84.4% (38 out of 45) of patients who showed poor response compared to 42.1% (8 out of 19) of patients who responded [223]. Finally, another report concluded that high plasma TGF-α levels predicted a lack of benefit from erlotinib treatment in NSCLC patients [224]. However, disparity in the number of patients with detectable serum TGFα, despite using similar methodology and the fact that some patients that responded still had detectable TGFα levels suggests that it may not be the most suitable predictive marker. Furthermore, others have shown that TGFα serum levels have no predictive value for response to combined cetuximab and celecoxib therapy in mCRC patients [225], while a more recent paper has shown the opposite findings to those above. Serum levels of TGFα were determined in un-resectable or metastatic gastric or esophagogastric junction adenocarcinoma treated with cisplatin, capecitabine and cetuximab. Patients with higher levels of TGFα, showed better response, longer PFS and improved OS compared to those with lower serum levels [226]. In addition, immunohistochemical staining for TGFα revealed the inverse correlative findings, where intratumoral TGFα expression associated with response to cetuximab or panitumumab in mCRC patients [217]. Gene expression analysis from 103 primary colon and rectum tumors was also recently performed for several potential predictive biomarkers including TGFα [227]. However, TGFα gene expression was not significantly associated with response to cetuximab, PFS nor OS in this study [227].

4.3. Epidermal Growth Factor (EGF)

Some reports have proposed that EGF may play a role in providing resistance in cell line based studies. Several tumor cell lines of SCCHN origin displayed increased cetuximab resistance upon the addition of EGF [228]. In addition, EGF silencing by specific siRNA was associated with an improved cetuximab response [228]. Similarly, cetuximab, erlotinib and gefitinib treated DU145 cells (a brain metastatic cell line from primary prostate cancer) also displayed significantly enhanced EGF expression [229]. Likewise, EGF expression was significantly up-regulated in the breast cancer cell line MDA-MB-468 following gefitinib treatment [230]. These findings led Ferrer-Soler and colleagues to propose that gefitinib-resistant breast cancer cells retain the ability to compensate for loss of

EGFR function by significantly up-regulating EGF-related ligands. Similarly, EGF serum levels were increased compared to baseline levels (prior to cetuximab treatment), after the administration of cetuximab in wt K-RAS mCRC patients. Importantly, this increase in serum EGF levels correlated to poorer clinical outcome [231]. However, colon cancer cell line responsiveness to the mitogenic stimulus provided by EGF was seen to correlate with cetuximab efficacy in another study [232]. Jhawer and colleagues found that EGF mediated cell cycle progression in 3 cell lines that were sensitive to cetuximab while no EGF-induced increase in cell cycle progression was seen in 3 cetuximab-refractory cell lines [232]. Thus, whether increase secretion of EGF after anti-EGFR treatment results in enhanced EGFR signaling and a refractory phenotype or more sensitive phenotype is currently not definitively determined.

The EGF 61A>G functional single nucleotide polymorphism is located in the 5'-untranslated region (UTR) of the EGF gene and has been associated with a greater risk of developing malignant melanoma [233], gastric cancer [234], hepatocellular carcinoma [235] and more aggressive disease in glioblastoma multiforme [236]. In addition, recent evidence suggests that this polymorphism may play a potential prognostic and predictive role mCRC. Garm-Spinder and colleagues determined the level of the genetic EGF 61 polymorphism variants in 71 mCRC patients who underwent cetuximab and irinotecan treatment (following failure to fluoropyrimidine, oxaliplatin and irinotecan regimes). Interestingly, patients with heterozygote EGF 61 A/G alleles were at a higher risk of early progression. Likewise these patients had significantly lower progression free survival and OS compared to patients with either homozygous alleles (EGF 61 A/A and EGF61 G/G) indicating differences in treatment response in these two sub-populations of patients [237]. Another sub-population of mCRC patients with the homozygous EGF 61 G/G were also shown to have favourable OS [238]. However, no correlation with the EGF 61 polymorphism variants was seen with RR in these patients who were treated with cetuximab and irinotecan salvage therapy after disease progression [238]. The EGF 61 G/G allele however, was found to associate with complete pathological response when analysing patients with rectal cancer who were enrolled in phase I/II clinical trials treated with cetuximab-based chemoradiation in 4 independent cancer centers [239]. From the 118 combined patients tested, 45.5% (5 out of 11) patients with the EGF 61 G/G genotype has a complete pathological response compared to 20.8% (11 out of 53) with the EGF 61 A/A genotype and 1.9% (1 out of 54) with EGF 61 A/G genotype [239]. Finally, despite finding a trend in association with OS, another study found no association between EGF 61 polymorphism and response to cetuximab monotherapy in 39 mCRC patients (who had failed either two regimens of chemotherapy or adjuvant therapy plus one chemotherapy regimen for metastatic disease) [240]. Importantly, the presence of the EGF 61 A/G and G/G alleles results in up-regulation of EGF levels thereby allowing for the possibility of evaluating EGF expression as a possible biomarker for response to treatment, PFS and OS in mCRC patients. However, in contrast to the above studies, EGF expression has been consistently shown to have no prognostic or predictive value clinically in assessing response to EGFR targeted therapy in several studies [212, 214, 217, 223, 227]. However, these studies did not distinguish patient EGF 61 polymorphism variants when determining whether overall EGF expression both in serum and/or intratumorally correlated to treatment response. Indeed, analysis of EGF 61 polymorphism variants, EGF serum levels and a correlation with response to cetuximab or any other anti-EGFR therapeutic in the same cohort of patients has not currently been published.

4.4. Heparin-Binding EGF-LIKE Growth Factor (HB-EGF)

Very little has been reported discuss a possible role in HB-EGF in mediating resistance to anti-EGFR agents in laboratory-based and clinical research. A small cohort of 26 mCRC patient samples were analysed for HB-EGF expression by immunohistochemistry [217]. In this study it was found that of the patient's with tissue that had detectable HB-EGF immunostaining disease RR was 84.6% (11 out of 13) and RR to cetuximab or panitumumab-based treatment was 46.2% (6 out of 13). In contrast patients with negative staining tumor tissue had a significantly lower disease RR of 31% (4 out of 13) and response rate of 15.4% (2 out of 13), indicating that HB-EGF expression may correlate with a favourable RR and overall outcome [217]. HB-EGF gene expression intratumorally in mCRC did not however correlate to response to cetuximab or OS in another larger cohort of mCRC treated with chemotherapy only *versus* cetuximab and chemotherapy [227]. Another study showed that HB-EGF serum levels may also predict response in cetuximab and irinotecan treated chemo-refractory mCRC patients [231]. However, this study was contradictory to the above study where HB-EGF expression was a negative predictor of response. Serum was taken from 45 patients prior and during several rounds of cetuximab infusion and then assessed for HB-EGF expression by ELISA. Interestingly, HB-EGF levels at day 57 (before the 5th cetuximab infusion) were associated with response in patients with tumors harbouring wt K-RAS, where non-responders had significantly higher levels compared to responders. Serum levels of HB-EGF taken earlier during the cetuximab treatment or pre-treated serum however did not significantly correlate with response nor OS. No correlation of HB-EGF serum expression with response to cetuximab was also observed in another cohort of mCRC patients [213]. However, another study found that HB-EGF expression in plasma samples was higher in SCCHN patients with recurrent disease compared to those from patients with newly diagnosed SCCHN, indicating that HB-EGF may play a role in disease progression [241]. Interestingly, these authors went on to demonstrate that addition of exogenous HB-EGF to 3 cetuximab sensitive SCCHN cell lines (SCC1, SCC25 and SCC15) enhanced the level of resistance to cetuximab in MTT and colony formation assays [241]. Furthermore, these authors then compared HB-EGF expression levels in the SCC1 (cetuximab sensitive) cell line compared to a cetuximab-refractory sub-population of the SCC1 cells called 1Cc8 generated after long-term continuous exposure to cetuximab generated previously from the same group [242]. As expected the 1Cc8 cetuximab refractory cell line displayed greater HB-EGF gene expression and a 27-fold decrease in miR-212 expression (a direct regulator of HB-EGF expression) compared to the cetuximab-sensitive parental SCC1 cell line. Importantly, knockdown of HB-EGF in the 1Cc8 cell line resulted in re-sensitizing these cells to the inhibitory effects of cetuximab suggesting that HB-EGF plays a causative role in promoting resistance to cetuximab in SCCHN cell lines [241]. Interestingly, HB-EGF blockade also resulted in breast cancer cell apoptosis in cells resistant to trastuzumab, an FDA approved anti-HER2 humanised antibody [243].

4.5. Betacellulin (BTC) and Epigen (EPGN)

There have been very few reports describing a potential role for betacellulin (BTC) or epigen (EPGN) in mediating resistance to anti-EGFR therapy. One report found that erlotinib and gefitinib treatment of DU145 cells for 24 hours resulted in a 2-fold increase in BTC mRNA [229]. This increase in BTC (along with an increase in EGF, neuregulin, HER2, HER3 and HER4) led the authors to hypothesise that these increases could allow for continued EGFR signaling and refractory outcomes. However, BTC expression was not increased in the other prostate cancer cell line tested when treated with erlotinib and gefitinib. Furthermore, BTC expression was similar comparing parental DU145 and a sub-population of DU145-erlotinib resistant cells [229]. A study by Cushman *et al.* failed to find any predictive value in mRNA expression of BTC and EPGN in mCRC patients treated with cetuximab and chemotherapy compared to chemotherapy alone [227].

Likewise, intratumoral BTC gene expression and serum BTC expression levels did not predict response to cetuximab monotherapy in 2 independent mCRC cohorts [212, 213]. Finally, despite detecting BTC protein expression in 80.8% (21 out of 26) and EPGN in 23.1% (6 out of 26) of mCRC patients by immunohistochemistry, BTC nor EPGN correlated with response to either cetuximab or panitumumab [217].

Other growth factors outside those that bind the EGFR have also been implicated in providing resistance to EGFR targeted therapy including Neuregulins, IGF, HGF, VEGF and several cytokines. We will discuss these ligands in conjunction with the role their associated receptor(s) may play in EGFR therapy in the next two sections.

5. BIOMARKERS PREDICTING SENSITIVITY AND RESISTANCE TO ANTI-EGFR THERAPIES - ALTERATIONS IN ERBB RECEPTORS FAMILY MEMBERS

In this section we will review the extensive current literature examining the changes in expression, mutational status and compensatory cross-talk of the HER receptors as possible predictive markers of tumor sensitivity and resistance to anti-EGFR agents. We will discuss each HER receptor in turn.

5.1. Epidermal Growth Factor Receptor (EGFR)

5.1.1. EGFR Gene and Protein Expression

Pioneering clinical trials evaluating anti-EGFR monotherapy led to modest overall outcomes due to tumor resistance, drawing researchers to begin the search for potential predicative biomarkers for treatment response. Several lines of evidence aided in the formulation of the hypothesis that levels of EGFR expression itself would act as a predictor of response, and thus was one of the first biomarkers evaluated. This hypothesis was based on the reasoning that the greater level of EGFR expression, the more tumor reliance or addiction towards EGFR signaling would be present and hence the greater anti-tumor effect would be seen when EGFR was blocked. Secondly, as reported in section 4, concurrent evidence was beginning to prove that ligands of the EGFR may predict response to anti-EGFR agents and thus it was fair to speculate that EGFR expression may also. Finally, significant reports published around the same time as these pivotal EGFR targeted clinical trials were on-going, demonstrated that the efficacy of the anti-HER2 mAb trastuzumab was dependent on the level of HER2 expression in metastatic breast cancer [244, 245]. Indeed, more recently, screening for the expression of HER2 is now routinely performed and only metastatic breast cancer patients with high HER2 levels are recommended as suitable candidates for trastuzumab-based therapies [246], although others have shown that patients with low levels of HER2 may also respond to trastuzumab [247]. Thus, similar correlations were anticipated with EGFR expression and response to treatment. A multitude of studies examining EGFR expression in patient tumor tissue have produced inconsistent findings somewhat refuting this hypothesis. A large, randomised, multi-center Phase II trial (IDEAL-1) was published in 2003, assessed single-agent gefitinib in patients with recurrent or refractory NSCLC who failed one or two prior chemotherapy regimens that included a platinum agent [155]. In this study they observed objective tumor responses in approximately 18-19% of patients treated with either 250 or 500mg gefitinib daily. However, analysis of the EGFR status by immunohistochemistry in 157 tumor specimens taken from this trial revealed no consistent correlation between EGFR expression and radiographic or symptomatic response [155, 156].

A series of similar studies have also shown no correlation between EGFR expression and gefitinib response in other cohort of advanced NSCLC patients [248 - 250]. High EGFR expression was not a predictive factor in gefitinib response in a small cohort of NSCLC patients [248]. Likewise, there was no significant correlation between response to gefitinib and EGFR staining intensity by immunohistochemistry in two other independent studies by Parra and colleagues and Cappuzzo *et al.* [249, 250]. However, another study has shown opposing findings to the reports described above [251]. In this study positive EGFR expression in NSCLC tissue from chemotherapy refractory advanced NSCLC did associate with response to gefitinib. Patients with EGFR positive protein expression as detected by immunohistochemistry displayed a 8.2% (13 out of 158) ORR compared to the 1.5% (1 out of 69) ORR of patients who had EGFR negative protein expression [251]. The same group subsequently found that EGFR gene expression as determined by PCR can also predict response to gefitinib in advanced NSCLC patients [252]. Furthermore, a follow up study by Cappuzzo and colleagues published contradictory findings regarding EGFR expression levels in advanced NSCLC patients treated with gefitinib compared to their earlier study [253]. EGFR protein expression levels as detected by immunohistochemistry was determined in 98 NSCLC tumors and grouped into high and low EGFR expression. Patients with high EGFR staining displayed significantly greater ORR to gefitinib (20.7%; 12 out of 58) compared to patients with low EGFR tumors (5.0%; 2 out of 40). Paradoxically, this study did not see a similar association between patient response and EGFR gene expression levels to that observed with patient EGFR protein expression levels. Patients with high EGFR expression also displayed greater TTP, longer survival and lower progression rate compared to patients with negative EGFR expression [253]. The authors speculated as to why a discrepancy was observed in regards to the predictive value of EGFR expression between their earlier study and other studies with this present study. Possible explanations included differences in staining techniques based on variations in antibodies and staining kits used and differences in cut off criteria interpreting or scoring EGFR expression status as high *versus* low (or positive *versus* negative) across various studies [253]. In fact, a follow-up report compared antibody kits highlights the importance of standardised techniques and how laboratory and research center differences can lead to varied outcomes [254]. Two often used immunohistochemistry compatible anti-EGFR antibody detection kits were compared against the same set of 296 NSCLC patient tumor tissues. Despite, both showing similar positivity for EGFR staining (69 *vs.* 72%), 24% of tumors showed a disparity in staining where one antibody system showed positive staining while the other showed negative staining as determined by the cut-off for EGFR positivity set by the authors. Furthermore, adjustable variations for EGFR positivity set by the authors to obtain the best "cut-off" EGFR positivity with respects to correlative power and gefitinib response was also assessed. These authors identified that a lower cut-off point (lower EGFR staining required to be considered a EGFR positive tumor specimen) are better predictors of survival outcomes compared to higher cut-off points [254]. Subsequently, a more recent article used another antibody, 5B7 that detects a region in the intracellular domain of the EGFR [255]. This study by Mascaux and colleagues found that EGFR expression as detected by 5B7 using immuno-histochemistry did indeed predict response to gefitinib monotherapy in 98 patients with recurrent NSCLC [255]. These authors suggest based on their data that the 5B7 antibody that recognised the intracellular region of the EGFR may be a more sensitive and selective antibody for immunohistochemistry compared to current antibodies that detect the extracellular region of the receptor. Until these criteria can be standardised across studies and research groups, (which is highly unlikely) discrepancies will continue to emerge and curtail possible movement of identified predictive markers from translational research to clinical management and practice. Pre-clinical studies have also showed that the efficacy of gefitinib was not related to EGFR expression on a series of human patient derived cells in tissue culture and animal xenograft experiments [85, 256].

A series of studies assessing the predictive value of EGFR expression in cetuximab-based or erlotinib-based treatment of NSCLC patients also report opposing findings. The EGFR expression levels were assessed in NSCLC patients enrolled in the multicenter randomised Phase III First Line ErbituX (FLEX) trial [257]. This study observed significantly improved OS in patients with advanced NSCLC treated with cetuximab plus cisplatin and vinorelbine compared to patients treated with cisplatin and vinorelbine without cetuximab [258]. Subsequent analysis of EGFR expression by immunohistochemistry allowed for stratification of patients into 2 groups; those that had tumors with high EGFR expression (n = 345) and those that expressed low EGFR expression in their NSCLC tumors (n = 763) [257]. A greater RR and OS was observed in patients treated with cetuximab plus chemotherapy compared to patients treated with chemotherapy only in the high EGFR expressing subgroup. This finding was not observed in patients with low EGFR expressing tumors indicating that high EGFR expression may predict response for this treatment regimen in NSCLC patients. These results led the authors to suggest that prospective identification of high EGFR expression can be used to select advanced NSCLC patients who are most likely to derive a greater survival benefit from the treatment of cetuximab plus chemotherapy. Furthermore, these findings should result in a change in routine clinical practice in the NSCLC setting [257]. Conversely, findings from another study assessing the predictive feasibility of EGFR expression in another large scale randomised Phase III (BMS099) study showed otherwise [259]. This study evaluated the use of first-line taxane/carboplatin treatment with or without cetuximab on stage IIIB or IV NSCLC patients without restriction of validated EGFR expression. No significant differences in overall RR were seen between treatment arms in either patients with EGFR positive staining or EGFR negative staining by immunohistochemistry [259]. Thus unlike the study by Pirker *et al.* this study showed no significant association between EGFR expression and response to cetuximab.

Several studies have also assessed the predictive value of EGFR expression in erlotinib based treatment of NSCLC. The important BR.21 phase III trial published a decade ago demonstrated a survival benefit for erlotinib compared to placebo in NSCLC patients who had progressed after standard chemotherapy [181]. Subsequent multivariate analysis revealed that positive EGFR expression, defined as greater than 10% of positive cell staining, was associated with a better RR (11.1%, 12 out of 108) compared to those with low EGFR expression (3.8%, 3 out of 80) [186]. However, other studies have reported opposing findings. A 12.3% ORR was observed in stage IIIB or IV advanced or recurrent metastatic NSCLC patients who had disease progression or relapse to platinum-based therapy when treated with erlotinib [179]. Analysis of EGFR status was found to be not associated to response in this trial of 57 tested patients [179]. Assessment of EGFR expression as a biomarker for erlotinib response have also been performed in two randomized multicenter Phase III trials evaluating the efficacy of erlotinib plus chemotherapy *versus* chemotherapy only in the NSCLC setting. The first study found that erlotinib with concurrent paclitaxel and carboplatin did not confer a survival advantage with or without erlotinib in chemotherapy-naïve patients with advanced NSCLC [260]. The second study also showed that erlotinib with concurrent cisplatin and gemcitabine did not provide a greater survival benefit compared to cisplatin and gemcitabine alone in chemotherapy-naïve patients with advanced, recurrent or metastatic NSCLC [261]. In addition, there was no correlation between the level of EGFR expression with RR and clinical outcome in either trial [260, 261]. Similarly, comparable RR to erlotinib were seen in bronchioloalveolar carcinoma patients that had tumors that were EGFR positive compared to those with EGFR negative expression [262].

Two landmark mCRC clinical studies in 2004 by Saltz *et al.* and Cunningham and colleagues also showed that the level of EGFR expression as assessed by immunohistochemistry scoring had no correlation to response to cetuximab in mCRC patients [111, 113]. Saltz and colleagues enrolled 57 mCRC patients, all of which were positive for EGFR expression and had failed irinotecan or an irinotecan-based treatment, into a phase II trial examining the efficacy of single-agent cetuximab [113]. They examined EGFR expression by immuno-histochemistry grading tumor tissue 1+ to 3+ based on increasing intensity of EGFR expression. Response to cetuximab was found to be 5.9% (1 out of 17) in patients with tumors with weak staining; 13.3% (4 out of 30) in patients with tumors with moderate staining; and 0% (0 out of 10) in patients with strong staining [113]. Similarly, the study by Cunningham *et al.* found that the degree of EGFR expression either as a percentage of cells with EGFR-positive staining or as the maximal staining intensity per cell did not correlate significantly to the clinical response of cetuximab [111]. Likewise, a large Phase II study by Lenz *et al.* subsequently confirmed these findings where EGFR expression as measured by immunohistochemistry did not correlate with response to cetuximab in mCRC patients refractory to irinotecan, oxaliplatin, and fluoropyrimidines [263]. Intratumoral EGFR gene expression in mCRC did not correlate to response to cetuximab treatment in another study of 39 mCRC patients refractory to irinotecan and oxaliplatin [264]. In fact, cetuximab achieved response in some mCRC patient despite EGFR being undetectable in their tumors by immuno-histochemistry indicating that very low levels of EGFR expression was adequate for cetuximab to illicit an inhibitory effect [264 - 266]. Gefitinib has also achieved response in NSCLC patients with little to no intratumoral EGFR expression [267]. However, these initial studies in mCRC were performed prior to stratifying patients into wt and mutated K-RAS groups. Nonetheless, several subsequent reports show EGFR expression has no predictive value in response to cetuximab in wt K-RAS mCRC tumors [212 - 214, 268]. A similar study assessing the *in vitro* efficacy of cetuximab against a large panel of colon cancer cell lines also supported the notion that EGFR expression does not correlate with response to anti-EGFR agents [232]. Likewise, EGFR amplification did not significant correlate with tumor response or survival following cetuximab monotherapy in recurrent high-grade glioma patients who had previous surgery, radiotherapy and chemotherapy [269].

EGFR expression has also provided little predictive value for response to anti-EGFR treatment in the SCCHN setting. Conflicting studies have been reported in regards to EGFR expression and efficacy of anti-EGFR agents in *in vitro* cell line based assays. The study by Jedlinski and colleagues showed that EGFR copy number, mRNA and protein expression did not correlate with sensitivity to cetuximab treatment in 25 SCCHN primary cell lines [220]. However, EGFR mRNA and protein expression was found to correlate with the IC_{50} values of gefitinib in a different series of 16 SCCHN cell lines [270]. Furthermore, stable knockdown of the EGFR in another independent set of 4 poorly responding SCCHN cell lines, re-sensitized these cells to the inhibitory effects of cetuximab and panitumumab suggesting that EGFR expression levels may indeed predict response [271]. Clinical studies however show differing outcomes. Psyrri and colleagues determined the EGFR expression level in operable stage III/IV SCCHN samples taken from 42 patients [272]. These patients were treated with carboplatin and paclitaxel followed by cetuximab, carboplatin and paclitaxel concurrently with radiation. EGFR expression did not correlate with clinical outcome in this study [272]. A large study evaluating EGFR expression in 411 recurrent or metastatic SCCHN tissue was performed assessing clinical response to cetuximab in combination with first-line cisplatin or carboplatin and 5-fluorouricil [268]. Similarly to the report by Psyrri, this study showed that clinically meaningful survival benefit was achieved independent of EGFR expression in recurrent and metastatic SCCHN [268]. However, another group reported that high levels of EGFR expression as determined by immunohistochemistry were associated with PFS of SCCHN patients treated with cetuximab [273]. Finally, Moehler *et al.* found that greater EGFR expression was associated with increased RR to cetuximab based treatment, but not with TTP or OS in advanced gastroesophageal cancer patients [274].

5.1.2. EGFR Gene Copy Number (GCN)

Conflicting findings have also been seen when analysing EGFR gene copy number (GCN) as a predictive marker for response to therapy targeting the EGFR. Nonetheless, EGFR GCN has been proposed by some as a reliable predictor of response. In fact many studies utilising clinical samples have identified an association between EGFR GCN and response to anti-EGFR therapies. EGFR GCN in mCRC tissue as detected by fluorescence in-situ hybridization (FISH) was seen to correlate to response to cetuximab or panitumumab. Increased EGFR GCN was detected in 88.9% (8 out of 9) patients with objective responses compared to only 4.8% (1 out of 21) patients who did not response [275]. Two years later, the same group confirmed these preliminary results in a larger cohort of mCRC patients identifying that non-increased EGFR GCN associated with failure to respond to panitumumab treatment [276]. Lievre *et al.* also reported that increased EGFR GCN also correlated to response to cetuximab in a smaller cohort of mCRC patients [277], while high EGFR GCN also correlated to response to cetuximab, paclitaxel and carboplatin in chemo-naïve advanced NSCLC patients [278] and increased EGFR GCN was significantly associated with better OS in metastatic gastric and oesophago-gastric junction cancer patients treated with cetuximab, 5-fluorouracil, oxaliplatin and leucovorin (FOLFOX) in first-line therapy [279].

Others have also seen correlations between EGFR GCN with survival response to gefitinib. An important study by Cappuzzo and colleagues published in 2005 developed an EGFR FISH scoring system which is often currently used to define

EGFR FISH positivity in retrospective tumor tissue [253]. This scoring system was established by assessing 102 advanced NSCLC patients treated with gefitinib, classifying 6 FISH groups with increasing EGFR GCN per cell based on the frequency of tumor cells with specific number of gene copies of the EGFR gene and chromosome 7 centromeres [253]. Essentially, patients are considered EGFR FISH positive if they display gene amplification as defined by the presence of tight gene clusters with ratios ≥ 2 genes/chromosome/cell or ≥ 15 gene copies/cell in more than 10% of cells or ≥ 4 gene copies in ≥ 40 of cells. Negative EGFR FISH is defined as no amplification with ≥ 4 gene copies in <40% of cells. Based on this criterion, Cappuzzo *et al.* found that NSCLC patients who were EGFR FISH positive had significantly higher RR to gefitinib (36.4%, 12 out of 33) compared to FISH negative patients (2.9%, 2 out of 69). These patients also had lower progression rate, longer TTP and longer survival compared to EGFR FISH negative patients [253]. Utilising this scoring system, other studies have observed similar associations with EGFR GCN and response to gefitinib. EGFR FISH positive NSCLC patients (16.4%, 11 out of 67) enrolled in the Phase III ISEL trial had a better ORR to gefitinib compared to patients with negative EGFR FISH (3.2%, 5 out of 155) [251]. Furthermore, this study also showed that gefitinib enhanced survival compared to placebo in the EGFR FISH positive patients only and not the FISH negative patients [251]. Similarly, findings were seen in patients from a randomised Phase II study evaluating gefitinib in chemo-naïve NSCLC patients [280]. EGFR FISH positivity also predicted a better survival outcome in bronchioloalveolar carcinoma patients treated with gefitinib [281]. Response to gefitinib was also associated with EGFR GCN, with disease control was seen in 63.2% (12 out of 19) patients in EGFR FISH positive patients compared to 38.9% (14 out of 36) FISH-negative patients [281]. Another study combining patient data from 2 independent trials for gefitinib also showed similar predictive value of EGFR FISH positivity [282]. Patients who were EGFR FISH positive had a RR of 33% to gefitinib *versus* patients who were EGFR FISH negative (6%) [282].

EGFR GCN has also been shown to predict response in trials evaluating erlotinib efficacy. Similarly, to the studies above with gefitinib, FISH positive patients enrolled in the BR-21 study also showed better OS when treated with erlotinib compared to placebo, while no significant difference in survival was seen between erlotinib or placebo treated EGFR FISH negative patients [283]. In addition, the overall RR to erlotinib in these advanced NSCLC patients with EGFR FISH positivity was 21.4% (6 out of 28) compared to 4.8% (3 out of 63) EGFR FISH negative patients [283]. Another study also tested EGFR GCN as a predictive marker for response to erlotinib or gefitinib in patients with squamous cell lung carcinoma (SCLC). In this study, patients with EGFR FISH positivity displayed an ORR of 26.3% (5 out of 19) compared to 2.0% (1 out of 50) seen in patients with EGFR FISH negative tumors [284].

More recently, systematic review and meta-analyses have proposed a role of EGFR GCN and patient outcomes following treatment with EGFR-targeted agents. One study showed that increased EGFR GCN as detected by FISH or chromogenic *in situ* hybridization (CISH) was associated with increased OS, progression free survival and TTP in patients with advanced or recurrent NSCLC treated with either gefitinib or erlotinib as monotherapy [285]. Another study also undertook a meta-analysis of 19 independent studies evaluating a potential correlation between EGFR GCN and overall RR to anti-EGFR therapy [286]. Findings from this systematic review supported the initial reports showing that there was a general association between higher overall RRs in patients with increased EGFR GCN. Interestingly, the difference in overall RR between mCRC patients with increase copy number compared to normal or reduced copy number was greater in K-RAS wild-type patients, while in K-RAS mutated patients the difference often did not exist. However, the authors of this report cautioned that although increased EGFR GCN is generally associated with a better outcome to anti-EGFR treatment, the clinical utility of this biomarker for selecting recipients for anti-EGFR treatment would be severely limited for several reasons. These include poor reproducibility of EGFR GCN enumeration due to highly heterogeneous EGFR GCN within a tumor and drastically variable determination of EGFR GCN despite using standardised methodology [286]. Furthermore, another study examining EGFR GCN by PCR showed no association between increased EGFR GCN with objective response to cetuximab in another cohort of mCRC who had failed irinotecan, oxaliplatin, and fluoropyrimidines-based treatments [263]. Likewise, no correlation with EGFR FISH status and PFS and OS was reported by two studies in SCCHN patients treated with cetuximab-based treatment [287, 288].

Others have also found no correlation. The study by Kim and colleagues reported the findings of a Phase III randomised trial (INTEREST) evaluating gefitinib *versus* docetaxel in locally advanced or metastatic NSCLC patients who had been pre-treated with platinum-based therapy [289]. This study showed no significant difference in OS of these patients treated with gefitinib *versus* docetaxel. Further classification of patients showed that patients with high EGFR GCN did not have longer survival when treated with gefitinib compared to docetaxel. However, despite not being discussed at length, the authors tabulated that patients with high EGFR GCN and treated with gefitinib displayed a slightly better median OS rate of 8.4 months compared to the 6.4 months OS seen in patients treated with gefitinib with low EGFR GCN [289]. EGFR copy number as determined by RT-qPCR also showed no correlation to gefitinib response in NSCLC tumor tissue from patients enrolled in the IDEAL and INTACT clinical trials [290]. Two independent studies also assessed the predictive value of EGFR GCN in Japanese patients with NSCLC following gefitinib treatment. In the first study an increase in gefitinib RR was observed between NSCLC patients who were EGFR FISH positive (30.8%, 8 out of 26) and EGFR FISH negative (21.4%; 6 out of 28) [291]. However, this increase was not-significant, and no significant difference was also seen in OS and TTP between EGFR FISH positive and EGFR FISH negative patients [291]. Similarly, the second study showed that EGFR FISH positivity had no significant association with OS and prolonged PFS of advanced or recurrent NSCLC patients treated with gefitinib [292]. Finally, EGFR GCN FISH positivity was not predictive of a survival benefit in advanced pancreatic cancer patients treated with first-line therapy of erlotinib with gemcitabine [293].

Despite some reports showing significant correlation with EGFR protein expression and EGFR GCN and response to treatment, the utility of these markers clinically are limited for several reasons. Firstly, there are many contradictory reports suggesting that they do not predict patient response or outcome. Secondly, the studies discussed above showing an association between response and EGFR expression or EGFR GCN still only predicts response in no more than 25% of patients and thus the majority of patients do not response despite falling into the "correct" sub-population of patients that should response. Encouragingly, however, the identification of EGFR mutations (summarised schematically in Fig (**3**) have led to greater predictive value when these mutations are present compared to EGFR expression and GCN, as will be discussed in the next section.

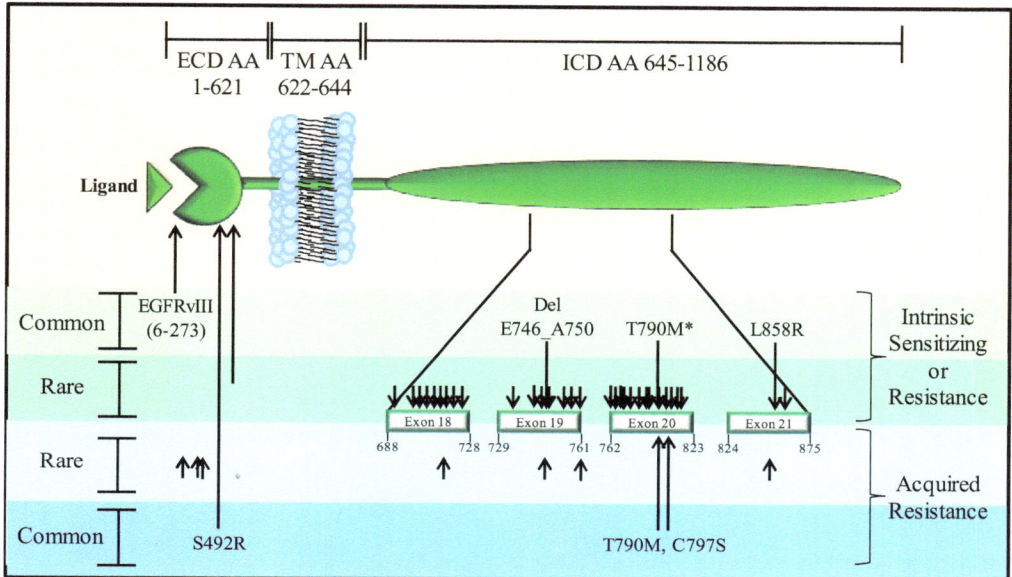

Fig. (3). Schematic of sensitizing and resistance inducing mutations in the EGFR. The common intrinsic sensitizing or resistance mutations (>5% in prevalence in at least one tumor type; shaded light green) include the EGFRvIII deletion, the Exon 19 deletion E746_A750) and the exon 21 L858R point mutation. *The EGFR T790M mutation has also been identified as a common intrinsic resistance mediator, although there are inconsistent studies presenting opposing views. The rare intrinsic sensitizing or resistance mutations (<5% in prevalence in at least one tumor type; shaded darker green) include P546S, V689M, P699S, N700D, R705G, E709Q, L718P, G719A/C/D/S/X, S720P/F, G721A, G724S, P733L/S, V740A, other deletions between residues 746-753, L747F/P, E749K, N756D, E758G, S761I, E762G, V765A/M, A767T, V769A/L, V774A, R776C/H, G779C/F/S, T783A/I, S784P, L798F/H/, K806E, Q812R, L814P, L861Q and insertion in exon 19 and 20. The common acquired resistance mutations (>5% in prevalence in at least one tumor type; shaded dark blue) include the S492R, T790M, C797S point mutations. The rare acquired resistance mutations (<5% in prevalence in at least one tumor type; shaded light blue) include R451C, K467T, G465R, G465E, E709A, L747S, D761Y, T854 and exon 20 insertions.

5.1.3. EGFR Mutations

5.1.3.1. Sensitizing EGFR Mutations

One of the most significant findings in the EGFR therapeutics field was discovered by 2 independent groups simultaneously and published in *The New England Journal of Medicine* and *Science* respectively in 2004 [159, 160]. The first study by Lynch and colleagues discovered heterozygous somatic mutations in the tyrosine kinase domain of the EGFR after sequencing the whole coding region of the EGFR from NSCLC patients. Specifically, these mutations included a range of in-frame deletions from amino acids 746 to 753 and substitutions L858R, L861Q and G719C. Importantly, at least one of these mutations was found in 88.9% (8 out of 9) of patients that showed gefitinib response whereas the mutations were not seen in the tumor tissue of 7 patients that did not respond to gefitinib. Transfection of wt EGFR, EGFR harbouring a deletion of residues 747–753 or L858R point mutation into Cos-7 cells demonstrated that these mutations were activated at least 2-fold greater than the wt EGFR when stimulated with EGF and this activation was far more sustained than that of the wt EGFR [159]. Furthermore, both EGFR mutants were more sensitive to the inhibitory effects of gefitinib compared to the wt receptor as measured by EGFR phosphorylation differences. Lynch and colleagues postulated based on their findings that these mutations (all found near the ATP binding cleave of the tyrosine kinase domain of the receptor) led to a conformational change that subsequently increases stabilisation of ATP binding and an enhanced, activated receptor. In addition, this hypothesised conformational change also led to increased stability of gefitinib binding to the ATP region and hence was proposed to be the mechanism of enhanced gefitinib sensitivity [159]. However, despite several reports aiming to confirm these hypothesis by structural analysis [294 - 298], there is no clear evidence to explain why gefitinib and erlotinib bind so firmly to the activated mutant receptor [299].

The second study by Paez and co-workers also identified mutations in the EGFR kinase domain following sequencing of exons 18 to 24 of the EGFR gene from NSCLC tumor tissue [160]. Importantly, these mutations were found in 5 out of 5 patients that responded to gefitinib while EGFR mutations were not seen in 4 patients that progressed on gefitinib. Furthermore, these mutations included the same L858R point mutation and in frame deletions within amino acids 747–753 to those observed by the study by Lynch. *In vitro* studies subsequently showed that the patient derived lung carcinoma cell line H3255, that also harboured the L858R

EGFR mutation was 50 times more sensitive to gefitinib inhibition of growth and inhibition of EGFR, Erk1/2 and Akt phosphorylation compared to 3 other patient-derived lung carcinoma cell lines with wt EGFR expression. The study by Paez also assessed the EGFR mutational status in NSCLC tumor tissue taken from patients who were not treated with gefitinib. Intriguingly, mutations in the kinase domain of the EGFR was far more frequent in adenocarcinomas (21.4%; 15 out of 70 patients) compared to other NSCLC (2.0%; 1 out of 49); observed more in women (20.0%; 9 out of 45) compared to men (9.5%; 7 out of 74) and more frequent in patients from Japan (29.3%, 29 out of 99) *versus* those from the United States (2.2%; 2 out of 90) [160]. An ensuing study using a larger number of NSCLC patients (n=519) concurred with the findings of Paez *et al.* observing that EGFR TK domain mutations were statistically significantly more frequent in adenocarcinomas *versus* cancer of other histologies (39.4%; 114 out of 289 *versus* 2.6%; 6 out of 230), in patients of East Asian ethnicity *versus* other ethnicities (29.6%; 107 out of 361 *versus* 8.2%; 13 out of 158), and in females *versus* males (42.1%; 72 out of 171 *versus* 13.8%; 48 out of 348) and also in individuals who had never smoked *versus* those that had previous or currently smoked (51.2%; 85 out of 166 *versus* 9.9%; 35 out of 353) [300]. Although not determined by Paez and colleagues nor Shigematsu *et al.* in their respective studies from the same cohort of patients Paez and co-workers noted that patients with adenocarcinoma, who are female or of East-Asian ethnicity have all been previously shown to be more responsive to EGFR inhibitors [155, 156], and thus postulated that the cause for this increase sensitivity may be due to the presence of these EGFR mutations.

Following these landmark papers, a large series of subsequent reports confirmed these findings in larger and independent NSCLC patient populations with varying ethnicities as summarised by Table **1**. Consistently, patients harbouring these EGFR mutations were significantly better responders to either gefitinib or erlotinib in almost all the studies outlined in Table **1**. Combined patient response in all these studies found that RR for patients with mutations was 68.9% (426 out of 618; ranging from 16-100%), while the RR of patients without EGFR mutations was 11.3% (109 out of 965; ranging from 0-59%).

Cetuximab is also effective against tumors in transgenic mice or xenograft models expressing the L858R EGFR mutation [301 - 304] and has been proposed as a possible mechanism of the observed response of NSCLC patients to the combined cetuximab and chemotherapy treatment [258, 305]. Panitumumab was also shown to inhibit the proliferation and *in vivo* tumor growth of cells harbouring the sensitizing EGFR mutations [306]. Due to this important discovery in NSCLC, many groups set out to identify EGFR mutations in other tumor types and decipher if these mutations could also predict response to anti-EGFR therapy. Interestingly, the presence of EGFR mutations have been detected in brain tumor metastases originating from NSCLC [47, 307 - 310], although other reports have shown no or very low presence of EGFR mutations [311, 312]. Nonetheless, similarly to NSCLC, EGFR tyrosine kinase inhibitors are also effective in treating brain metastasis harbouring EGFR mutations that originated from primary NSCLC tumors [310, 313 - 316].

However, the high mutational rates of exons 18-21 of the EGFR appear to be unique to patient tissue in the NSCLC setting. In fact, the original report by Lynch and colleagues describing these EGFR mutations, did not identify any mutations in the tyrosine kinase domain of the EGFR in 95 primary tumors from non-NSCLC patients (15 breast, 20 colon, 16 kidney, 40 pancreatic and 4 brain) and 108 cancer derived cell lines representing diverse histological types [159]. Similarly, a subsequent study by Shigematsu and colleagues using larger sample sizes found comparable EGFR mutational rates to those seen by Lynch *et al.* [300]. They detected EGFR tyrosine kinase domain mutations in 21.1% (130 out of 617) of NSCLC tumor tissue but did not detect any EGFR mutations in any of the 243 prostate, bladder, breast, colorectal and gallbladder cancers tested [300]. Likewise, mutational analysis of the tyrosine kinase domain of the EGFR from 9 glioblastoma patients also did not reveal the presence of any mutations affecting the amino acid sequence of the EGFR [317]. No EGFR mutations in exon 17-24 were detected in 59 glioblastomas in another study. This study also found only one EGFR mutation (G719S) in 293 colorectal tumors assessed [318]. The presence of any EGFR activating mutations in exon 19 and 21 were also not observed in breast cancer tissue [319] and whole-exome sequencing from patient-matched tumor-normal pairs also found that EGFR mutations were extremely rare in SCCHN [320]. Another report found no mutations in exon 18-24 of the EGFR gene in 82 SCCHN tumors [321], however another group found 7.3% (3 out of

41) of SCCHN tumors contained the exon 19 (del746_A750) commonly seen in NSCLC tumors [322]. Other analysis have shown low levels of EGFR mutations in the tyrosine kinase domain in 12.1% (4 out of 33) of colorectal [323], 12.5% (3 out of 24) of small intestinal adenocarcinoma [324], 10.2-13.0% (9 out of 88 - 13 out of 100) of prostate tumor tissue [325, 326] and 2.0% (1 out of 50) of oesophageal cancer [327]. Introduction of three of these point mutations (E749K, E762G and A767T) into the colorectal cell line LS174T led to differential sensitivity to gefitinib compared to cells with wt EGFR expression [328]. A large study evaluated the presence of EGFR mutations in exons 18-21 from 958 advanced tumors of various origins. Excluding NSCLC tumors, which were found to have EGFR mutations in 16.0% (21 out of 131), only 1.6% (13 out of 827) of non-NSCLC tumors contained an EGFR mutation [329]. Although relatively rare, EGFR point mutations G719S and G724S have been identified in colorectal adenocarcinoma [318, 330, 331]. Introduction of these EGFR mutations into the BaF/3 cell line led to significantly enhanced sensitivity to cetuximab *in vitro* [330], however one patient found to express the G719S mutation failed to respond to gefitinib treatment [331]. Thus, whether these mutations lead to increased sensitivity to anti-EGFR therapy in cancer patients with tumors other than NSCLC is yet to be fully determined.

Nonetheless, identifying EGFR mutations in the tyrosine kinase domain of the EGFR as a positive predictor of response to gefitinib and erlotinib in NSCLC led to attempts to screen for these mutations to improve selection of patients that would most benefit from anti-EGFR therapy. In particular, two of these EGFR activating mutations; micro-deletions in exon 19 (del746_A750) which lead to the removal of a leucine-arginine-glutamic acid-alanine motif and the L858R point mutation in exon 21 make up approximately 85-90% of the known EGFR mutations and hence have drawn the most focus for pre-treatment prospective testing [332, 333]. The first prospective trials evaluating gefitinib treatment of NSCLC patient sub-populations specifically harbouring EGFR activating mutations were reported in 2006, only 2 years after the initial discovery of the EGFR tyrosine kinase domain mutations. Eligibility criteria for these initial trials included patients with confirmed stage IIIB and IV, chemo-naïve NSCLC, Eastern Cooperative Oncology Group (ECOG) performance status of 0-2 and the presence of EGFR mutations in exons 18-21. In the first trial by Inoue *et al.* patients were found to harbour EGFR mutations and were subsequently given first-line gefitinib treatment resulted in a RR and disease control rate of 75.0% (12 out of 16) and 87.5% (14 out of 16) respectively [334]. Another phase II trial enrolled 16 NSCLC patients following positive detection of EGFR mutations and observed identical overall RR of 75.0% (12 out of 16) as that of Inoue and colleagues after first-line gefitinib treatment [335]. In another Phase II trial, 27 patients with confirmed EGFR mutations were given gefitinib as either first (n=4) or second-line (n=23) treatment following chemotherapy resulting in an overall RR of 77.7% (21 out of 27) [336]. A series of trials for NSCLC patients selected for positive EGFR mutation status followed including trials evaluating gefitinib in patients in first, second-line or greater therapy, poorer ECOG performance status, Caucasian patient populations and in elderly patients [337 - 347]. In all these studies, the overall response rates to gefitinib treatment ranged from 46 - 76%, significantly better than observed in unselected patient populations.

Erlotinib as monotherapy in prospective studies of patients with NSCLC and EGFR mutations have also been performed. The study by Rosell and colleagues screened 2105 Spanish NSCLC patients and found that 350 were positive for either the exon 19 deletion of L858R EGFR mutation. Of these 350 patients, 217 were enrolled into a trial evaluating erlotinib treatment and 197 were assessed for erlotinib response. Overall, the RR was 70.6% (139 out of 197), median PFS was 14.0 months and OS was 27.0 months [348]. Other prospective studies have also been performed assessing gefitinib and erlotinib in patients with pathologically confirmed NSCLC harbouring activating EGFR mutations and measurable brain metastases. In the open-labelled phase II study evaluating gefitinib or erlotinib as first, second or third-line treatment by Park and colleagues, a RR of 82.1% (23 out of 28) and a disease control rate of 92.9% (26 out of 28) was seen [349].

Importantly, comparisons between treatment efficacy of chemotherapy and gefitinib have been performed as first-line therapy for EGFR mutation positive NSCLC patients with gefitinib showing more favourable response compared to chemotherapy. Maemondo and colleagues performed a multicenter, randomised Phase III trial comparing first-line gefitinib *versus* carboplatin/paclitaxel in patients with metastatic NSCLC with EGFR mutations [161]. Patients treated with gefitinib compared to chemotherapy had a better ORR (73.7% *vs.* 30.7%), PFS (10.8 months *vs.* 5.4 months) and OS rate (30.5 months *vs.* 23.6 months) [161]. A similar study also showed greater 12 month PFS in EGFR mutation positive advanced pulmonary adenocarcinoma patients treated with gefitinib (24.9%) *versus* carboplatin/paclitaxel (6.7%) [350]. Another phase III trial showed that gefitinib treatment resulted in a significantly greater PFS rate in EGFR mutation positive NSCLC patients compared to those treated with cisplatin plus docetaxel as first line therapy [162]. Likewise, a European randomised phase III trial (EURTAC) compared the efficacy of cisplatin plus docetaxel this time *versus* erlotinib as first-line therapy for Caucasian patients with NSCLC harbouring EGFR mutations [185]. Similarly to the results seen with gefitinib, PFS was enhanced in the erlotinib group *versus* the chemotherapy treated group (9.7 months *vs.* 5.2 months) [185]. Finally, another study evaluated erlotinib compared to carboplatin plus gemcitabine in a randomised, open-label phase III trial for Asian NSCLC patients with EGFR mutations and found that PFS was longer in erlotinib treated patients than chemotherapy treated patients (13.1 months *vs.* 4.6 months) [187]. However, a follow-up article of this study reported that there was no significant difference between OS of patients treated with erlotinib or chemotherapy (22.8 months *vs.* 27.2 months) [188]. More recently, Yang and colleagues showed that Afatinib produced a better OS compared to cisplatin-based chemotherapy in NSCLC patients with the exon 19 mutation but no significant difference in OS was seen between afatinib and chemotherapy treated patients with L858R mutations [201].

Further analysis has been performed examining possible differences in response of NSCLC patients based on which EGFR mutation they harbour across exons 18-21. Mitsudomi and colleagues showed that NSCLC patients with the exon 19 deletion are more responsive to gefitinib compared to those with the L858R mutation [351]. Rosell and colleagues observed similar findings with erlotinib [348]. In another study, NSCLC patients with exon 18 mutations showed a 100% (4 out of 4) response and patients with exon 19 mutations showed a 85.7% (6 out of 7) response. This RR was decidedly better than the RR of patients with exon 20 (50%; 2 out of 4) and exon 21 mutations (62.5%; 5 out of 8) [352]. Another more recent report examined exon 18-21 EGFR mutations in a large number of French

NSCLC patients and found that patients with exon 18 sensitizing mutations had a worse PFS than those with exon 19 or 21 mutations [353]. Finally, 2 studies from the same group also examined differences in patient outcome stratifying patients into groups based on which EGFR mutations they harboured. In one study, the clinical outcomes of gefitinib treatment in NSCLC patients with either the two most common mutations (exon 19 deletions or L585R) was compared with those with rarer mutations. Interestingly, those patients with the common mutations had a higher response rate (83.3%; 10 out of 12 *vs.* 28.6%; 2 out of 7), longer median PFS (12.7 *vs.* 4.9 months) and longer OS (24.7 *vs.* 12.3 months) compared to those with uncommon mutations [354]. In the other study, the RR, TTF and OS of patients with exon 19 deletion or the exon 21 L858R mutation were 83.7% (36 out of 43), 8.9 months and 24.1 months; while for patients with other EGFR mutations the outcomes were significantly lower (RR= 16.7%; 2 out of 12; TPP = 2.1 months; OS = 6.7 months). Interestingly, the RR and survival rates in these patients with less common EGFR mutations were lower than those patients with wild-type EGFR, suggesting that these mutations may predict less favourable outcomes to gefitinib [355].

The majority of research and clinical studies have focused on the exon 19 deletions and L858R point-mutation due to being the most common EGFR mutations seen clinically. However, others have assessed the role of the L861Q mutation (originally found by Lynch *et al.*) in predictive response, although inconclusive data has been reported [353, 355, 356]. Meanwhile, several other mutations may also predict favourable or poorer response to anti-EGFR based therapy as specifically reviewed by Massarelli and colleagues [357]. These mutations include G719A/C/D/S/X [297, 358], V689M, S720P/F, P699S [348, 359], N700D, E709Q [360], G721A, V740A [361], V769A/L [362, 363], L718P [251], P733L/S, L747F/P, N756D, E758G [364, 365], S761I [356, 363, 366, 367], insertion in exon 20 [368 - 371], V765A/M [332, 364, 372], T783A/I [348, 364], V774A [358], S784P [361], R776C/H, G779C/F/S, L798F/H/, K806E, Q812R, L814P [364]. Another study identified 2 novel point-mutations (R705G and P546S) in the EGFR gene of a patient's head and neck tumor that had complete regression following cetuximab monotherapy post-surgery and radiotherapy. NIH3T3 cells stably transfected with the EGFR containing the P546S mutation were significantly more sensitive to cetuximab inhibition compared to cells with wildtype EGFR suggesting that this mutation may also provide sensitivity to EGFR inhibitors [373]. Likewise, a polymorphism of EGFR R521K correlated with improved cetuximab and FOLFOX-4 (oxaliplatin, folinic acid and 5-FU) response and associated with a longer PFS period and OS in mCRC patients [374]. However, due to the fact that many of these mutations have only been reported in case studies of one or few patients, they may not have much clinical significance in the treatment of patients as these EGFR mutations are relatively rare.

Despite these promising findings that several EGFR mutations can predict sensitivity to anti-EGFR therapy, most patients who initially respond commonly and rapidly relapse, presenting with reoccurrence of tumors that are frequently resistant to the original therapy. In our next section we will examine the EGFR mutations that confer resistance to anti-EGFR therapy.

5.1.3.2. EGFR Mutations that Lead to Resistance

The excitement generated by the discovery that specific EGFR mutations could predict enhanced sensitivity to gefitinib in NSCLC patients in 2004 was dampened somewhat by the equally important discovery in 2005 that other EGFR mutations acquired during and post treatment could confer resistance and ultimately lead to a lack of patient response. The initial discovery of an EGFR point-mutation that confers acquired resistance to EGFR tyrosine kinase inhibitors was made in a small set of NSCLC patients who originally responded well to gefitinib or erlotinib but subsequently presented with tumor progression [192]. Examination of pre-treated lung tumor biopsies revealed an EGFR mutation that predicts gefitinib or erlotinib sensitivity including the most common L858R in one patient and the exon 19 delE746-A750 in another patient. Analysis of subsequent biopsies from these patients after treatment and tumor progression also revealed the same patient matched sensitizing EGFR mutations. This suggests that these mutations are maintained during treatment response and acquired tumor resistance and supports the notion that relapsed or metastatic tumors are derived from progenitor cells within the original tumor. However, in addition to these sensitizing mutations, Pao and colleagues sequenced exon 18-24 of the EGFR in the secondary biopsies or from cells in pleural effusion taken after tumor progression, and found that all 3 patients contained a nucleotide change predicting a threonine to methionine change at position 790 (T790M). Importantly, Pao and colleagues did not find the T790M mutation in any of 155 NSCLC tumors resected prior to treatment with EGFR tyrosine kinase inhibitors suggesting that the T790M was a secondary, acquired mutation arising during or post administration of gefitinib or erlotinib into the patient [192]. This notion was supported by other reports [350, 375 - 377] including a study by Vikis *et al.* who did not find the T790M mutation in any of the 282 lung and bronchoalveolar tumor tissue their screened [376] and a study by Mok and colleagues who found the T790M mutation in only 2.5% (11 out of 437) of patients prior to gefitinib treatment [350].

However, the study by Rosell and colleagues report opposing findings to the studies above. In this study, 36.2% (75 out of 207) of NSCLC patients samples prior to anti-EGFR treatment from two independent cohorts contained the T790M suggesting that the T790M mutation is present in relatively high levels in baseline NSCLC tumors and is not an acquired mutation as a result of treatment [378]. Similarly, another study identified the T790M mutation in circulating tumors cells from 38.5% (10 out of 26) of NSCLC patients taken prior to treatment of anti-EGFR agents [379]. Analysis of plasma DNA from patients with advanced stage NSCLC also found that 8.2% (4 out of 49) harboured de novo EGFR T790M mutations in another study [380]. The large discrepancy between the T790M mutational rates in pre-treated NSCLC patient samples across several reports has been explained by the use of differing techniques with varying sensitivity thresholds. Indeed, using the Scorpion Amplification Refractory Mutation System (SARMS) technology test, Maheswaran and colleagues were able to identify rare *EGFR* mutant alleles below the detection limit of standard sequencing. Furthermore, verifying this point of superior detection techniques, Su and colleagues directly compared the ability of direct sequencing *versus* matrix-assisted laser desorption ionization–time of flight mass spectrometry (MALDI-TOF MS) in detecting the EGFR T790M mutation in treatment naïve and pre-treated NSCLC tumor tissue [381]. In this report, MALDI-TOF MS was highly sensitive in detecting and quantifying the frequency of EGFR T790M mutations identifying the T790M mutation in 25.2% (27 out of 107) of EGFR TKI-naive patients and 31.5% (23 out of 73) of pre-treated NSCLC patients. In contrast, direct sequencing only detected T790M mutations in 2.8% (3 out of 107) and 2.7% (2 out of 73) of treatment naïve and pre-treated patients respectively [381]. This study clearly highlights the need to use the most sensitive techniques available to truly determine the levels of biomarker expression to form accurate correlative predictions. Importantly, these studies showed that T790M conferred intrinsic resistance to anti-EGFR inhibitors (gefitinib or erlotinib). In each of the reports by Rosell, Maheswaran and Su, the presence of EGFR T790M mutations correlated with reduced PFS in patients with NSCLC who received TKI treatment indicating a possible role of the T90M mutation in mediating intrinsic resistance along with its accepted role in acquired resistance [378, 379, 381]. Furthermore, germline T790M mutations have been reported in familial NSCLC patients and family members of these patients suggesting a greater susceptibility of NSCLC development in individuals with this mutation [382 - 384].

In addition, to their initial findings, Pao and colleagues also observed that a patient derived NSCLC cell line (H1975) with both the sensitizing L585R mutation and the T790M mutation was far more resistant to the anti-proliferative effects of gefitinib and erlotinib compared to another NSCLC patient derived cell line (H3255) that harbours only the L858R mutation somewhat proving that the T790M mutation can mediate resistance to EGFR tyrosine kinase inhibitors [192].

Another study published 2 days after the Pao *et al.* paper also identified the T790M EGFR point-mutation that confers acquired resistance to gefitinib in a relapsed NSCLC tumor post gefitinib treatment. In this study, Kobayashi and colleagues documented a case study of a NSCLC patient who harboured the EGFR sensitizing deletion del747-S752 in his primary tumor and responded as expected to gefitinib [191]. However, following 24 months of remission, tumor reoccurrence was detected and exon 18-21 of the EGFR gene was sequenced from a biopsy taken from the recurrent tumor. The original EGFR sensitizing deletion (del747-S752) found in his primary biopsy was maintained in the recurrent tumor (as also seen by Pao and colleagues); however a second mutation predicting the T790M mutation was also detected. Interestingly, subsequent reports have assessed the continued presence of EGFR sensitizing mutations in NSCLC patients who developed resistance to gefitinib or erlotinib. One report found that 98.4% (61 out of 62) of these patients maintained their EGFR sensitizing mutation in a follow-up biopsy taken after observed tumor progression [375] while another found that 100% (37 out of 37) of resistant tumors retained their original activating EGFR mutations [385]. Other studies concurred with those of Pao and colleagues and Kobayashi and co-workers finding that approximately 43 - 63% of patients with acquired resistance to EGFR tyrosine kinase inhibitors harbour the T790M mutation in relapsed tumors [375, 377, 385 - 387].

In addition, Kobayashi and colleagues went on to show that gefitinib was far less effective in inhibiting EGFR phosphorylation in COS-7 and NIH3T3 cells transfected with EGFR containing the T790M mutation compared to wt EGFR. These authors also speculated that the methionine substitution led to a bulkier side chain compared to threonine and a greater steric hindrance to tyrosine kinase inhibitor binding [191]. Another study however further examined the structural change resulting from the T790M mutation. They concluded that this mutation enhances ATP binding affinity resulting in resistance through a mechanism where ATP successfully competes with either gefitinib or erlotinib for the binding to the Lysine 721 residue and not through steric hindrance [388]. Further supporting this conclusion is evidence showing that irreversible EGFR inhibitors can overcome the presence of the T790M mutation in NSCLC by forming covalent bonds with Cys-797 at the edge of the ATP-binding cleft of the EGFR therefore suggesting that steric hindrance is not the major mechanism of resistance mediated by the T790M mutation [388]. Interestingly, there is also evidence from animal xenograft and patient derived xenograft models that cetuximab and panitumumab can inhibit tumors harbouring the T790M mutation [301, 302, 304, 306, 389].

Importantly, the observation that other EGFR inhibitors could overcome T790M mediated resistance to gefitinib and erlotinib in cell lines have led to the clinical development and application of second and third-generation EGFR family tyrosine kinase inhibitors in the attempt to specifically treat NSCLC tumors that harbour the T790M mutation. The second-generation agents that specifically inhibit the EGFR and at least one other EGFR family member (HER2, HER3 or HER4) include pelitinib/EKB569 [390, 391], neratinib/HKI-272 [392, 393], cancertinib/CI-1033 [394, 395], lapatinib/GW-572016 [396], decomitinib/

PF00299804 [397, 398], icotinib/BPI-2009H [399, 400] and afatinib/ BIBW2992 [401]. All of these inhibitors have entered clinical trials for NSCLC, often after disease progression following gefitinib or erlotinib treatment and have shown some level of clinical efficacy. Lapatinib, which is approved for the treatment of HER2-positive metastatic breast cancer patients, produced a lack of response in 8 patients with EGFR mutations in patients with recurrent or metastatic NSCLC [396]. Afatinib is the only second-generation agent approved in the NSCLC setting (as outlined in section 3.6 of this review). Cetuximab in combination with vinorelbine was also effective in one NSCLC patient following the acquisition of resistance to second-line erlotinib and fourth-line gefitinib therapy [402].

Several adverse effects of agents that target the wt EGFR have been reported include diarrhoea, nausea and skin toxicities and as such third generation anti-EGFR inhibitors have been developed to alleviate these effects by only inhibiting EGFR mutations and not wild-type EGFR expressed on normal tissue. Two of these agents, AZD9291 and Rociletinib/CO1686 have shown encouraging pre-clinical evaluation specifically inhibiting tumors with either EGFR activating and acquired resistance mutations and showing reduced efficacy for tumors with wildtype EGFR only [403 - 406]. Currently three agents AZD9291, Rociletinib/ CO-16886 and HM61713 are under clinical evaluation for the treatment of NSCLC patients with T790M mutations [407, 408]. Based on data from these trials both AZD9291 and Rociletinib have been granted breakthrough therapy designation by the US FDA for the treatment of patients with EGFR T790M positive NSCLC whose disease has progressed during treatment with a previous EGFR tyrosine kinase inhibitor [407]. Whether these inhibitors will provide greater response and OS rates in NSCLC patients harbouring EGFR mutations in either first-line treatment or after resistance has been acquired is yet to be fully determined.

Similarly to that seen with EGFR sensitizing mutations, a small percentage of NSCLC tumors express EGFR mutations, other than the T790M mutation, which correlate with acquired resistance. These mutations include E709A [409, 410], L747S [411], D761Y [387], exon 20 insertions [361, 370], [392, 397], [412 - 415] and T854A [416]. Despite the emergence of second and third line EGFR tyrosine kinase inhibitors that may overcome the resistance observed to gefitinib and erlotinib many researchers speculate that treatment of patients with these inhibitors may also eventually yield acquired EGFR mutations that lead to refractory long-term outcomes, similar to that currently observed when treated with currently approved anti-EGFR therapies. As such, cell-based mutagenesis screens and crystallography studies have identified predicted mutations that promote resistance by blocking covalent biding of irreversible second and third-generation EGFR tyrosine kinase inhibitors [417 - 421]. These mutations included E931G, H773L, L658P, L655H, C797S, L718Q, G796X and L844V. Importantly, one of these mutation, C797S, was recently discovered in 40.0% (6 out of 15) of cell-free plasma samples from NSCLC patients taken after they developed resistance to the third-generation EGFR inhibitor AZD9291 [422]. This point-mutation was not seen in pre-treatment samples indicating that the C797S mutation had been acquired during AZD9291 treatment. Ba/F3 and NSCLC cells expressing the C797S-mutant were more resistant to AZD9291-mediated cell growth inhibition compared to parental cells [421, 422].

A study by Montagut and colleagues also identified another point-mutation, S492R, (not seen in resistant NSCLC tumors) in the ectodomain of the EGFR in biopsies from two out of 10 mCRC patients taken following disease progression after a prior response to cetuximab with chemotherapy [423]. This mutation was not seen in the pre-treatment tumor samples of these 2 patients or in 156 mCRC tumors from chemotherapy-naive and cetuximab–naive patients [423]. A subsequent study analysing 37 mCRC patient matched samples pre-cetuximab treatment and post acquired resistance to cetuximab revealed EGFR mutations in the post cetuximab treated tumors. These included the same mutation (S492R) in 3 patient samples as previously identified by Montagut and colleagues and 2 novel mutations, R451C identified in one patient and K467T seen in another patient [424]. Analysis of EGFR mutations in 5 colon cancer cell lines with acquired resistance to cetuximab after long-term culturing in the presence of cetuximab also identified 3 EGFR mutations (S464L, G465R and I491M). The resistant cell lines did not however acquire the 3 mutations Arena and colleagues identified in patient tumor tissue while the mutations seen in patient tissue were not replicated in the resistant cell lines [424]. However, more recently, one of these mutations (G465R) identified in the acquired cetuximab resistant cell lines by Arena *et al.*

was identified in the post cetuximab treated biopsy of one that was not present in the pre-treated patient matched specimens. A novel EGFR G465E mutation was also observed in the post but not the pre-treated mCRC biopsy of another patient [425]. Interestingly, the study by Montagut and colleagues also created cetuximab-refractory DIFI colon cancer cells (similarly to Arena *et al.*) and found that the EGFR mutation status in there resistant clones did in fact contain the EGFR S492R mutation observed in patients. Further experiments showed that this mutation leads to a confirmation that blocks cetuximab binding and thus it was speculated that acquired resistance to cetuximab occurs in some patients by the S492R mutation blocking cetuximab-EGFR association. However, this mechanism of acquired resistance is only seen in a small percentage of patients (11-20%) [423, 424] and was not seen in another recent study examining 16 mCRC patients with matched pre and post cetuximab or panitumumab treated tumors [426]. Furthermore, the acquired cetuximab-refractory DIFI cell line models emphasises that acquired resistance can occur by several mechanisms and mutational heterogeneity readily occurs to provide resistance as seen in the reports by Arena and Montagut and another study by Yu and colleagues. In this study, examination of EGFR mutations was not performed however they observed that acquired cetuximab-refractory DIFI cells expressed significantly less EGFR potentially through enhanced receptor ubiquitination [427]. Most recently, next-generation sequencing was performed on mCRC tumor tissue from patients' pre and post cetuximab or panitumumab treated to identify EGFR ectodomain mutations [426]. None of the pre-treatment or control samples showed *EGFR* ectodomain mutations, however a sample from one patient treated with panitumumab contained an acquired EGFR G465R mutation (the same point mutation identified by Arena *et al.* and Bertotti *et al.*) [424, 425]. Further analysis showed that this mutation is located in the binding epitope of both panitumumab and cetuximab and thus could block biding of both antibodies providing cross-resistance to both anti-EGFR agents [426]. This is in contrast to the S492R mutation that inhibits cetuximab binding but does not significantly alter the binding of panitumumab [423]. In accordance with the notion that these mutations are acquired, another study found that only 1.5% (1 out of 65) of EGFR inhibitor treatment naïve mCRC patients were positive to point-mutations in the EGFR binding region (L2 domain) and thus these mutations may only be predictive of acquired resistance [428].

However, besides the T790M mutation seen in approximately 50% of EGFR tyrosine kinase inhibitor refractory NSCLC tumors these other mutations that predict or confer resistance to anti-EGFR therapy may not be of substantial abundance to provide changes in clinical management of patients and thus do not provide high clinical significance.

5.1.3.3. EGFRvIII

The EGFRvIII (also known as ΔEGFR and Δ2-7EGFR) is formed from the loss of exons 2 to 7 of the EGFR gene, resulting in an in-frame deletion of 267 amino acids in the extracellular domain and a truncated protein similar to the v-erb-B transforming protein of avian erythroblastosis virus [54, 429]. Although the truncated EGFRvIII is unable to bind any known EGFR ligand [430, 431] the receptor shows constitutive tyrosine kinase activity which is believed to confer enhanced downstream pro-oncogenic signaling [65, 432, 433]. Although most studies focused on EGFRvIII are in glioblastoma, where it is expressed in approximately 30-40% of primary glioblastoma tissue [65, 68, 434], others have identified EGFRvIII expression in a number of cancer types including SCCHN, lung and breast [435 - 438].

The EGFRvIII expression has been associated with resistance to anti-EGFR therapy due to its constitutively active pro-proliferative and pro-survival/ant--apoptotic signaling characteristics, although many contradictory studies show no correlation or the opposite findings. Cetuximab treatment of glioblastoma cell lines stably expressing EGFRvIII produced mixed results with some studies showing little to no effect while others observed significant inhibitory effects *in vitro* and in animal xenograft models [439 - 444]. Gefitinib and erlotinib also exhibit a range of inhibitory effects against EGFRvIII expressing glioblastoma cells [445 - 451]. Interestingly, panitumumab however, could significantly reduce the *in vivo* subcutaneous growth of EGFRvIII positive glioblastoma cells [452, 453]. EGFRvIII expression was also determined as a potential predictive marker in a study evaluating cetuximab in patients with recurrent glioblastoma [454]. In this study, although not statistically significant patients with EGFRvIII positive tumors (n=11) had worst PFS (1.6 *vs.* 1.9 months) and OS (3.3 *vs.* 4.9 months) compared to patients without EGFRvIII (n=24) following cetuximab treatment. However, further analysis of a subpopulation of patients with amplification of the EGFR gene found that patients with EGFR amplification and EGFRvIII expression (n=11) had significantly worst PFS (1.6 *vs.* 3.0 months) and OS (3.3 *vs.* 5.6 months) compared to patients with EGFR amplification without EGFRvIII expression (n=8) following cetuximab treatment [454].

Other studies have examined the tumor expression levels of EGFRvIII expression as a predictive biomarker in gefitinib or erlotinib based glioblastoma therapy in clinical samples with inconsistent findings. Mellinghoff and colleagues determined the EGFRvIII expression in recurrent high-grade glioma patients treated with either gefitinib or erlotinib [455]. Combined data from independent test and validation set of tumor tissue found that 86.7% (13 out of 15) patients who responded to gefitinib or erlotinib expressed EGFRvIII, whereas only 38.6% (17 out of 44) of non-responders expressed EGFRvIII, suggesting that EGFRvIII expression may somewhat predict positive response. Further molecular analysis of these tumors revealed that expression of both EGFRvIII and PTEN expression correlated significantly to response to either gefitinib or erlotinib. Specifically, of the 15 patients who responded, 13 were positive for both EGFRvIII and PTEN, while of the 44 patients who did not respond, only 3 patients expressed both markers [455]. Several studies have subsequently failed to recapitulate these findings in other retrospective studies involving anti-EGFR therapy in the glioma patient setting. In a phase I/II study, Brown and colleagues evaluated erlotinib and temozolomide treatment in newly diagnosed glioblastoma patients who had recently had maximal surgical resection. In this study neither EGFRvIII expression alone nor EGFRvIII and PTEN co-expression significantly correlated with PFS and OS [456]. In another study, the presence of EGFRvIII expression was in fact correlated to poor PFS in patients with progressive glioblastoma who were treated with erlotinib [457]. Patients with co-expression of EGFRvIII and PTEN also showed poorer PFS and RR. In addition, a phase II trial evaluating gefitinib in recurrent glioblastoma patients found that EGFRvIII protein expression did not predict either disease control or survival [317]. Others have also observed no correlation with EGFRvIII expression and response to gefitinib or erlotinib and patient outcome, however some of these studies report only small numbers of EGFRvIII positive samples and thus statistical analysis is limited [458 - 460].

EGFRvIII expression has also been associated with refractory outcomes in the SCCHN setting. SCCHN cells stably transfected with EGFRvIII were more resistant to cetuximab inhibition compared with control cells in both cell culture and animal xenograft models [436]. Likewise, patients with recurrent or metastatic SCCHN treated with cetuximab and docetaxel and displaying high EGFRvIII expression correlated with a worst disease control rates (12.5; 1 out of 8 *vs.* 64.9%; 24 out of 37) and shorter PFS (2.0 *vs.* 5.4 months) compared to low EGFRvIII expression [221]. Although EGFRvIII expression did not significantly associate with OS in this study [221] and EGFRvIII gene expression did not correlate with cetuximab response in another cohort of loco-regional advanced SCCHN patients [461]. Conversely, another study by Chau and colleagues found that EGFRvIII expression was associated with better disease control in recurrent and metastatic SCCHN patients who had been treated with erlotinib or other non EGFR inhibitors in separate trials [462].

Finally, lung cancer models expressing EGFRvIII are also refractory to cetuximab, gefitinib and erlotinib but may be inhibited by new generation anti-EGFR inhibitors such as HKI-272 [438, 463]. However, as EGFRvIII expression in lung cancer is relatively rare (approximately 5%), screening or selecting patients based on EGFRvIII expression may not be clinically feasible and useful for selective treatment. The EGFRvIII has been associated with clinical response to anti-EGFR inhibitors. However, until a clearer understanding of the exact role this mutant receptor plays in tumor resistance (or sensitivity) is established, the detection of its expression in patient tumor tissue may not be of much clinical benefit in patient management and treatment selection.

5.2. HER2 (ErbB2)

The development of targeted therapies that could successfully inhibit EGFR activation subsequently led to the now common discovery that other tyrosine receptor kinases could trigger compensatory downstream signals ultimately leading to continued proliferation and resistance to anti-EGFR therapeutic agents. Naturally, it was discovered that each of the EGFR family members could provide these compensatory signal transduction. In the next sections of this review we will focus on the role of HER2, HER3 and HER4 in mediating resistance to anti-EGFR therapy.

Several clinical and laboratory based studies have identified HER2 as a potential initiator of resistance to anti-EGFR therapy. The study by Bertotti and colleagues examined potential resistance mediators to cetuximab in 85 independent patient-derived xenograft (PDX) lines originally resected from the liver metastases of mCRC patients [464]. Of these PDX models, 22.9% (11 out of 48) were resistant to cetuximab in a sub-population of samples that contained only wt K-RAS, N-RAS, B-RAF and PIK3CA (4 known markers of resistance when mutated in mCRC) indicating other resistance drivers in these tumors. Importantly, genomic amplification of HER2 was identified in 4 of the 11 resistant PDX. Furthermore, analysis of K-RAS wild-type mCRC tumor tissue from patients who did not respond to cetuximab or panitumumab revealed 17.6% (3 out of 17) expressed high HER2 expression whereas in the contrary 0% (0 out of 14) expressed high HER2 expression in K-RAS wildtype mCRC from patients who did response to anti-EGFR therapy [464]. Furthermore, introduction of HER2 mutations found in mCRC patient tissue, into colon cancer cell lines resulted in enhanced resistance to cetuximab and panitumumab [465]. Similarly, another study evaluated HER2 amplification in a cohort of 233 mCRC tissue taken from patients prior to their treatment with cetuximab monotherapy or in combination with chemotherapy [466]. In agreement with the study by Bertotti *et al.* a small number of tumors contained HER2 amplification (5.6%; 13 out of 233) however the median PFS (149 *vs.* 89 days) and OS (515 *vs.* 307 days) was significantly longer in the non-HER2 amplification group *versus* the HER2 amplified group. Parallel significant results were obtained when only K-RAS wildtype tumors were reassessed [466] suggesting that HER2 amplification may provide an alternative resistance mechanism to cetuximab to that of K-RAS mutation (and perhaps N-RAS, B-RAF and PIK3CA mutations).

In addition, Yonesaka and colleagues observed that HER2 amplification may also play a role in acquired resistance to cetuximab. Assessment of HER2 amplification in mCRC tumor tissue was significantly increased in post-cetuximab treated tissue compared to pre-cetuximab treated tissue from 2 mCRC patients. Likewise, levels of HER2 extracellular domain was increased in the post-cetuximab treated serum taken at the time of disease progression compared the levels detected in serum taken from the same patients prior to treatment. Finally, continuous co-culturing of cetuximab-sensitive cell lines to cetuximab led to the acquisition of resistant clones. Many of these resistant clones contained enhanced HER2 or phosphorylated HER2 expression compared to the cetuximab-sensitive parental cell lines [466]. Wheeler and colleagues had previously observed similar findings when generating cetuximab resistant NSCLC and SCCHN cell lines. HER2 phosphorylation was increased in both resistant cell lines compared to the cetuximab-sensitive parental cell lines [242].

HER2 expression has also been shown to play a role in an acquired resistance to gefitinib and erlotinib. In one study HER2 amplification was observed in 11.5% (3 out of 26) of NSCLC tumor tissue taken after patients had developed acquired resistance to either gefitinib or erlotinib [467]. HER2 amplification was detected in only 1.0% (1 out of 99) of lung adenocarcinoma of untreated patients suggesting that HER2 amplification may be acquired during or after treatment or that cells containing HER2 amplification be enriched by treatment up to detectable levels [467]. However, in complete contrast to the above data, some studies suggest that HER2 amplification is a positive biomarker for response to anti-EGFR therapy. Cappuzzo and colleagues evaluated HER2 GCN by FISH in tumors from NSCLC patients treated with gefitinib [468]. Patients with HER2 FISH positive tumors displayed an overall RR of 34.8% (8 out of 23), median TTP of 9 months and median OS of 21 months. These outcomes were significantly better than patients with HER2 FISH negative tumors where this group displayed an overall RR of only 6.4% (5 out of 78), median TTP of 3 months and median OS of 8 months [468]. Other study also correlated HER2 GCN with response to gefitinib using either FISH or CISH [282, 469]. Similarly, patients with HER2 FISH positive expression in K-RAS wildtype mCRC tumors who were treated with either cetuximab or panitumumab had significantly greater PFS and OS *versus* patients with HER2 FISH negative tumors [470]. High HER2 gene expression also correlated with better PFS of mCRC patients treated with cetuximab and chemotherapy [227].

However, several other reports have shown that HER2 amplification or high levels of gene expression have no significant positive or negative correlation with response to anti-EGFR treatment in several tumor types clinically [155, 212, 249, 471 - 474]. The lack of consistency in determining whether HER2 expression correlates with response suggests that it is not a reliable biomarker for at least EGFR-based therapies. Further assessment and greater understanding elucidating the reasons behind how such contradictory findings arise are required before HER2 expression status can become a dependable predictive biomarker clinically.

Somatic mutations of the HER2 gene have also been proposed to influence tumor response to anti-EGFR inhibitors. A point mutation in HER2 (A773V) was also identified in 25.0% (1 out of 4) SCCHN tumors from patients who responded to gefitinib. This mutation was not seen in any of the tumor tissue from 9 non-responders [321]. A series of somatic mutations in HER2 have also been isolated in breast cancer, some of which enhance sensitivity and other confers resistance to lapatinib [475 - 477]. Whether these mutations also affect efficacy of inhibitors that specifically inhibit the EGFR (unlike lapatinib that inhibits both EGFR and HER2) is unclear. Likewise, whether low levels of somatic HER2 mutations found in lung, hepatocellular, gastric and colorectal cancers [478 - 482] have any bearing on response to anti-EGFR therapy is yet to be determined.

5.3. HER3, HER4 and Neuregulins (NRG)

Neuregulin (NRG; also known as heregulin, Neu differentiation factor and glial growth factors) are encoded by 4 genes and due to alternative splicing are present in many isoforms all of which bind the HER family of receptors, most commonly HER3 (ErbB3) and HER4 (ErbB4) [483 - 487].

Along with increased HER2 amplification as discussed above, Yonesaka and colleagues also found that increased levels of neuregulin (NRG) was predictive of patient response to cetuximab [466]. Low levels of NRG in the plasma of mCRC patients taken prior to cetuximab treatment correlated with patient response, improved PFS (161 *vs.* 59 days) and OS (366 *vs.* 137 days) compared to patients with high NRG plasma levels. Similarly, NRG gene expression levels in the tumor of mCRC patients also correlated to better patient response. This result was similar in all patients and K-RAS wildtype only sub-groups. In addition, NRG plasma levels were significantly higher in plasma taken from patients after the acquisition of cetuximab resistance compared to plasma levels taken from the same patients prior to cetuximab treatment. This suggests that cetuximab-refractory tumors may express and secrete greater NRG levels and that NRG may represent a novel biomarker for cetuximab efficacy in mCRC patients. In addition, a cell line with acquired resistance to cetuximab following continuous long-term exposure to cetuximab in culture secreted greater levels of NRG and had subsequently higher levels of phosphorylated HER3 and HER4 compared to the cetuximab-sensitive parental cell line [466]. Similarly, colon cancer cells stably expressing NRG (and subsequently secreting greater levels of NRG) were significantly more resistant to cetuximab compared to the parental cell line [488]. Another report found that breast cancer cell lines that were intrinsically resistant to gefitinib produced significantly greater levels of NRG following gefitinib treatment [230]. In the contrary, gefitinib-sensitive cells did the opposite, significantly expressed much less NRG when challenged with gefitinib [230], suggesting that resistance may come about through the ability of a cell to increased production of ligands that stimulate activation of compensatory receptors such as HER3 and HER4 in this case and thus overcoming the inhibition of EGFR activity. Further supporting this hypothesis is data from Sergina and colleagues who show that several breast cancer cell lines treated with gefitinib or erlotinib display a delayed yet sustained HER3 re-phosphorylation [489]. Although, not evaluated in this report, one can speculate that enhanced NRG expression following gefitinib treatment as reported in the studies described above could be the reason for this restored HER3 activity. Similarly, NRG expression was dramatically increased in prostate cancer cells following erlotinib treatment [229]. Likewise, NRGβ1 could overcome the inhibitory effects of gefitinib when tested on breast cancer cells [490], further strengthening this notion. NRG has also been shown to promote resistance to lapatinib in gastric, gastroesophageal and breast cancer settings [491 - 494]. However, other laboratory and clinical based studies evaluating NRG expression showed no correlation with NRG expression and patient response to anti-EGFR therapies [205, 219].

Along with differential expression of NRG, alterations in its receptors, HER3 and HER4 have also been implicated in differential response to anti-EGFR therapies. As discussed above, Sergina and colleagues found a delayed yet sustained HER3 re-phosphorylation after gefitinib or erlotinib treatment, which correlated with lack of long-term efficacy of these agents [489]. Likewise, gefitinib and erlotinib enhanced the expression of HER3 in breast cancer cell lines [495]. Another study showed that HER3 expression correlated with reduced gefitinib response in 10 SCCHN cell lines [496]. Other studies evaluating a role of HER3 in resistance to anti-EGFR therapy have been performed using acquired resistant cell line models. Two studies by the same group found that NSCLC and SCCHN cells with acquired cetuximab-resistance had increased HER3 expression and activity and greater EGFR-HER3 association compared to cetuximab-sensitive matched parental cell lines [242, 497]. Another study evaluated resistance mechanisms in an acquired gefitinib NSCLC cell line following continuous, long-term co-culturing with gefitinib [498]. Receptor tyrosine kinase arrays established that gefitinib could inhibit EGFR, HER3 and MET in the parental cell lines but had little effect on the acquired resistant matched cell lines. Furthermore, they determined that the acquired resistance to gefitinib in these cells was driven through HER3 activation *via* MET amplification. Importantly, MET amplification was also detected in 22.2% (4 out of 18) NSCLC tumor tissue from patients whom had shown PR initially to gefitinib or erlotinib but had developed resistance. In addition, 2 out of 8 paired tumor samples showed MET amplification in post-treatment samples but not in the pre-treated samples. However, whether these tumors with MET amplification (as determined by FISH) also expressed greater HER3 activity was not reported in this article [498]. Supporting these findings is a recent study by Cushman and co-workers who determined whether HER3 gene expression correlated to reduced response to cetuximab in mCRC treated with FOLFOX or FOLFIRI with or without cetuximab [227]. Higher HER3 gene expression was found to be predictive for a lack of benefit from cetuximab treatment in the K-RAS wildtype subgroup (but not in the K-RAS mutated subgroup) [227].

A series of studies by Scartozzi and colleagues have also evaluated the role of HER3 in resistance and poor clinical outcomes in mCRC patients treated with cetuximab based regimens. In the first study, HER3 protein expression by immunohistochemistry was determined in 84 patients with K-RAS wildtype advanced mCRC who were subsequently treated with cetuximab and irinotecan after at least one line of previous chemotherapy [499]. Patients with HER3 positive staining displayed worst response rates (18.2%; 8 out of 44 *vs.* 42.5%; 17 out of 40), poorer median PFS (2.8 *vs.* 6.3 months) and OS (10.5 *vs.* 13.6 months) compared to patients with undetectable intratumoral HER3 expression [499]. Similar data was reported in another paper by Scartozzi and co-workers confirming that HER3 expression were predictive of poor response and worst outcome in mCRC treated with cetuximab and irinotecan [500]. Subsequently, a most recent prospective study by these researchers has included HER3 expression as a biomarker that places patients in an unfavourable group (*i.e.*: those that are expected to have poorer response and overall outcomes to cetuximab). This report provided proof of principle evidence that a prospective molecular signature is feasible for further selection of K-RAS wildtype mCRC patients into those that would and would not benefit from cetuximab treatment based on the expression status of HER3 and other biomarkers [501].

Other studies assessing the correlation of HER3 with the reduced efficacy of anti-EGFR therapy, present opposing results however to the reports above. The study by Gandhi *et al.* did not find any significant correlation with HER3 gene expression with gefitinib or erlotinib sensitivity in a panel of 112 lung cell lines including 77 NSCLC and 32 SCLC [502]. The study by Hickinson *et al.* also observed contradictory findings to those above, reporting that high HER3 expression correlated with increased gefitinib sensitivity in a series of 20 head & neck cancer cell lines [209]. Another report observed that high HER3 expression in conjunction with high e-cadherin expression correlated with improved *in vitro* response to gefitinib in 21 NSCLC cell lines [503]. Furthermore, these authors observed that the co-expression of HER3 and e-cadherin correlated significantly in NSCLC patient tumor tissue. However, the tissue used for this study was not from patients treated with gefitinib (or another anti-EGFR agent) and thus whether HER3 and e-cadherin expression correlated with improved gefitinib response was not established clinically in this study [503]. Nonetheless, another study had evaluated HER3 expression as a predictive biomarker to gefitinib response in NSCLC. In this study by Cappuzzo and colleagues, patients with advanced NSCLC with HER3 FISH positive did not have a significantly better RR to gefitinib or improved OS rate, but did display a significantly longer TTP compared to NSCLC patients with HER3 FISH negative tumors [504]. Interestingly, in this study, patients with both FISH positive EGFR and HER3 or FISH positive HER2 and HER3 had no significant difference in OS compared to both EGFR/HER3 and HER2/HER3 FISH negative patient sub-populations respectively, suggesting that genomic gain of HER3 is not a biomarker for response to gefitinib in NSCLC patients [504]. Thus, taken together the predictive value of HER3 as a biomarker for tumor response to anti-EGFR therapy is still inconclusive and further research is required.

Only a few studies have implicated HER4 expression in the sensitivity of cancer cells to anti-EGFR. A study by Black *et al.* correlated the loss of expression of full-length HER4 and increased expression of cleaved HER4 with the inability of cetuximab to inhibit DNA synthesis in a panel of 11 human urothelial cancer cell lines [505]. The study by Baker and colleagues assessed 110 genes for their ability to predict response to cetuximab monotherapy in 144 K-RAS wildtype mCRC patients [212]. Increased expression of HER4 correlated with reduced PFS but did not significantly correlate with tumor ORR. Although, very few papers have assessed HER4 expression as a biomarker for anti-EGFR therapy, several new generation inhibitors target EGFR along with other HER family members and some evidence exists that blockade of more than one EGFR family member simultaneously may indeed be more effective than EGFR blockade alone [488, 497, 506, 507].

6. ALTERATIONS IN NON-ERBB RECEPTOR FAMILY MEMBERS

As with the other three members of the EGFR family, it is not surprising that other receptor tyrosine kinases can compensate for the blockade of the EGFR to maintain downstream signaling, continued cell proliferation and survival and subsequently provide resistance to EGFR inhibitors. Some evidence exist for several ligand/receptor systems such as integrin β1 [508, 509], ROS-1 [510], IL-6 [511 - 514], G protein-coupled receptors [515] and toll-like receptor 9 [516] in providing resistance mechanisms to EGFR inhibitors. However, we will not further discuss these systems. In this last section of our review we will summarise the current literature discussing the role of 6 ligand/receptor signaling families in mediating resistance to anti-EGFR therapy (as schematically shown in Fig (**4**)).

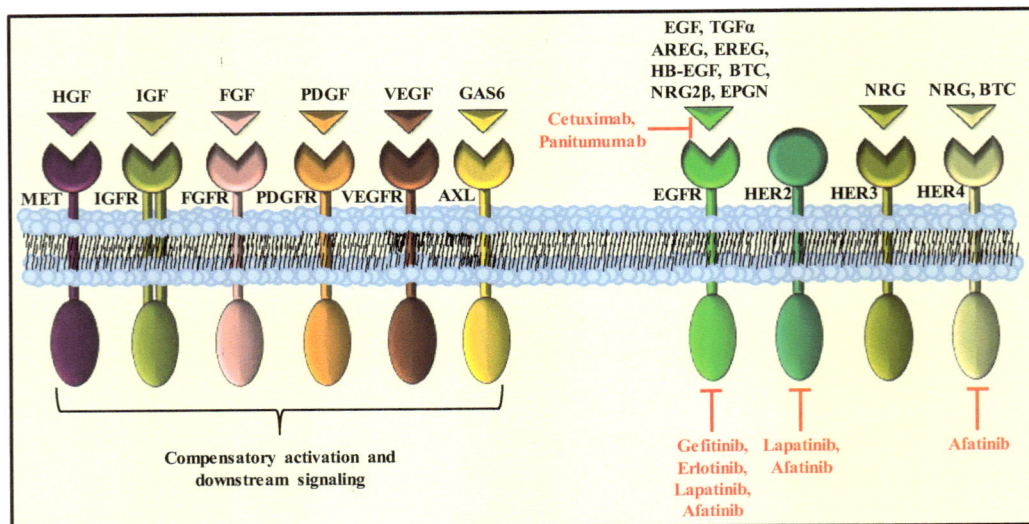

Fig. (4). Schematic of compensatory signaling from alternative ligand/receptor pairs following EGFR blockade. EGFR phosphorylation is blocked by either mAbs or TKI's. However, signaling from HGF/MET, IGF/IGFR, FGF/FGFR, PDGF/PDGFR, VEGF/VEGFR and GAS6/AXL leads to compensatory pathway activation and overall resistance to anti-EGFR therapy.

6.1. Hepatocyte Growth Factor/Scatter Factor (HGF)/MET

Met, also known as hepatocyte growth factor receptor (HGFR), is a receptor tyrosine kinase that drives many physiological processes and is often aberrantly activated in cancer [517 - 522]. There is strong evidence through a large body of laboratory and clinical based research for increased MET activity (through increased gene amplification and protein expression) in providing both *de novo* and acquired resistance to anti-EGFR therapy.

Increased MET expression has been associated with poorer outcomes in mCRC patients treated with cetuximab. In a study by Inno *et al.* mCRC patients with over-expressed MET expression as detected by immunohistochemistry had a significantly shorter median PFS (3.0 *vs.* 5.0 months) and median OS (10.0 *vs.* 11.0 months) compared to patients with lower levels of intra-tumoral MET expression. These patients also displayed greater objective response rates to cetuximab based treatments (14.3 *vs.* 29.4%), but this difference was not significant [523]. Very similar results were observed in another cohort of mCRC patients treated with cetuximab or panitumumab based therapies [524]. Analysis of MET expression by immunohistochemistry found that over-expressed MET correlated with lower disease control rates (53.9%; 14 out of 26 *vs.* 82.1%; 23 out of 28) and shorter PFS (4.7 *vs.* 6.8 months) in patients with mCRC K-RAS wildtype tumors. Similarly to the study by Inno *et al.* a worse, yet non-significant decrease in overall RR to cetuximab or panitumumab based treatment was reported comparing MET over-expression *versus* MET normal to low expression (34.6; 9 out of 26 *vs.* 42.9%; 12 out of 28) [524]. Serum levels of HGF, the ligand for MET has also been evaluated as a predictive marker for cetuximab and panitumumab efficacy in patients with K-RAS wildtype mCRC. High levels of HGF in the serum of K-RAS wildtype patients taken prior to cetuximab or panitumumab based treatment correlated with significantly lower PFS (4.4 *vs.* 6.4 months) and OS (8.0 *vs.* 15.3 months) compared to patients with low serum levels of HGF [222]. Just like the studies above assessing MET expression with overall response rate, there was no significant difference in overall RR between subgroups of high *versus* low HGF serum levels (30.8; 16 out of 52 *vs.* 35.3%; 18 out of 51) [222]. Similarly, HGF detection in serum correlated significantly with poorer PFS in patients with advanced NSCLC and wildtype EGFR treated with gefitinib or erlotinib [525]. Higher levels of HGF in the serum of NSCLC patients was also found to correlated with progressive disease and significantly associated with shorter PFS and OS in another study [526].

Another study assessed whether phosphorylated MET correlated to gefitinib treatment outcomes in NSCLC patients [527]. Patients with high phospho-(Y1003) MET staining by immunohistochemistry displayed significantly lower objective response rates (0%; 0 out of 4 *vs.* 7.7%; 3 out of 39) and lower TTP (1.2 *vs.* 3.2 months) compared to patient with low to moderate phospho-(Y1003) MET staining [527]. The study by Benedettini and co-workers observed similar results in a cohort of NSCLC patients harbouring EGFR sensitizing mutations that were treated with EGFR TKI's. Both Met phosphorylation and expression were strongly associated with shorter PFS [528]. However, MET expression was not a predictive biomarker for cetuximab based treatment in a cohort of SCCHN patients [272].

Several, laboratory studies have also implicated MET in providing primary resistance to anti-EGFR therapy. In one study, Met overexpression and constitutive activation was thought to provide primary resistance to cetuximab in 2 NSCLC patient-derived xenografts [529]. Another study by Bardelli and colleagues ectopically over-expressed MET into two anti-EGFR agent sensitive colon cancer cell lines (DIFI and LIM1215) and found that over-expression resulted in reduced cetuximab and panitumumab efficacy [530], While acquired resistance to cetuximab was associated with up-regulation of MET expression [242]. Furthermore, HGF stimulated or transduced cells also displayed cetuximab-refractory outcomes in culture and in subcutaneous xenograft models [530, 531]. This HGF mediated rescue of cancer cells from cetuximab inhibition *via* MET activation have also been reported by other groups [532, 533]. Similarly, addition of HGF secreted from colorectal cancer associated fibroblasts led to enhanced resistance to cetuximab in colon cancer stem-like cells [534]. HGF also conferred resistance to lapatinib in breast cancer resistance [535] and resistance to gefitinib in kidney, liver and tongue-derived cancer cells [536]. Several studies by Yano and colleagues also reported similar findings with HGF/MET activation through HGF stimulation or from co-culturing with HGF secreting fibroblasts providing resistance to gefitinib in adenocarcinoma cells with activating EGFR mutations [537 - 539]. In one of these studies higher HGF expression was also identified in 3 out of 3 lung adenocarcinoma patients who showed no response to gefitinib suggesting a mechanism for intrinsic resistance [537].

Met amplification was not identified in these 3 tumors. In conjunction with this report, others have observed that MET amplification is uncommon in untreated NSCLC patient tumors [540 - 543]. Likewise, MET amplification is rare in untreated mCRC patients [523, 544, 545] and thus its role in primary resistance to anti-EGFR therapy is minimal. However, several studies have identified an increase in MET amplification in patient tumor tissue following treatment with EGFR inhibitors suggesting a role for MET amplification in acquired resistance. As mentioned earlier in section 5.3, the study by Engelman and colleagues evaluated resistance mechanisms in an acquired gefitinib NSCLC cell line following continuous, long-term co-culturing with gefitinib [498]. The acquired resistance sub-cell lines contained 5-10 fold MET amplification and the acquired resistance to gefitinib in these cells was driven through HER3 activation *via* MET amplification. MET amplification was not seen in the gefitinib-sensitive parental cell line. Importantly, 22.2% (4 out of 18) of NSCLC tumor tissue taken from patients whom had shown initial response to gefitinib or erlotinib but had developed resistance contained MET amplification. In addition, 25.0% (2 out of 8) of post-treatment tumors contained MET amplification that was not observed in the patient matched pre-treatment tumor tissue [498]. The study by Bean and colleagues support the above findings [546]. In this report, assessment of MET amplification was performed in NSCLC samples that had never received treatment with kinase inhibitors and NSCLC samples from patients treated with gefitinib or erlotinib who had developed resistance. MET amplification was identified in only 3.2% (2 out of 62) of untreated tumors compared to 20.9% (9 out of 43) of patients with acquired resistance to gefitinib and erlotinib [546]. However, the evaluation of patient matched tumors prior to treatment of gefitinib and erlotinib was not reported in this study and thus it is unsure how many of these patients with acquired resistance obtained MET amplification during treatment. The study by Chen and co-workers also assessing MET amplification in treatment naïve and EGFR TKI-refractory NSCLC patients obtained similar results [547]. MET was amplified in 3.8% (2 out of 53) of treatment naïve NSCLC patients and in 17.2% (5 out of 29) of patients with gefitinib or erlotinib resistance. Importantly, Chen and colleagues also examined MET amplification in pre and post treatment samples from the same patient. Three out of nine patients with paired tumor specimens showed c-MET amplification in the resistant tumor tissue but not in the pre-treatment specimens [547]. However, another study also assessing pre and post treatment patient matched NSCLC tumor tissue for MET amplification only found 5% (2 out of 38) of samples in the post-treatment group contained MET amplification. Finally, the study by Bardelli and colleagues also supports the notion that MET amplification may provide resistance to cetuximab in patients with mCRC [530]. In this report, pre and post cetuximab and panitumumab-based treated mCRC samples were analysed for MET amplification from 7 patients who initially responded but had subsequently relapsed. MET amplification was detected in 3 out these 7 post-treatment specimens but was not seen in 2 of the matched pre-treated samples. Interestingly, a very low level of chromosomal rearrangement associated with MET amplification was detected in the pre-treated sample of the other patient that exhibited MET amplification in their post-treatment sample [530]. This is in accordance with another report that observed low level pre-existing MET amplification in pre-treated tumor cells that were resistance to anti-EGFR therapy [548]. Thus, these cells with MET amplification are positively selected for by EGFR inhibitors ultimately leading to larger populations of resistance cells with MET amplification. This allows one to speculate that post-treated MET amplification positive tumors may have originated from tumors containing low levels of MET amplification albeit undetectable, prior to treatment which are enriched during and following anti-EGFR agent exposure. Importantly, the study by Bardelli *et al.* also reported that MET amplification could be detected in the circulating DNA in patient serum prior to relapse being clinically evident [530]. The early detection of amplified MET by non-invasive means may allow for earlier implementation of suitable treatment strategies such as combinational anti-EGFR and anti-HGF/MET therapies. Indeed this strategic combination of agents targeting both EGFR and HGF/MET signaling has been assessed in pre-clinical models [136, 530, 534, 549 - 553] and tested clinically [554 - 557].

6.2. Insulin-like Growth Factor (IGF)/IGF-R

Another well described growth factor system is the Insulin-like growth factor (IGF) receptor signaling family which is involved in cancer cell growth, survival, metabolism and transformation [558 - 561]. The IGF signalling network also interacts and contains common downstream substrates with the EGFR [562, 563]. Thus, not surprisingly, the IGF family has been implicated in providing compensatory signaling to cells upon EGFR blockade and promotes tumor resistance to EGFR targeted therapy.

Both IGF ligands have been shown to provide resistance to anti-EGFR therapy. In a report by Liu and colleagues, IGF-1 could partially rescue DIFI colon cancer cells from the inhibitory and pro-apoptotic effects of cetuximab [564]. Similarly, IGF-1 stimulation of SCCHN cells could block the inhibitory effects of an anti-EGFR agent [565]. The presence of IGF-1 in the serum of gefitinib treated advanced NSCLC patients was also found to be a negative predictive factor for gefitinib treatment [566]. Likewise, a prostate cancer cell line (DU-145) with acquired resistance to gefitinib expressed higher levels of IGF-2 compared to the gefitinib-sensitive parental cell line. However, this increase in IGF-2 gene expression was not seen in a gefitinib-acquired resistant breast cancer cell line (MCF-7), although IGF-1R phosphorylation was enhanced [567]. Importantly, IGF-1 was associated to clinical response to cetuximab and irinotecan in mCRC patients. IGF-1 positive staining as determined by immunohistochemistry correlated with decreased partial remission (22.0%; 13 out of 59 *vs.* 64.5%; 20 out of 31), reduced median PFS (2.5 *vs.* 9.0 months) and median OS (8.0 *vs.* 25.0 months) compared to patients with IGF-1 negative tumors [500]. IGF-1 and IGF-1R germline polymorphisms were also significantly associated with response to cetuximab and survival outcomes in patients with mCRC [568]. The recent study by Zanella and colleagues found that high IGF2 gene expression was observed in 23.2% (14 out of 60) of PDX in mice that showed SD after cetuximab treatment compared to only 6.4% (2 out of 31) PDX where tumor shrinkage was observed [569]. However, this association was not significant. Nonetheless, analysis of a public data based and of their own institutional mCRC specimens (that did not have mutations in K-RAS, N-RAS, B-RAF or PIK3CA) also showed that IGF2 expression was greater in patients with SD compared to patients showing overall response to cetuximab. Interestingly, lower levels of IGF2 was seen in PDXs and mCRC patient samples who had progressive disease compared to those with SD prompting the authors to speculate that IGF2 expression maybe a response modifier and not a conventional resistance biomarker and that expression of IGF2 may distinguish between partially sensitive and totally sensitive mCRC and not between fully resistant *versus* responsive cases [569].

The majority of laboratory evidence indicating resistance to anti-EGFR therapy has arisen from studies evaluating IGF-1R. One of the original reports regarding this notion was published by Chakravarti and colleagues who showed that IGF-1R mediated resistance to the anti-EGFR inhibitor, AG1478 in glioblastoma cells *in vitro* [563]. The study by Yang *et al.* demonstrated a correlation of phosphorylated IGF-1R with efficacy of gefitinib in colon cancer cell lines, where IGF-1R phosphorylation was undetectable or present at very low levels in highly gefitinib-sensitive cell lines and was present at high levels in less responsive cell lines [570]. Another report also demonstrated that IGF-1R mediated resistance to erlotinib in several NSCLC cell lines. In this study, erlotinib induced IGF-1R phosphorylation upon erlotinib treatment in erlotinib refractory cells and a cell line with acquired erlotinib resistance compared to erlotinib sensitive cell lines. The acquired erlotinib resistant cell line also displayed greater hetero-dimerization with the EGFR compared to the erlotinib sensitive parental cell line suggesting that erlotinib resistance arises from compensatory increased IGF-1R hetero-dimerization and activity [571]. Similar cross-talk was seen in gefitinib treated NSCLC cells [572]. Others also reported increased phosphorylated IGF-1R in NSCLC and hepatocellular carcinoma cells with acquired resistance to gefitinib, erlotinib or irreversible EGFR tyrosine kinase inhibitors [573 - 578]. Another *in vitro* model for acquired resistance to gefitinib has also identified increased IGF-1R phosphorylation in resistant cells. In the study by Guix *et al.* A431 cells were treated long-term with gefitinib to generate gefitinib refractory cells. These resistant cells had greater phosphorylated IGF-1R and decreased gene expression of the IGF ligand regulating IGF binding proteins 3 and 4 (IGFBP3 and IGFBP4). Addition of recombinant IGFBP3 re-sensitized the gefitinib-resistant A431 cells to the inhibitory effects of gefitinib [579]. Similarly, IGFBP3 expression and secretion was reduced in other NSCLC cells with gefitinib and erlotinib-acquired resistance [580]. However, analysis of serum of 20 NSCLC patients that had shown PR to gefitinib and erlotinib but then developed resistance showed that IGFBP3 levels were similar in serum taken before treatment and in serum taken after the development of resistance [580]. This suggests that unlike that seen in acquired resistance models in the laboratory, acquired resistance in patients was not due to loss of IGFBP3 expression and secretion and may not be a significant molecular mechanism in NSCLC patients. A recent report also showed that stable knockdown of IGF-1R in NSCLC cells also led to increased sensitivity to gefitinib and erlotinib compared to control cells [581]. Another study by Hurbin and co-workers evaluated a possible association with IGF-1R expression and gefitinib response in patients with mucinous adenocarcinomas. In this study, increased expression of IGF-1R was observed in 92.3% (12 out of 13) patients with disease progression, although the only mucinous adenocarcinoma patient to show disease control also had high IGF-1R expression [582]. Likewise, another study demonstrated that mCRC patients with intratumoral phosphorylated IGF-1R and co-expression of matrix metalloproteinase-7 (MMP-7) were associated with poor response to either cetuximab or panitumumab. Furthermore, in patients with K-RAS wildtype tumors, expression of activated IGF-1R and MMP-7 correlated with poorer PFS (2.7 *vs.* 3.5 months) and OS (6.4 *vs.* 8.6 months) compared to those that did not [583].

However, other clinical observations observe contradictory results to those described above in several independent studies that suggest that over-expression of IGF-1R is a favourable prognostic factor in mCRC treated with cetuximab. Cappuzzo and colleagues examined the association between IGF-1R expression and mCRC patient outcomes following cetuximab based treatment. In this study, they observed no significant correlation between IGF-1R expression with RRor TTP survival but found that OS was significantly better in patients with positive IGF-1R expression compared to patients with negative expression (16.1 *vs.* 6.7 months) [545]. These results are in accordance with the study by Inno *et al.* who also evaluating IGF-1R expression in mCRC patients that were treated with cetuximab based therapies. In this study IGF-1R again did not correlate with ORR or PFS but similarly to Cappuzzo's study, patients with higher IGF-1R expression displayed a significantly greater median OS (14.0 *vs.* 8.0 months) in both the overall and K-RAS wildtype patient populations [523]. A third study evaluated gene expression in tumor tissue of chemorefractory mCRC patients taken prior to cetuximab monotherapy. In this study by Huang *et al.* elevated IGF-1R expression levels was associated with an improved disease control rate and PFS in the K-RAS wildtype sub-population of patients compared to patients with lower IGF-1R expression. Inversely, lower IGF-1R gene expression was associated with a lack of cetuximab benefit across the whole patient population [584]. Two other studies evaluating IGF-1R expression by immunohistochemistry in gefitinib treated NSCLC patients also found no correlation with IGF-1R expression and gefitinib resistance [585, 586]. Likewise, gefitinib treatment of locally advanced SCCHN patients produced similar disease-free survival irrespective of IGF-1R expression levels [587].

Overall, the current literature suggests that the IGF/IGFR signaling axis may play a role in compensatory signaling upon EGFR blockade, although clearly contradictory evidence exists. Nonetheless, combinational therapy targeting both pathways has been tested clinically [588 - 590]. However, these trials have failed to demonstrate sufficient benefit as combined therapies.

6.3. Fibroblast Growth Factor (FGF)/FGFR

Similarly to other receptor tyrosine kinase systems, components of the fibroblast growth factor signaling family are dys-regulated in various cancers [591 - 595]. However, there is only a relatively small body of research supporting the notion that FGF/FGFR signaling can elicits resistance to anti-EGFR therapy. A recent study demonstrated that lapatinib sensitivity in oesophageal squamous cell carcinoma cell lines was reduced when cells were co-treated with lapatinib and supernatant containing FGF ligands from fibroblasts compared to lapatinib treatment alone [596]. Similarly, the study by Zhang and colleagues described the establishment of a cetuximab acquired-resistant oesophageal squamous cell carcinoma (TE-6) xenograft model established through continued cetuximab treatment *in vivo*. In this study, the acquired resistant xenograft contained significantly greater *FGFR2* gene amplification and overexpression compared to the cetuximab-sensitive TE-6 parental xenografts [597]. In another study, FGF stimulation of pancreatic carcinoma cells compensated for EGFR blockade with cetuximab and may assist in providing resistance to these cells [598].

An important report by Lee and colleagues recently identified feedback FGFR signaling as a mediator of resistance to erlotinib in NSCLC. Short-term (24 h) erlotinib exposure of NSCLC cells with sensitizing EGFR mutations resulted in increased gene expression of several family members of the FGF signaling pathway including FGFR2, FGFR3, FRS2, FGF13 and HSPG2 and enhanced secretion of FGF16 [511]. This enhancement in FGF/FGFR signaling and subsequent activation of downstream compensatory signals as a response to EGFR inhibition may significantly contribute to acquire resistance thereby limiting the efficacy of anti-EGFR TKIs. Whether this is a resistance mechanism observed in patients with activating EGFR mutations is yet to be clearly determined but warrants further evaluation. Short-term (4 days) gefitinib exposure of several NSCLC cell lines with EGFR mutations also generated similar results to those seen above by Lee *et al.* In this study by Ware and colleagues, microarray analysis revealed increased FGFR2 and FGFR3 expression in gefitinib-treated cells compared to their control-treated counterparts [599]. In a follow-up paper by the same group, long-term gefitinib exposure generating gefitinib-resistant clones also resulted in increased FGF/FGFR family members. Several cell lines with acquired gefitinib-resistance expressed greater FGF2 and FGFR1 gene and protein levels compared to the gefitinib-sensitive parental cell lines suggesting that FGF/FGFR signaling may compensate for EGFR blockade by gefitinib in NSCLC tumors [600]. Finally, another study showed that long-term exposure of A431 cells to cetuximab, resulting in the selection of a cetuximab-resistant A431 sub-population which contained increased FGFR3 activity compared to the control cells [218]. These findings overall provide greater insight into FGF/FGFR signaling as an alternative mechanism of tumor resistance to anti-EGFR therapy. However, verification of these findings and clinical relevance and application is still yet to be established.

6.4. Platelet-derived Growth Factor (PDGF)/PDGFR

The family of PDGF ligands and PDGFRα/β receptors have been strongly implicated in cancer progression in several tumor types [601 - 605]. However, only a few reports have associated its aberrant expression with resistance to anti-EGFR therapy and most of these studies have been described using cell lines with little clinical evidence supporting these laboratory findings. Kassouf and colleagues showed that PDGFRβ expression negatively correlated with the efficacy of gefitinib in inhibiting transitional cell carcinoma of the bladder cell lines [606]. Likewise, PDGFRβ expression also negatively correlated with erlotinib efficacy in a series of NSCLC cell lines *in vitro* [607].

In parallel, to studies discussed above showing EGFR inhibition increases the expression of HER3 and MET, Akhavan and colleagues recently observed that EGFR TKI treatment de-represses PDGFRβ, leading to enhanced expression and resistance to erlotinib in glioma cells and PDX models [608]. Furthermore, glioma tumor progression switched from EGFR to PDGFRβ driven when tumors were challenged with erlotinib. PDGFRβ expression was also elevated in a glioma patient's post lapatinib treated specimen compared to the patient's pre-treated specimen [608]. Despite only one set of pre and post-treatment patient matched samples reported here, these findings suggest that resistance to EGFR TKIs may occur through enhanced PDGFRβ expression in glioma patients. Likewise, an earlier study identified a significant increase in PDGFRβ gene expression levels in post-cetuximab treated samples compared to pre-treated specimens from patients with locally advanced rectal cancer [609]. Another study showed that a gefitinib acquired resistant glioblastoma cell line expressed increased levels of PDGFRα compared to the parental gefitinib-sensitive counterpart [510].

6.5. Vascular Endothelial Growth Factor (VEGF)/VEGFR

The VEGF family is made up of 6 ligands and 3 receptors and is intimately associated with angiogenesis, proliferation, survival and wound healing [610 - 614]. VEGF expression is induced by hypoxic stimuli, growth factor and cytokine signaling including the EGFR [102, 615, 616]. The expression of VEGF has also been identified as a possible predictor of resistance to anti-EGFR inhibitors.

One of the first studies to identify VEGF expression as a potential biomarker for resistance to anti-EGFR therapy came from Viloria-Petit and colleagues who generated cetuximab resistance A431 xenografts *in vivo* [617]. In this study, A431 xenografts treated with cetuximab (or two other EGFR monoclonal antibodies) led to tumor regression followed by re-establishment of refractory tumors following treatment withdrawal. *Ex vivo* analysis of these refractory tumors revealed that 5 out of 6 resistant variants expressed at least 2-fold more VEGF mRNA and protein compared to control treated A431 cells. Importantly, A431 cells stably transfected with VEGF were more resistant to cetuximab treatment *in vivo* compared to parental xenografts suggesting that VEGF over-expression correlated with cetuximab efficacy [617]. Likewise, GEO colon cancer cell xenografts with acquired resistance to either cetuximab or gefitinib generated in similar *in vivo* fashion to Viloria-Petit *et al.* also expressed and secreted increased levels of VEGF compared to the parental cell line. This resistance could be overcome by VEGFR targeting suggesting that VEGF signaling may indeed play a role in resistance to anti-EGFR inhibitors [618]. In another study, these GEO resistant cells, along with gefitinib acquired resistant PC3 prostate cancer cells were found to also expressed increased gene expression and protein levels of VEGFR-1 compared to parental sensitive cells, while VEGFR-1 overexpression (by transfection) in gefitinib-sensitive prostate PC3 cells and colon SW480 cells reduced sensitivity to gefitinib [619]. Interestingly, the study by Li and colleagues identified that the efficacy of bevacizumab (an FDA-approved anti-VEGF monoclonal antibody) in combination with erlotinib is dependent on the level of VEGF secreted in NSCLC cells. NSCLC cells that were resistant to erlotinib monotherapy and secreted high VEGF levels could be inhibited by combined bevacizumab and erlotinib treatment, but those that secreted low levels could not [620]. However, whether this hypothesis translates to clinical application was not tested in this report. Intriguingly, another report found a significant association between increased VEGF levels in tumor tissue with higher odds of progression in patients with ovarian cancer that were treated with a combination of bevacizumab and erlotinib [621]. Another study also found that the ratio of phosphorylated VEGFR2: total VEGFR2 was significantly greater in recurrent or metastatic SCCHN patients with complete response compared to patients who had stable or progressive disease following combined erlotinib and bevacizumab treatment [622].

Evaluation of other clinical samples has shown mixed outcomes regarding the predictive value of VEGF/VEGFR expression to patient response to anti-EGFR inhibitors. The study by Vallbohmer and co-workers analysed the levels of VEGF gene expression in tumor tissue of mCRC patients who had previously failed at least two prior chemotherapy regimens or adjuvant therapy plus one chemo-therapy regimen for metastatic disease, and were treated with cetuximab monotherapy. Significantly less VEGF gene expression was found in tumor samples from patients with PR or SD compared to patients with progressive disease suggesting that higher VEGF gene expression were associated with resistance to cetuximab. However, VEGF gene expression did not significantly correlate with OS in this mCRC patient cohort [264]. In another study, protein expression by immunohistochemistry analysis of VEGF/VEGFR family components was performed in tumor specimens taken from patients with advanced or metastatic adenocarcinoma of the stomach or gastroesophageal junction who were treated with cetuximab. In this study, patients whose tumors expressed VEGF-C tended to have longer OS times (17.1 *vs.* 12.2 months) than those whose tumors were negative for VEGF-C, although this difference was not significant. No significant difference was seen in PFS of these patients either. Analysis of VEGF-D and VEGFR3 tumor expression also found that they did not correlate with any clinical outcomes [274].

Assessment of VEGF levels in the serum of patients has also yielded varying results in regards to predictive value for clinical utility of anti-EGFR agents. In a study by Byers *et al.* 38 cytokines and angiogenic factors were assessed by ELISA in the serum of SCCHN patients treated with cetuximab, carboplatin and paclitaxel. In this study, higher levels of VEGF (and IL-8, Gro-α, IL-4, osteopontin, eotaxin, G-CSF, and SDF-1α) significantly correlated with patients who had progressive disease [623]. However, the study by Argiris and colleagues found that serum VEGF levels were not significantly associated with tumor response or PFS in patients with locally advanced stage III–IVB head and neck cancer treated with cetuximab, chemotherapy and radiotherapy [512]. Likewise, serum levels of VEGF did not significantly correlate with response, PFS and OS of patients with un-resectable or metastatic gastric or esophagogastric junction adenocarcinoma treated with cetuximab, cisplatin and capecitabine [226]. Similarly, no significant associations between median PFS and progression rates and urinary levels of VEGF (or intratumoral VEGFR-1 levels) were observed in ovarian cancer patients treated with bevacizumab and erlotinib [621].

Vincenzi and colleagues evaluated the differences in VEGF serum levels in cetuximab and irinotecan third-line treated mCRC patients prior to and at days 1, 21, 50 and 92 after treatment. In this study, patients were divided into two groups, those that had at least 50% reduction of VEGF levels at day 92 compared to levels prior to treatment and those that did not. Patients with at least 50% reduction of VEGF with respect to the basal value (n=22) demonstrated a statistically significant higher RR(45.5%; 10 out of 22 *vs.* 8.7%; 2 out of 23), longer TTP rate (6.0 *vs.* 3.9 months) and greater OS rate (11.0 *vs.* 9.6 months) compared to patients that did not have at least a 50% reduction in VEGF levels after treatment (n=23) [624]. Thus, these authors speculate that a VEGF reduction of at least 50% may represent an important prognostic factor for TTP and OS in mCRC patients treated with cetuximab-based therapies.

However, despite some evidence suggesting that VEGF expression may be of prognostic and predictive value to anti-EGFR treatment, and that the dual blockade of EGFR and VEGF/VEGFR may provide greater anti-tumor effects, combination treatments clinically have yield only modest results. Erlotinib did not increase the efficacy of bevacizumab in metastatic renal cancer patients [625] or ovarian patients, with erlotinib increasing toxicity in the ovarian cancer trial [621]. The combination of erlotinib or gefitinib with bevacizumab has displayed mixed results in the NSCLC setting [626 - 631]. Cetuximab combined with bevacizumab and chemotherapy resulted in a significantly worse PFS and a decrease in quality of life compared with the combination of bevacizumab and chemotherapy alone in mCRC patients [632].

6.6. GAS6/AXL

AXL, also named UFO, Ark and Tyro7, belongs to the TAM (Tyro-Axl-Mer) receptor tyrosine kinase family and is involved in cell migration, invasion and cancer metastasis [633 - 635]. Several laboratory and clinical based studies have implicated AXL as a driver of resistance to anti-EGFR therapy.

The study by Byers and colleagues separated a large number of NSCLC cell lines into either epithelial or mesenchymal sub-groups based on the expression of a 76 gene signature [636]. Strikingly, NSCLC cells (n=20) that were characterised as mesenchymal expressed significantly greater gene and protein levels of AXL and were significantly more resistant to both gefitinib and erlotinib compared to the NSCLC (N=34) classified as epithelial cells. AXL inhibition could re-sensitize these mesenchymal cells to EGFR inhibition suggesting that AXL may play a role in resistance to anti-EGFR agents in NSCLC cells. Furthermore, Byers *et al.* went on to characterise patients from the Biomarker-Integrated Approaches of Targeted Therapy for Lung Cancer Elimination (BATTLE) clinical trial [637] into epithelial or mesenchymal tumors and found that EGFR/KRAS wild-type tumors with the mesenchymal-like signature were less responsive to erlotinib and expressed significantly greater levels of both AXL and Gas6 a ligand for AXL suggesting that Gas6 and AXL may represent novel negative predictors of erlotinib response in NSCLC patients [636]. Another study also showed that expression of AXL inversely correlated with NSCLC cell line sensitivity to erlotinib [638], while others found that down-regulation of AXL enhanced

NSCLC cell sensitivity to erlotinib [639]. These findings are also in agreement with another study where bioinformatics analysis of public databases identified AXL expression as an exceptionally strong predictor of intrinsic resistance to erlotinib and lapatinib in triple negative breast cancer cells [640]. Finally, another study showed that the treatment of glioblastoma xenografts with erlotinib also led to increased phosphorylated AXL [608].

Several studies have evaluated the role of AXL in acquired resistance. The study by Zhang and colleagues evaluated AXL expression by immunohistochemistry in 35 matched *EGFR*-mutant NSCLC specimens obtained from patients pre-treatment with EGFR inhibitors gefitinib or erlotinib and post-treatment after the development of resistance [641]. Of these 35 matched tumors, 20 were negative for AXL expression in both the pre and post treatment samples. Of the remaining 15 matched sections, 11 post treatment samples expressed greater AXL expression than the pre-treated samples. Furthermore, of the remaining 4 matched tumor pairs that were positive and equally immunostained for AXL expression in both pre and post treatment specimens, greater expression of Gas6 was observed in the post-treatment samples suggesting that resistance may have occurred through enhanced activity of AXL in these tumors. The study by Ji and co-workers also assessed the expression of AXL in NSCLC tumor tissue with EGFR mutations from patients who had showed initial PR to gefitinib but subsequently progressed with gefitinib refractory outcomes. In this study, AXL expression was increased in 19.2% (5 out of 26) patient tumor tissue post-treatment compared to pre-treatment patient matched tumor tissue. Thus in accordance with the study by Zhang *et al.* increased AXL expression may be a mechanism of acquired resistance to EGFR TKI's in the NSCLC setting [642].

The study of Zhang also examined AXL expression in erlotinib acquired resistant NSCLC cell lines. Erlotinib sensitive HCC827 cells were injected subcutaneously into mice and treated with vehicle or with increasing doses of erlotinib for 5 months to derive erlotinib-resistant tumors. AXL and Gas6 gene expression was increased in 88.2% (15 out of 17) and 47.1% (8 out of 17) of the erlotinib resistant tumors respectively compared to vehicle control treated sensitive HCC827 tumors. Higher levels of phosphorylated and AXL protein expression was also observed in the erlotinib resistant tumors and AXL expression was also elevated in erlotinib acquired resistant H3255 sub-clones compared to erlotinib sensitive H3255 parental cell [641]. Another study also observed elevated AXL expression in HCC827 erlotinib resistant cells after *in vitro* acquired resistance [643]. Similarly, increased AXL activity and/or expression was observed in a head and neck carcinoma cell line (HN5) with acquired resistance to erlotinib, in a breast cancer cell line (BT474) with acquired resistance to lapatinib and in NSCLC cell lines (PC9 and H292) with acquired resistance to gefitinib and afatinib compared to the respective parental EGFR inhibitor sensitive cell lines [644 - 647]. The AXL mediated resistance to gefitinib in NSCLC cells may be somewhat due to changes in AXL-regulated miRNA expression [648].

AXL expression has also been implicated in intrinsic and acquired resistance to cetuximab. Brand *et al.* generated acquired cetuximab resistant H226 NSCLC cancer cells through long-term culturing in the presence of cetuximab *in vitro* or by cetuximab treatment of H226 xenografts *in vivo* until tumors were refractory to cetuximab treatment [649]. All cetuximab resistant clones generated from both *in vitro* and *in vivo* methodologies expressed greater levels of phosphorylated and total AXL levels compared to the cetuximab sensitive parental H226 cell line. In addition, stable transfection of AXL led to increased resistance to cetuximab in parental H226 cells compared to cells transfected with vector control. Brand and colleagues went on to show similar results in the cetuximab sensitive SCCHN cell line UM-SCC1. Once more acquired cetuximab resistant clones (generate *in vitro*) expressed greater levels of AXL compared to the UM-SCC1 parental cell line. Finally, tumors from 6 SCCHN patients were resected and injected into mice to create PDX models. Three of these PDXs were responsive to cetuximab treatment *in vivo* while the other three were refractory to cetuximab. Consistently, the 3 refractory PDX tumors expressed greater levels of phosphorylated and total AXL compared to the three cetuximab-sensitive PDX tumors [649]. Although this sample size is very small, the findings by Brand *et al.* may be of great significance and offer proof-of-principle evidence for a larger scaled retrospective evaluation of SCCHN (and other tumor types) to determine whether phosphorylated and/or total AXL levels are potential predictive biomarkers of cetuximab response.

CONCLUDING REMARKS

Tremendous advances have been made over the last 2 decades in elucidating the molecular mechanisms of tumour resistance to anti-EGFR based treatment. Nonetheless, despite our enhanced comprehension of the complexity of tumor signaling in regards to tumor progression and resistance to therapy, only modest progress has been made to overcome the lack of overall effectiveness of EGFR targeted therapy. Our review summarises the evidence of numerous potential biomarkers including ligand and receptors of the EGFR family and alternative families. However, despite a multitude of articles reporting the predictive value of each of these candidates, contradictory data exists for most of these molecular markers. Our review has also highlighted the variation of potential biomarker identification based on differing techniques used, raising the requirement of standardised screening using the most sensitive detection methods to perform biomarker validation. In spite of this, logistically these universally used protocols will be extremely difficult to implement leading to continued inconsistent outcomes being reported which will ultimately hinder the development of optimised treatment strategies.

Thus to date, only the EGFR sensitizing mutations L858R and delE746_A750 and the resistance inducing EGFR T790M mutation can be identified and used with any confidence as prospective predictors of response to anti-EGFR therapeutics. Furthermore, it is abundantly clear that patient populations are extremely heterogeneous in nature and thus patients must be divided into various sub-populations before any predictive biomarker can be of any use clinically. Indeed, one of the most accurate predictors of response to EGFR therapy, the EGFR sensitizing mutations are only present in a relatively small number of patients (10-15%), generally of Asian ethnicity and are exclusive to the NSCLC setting only. This limits the effectiveness of even the better predictive biomarkers currently identified to small sub-populations of patients.

In addition, heterozygosity within each individual tumor will almost always allow for tumor recurrence (if an initial response is even observed), leading to the re-establishment of a tumor that is mostly refractory to the original treatment regimen. Many trials have been performed targeting 2 or more signaling networks either simultaneously or in succession with the goal to overcome both intrinsic and acquired resistance. However, most of these trials have failed to produce significant improvements compared to single agents alone and have often enhanced toxicity. Clearly, the major challenge of tumor resistance that arose when first using anti-EGFR therapy clinically many years ago remains a significant obstacle of successful cancer treatment today.

We have broken down potential biomarkers into individual molecular mediators to reduce confusion and increase coherence in writing this review. However, in many of the cited reports here, a combination of biomarkers or a distinct signature have been presented and will represent a greater predictive value of tumor response. It is evident from our extensive review that very few biomarkers can be used in isolation to predict sensitivity or resistance to anti-EGFR therapy and thus studies identifying predictive clusters or signatures should now be a research focus. In addition, despite this review only summarising the role of ligand and receptors in resistance, these signatures should include downstream signaling molecules and positive and negative regulators of signaling, transcription factors and other molecules involved in cellular phenotype and behaviour in which we focus on in our adjoining review (Part II of this series).

CONFLICT OF INTEREST

The author confirms that author has no conflict of interest to declare for this publication.

ACKNOWLEDGEMENTS

I acknowledge the NH&MRC for funding for Project grant #APP1080498.

ABBREVIATIONS

AREG	=	Amphiregulin
BTC	=	Betacellulin
EGF	=	Epidermal growth factor
EGFR	=	Epidermal growth factor receptor
EPGN	=	Epigen
EREG	=	Epiregulin

FISH	=	Fluorescence *in-situ* hybridization
GCN	=	Gene copy number
HB-EGF	=	Heparin-binding EGF
mCRC	=	Metastatic colorectal carcinoma
NSCLC	=	Non-small cell lung carcinoma
ORR	=	Objective response rate
OS	=	Overall survival
PDX	=	Patient-derived xenografts
PFS	=	Progression-free survival
PR	=	Partial response
RR	=	Response rate
SCCHN	=	Squamous cell carcinoma of the head and neck
SD	=	Stable disease
TGFα	=	Transforming growth factor-alpha
TKI's	=	Tyrosine kinase inhibitors
TTP	=	Time-to-progression

REFERENCES

[1]   Cohen S. Isolation of a mouse submaxillary gland protein accelerating incisor eruption and eyelid opening in the new-born animal. J Biol Chem 1962; 237(5): 1555-62.
[PMID: 13880319]

[2]   Fry DW. Inhibition of the epidermal growth factor receptor family of tyrosine kinases as an approach to cancer chemotherapy: progression from reversible to irreversible inhibitors. Pharmacol Ther 1999; 82(2-3): 207-18.
[PMID: 10454198]

[3]   Carpenter G, King L Jr, Cohen S. Epidermal growth factor stimulates phosphorylation in membrane preparations *in vitro*. Nature 1978; 276(5686): 409-10.
[PMID: 309559]

[4]   Schechter AL, Stern DF, Vaidyanathan L, *et al.* The neu oncogene: an erb-B-related gene encoding a 185,000-Mr tumour antigen. Nature 1984; 312(5994): 513-6.
[PMID: 6095109]

[5]   Plowman GD, Whitney GS, Neubauer MG, *et al.* Molecular cloning and expression of an additional epidermal growth factor receptor-related gene. Proc Natl Acad Sci USA 1990; 87(13): 4905-9.
[PMID: 2164210]

[6]   Plowman GD, Culouscou JM, Whitney GS, *et al.* Ligand-specific activation of HER4/p180erbB4, a fourth member of the epidermal growth factor receptor family. Proc Natl Acad Sci USA 1993; 90(5): 1746-50.
[PMID: 8383326]

[7]   Riese DJ II, Stern DF. Specificity within the EGF family/ErbB receptor family signaling network. BioEssays 1998; 20(1): 41-8.
[PMID: 9504046]

[8]   Olayioye MA, Neve RM, Lane HA, Hynes NE. The ErbB signaling network: receptor heterodimerization in development and cancer. EMBO J 2000; 19(13): 3159-67.
[PMID: 10880430]

[9]   Davies RL, Grosse VA, Kucherlapati R, Bothwell M. Genetic analysis of epidermal growth factor action: assignment of human epidermal growth factor receptor gene to chromosome 7. Proc Natl Acad Sci USA 1980; 77(7): 4188-92.
[PMID: 6254014]

[10]   Shimizu Y, Shimizu N. Genetics of cell-surface receptors for bioactive polypeptides: a variant of mouse BALBc/3T3 fibroblasts possessing altered insulin-binding ability. Somatic Cell Genet 1980; 6(5): 583-601.
[PMID: 7001653]

[11]   Ushiro H, Cohen S. Identification of phosphotyrosine as a product of epidermal growth factor-activated protein kinase in A-431 cell membranes. J Biol Chem 1980; 255(18): 8363-5.
[PMID: 6157683]

[12]   Cummings RD, Soderquist AM, Carpenter G. The oligosaccharide moieties of the epidermal growth factor receptor in A-431 cells. Presence of complex-type N-linked chains that contain terminal N-acetylgalactosamine residues. J Biol Chem 1985; 260(22): 11944-52.
[PMID: 2995354]

[13]   Mayes EL, Waterfield MD. Biosynthesis of the epidermal growth factor receptor in A431 cells. EMBO J 1984; 3(3): 531-7.
[PMID: 6325174]

[14]   Bajaj M, Waterfield MD, Schlessinger J, Taylor WR, Blundell T. On the tertiary structure of the extracellular domains of the epidermal growth factor and insulin receptors. Biochim Biophys Acta 1987; 916(2): 220-6.
[PMID: 3676333]

[15]   Lax I, Johnson A, Howk R, *et al.* Chicken epidermal growth factor (EGF) receptor: cDNA cloning, expression in mouse cells, and differential binding of EGF and transforming growth factor alpha. Mol Cell Biol 1988; 8(5): 1970-8.
[PMID: 3260329]

[16]   Cadena DL, Chan CL, Gill GN. The intracellular tyrosine kinase domain of the epidermal growth factor receptor undergoes a conformational change upon autophosphorylation. J Biol Chem 1994; 269(1): 260-5.
[PMID: 8276804]

[17]   de Larco JE, Todaro GJ. Growth factors from murine sarcoma virus-transformed cells. Proc Natl Acad Sci USA 1978; 75(8): 4001-5.
[PMID: 211512]

[18]   Shoyab M, McDonald VL, Bradley JG, Todaro GJ. Amphiregulin: a bifunctional growth-modulating

glycoprotein produced by the phorbol 12-myristate 13-acetate-treated human breast adenocarcinoma cell line MCF-7. Proc Natl Acad Sci USA 1988; 85(17): 6528-32.
[PMID: 3413110]

[19]   Higashiyama S, Abraham JA, Miller J, Fiddes JC, Klagsbrun M. A heparin-binding growth factor secreted by macrophage-like cells that is related to EGF. Science 1991; 251(4996): 936-9.
[PMID: 1840698]

[20]   Shing Y, Christofori G, Hanahan D, *et al.* Betacellulin: A mitogen from pancreatic beta cell tumors. Science 1993; 259(5101): 1604-7.
[PMID: 8456283]

[21]   Toyoda H, Komurasaki T, Uchida D, *et al.* Epiregulin. A novel epidermal growth factor with mitogenic activity for rat primary hepatocytes. J Biol Chem 1995; 270(13): 7495-500.
[PMID: 7706296]

[22]   Pinkas-Kramarski R, Shelly M, Guarino BC, *et al.* ErbB tyrosine kinases and the two neuregulin families constitute a ligand-receptor network. Mol Cell Biol 1998; 18(10): 6090-101.
[PMID: 9742126]

[23]   Strachan L, Murison JG, Prestidge RL, Sleeman MA, Watson JD, Kumble KD. Cloning and biological activity of epigen, a novel member of the epidermal growth factor superfamily. J Biol Chem 2001; 276(21): 18265-71.
[PMID: 11278323]

[24]   Massagué J, Pandiella A. Membrane-anchored growth factors. Annu Rev Biochem 1993; 62: 515-41.
[PMID: 8394682]

[25]   Moolenaar WH, Bierman AJ, Tilly BC, *et al.* A point mutation at the ATP-binding site of the EGF-receptor abolishes signal transduction. EMBO J 1988; 7(3): 707-10.
[PMID: 3260862]

[26]   Wells A, Welsh JB, Lazar CS, Wiley HS, Gill GN, Rosenfeld MG. Ligand-induced transformation by a noninternalizing epidermal growth factor receptor. Science 1990; 247(4945): 962-4.
[PMID: 2305263]

[27]   Cohen S, Ushiro H, Stoscheck C, Chinkers M. A native 170,000 epidermal growth factor receptor-kinase complex from shed plasma membrane vesicles. J Biol Chem 1982; 257(3): 1523-31.
[PMID: 6276390]

[28]   Wada T, Qian XL, Greene MI. Intermolecular association of the p185neu protein and EGF receptor modulates EGF receptor function. Cell 1990; 61(7): 1339-47.
[PMID: 1973074]

[29]   Yarden Y, Schlessinger J. Self-phosphorylation of epidermal growth factor receptor: evidence for a model of intermolecular allosteric activation. Biochemistry 1987; 26(5): 1434-42.
[PMID: 3494472]

[30]   Burgess AW. EGFR family: structure physiology signalling and therapeutic targets. Growth Factors 2008; 26(5): 263-74.
[PMID: 18800267]

[31]   Miettinen PJ, Berger JE, Meneses J, *et al.* Epithelial immaturity and multiorgan failure in mice lacking

epidermal growth factor receptor. Nature 1995; 376(6538): 337-41.
[PMID: 7630400]

[32]   Sibilia M, Steinbach JP, Stingl L, Aguzzi A, Wagner EF. A strain-independent postnatal neurodegeneration in mice lacking the EGF receptor. EMBO J 1998; 17(3): 719-31.
[PMID: 9450997]

[33]   Sibilia M, Wagner EF. Strain-dependent epithelial defects in mice lacking the EGF receptor. Science 1995; 269(5221): 234-8.
[PMID: 7618085]

[34]   Threadgill DW, Dlugosz AA, Hansen LA, *et al.* Targeted disruption of mouse EGF receptor: effect of genetic background on mutant phenotype. Science 1995; 269(5221): 230-4.
[PMID: 7618084]

[35]   Abbott BD, Pratt RM. Retinoic acid alters epithelial differentiation during palatogenesis. J Craniofac Genet Dev Biol 1991; 11(4): 315-25.
[PMID: 1812132]

[36]   Warburton D, Seth R, Shum L, *et al.* Epigenetic role of epidermal growth factor expression and signalling in embryonic mouse lung morphogenesis. Dev Biol 1992; 149(1): 123-33.
[PMID: 1728582]

[37]   den Hertog J, de Laat SW, Schlessinger J, Kruijer W. Neuronal differentiation in response to epidermal growth factor of transfected murine P19 embryonal carcinoma cells expressing human epidermal growth factor receptors. Cell Growth Differ 1991; 2(3): 155-64.
[PMID: 2059566]

[38]   Joh T, Darland T, Samuels M, Wu JX, Adamson ED. Regulation of epidermal growth factor receptor gene expression in murine embryonal carcinoma cells. Cell Growth Differ 1992; 3(5): 315-25.
[PMID: 1633114]

[39]   Ignar-Trowbridge DM, Nelson KG, Bidwell MC, *et al.* Coupling of dual signaling pathways: epidermal growth factor action involves the estrogen receptor. Proc Natl Acad Sci USA 1992; 89(10): 4658-62.
[PMID: 1584801]

[40]   Nelson KG, Takahashi T, Bossert NL, Walmer DK, McLachlan JA. Epidermal growth factor replaces estrogen in the stimulation of female genital-tract growth and differentiation. Proc Natl Acad Sci USA 1991; 88(1): 21-5.
[PMID: 1986369]

[41]   Reynolds BA, Weiss S. Generation of neurons and astrocytes from isolated cells of the adult mammalian central nervous system. Science 1992; 255(5052): 1707-10.
[PMID: 1553558]

[42]   Engelman JA, Settleman J. Acquired resistance to tyrosine kinase inhibitors during cancer therapy. Curr Opin Genet Dev 2008; 18(1): 73-9.
[PMID: 18325754]

[43]   Mendelsohn J, Baselga J. The EGF receptor family as targets for cancer therapy. Oncogene 2000; 19(56): 6550-65.

[PMID: 11426640]

[44] Salomon DS, Brandt R, Ciardiello F, Normanno N. Epidermal growth factor-related peptides and their receptors in human malignancies. Crit Rev Oncol Hematol 1995; 19(3): 183-232.
[PMID: 7612182]

[45] Baselga J, Norton L, Masui H, *et al.* Antitumor effects of doxorubicin in combination with anti-epidermal growth factor receptor monoclonal antibodies. J Natl Cancer Inst 1993; 85(16): 1327-33.
[PMID: 8340945]

[46] Fan Z, Baselga J, Masui H, Mendelsohn J. Antitumor effect of anti-epidermal growth factor receptor monoclonal antibodies plus cis-diamminedichloroplatinum on well established A431 cell xenografts. Cancer Res 1993; 53(19): 4637-42.
[PMID: 8402640]

[47] Barnes D, Sato G. Serum-free cell culture: a unifying approach. Cell 1980; 22(3): 649-55.
[PMID: 7460009]

[48] Sporn MB, Todaro GJ. Autocrine secretion and malignant transformation of cells. N Engl J Med 1980; 303(15): 878-80.
[PMID: 7412807]

[49] Kawamoto T, Sato JD, Le A, Polikoff J, Sato GH, Mendelsohn J. Growth stimulation of A431 cells by epidermal growth factor: identification of high-affinity receptors for epidermal growth factor by an anti-receptor monoclonal antibody. Proc Natl Acad Sci USA 1983; 80(5): 1337-41.
[PMID: 6298788]

[50] Sato JD, Kawamoto T, Le AD, Mendelsohn J, Polikoff J, Sato GH. Biological effects *in vitro* of monoclonal antibodies to human epidermal growth factor receptors. Mol Biol Med 1983; 1(5): 511-29.
[PMID: 6094961]

[51] Schreiber AB, Lax I, Yarden Y, Eshhar Z, Schlessinger J. Monoclonal antibodies against receptor for epidermal growth factor induce early and delayed effects of epidermal growth factor. Proc Natl Acad Sci USA 1981; 78(12): 7535-9.
[PMID: 6278478]

[52] Waterfield MD, Mayes EL, Stroobant P, *et al.* A monoclonal antibody to the human epidermal growth factor receptor. J Cell Biochem 1982; 20(2): 149-61.
[PMID: 6188757]

[53] Gill GN, Kawamoto T, Cochet C, *et al.* Monoclonal anti-epidermal growth factor receptor antibodies which are inhibitors of epidermal growth factor binding and antagonists of epidermal growth factor binding and antagonists of epidermal growth factor-stimulated tyrosine protein kinase activity. J Biol Chem 1984; 259(12): 7755-60.
[PMID: 6330079]

[54] Downward J, Yarden Y, Mayes E, *et al.* Close similarity of epidermal growth factor receptor and v-erb-B oncogene protein sequences. Nature 1984; 307(5951): 521-7.
[PMID: 6320011]

[55] Ullrich A, Coussens L, Hayflick JS, *et al.* Human epidermal growth factor receptor cDNA sequence and aberrant expression of the amplified gene in A431 epidermoid carcinoma cells. Nature 1984;

309(5967): 418-25.
[PMID: 6328312]

[56]   Hendler FJ, Ozanne BW. Human squamous cell lung cancers express increased epidermal growth
         factor receptors. J Clin Invest 1984; 74(2): 647-51.
         [PMID: 6086719]

[57]   Velu TJ, Beguinot L, Vass WC, *et al.* Epidermal-growth-factor-dependent transformation by a human
         EGF receptor proto-oncogene. Science 1987; 238(4832): 1408-10.
         [PMID: 3500513]

[58]   Luwor RB, Zhu HJ, Walker F, *et al.* The tumor-specific de2-7 epidermal growth factor receptor
         (EGFR) promotes cells survival and heterodimerizes with the wild-type EGFR. Oncogene 2004;
         23(36): 6095-104.
         [PMID: 15221011]

[59]   Pierce JH, Ruggiero M, Fleming TP, *et al.* Signal transduction through the EGF receptor transfected in
         IL-3-dependent hematopoietic cells. Science 1988; 239(4840): 628-31.
         [PMID: 3257584]

[60]   Riese DJ II, van Raaij TM, Plowman GD, Andrews GC, Stern DF. The cellular response to
         neuregulins is governed by complex interactions of the erbB receptor family. Mol Cell Biol 1995;
         15(10): 5770-6.
         [PMID: 7565730]

[61]   Wang HM, Collins M, Arai K, Miyajima A. EGF induces differentiation of an IL-3-dependent cell line
         expressing the EGF receptor. EMBO J 1989; 8(12): 3677-84.
         [PMID: 2531081]

[62]   Santon JB, Cronin MT, MacLeod CL, Mendelsohn J, Masui H, Gill GN. Effects of epidermal growth
         factor receptor concentration on tumorigenicity of A431 cells in nude mice. Cancer Res 1986; 46(9):
         4701-5.
         [PMID: 3015393]

[63]   Filmus J, Trent JM, Pollak MN, Buick RN. Epidermal growth factor receptor gene-amplified MDA-
         468 breast cancer cell line and its nonamplified variants. Mol Cell Biol 1987; 7(1): 251-7.
         [PMID: 3494191]

[64]   Bartlett JM, Langdon SP, Simpson BJ, *et al.* The prognostic value of epidermal growth factor receptor
         mRNA expression in primary ovarian cancer. Br J Cancer 1996; 73(3): 301-6.
         [PMID: 8562334]

[65]   Ekstrand AJ, James CD, Cavenee WK, Seliger B, Pettersson RF, Collins VP. Genes for epidermal
         growth factor receptor, transforming growth factor alpha, and epidermal growth factor and their
         expression in human gliomas *in vivo.* Cancer Res 1991; 51(8): 2164-72.
         [PMID: 2009534]

[66]   Hollstein MC, Smits AM, Galiana C, *et al.* Amplification of epidermal growth factor receptor gene but
         no evidence of ras mutations in primary human esophageal cancers. Cancer Res 1988; 48(18): 5119-
         23.
         [PMID: 3044581]

[67] Ishitoya J, Toriyama M, Oguchi N, *et al.* Gene amplification and overexpression of EGF receptor in squamous cell carcinomas of the head and neck. Br J Cancer 1989; 59(4): 559-62.
[PMID: 2713242]

[68] Libermann TA, Nusbaum HR, Razon N, *et al.* Amplification, enhanced expression and possible rearrangement of EGF receptor gene in primary human brain tumours of glial origin. Nature 1985; 313(5998): 144-7.
[PMID: 2981413]

[69] Neal DE, Marsh C, Bennett MK, *et al.* Epidermal-growth-factor receptors in human bladder cancer: comparison of invasive and superficial tumours. Lancet 1985; 1(8425): 366-8.
[PMID: 2857420]

[70] Sainsbury JR, Farndon JR, Needham GK, Malcolm AJ, Harris AL. Epidermal-growth-factor receptor status as predictor of early recurrence of and death from breast cancer. Lancet 1987; 1(8547): 1398-402.
[PMID: 2884496]

[71] Veale D, Ashcroft T, Marsh C, Gibson GJ, Harris AL. Epidermal growth factor receptors in non-small cell lung cancer. Br J Cancer 1987; 55(5): 513-6.
[PMID: 3038157]

[72] Jaros E, Perry RH, Adam L, *et al.* Prognostic implications of p53 protein, epidermal growth factor receptor, and Ki-67 labelling in brain tumours. Br J Cancer 1992; 66(2): 373-85.
[PMID: 1503912]

[73] Mayer A, Takimoto M, Fritz E, Schellander G, Kofler K, Ludwig H. The prognostic significance of proliferating cell nuclear antigen, epidermal growth factor receptor, and mdr gene expression in colorectal cancer. Cancer 1993; 71(8): 2454-60.
[PMID: 8095852]

[74] Dazzi H, Hasleton PS, Thatcher N, *et al.* Expression of epidermal growth factor receptor (EGF-R) in non-small cell lung cancer. Use of archival tissue and correlation of EGF-R with histology, tumour size, node status and survival. Br J Cancer 1989; 59(5): 746-9.
[PMID: 2544220]

[75] Dittadi R, Gion M, Pagan V, *et al.* Epidermal growth factor receptor in lung malignancies. Comparison between cancer and normal tissue. Br J Cancer 1991; 64(4): 741-4.
[PMID: 1654986]

[76] Klijn JG, Berns PM, Schmitz PI, Foekens JA. The clinical significance of epidermal growth factor receptor (EGF-R) in human breast cancer: a review on 5232 patients. Endocr Rev 1992; 13(1): 3-17.
[PMID: 1313356]

[77] Ciardiello F, Caputo R, Bianco R, *et al.* Antitumor effect and potentiation of cytotoxic drugs activity in human cancer cells by ZD-1839 (Iressa), an epidermal growth factor receptor-selective tyrosine kinase inhibitor. Clin Cancer Res 2000; 6(5): 2053-63.
[PMID: 10815932]

[78] Perera SA, Li D, Shimamura T, *et al.* HER2YVMA drives rapid development of adenosquamous lung tumors in mice that are sensitive to BIBW2992 and rapamycin combination therapy. Proc Natl Acad

Sci USA 2009; 106(2): 474-9.
[PMID: 19122144]

[79]   Pollack VA, Savage DM, Baker DA, *et al.* Inhibition of epidermal growth factor receptor-associated tyrosine phosphorylation in human carcinomas with CP-358,774: dynamics of receptor inhibition *in situ* and antitumor effects in athymic mice. J Pharmacol Exp Ther 1999; 291(2): 739-48.
[PMID: 10525095]

[80]   Rusnak DW, Affleck K, Cockerill SG, *et al.* The characterization of novel, dual ErbB-2/EGFR, tyrosine kinase inhibitors: potential therapy for cancer. Cancer Res 2001; 61(19): 7196-203.
[PMID: 11585755]

[81]   Rusnak DW, Lackey K, Affleck K, *et al.* The effects of the novel, reversible epidermal growth factor receptor/ErbB-2 tyrosine kinase inhibitor, GW2016, on the growth of human normal and tumor-derived cell lines *in vitro* and *in vivo.* Mol Cancer Ther 2001; 1(2): 85-94.
[PMID: 12467226]

[82]   Yang XD, Jia XC, Corvalan JR, Wang P, Davis CG, Jakobovits A. Eradication of established tumors by a fully human monoclonal antibody to the epidermal growth factor receptor without concomitant chemotherapy. Cancer Res 1999; 59(6): 1236-43.
[PMID: 10096554]

[83]   Balaban N, Moni J, Shannon M, Dang L, Murphy E, Goldkorn T. The effect of ionizing radiation on signal transduction: antibodies to EGF receptor sensitize A431 cells to radiation. Biochim Biophys Acta 1996; 1314(1-2): 147-56.
[PMID: 8972728]

[84]   Huang SM, Bock JM, Harari PM. Epidermal growth factor receptor blockade with C225 modulates proliferation, apoptosis, and radiosensitivity in squamous cell carcinomas of the head and neck. Cancer Res 1999; 59(8): 1935-40.
[PMID: 10213503]

[85]   Sirotnak FM, Zakowski MF, Miller VA, Scher HI, Kris MG. Efficacy of cytotoxic agents against human tumor xenografts is markedly enhanced by coadministration of ZD1839 (Iressa), an inhibitor of EGFR tyrosine kinase. Clin Cancer Res 2000; 6(12): 4885-92.
[PMID: 11156248]

[86]   Wollman R, Yahalom J, Maxy R, Pinto J, Fuks Z. Effect of epidermal growth factor on the growth and radiation sensitivity of human breast cancer cells *in vitro.* Int J Radiat Oncol Biol Phys 1994; 30(1): 91-8.
[PMID: 8083133]

[87]   Atlas I, Mendelsohn J, Baselga J, Fair WR, Masui H, Kumar R. Growth regulation of human renal carcinoma cells: role of transforming growth factor alpha. Cancer Res 1992; 52(12): 3335-9.
[PMID: 1596891]

[88]   Fan Z, Baselga J, Masui H, Mendelsohn J. Antitumor effect of anti-epidermal growth factor receptor monoclonal antibodies plus cis-diamminedichloroplatinum on well established A431 cell xenografts. Cancer Res 1993; 53(19): 4637-42.
[PMID: 8402640]

[89]   Hofer DR, Sherwood ER, Bromberg WD, Mendelsohn J, Lee C, Kozlowski JM. Autonomous growth

of androgen-independent human prostatic carcinoma cells: role of transforming growth factor alpha. Cancer Res 1991; 51(11): 2780-5.
[PMID: 2032218]

[90] Karnes WE Jr, Weller SG, Adjei PN, *et al.* Inhibition of epidermal growth factor receptor kinase induces protease-dependent apoptosis in human colon cancer cells. Gastroenterology 1998; 114(5): 930-9.
[PMID: 9558281]

[91] Masui H, Kawamoto T, Sato JD, Wolf B, Sato G, Mendelsohn J. Growth inhibition of human tumor cells in athymic mice by anti-epidermal growth factor receptor monoclonal antibodies. Cancer Res 1984; 44(3): 1002-7.
[PMID: 6318979]

[92] Sato JD, Le AD, Kawamoto T. Derivation and assay of biological effects of monoclonal antibodies to epidermal growth factor receptors. Methods Enzymol 1987; 146: 63-81.
[PMID: 3500387]

[93] Fan Z, Shang BY, Lu Y, Chou JL, Mendelsohn J. Reciprocal changes in p27(Kip1) and p21(Cip1) in growth inhibition mediated by blockade or overstimulation of epidermal growth factor receptors. Clin Cancer Res 1997; 3(11): 1943-8.
[PMID: 9815583]

[94] Peng D, Fan Z, Lu Y, DeBlasio T, Scher H, Mendelsohn J. Anti-epidermal growth factor receptor monoclonal antibody 225 up-regulates p27KIP1 and induces G1 arrest in prostatic cancer cell line DU145. Cancer Res 1996; 56(16): 3666-9.
[PMID: 8706005]

[95] Liu B, Fang M, Schmidt M, Lu Y, Mendelsohn J, Fan Z. Induction of apoptosis and activation of the caspase cascade by anti-EGF receptor monoclonal antibodies in DiFi human colon cancer cells do not involve the c-jun N-terminal kinase activity. Br J Cancer 2000; 82(12): 1991-9.
[PMID: 10864208]

[96] Stampfer MR, Pan CH, Hosoda J, Bartholomew J, Mendelsohn J, Yaswen P. Blockage of EGF receptor signal transduction causes reversible arrest of normal and immortal human mammary epithelial cells with synchronous reentry into the cell cycle. Exp Cell Res 1993; 208(1): 175-88.
[PMID: 7689475]

[97] Tortora G, Caputo R, Pomatico G, *et al.* Cooperative inhibitory effect of novel mixed backbone oligonucleotide targeting protein kinase A in combination with docetaxel and anti-epidermal growth factor-receptor antibody on human breast cancer cell growth. Clin Cancer Res 1999; 5(4): 875-81.
[PMID: 10213224]

[98] Wu X, Fan Z, Masui H, Rosen N, Mendelsohn J. Apoptosis induced by an anti-epidermal growth factor receptor monoclonal antibody in a human colorectal carcinoma cell line and its delay by insulin. J Clin Invest 1995; 95(4): 1897-905.
[PMID: 7706497]

[99] Wu X, Rubin M, Fan Z, *et al.* Involvement of p27KIP1 in G1 arrest mediated by an anti-epidermal growth factor receptor monoclonal antibody. Oncogene 1996; 12(7): 1397-403.
[PMID: 8622855]

[100] Bruns CJ, Harbison MT, Davis DW, *et al.* Epidermal growth factor receptor blockade with C225 plus gemcitabine results in regression of human pancreatic carcinoma growing orthotopically in nude mice by antiangiogenic mechanisms. Clin Cancer Res 2000; 6(5): 1936-48.
[PMID: 10815919]

[101] Perrotte P, Matsumoto T, Inoue K, *et al.* Anti-epidermal growth factor receptor antibody C225 inhibits angiogenesis in human transitional cell carcinoma growing orthotopically in nude mice. Clin Cancer Res 1999; 5(2): 257-65.
[PMID: 10037173]

[102] Petit AM, Rak J, Hung MC, *et al.* Neutralizing antibodies against epidermal growth factor and ErbB-2/neu receptor tyrosine kinases down-regulate vascular endothelial growth factor production by tumor cells *in vitro* and *in vivo*: angiogenic implications for signal transduction therapy of solid tumors. Am J Pathol 1997; 151(6): 1523-30.
[PMID: 9403702]

[103] Fan Z, Lu Y, Wu X, Mendelsohn J. Antibody-induced epidermal growth factor receptor dimerization mediates inhibition of autocrine proliferation of A431 squamous carcinoma cells. J Biol Chem 1994; 269(44): 27595-602.
[PMID: 7961676]

[104] Sunada H, Magun BE, Mendelsohn J, MacLeod CL. Monoclonal antibody against epidermal growth factor receptor is internalized without stimulating receptor phosphorylation. Proc Natl Acad Sci USA 1986; 83(11): 3825-9.
[PMID: 2424012]

[105] Naramura M, Gillies SD, Mendelsohn J, Reisfeld RA, Mueller BM. Therapeutic potential of chimeric and murine anti-(epidermal growth factor receptor) antibodies in a metastasis model for human melanoma. Cancer Immunol Immunother 1993; 37(5): 343-9.
[PMID: 8402738]

[106] Divgi CR, Welt S, Kris M, *et al.* Phase I and imaging trial of indium 111-labeled anti-epidermal growth factor receptor monoclonal antibody 225 in patients with squamous cell lung carcinoma. J Natl Cancer Inst 1991; 83(2): 97-104.
[PMID: 1988695]

[107] Goldstein NI, Prewett M, Zuklys K, Rockwell P, Mendelsohn J. Biological efficacy of a chimeric antibody to the epidermal growth factor receptor in a human tumor xenograft model. Clin Cancer Res 1995; 1(11): 1311-8.
[PMID: 9815926]

[108] Baselga J, Pfister D, Cooper MR, *et al.* Phase I studies of anti-epidermal growth factor receptor chimeric antibody C225 alone and in combination with cisplatin. J Clin Oncol 2000; 18(4): 904-14.
[PMID: 10673534]

[109] Robert F, Ezekiel MP, Spencer SA, *et al.* Phase I study of anti--epidermal growth factor receptor antibody cetuximab in combination with radiation therapy in patients with advanced head and neck cancer. J Clin Oncol 2001; 19(13): 3234-43.
[PMID: 11432891]

[110] Shin DM, Donato NJ, Perez-Soler R, *et al.* Epidermal growth factor receptor-targeted therapy with

C225 and cisplatin in patients with head and neck cancer. Clin Cancer Res 2001; 7(5): 1204-13.
[PMID: 11350885]

[111] Cunningham D, Humblet Y, Siena S, *et al.* Cetuximab monotherapy and cetuximab plus irinotecan in irinotecan-refractory metastatic colorectal cancer. N Engl J Med 2004; 351(4): 337-45.
[PMID: 15269313]

[112] Saltz LB. Can the addition of cetuximab to irinotecan improve outcome in colorectal cancer? Nat Clin Pract Oncol 2005; 2(1): 20-1.
[PMID: 16264850]

[113] Saltz LB, Meropol NJ, Loehrer PJ Sr, Needle MN, Kopit J, Mayer RJ. Phase II trial of cetuximab in patients with refractory colorectal cancer that expresses the epidermal growth factor receptor. J Clin Oncol 2004; 22(7): 1201-8.
[PMID: 14993230]

[114] Lyseng-Williamson KA. Cetuximab: a guide to its use in combination with FOLFIRI in the first-line treatment of metastatic colorectal cancer in the USA. Mol Diagn Ther 2012; 16(5): 317-22.
[PMID: 23055389]

[115] Van Cutsem E, Köhne CH, Hitre E, *et al.* Cetuximab and chemotherapy as initial treatment for metastatic colorectal cancer. N Engl J Med 2009; 360(14): 1408-17.
[PMID: 19339720]

[116] Van Cutsem E, Köhne CH, Láng I, *et al.* Cetuximab plus irinotecan, fluorouracil, and leucovorin as first-line treatment for metastatic colorectal cancer: updated analysis of overall survival according to tumor KRAS and BRAF mutation status. J Clin Oncol 2011; 29(15): 2011-9.
[PMID: 21502544]

[117] Bokemeyer C, Bondarenko I, Hartmann JT, *et al.* Efficacy according to biomarker status of cetuximab plus FOLFOX-4 as first-line treatment for metastatic colorectal cancer: the OPUS study. Ann Oncol 2011; 22(7): 1535-46.
[PMID: 21228335]

[118] Bokemeyer C, Bondarenko I, Makhson A, *et al.* Fluorouracil, leucovorin, and oxaliplatin with and without cetuximab in the first-line treatment of metastatic colorectal cancer. J Clin Oncol 2009; 27(5): 663-71.
[PMID: 19114683]

[119] Cohen MH, Chen H, Shord S, *et al.* Approval summary: Cetuximab in combination with cisplatin or carboplatin and 5-fluorouracil for the first-line treatment of patients with recurrent locoregional or metastatic squamous cell head and neck cancer. Oncologist 2013; 18(4): 460-6.
[PMID: 23576486]

[120] Cohen RB. Current challenges and clinical investigations of epidermal growth factor receptor (EGFR)- and ErbB family-targeted agents in the treatment of head and neck squamous cell carcinoma (HNSCC). Cancer Treat Rev 2014; 40(4): 567-77.
[PMID: 24216225]

[121] Bonner JA, Harari PM, Giralt J, *et al.* Radiotherapy plus cetuximab for squamous-cell carcinoma of the head and neck. N Engl J Med 2006; 354(6): 567-78.
[PMID: 16467544]

[122] Bonner JA, Harari PM, Giralt J, *et al.* Radiotherapy plus cetuximab for locoregionally advanced head and neck cancer: 5-year survival data from a phase 3 randomised trial, and relation between cetuximab-induced rash and survival. Lancet Oncol 2010; 11(1): 21-8.
[PMID: 19897418]

[123] Vermorken JB, Trigo J, Hitt R, *et al.* Open-label, uncontrolled, multicenter phase II study to evaluate the efficacy and toxicity of cetuximab as a single agent in patients with recurrent and/or metastatic squamous cell carcinoma of the head and neck who failed to respond to platinum-based therapy. J Clin Oncol 2007; 25(16): 2171-7.
[PMID: 17538161]

[124] Baselga J, Trigo JM, Bourhis J, *et al.* Phase II multicenter study of the antiepidermal growth factor receptor monoclonal antibody cetuximab in combination with platinum-based chemotherapy in patients with platinum-refractory metastatic and/or recurrent squamous cell carcinoma of the head and neck. J Clin Oncol 2005; 23(24): 5568-77.
[PMID: 16009950]

[125] Herbst RS, Arquette M, Shin DM, *et al.* Phase II multicenter study of the epidermal growth factor receptor antibody cetuximab and cisplatin for recurrent and refractory squamous cell carcinoma of the head and neck. J Clin Oncol 2005; 23(24): 5578-87.
[PMID: 16009949]

[126] Vermorken JB, Mesia R, Rivera F, *et al.* Platinum-based chemotherapy plus cetuximab in head and neck cancer. N Engl J Med 2008; 359(11): 1116-27.
[PMID: 18784101]

[127] Mesía R, Rivera F, Kawecki A, *et al.* Quality of life of patients receiving platinum-based chemotherapy plus cetuximab first line for recurrent and/or metastatic squamous cell carcinoma of the head and neck. Ann Oncol 2010; 21(10): 1967-73.
[PMID: 20335368]

[128] Rivera F, García-Castaño A, Vega N, Vega-Villegas ME, Gutiérrez-Sanz L. Cetuximab in metastatic or recurrent head and neck cancer: the EXTREME trial. Expert Rev Anticancer Ther 2009; 9(10): 1421-8.
[PMID: 19828002]

[129] Mendez MJ, Green LL, Corvalan JR, *et al.* Functional transplant of megabase human immunoglobulin loci recapitulates human antibody response in mice. Nat Genet 1997; 15(2): 146-56.
[PMID: 9020839]

[130] Yang XD, Jia XC, Corvalan JR, Wang P, Davis CG, Jakobovits A. Eradication of established tumors by a fully human monoclonal antibody to the epidermal growth factor receptor without concomitant chemotherapy. Cancer Res 1999; 59(6): 1236-43.
[PMID: 10096554]

[131] Hecht JR, Patnaik A, Berlin J, *et al.* Panitumumab monotherapy in patients with previously treated metastatic colorectal cancer. Cancer 2007; 110(5): 980-8.
[PMID: 17671985]

[132] Muro K, Yoshino T, Doi T, *et al.* A phase 2 clinical trial of panitumumab monotherapy in Japanese patients with metastatic colorectal cancer. Jpn J Clin Oncol 2009; 39(5): 321-6.

[PMID: 19287023]

[133] Van Cutsem E, Peeters M, Siena S, *et al.* Open-label phase III trial of panitumumab plus best supportive care compared with best supportive care alone in patients with chemotherapy-refractory metastatic colorectal cancer. J Clin Oncol 2007; 25(13): 1658-64.
[PMID: 17470858]

[134] Goozner M. Accelerated drug approval: FDA may get tougher; companies cite hurdles. J Natl Cancer Inst 2011; 103(6): 455-7.
[PMID: 21393609]

[135] Konecny GE, Pegram MD, Venkatesan N, *et al.* Activity of the dual kinase inhibitor lapatinib (GW572016) against HER-2-overexpressing and trastuzumab-treated breast cancer cells. Cancer Res 2006; 66(3): 1630-9.
[PMID: 16452222]

[136] Xia W, Mullin RJ, Keith BR, *et al.* Anti-tumor activity of GW572016: a dual tyrosine kinase inhibitor blocks EGF activation of EGFR/erbB2 and downstream Erk1/2 and AKT pathways. Oncogene 2002; 21(41): 6255-63.
[PMID: 12214266]

[137] Zhou H, Kim YS, Peletier A, McCall W, Earp HS, Sartor CI. Effects of the EGFR/HER2 kinase inhibitor GW572016 on EGFR- and HER2-overexpressing breast cancer cell line proliferation, radiosensitization, and resistance. Int J Radiat Oncol Biol Phys 2004; 58(2): 344-52.
[PMID: 14751502]

[138] Blackwell KL, Pegram MD, Tan-Chiu E, *et al.* Single-agent lapatinib for HER2-overexpressing advanced or metastatic breast cancer that progressed on first- or second-line trastuzumab-containing regimens. Ann Oncol 2009; 20(6): 1026-31.
[PMID: 19179558]

[139] Toi M, Iwata H, Fujiwara Y, *et al.* Lapatinib monotherapy in patients with relapsed, advanced, or metastatic breast cancer: efficacy, safety, and biomarker results from Japanese patients phase II studies. Br J Cancer 2009; 101(10): 1676-82.
[PMID: 19844234]

[140] Chu QS, Schwartz G, de Bono J, *et al.* Phase I and pharmacokinetic study of lapatinib in combination with capecitabine in patients with advanced solid malignancies. J Clin Oncol 2007; 25(24): 3753-8.
[PMID: 17704424]

[141] Cameron D, Casey M, Press M, *et al.* A phase III randomized comparison of lapatinib plus capecitabine *versus* capecitabine alone in women with advanced breast cancer that has progressed on trastuzumab: updated efficacy and biomarker analyses. Breast Cancer Res Treat 2008; 112(3): 533-43.
[PMID: 18188694]

[142] Geyer CE, Forster J, Lindquist D, *et al.* Lapatinib plus capecitabine for HER2-positive advanced breast cancer. N Engl J Med 2006; 355(26): 2733-43.
[PMID: 17192538]

[143] Jelovac D, Emens LA. HER2-directed therapy for metastatic breast cancer. Oncology (Huntingt) 2013; 27(3): 166-75.
[PMID: 23687784]

[144] Ryan Q, Ibrahim A, Cohen MH, *et al.* FDA drug approval summary: lapatinib in combination with capecitabine for previously treated metastatic breast cancer that overexpresses HER-2. Oncologist 2008; 13(10): 1114-9.
[PMID: 18849320]

[145] Bachelot T, Romieu G, Campone M, *et al.* Lapatinib plus capecitabine in patients with previously untreated brain metastases from HER2-positive metastatic breast cancer (LANDSCAPE): a single-group phase 2 study. Lancet Oncol 2013; 14(1): 64-71.
[PMID: 23122784]

[146] Woodburn JR. The epidermal growth factor receptor and its inhibition in cancer therapy. Pharmacol Ther 1999; 82(2-3): 241-50.
[PMID: 10454201]

[147] Chan KC, Knox WF, Gandhi A, Slamon DJ, Potten CS, Bundred NJ. Blockade of growth factor receptors in ductal carcinoma *in situ* inhibits epithelial proliferation. Br J Surg 2001; 88(3): 412-8.
[PMID: 11260109]

[148] Ciardiello F, Caputo R, Bianco R, *et al.* Antitumor effect and potentiation of cytotoxic drugs activity in human cancer cells by ZD-1839 (Iressa), an epidermal growth factor receptor-selective tyrosine kinase inhibitor. Clin Cancer Res 2000; 6(5): 2053-63.
[PMID: 10815932]

[149] Baselga J, Rischin D, Ranson M, *et al.* Phase I safety, pharmacokinetic, and pharmacodynamic trial of ZD1839, a selective oral epidermal growth factor receptor tyrosine kinase inhibitor, in patients with five selected solid tumor types. J Clin Oncol 2002; 20(21): 4292-302.
[PMID: 12409327]

[150] Goss G, Hirte H, Miller WH Jr, *et al.* A phase I study of oral ZD 1839 given daily in patients with solid tumors: IND.122, a study of the Investigational New Drug Program of the National Cancer Institute of Canada Clinical Trials Group. Invest New Drugs 2005; 23(2): 147-55.
[PMID: 15744591]

[151] Herbst RS, Maddox AM, Rothenberg ML, *et al.* Selective oral epidermal growth factor receptor tyrosine kinase inhibitor ZD1839 is generally well-tolerated and has activity in non-small-cell lung cancer and other solid tumors: results of a phase I trial. J Clin Oncol 2002; 20(18): 3815-25.
[PMID: 12228201]

[152] Nakagawa K, Tamura T, Negoro S, *et al.* Phase I pharmacokinetic trial of the selective oral epidermal growth factor receptor tyrosine kinase inhibitor gefitinib ('Iressa', ZD1839) in Japanese patients with solid malignant tumors. Ann Oncol 2003; 14(6): 922-30.
[PMID: 12796031]

[153] Ranson M, Hammond LA, Ferry D, *et al.* ZD1839, a selective oral epidermal growth factor receptor-tyrosine kinase inhibitor, is well tolerated and active in patients with solid, malignant tumors: results of a phase I trial. J Clin Oncol 2002; 20(9): 2240-50.
[PMID: 11980995]

[154] Swaisland H, Laight A, Stafford L, *et al.* Pharmacokinetics and tolerability of the orally active selective epidermal growth factor receptor tyrosine kinase inhibitor ZD1839 in healthy volunteers. Clin Pharmacokinet 2001; 40(4): 297-306.

[PMID: 11368294]

[155] Fukuoka M, Yano S, Giaccone G, *et al.* Multi-institutional randomized phase II trial of gefitinib for previously treated patients with advanced non-small-cell lung cancer (The IDEAL 1 Trial) [corrected]. J Clin Oncol 2003; 21(12): 2237-46. [corrected].
[PMID: 12748244]

[156] Kris MG, Natale RB, Herbst RS, *et al.* Efficacy of gefitinib, an inhibitor of the epidermal growth factor receptor tyrosine kinase, in symptomatic patients with non-small cell lung cancer: a randomized trial. JAMA 2003; 290(16): 2149-58.
[PMID: 14570950]

[157] Giaccone G, Herbst RS, Manegold C, *et al.* Gefitinib in combination with gemcitabine and cisplatin in advanced non-small-cell lung cancer: a phase III trial--INTACT 1. J Clin Oncol 2004; 22(5): 777-84.
[PMID: 14990632]

[158] Herbst RS, Giaccone G, Schiller JH, *et al.* Gefitinib in combination with paclitaxel and carboplatin in advanced non-small-cell lung cancer: a phase III trial--INTACT 2. J Clin Oncol 2004; 22(5): 785-94.
[PMID: 14990633]

[159] Lynch TJ, Bell DW, Sordella R, *et al.* Activating mutations in the epidermal growth factor receptor underlying responsiveness of non-small-cell lung cancer to gefitinib. N Engl J Med 2004; 350(21): 2129-39.
[PMID: 15118073]

[160] Paez JG, Jänne PA, Lee JC, *et al.* EGFR mutations in lung cancer: correlation with clinical response to gefitinib therapy. Science 2004; 304(5676): 1497-500.
[PMID: 15118125]

[161] Maemondo M, Inoue A, Kobayashi K, *et al.* North-East Japan Study Group. Gefitinib or chemotherapy for non-small-cell lung cancer with mutated EGFR. N Engl J Med 2010; 362(25): 2380-8.
[PMID: 20573926]

[162] Mitsudomi T, Morita S, Yatabe Y, *et al.* West Japan Oncology Group. Gefitinib *versus* cisplatin plus docetaxel in patients with non-small-cell lung cancer harbouring mutations of the epidermal growth factor receptor (WJTOG3405): an open label, randomised phase 3 trial. Lancet Oncol 2010; 11(2): 121-8.
[PMID: 20022809]

[163] Chung C. Tyrosine kinase inhibitors for epidermal growth factor receptor gene mutation-positive non-small cell lung cancers: an update for recent advances in therapeutics. J Oncol Pharm Pract 2015; 1078155215577810.
[PMID: 25855240]

[164] Gaffney DC, Soyer HP, Simpson F. The epidermal growth factor receptor in squamous cell carcinoma: An emerging drug target. Australas J Dermatol 2014; 55(1): 24-34.
[PMID: 23425099]

[165] Moyer JD, Barbacci EG, Iwata KK, *et al.* Induction of apoptosis and cell cycle arrest by CP-358,774, an inhibitor of epidermal growth factor receptor tyrosine kinase. Cancer Res 1997; 57(21): 4838-48.
[PMID: 9354447]

[166] Pollack VA, Savage DM, Baker DA, *et al.* Inhibition of epidermal growth factor receptor-associated tyrosine phosphorylation in human carcinomas with CP-358,774: dynamics of receptor inhibition *in situ* and antitumor effects in athymic mice. J Pharmacol Exp Ther 1999; 291(2): 739-48.
[PMID: 10525095]

[167] Durkin AJ, Bloomston PM, Rosemurgy AS, *et al.* Defining the role of the epidermal growth factor receptor in pancreatic cancer grown *in vitro.* Am J Surg 2003; 186(5): 431-6.
[PMID: 14599602]

[168] Bruns CJ, Solorzano CC, Harbison MT, *et al.* Blockade of the epidermal growth factor receptor signaling by a novel tyrosine kinase inhibitor leads to apoptosis of endothelial cells and therapy of human pancreatic carcinoma. Cancer Res 2000; 60(11): 2926-35.
[PMID: 10850439]

[169] Ng SS, Tsao MS, Nicklee T, Hedley DW. Effects of the epidermal growth factor receptor inhibitor OSI-774, Tarceva, on downstream signaling pathways and apoptosis in human pancreatic adenocarcinoma. Mol Cancer Ther 2002; 1(10): 777-83.
[PMID: 12492110]

[170] Hanauske AR, Cassidy J, Sastre J, *et al.* Phase 1b dose escalation study of erlotinib in combination with infusional 5-Fluorouracil, leucovorin, and oxaliplatin in patients with advanced solid tumors. Clin Cancer Res 2007; 13(2 Pt 1): 523-31.
[PMID: 17255274]

[171] Iannitti D, Dipetrillo T, Akerman P, *et al.* Erlotinib and chemoradiation followed by maintenance erlotinib for locally advanced pancreatic cancer: a phase I study. Am J Clin Oncol 2005; 28(6): 570-5.
[PMID: 16317266]

[172] Van Cutsem E, Verslype C, Beale P, *et al.* A phase Ib dose-escalation study of erlotinib, capecitabine and oxaliplatin in metastatic colorectal cancer patients. Ann Oncol 2008; 19(2): 332-9.
[PMID: 17986625]

[173] Messersmith WA, Jimeno A, Jacene H, *et al.* Phase I trial of oxaliplatin, infusional 5-fluorouracil, and leucovorin (FOLFOX4) with erlotinib and bevacizumab in colorectal cancer. Clin Colorectal Cancer 2010; 9(5): 297-304.
[PMID: 21208844]

[174] Ma WW, Herman JM, Jimeno A, *et al.* A tolerability and pharmacokinetic study of adjuvant erlotinib and capecitabine with concurrent radiation in resected pancreatic cancer. Transl Oncol 2010; 3(6): 373-9.
[PMID: 21151476]

[175] Calvo E, Malik SN, Siu LL, *et al.* Assessment of erlotinib pharmacodynamics in tumors and skin of patients with head and neck cancer. Ann Oncol 2007; 18(4): 761-7.
[PMID: 17317676]

[176] Patnaik A, Wood D, Tolcher AW, *et al.* Phase I, pharmacokinetic, and biological study of erlotinib in combination with paclitaxel and carboplatin in patients with advanced solid tumors. Clin Cancer Res 2006; 12(24): 7406-13.
[PMID: 17189413]

[177] Hidalgo M, Siu LL, Nemunaitis J, *et al.* Phase I and pharmacologic study of OSI-774, an epidermal growth factor receptor tyrosine kinase inhibitor, in patients with advanced solid malignancies. J Clin Oncol 2001; 19(13): 3267-79.
[PMID: 11432895]

[178] Messersmith WA, Laheru DA, Senzer NN, *et al.* Phase I trial of irinotecan, infusional 5-fluorouracil, and leucovorin (FOLFIRI) with erlotinib (OSI-774): early termination due to increased toxicities. Clin Cancer Res 2004; 10(19): 6522-7.
[PMID: 15475439]

[179] Pérez-Soler R, Chachoua A, Hammond LA, *et al.* Determinants of tumor response and survival with erlotinib in patients with non--small-cell lung cancer. J Clin Oncol 2004; 22(16): 3238-47.
[PMID: 15310767]

[180] Giaccone G, Gallegos Ruiz M, Le Chevalier T, *et al.* Erlotinib for frontline treatment of advanced non-small cell lung cancer: a phase II study. Clin Cancer Res 2006; 12(20 Pt 1): 6049-55.
[PMID: 17062680]

[181] Shepherd FA, Rodrigues Pereira J, Ciuleanu T, *et al.* National Cancer Institute of Canada Clinical Trials Group. Erlotinib in previously treated non-small-cell lung cancer. N Engl J Med 2005; 353(2): 123-32.
[PMID: 16014882]

[182] Melosky B. Review of EGFR TKIs in Metastatic NSCLC, Including Ongoing Trials. Front Oncol 2014; 4: 244.
[PMID: 25309870]

[183] Eberhard DA, Johnson BE, Amler LC, *et al.* Mutations in the epidermal growth factor receptor and in KRAS are predictive and prognostic indicators in patients with non-small-cell lung cancer treated with chemotherapy alone and in combination with erlotinib. J Clin Oncol 2005; 23(25): 5900-9.
[PMID: 16043828]

[184] Pao W, Miller V, Zakowski M, *et al.* EGF receptor gene mutations are common in lung cancers from "never smokers" and are associated with sensitivity of tumors to gefitinib and erlotinib. Proc Natl Acad Sci USA 2004; 101(36): 13306-11.
[PMID: 15329413]

[185] Rosell R, Carcereny E, Gervais R, *et al.* Spanish Lung Cancer Group in collaboration with Groupe Français de Pneumo-Cancérologie and Associazione Italiana Oncologia Toracica. Erlotinib *versus* standard chemotherapy as first-line treatment for European patients with advanced EGFR mutation-positive non-small-cell lung cancer (EURTAC): a multicentre, open-label, randomised phase 3 trial. Lancet Oncol 2012; 13(3): 239-46.
[PMID: 22285168]

[186] Tsao MS, Sakurada A, Cutz JC, *et al.* Erlotinib in lung cancer - molecular and clinical predictors of outcome. N Engl J Med 2005; 353(2): 133-44.
[PMID: 16014883]

[187] Zhou C, Wu YL, Chen G, *et al.* Erlotinib *versus* chemotherapy as first-line treatment for patients with advanced EGFR mutation-positive non-small-cell lung cancer (OPTIMAL, CTONG-0802): a multicentre, open-label, randomised, phase 3 study. Lancet Oncol 2011; 12(8): 735-42.

[PMID: 21783417]

[188] Zhou C, Wu YL, Chen G, *et al.* Final overall survival results from a randomised, phase III study of erlotinib *versus* chemotherapy as first-line treatment of EGFR mutation-positive advanced non-smal--cell lung cancer (OPTIMAL, CTONG-0802). Ann Oncol 2015; 26(9): 1877-83.
       [PMID: 26141208]

[189] Moore MJ, Goldstein D, Hamm J, *et al.* National Cancer Institute of Canada Clinical Trials Group. Erlotinib plus gemcitabine compared with gemcitabine alone in patients with advanced pancreatic cancer: a phase III trial of the National Cancer Institute of Canada Clinical Trials Group. J Clin Oncol 2007; 25(15): 1960-6.
       [PMID: 17452677]

[190] Iyer R, Bharthuar A. A review of erlotinib--an oral, selective epidermal growth factor receptor tyrosine kinase inhibitor. Expert Opin Pharmacother 2010; 11(2): 311-20.
       [PMID: 20088749]

[191] Kobayashi S, Boggon TJ, Dayaram T, *et al.* EGFR mutation and resistance of non-small-cell lung cancer to gefitinib. N Engl J Med 2005; 352(8): 786-92.
       [PMID: 15728811]

[192] Pao W, Miller VA, Politi KA, *et al.* Acquired resistance of lung adenocarcinomas to gefitinib or erlotinib is associated with a second mutation in the EGFR kinase domain. PLoS Med 2005; 2(3): e73.
       [PMID: 15737014]

[193] Li D, Ambrogio L, Shimamura T, *et al.* BIBW2992, an irreversible EGFR/HER2 inhibitor highly effective in preclinical lung cancer models. Oncogene 2008; 27(34): 4702-11.
       [PMID: 18408761]

[194] Solca F, Dahl G, Zoephel A, *et al.* Target binding properties and cellular activity of afatinib (BIBW 2992), an irreversible ErbB family blocker. J Pharmacol Exp Ther 2012; 343(2): 342-50.
       [PMID: 22888144]

[195] Katakami N, Atagi S, Goto K, *et al.* LUX-Lung 4: a phase II trial of afatinib in patients with advanced non-small-cell lung cancer who progressed during prior treatment with erlotinib, gefitinib, or both. J Clin Oncol 2013; 31(27): 3335-41.
       [PMID: 23816963]

[196] Miller VA, Hirsh V, Cadranel J, *et al.* Afatinib *versus* placebo for patients with advanced, metastatic non-small-cell lung cancer after failure of erlotinib, gefitinib, or both, and one or two lines of chemotherapy (LUX-Lung 1): a phase 2b/3 randomised trial. Lancet Oncol 2012; 13(5): 528-38.
       [PMID: 22452896]

[197] Sequist LV, Yang JC, Yamamoto N, *et al.* Phase III study of afatinib or cisplatin plus pemetrexed in patients with metastatic lung adenocarcinoma with EGFR mutations. J Clin Oncol 2013; 31(27): 3327-34.
       [PMID: 23816960]

[198] Wu YL, Zhou C, Hu CP, *et al.* Afatinib *versus* cisplatin plus gemcitabine for first-line treatment of Asian patients with advanced non-small-cell lung cancer harbouring EGFR mutations (LUX-Lung 6): an open-label, randomised phase 3 trial. Lancet Oncol 2014; 15(2): 213-22.
       [PMID: 24439929]

[199] Yang JC, Sequist LV, Geater SL, *et al.* Clinical activity of afatinib in patients with advanced non-small-cell lung cancer harbouring uncommon EGFR mutations: a combined post-hoc analysis of LUX-Lung 2, LUX-Lung 3, and LUX-Lung 6. Lancet Oncol 2015; 16(7): 830-8. [PMID: 26051236]

[200] Yang JC, Shih JY, Su WC, *et al.* Afatinib for patients with lung adenocarcinoma and epidermal growth factor receptor mutations (LUX-Lung 2): a phase 2 trial. Lancet Oncol 2012; 13(5): 539-48. [PMID: 22452895]

[201] Yang JC, Wu YL, Schuler M, *et al.* Afatinib *versus* cisplatin-based chemotherapy for EGFR mutation-positive lung adenocarcinoma (LUX-Lung 3 and LUX-Lung 6): analysis of overall survival data from two randomised, phase 3 trials. Lancet Oncol 2015; 16(2): 141-51. [PMID: 25589191]

[202] Regales L, Gong Y, Shen R, *et al.* Dual targeting of EGFR can overcome a major drug resistance mutation in mouse models of EGFR mutant lung cancer. J Clin Invest 2009; 119(10): 3000-10. [PMID: 19759520]

[203] Janjigian YY, Smit EF, Groen HJ, *et al.* Dual inhibition of EGFR with afatinib and cetuximab in kinase inhibitor-resistant EGFR-mutant lung cancer with and without T790M mutations. Cancer Discov 2014; 4(9): 1036-45. [PMID: 25074459]

[204] Wheeler DL, Iida M, Kruser TJ, *et al.* Epidermal growth factor receptor cooperates with Src family kinases in acquired resistance to cetuximab. Cancer Biol Ther 2009; 8(8): 696-703. [PMID: 19276677]

[205] Kakiuchi S, Daigo Y, Ishikawa N, *et al.* Prediction of sensitivity of advanced non-small cell lung cancers to gefitinib (Iressa, ZD1839). Hum Mol Genet 2004; 13(24): 3029-43. [PMID: 15496427]

[206] Ishikawa N, Daigo Y, Takano A, *et al.* Increases of amphiregulin and transforming growth factor-alpha in serum as predictors of poor response to gefitinib among patients with advanced non-small cell lung cancers. Cancer Res 2005; 65(20): 9176-84. [PMID: 16230376]

[207] Masago K, Fujita S, Hatachi Y, *et al.* Clinical significance of pretreatment serum amphiregulin and transforming growth factor-alpha, and an epidermal growth factor receptor somatic mutation in patients with advanced non-squamous, non-small cell lung cancer. Cancer Sci 2008; 99(11): 2295-301. [PMID: 18811692]

[208] Yonesaka K, Zejnullahu K, Lindeman N, *et al.* Autocrine production of amphiregulin predicts sensitivity to both gefitinib and cetuximab in EGFR wild-type cancers. Clin Cancer Res 2008; 14(21): 6963-73. [PMID: 18980991]

[209] Hickinson DM, Marshall GB, Beran GJ, *et al.* Identification of biomarkers in human head and neck tumor cell lines that predict for *in vitro* sensitivity to gefitinib. Clin Transl Sci 2009; 2(3): 183-92. [PMID: 20443891]

[210] Khambata-Ford S, Garrett CR, Meropol NJ, *et al.* Expression of epiregulin and amphiregulin and K-

ras mutation status predict disease control in metastatic colorectal cancer patients treated with cetuximab. J Clin Oncol 2007; 25(22): 3230-7.
[PMID: 17664471]

[211] Jacobs B, De Roock W, Piessevaux H, *et al.* Amphiregulin and epiregulin mRNA expression in primary tumors predicts outcome in metastatic colorectal cancer treated with cetuximab. J Clin Oncol 2009; 27(30): 5068-74.
[PMID: 19738126]

[212] Baker JB, Dutta D, Watson D, *et al.* Tumour gene expression predicts response to cetuximab in patients with KRAS wild-type metastatic colorectal cancer. Br J Cancer 2011; 104(3): 488-95.
[PMID: 21206494]

[213] Tabernero J, Cervantes A, Rivera F, *et al.* Pharmacogenomic and pharmacoproteomic studies of cetuximab in metastatic colorectal cancer: biomarker analysis of a phase I dose-escalation study. J Clin Oncol 2010; 28(7): 1181-9.
[PMID: 20100964]

[214] Pentheroudakis G, Kotoula V, De Roock W, *et al.* Biomarkers of benefit from cetuximab-based therapy in metastatic colorectal cancer: interaction of EGFR ligand expression with RAS/RAF, PIK3CA genotypes. BMC Cancer 2013; 13: 49.
[PMID: 23374602]

[215] Saridaki Z, Tzardi M, Papadaki C, *et al.* Impact of KRAS, BRAF, PIK3CA mutations, PTEN, AREG, EREG expression and skin rash in ≥ 2 line cetuximab-based therapy of colorectal cancer patients. PLoS One 2011; 6(1): e15980.
[PMID: 21283802]

[216] Jonker DJ, Karapetis CS, Harbison C, *et al.* Epiregulin gene expression as a biomarker of benefit from cetuximab in the treatment of advanced colorectal cancer. Br J Cancer 2014; 110(3): 648-55.
[PMID: 24335920]

[217] Yoshida M, Shimura T, Sato M, *et al.* A novel predictive strategy by immunohistochemical analysis of four EGFR ligands in metastatic colorectal cancer treated with anti-EGFR antibodies. J Cancer Res Clin Oncol 2013; 139(3): 367-78.
[PMID: 23099994]

[218] Oliveras-Ferraros C, Cufi S, Queralt B, *et al.* Cross-suppression of EGFR ligands amphiregulin and epiregulin and de-repression of FGFR3 signalling contribute to cetuximab resistance in wild-type KRAS tumour cells. Br J Cancer 2012; 106(8): 1406-14.
[PMID: 22491422]

[219] Oliveras-Ferraros C, Massaguer Vall-Llovera A, Carrion Salip D, *et al.* Evolution of the predictive markers amphiregulin and epiregulin mRNAs during long-term cetuximab treatment of KRAS wild-type tumor cells. Invest New Drugs 2012; 30(2): 846-52.
[PMID: 21161326]

[220] Jedlinski A, Ansell A, Johansson AC, Roberg K. EGFR status and EGFR ligand expression influence the treatment response of head and neck cancer cell lines. J Oral Pathol Med 2013; 42(1): 26-36.
[PMID: 22643066]

[221] Tinhofer I, Klinghammer K, Weichert W, *et al.* Expression of amphiregulin and EGFRvIII affect

outcome of patients with squamous cell carcinoma of the head and neck receiving cetuximab-docetaxel treatment. Clin Cancer Res 2011; 17(15): 5197-204.
[PMID: 21653686]

[222] Takahashi N, Yamada Y, Furuta K, *et al.* Serum levels of hepatocyte growth factor and epiregulin are associated with the prognosis on anti-EGFR antibody treatment in KRAS wild-type metastatic colorectal cancer. Br J Cancer 2014; 110(11): 2716-27.
[PMID: 24800946]

[223] Rhee J, Han SW, Cha Y, *et al.* High serum TGF-α predicts poor response to lapatinib and capecitabine in HER2-positive breast cancer. Breast Cancer Res Treat 2011; 125(1): 107-14.
[PMID: 20936340]

[224] Addison CL, Ding K, Zhao H, *et al.* Plasma transforming growth factor alpha and amphiregulin protein levels in NCIC Clinical Trials Group BR.21. J Clin Oncol 2010; 28(36): 5247-56.
[PMID: 21079146]

[225] Chan E, Lafleur B, Rothenberg ML, *et al.* Dual blockade of the EGFR and COX-2 pathways: a phase II trial of cetuximab and celecoxib in patients with chemotherapy refractory metastatic colorectal cancer. Am J Clin Oncol 2011; 34(6): 581-6.
[PMID: 21217396]

[226] Zhang X, Xu J, Liu H, *et al.* Predictive biomarkers for the efficacy of cetuximab combined with cisplatin and capecitabine in advanced gastric or esophagogastric junction adenocarcinoma: a prospective multicenter phase 2 trial. Med Oncol 2014; 31(10): 226.
[PMID: 25234930]

[227] Cushman SM, Jiang C, Hatch AJ, *et al.* Gene expression markers of efficacy and resistance to cetuximab treatment in metastatic colorectal cancer: results from CALGB 80203 (Alliance). Clin Cancer Res 2015; 21(5): 1078-86.
[PMID: 25520391]

[228] Ansell A, Jedlinski A, Johansson AC, Roberg K. Epidermal growth factor is a potential biomarker for poor cetuximab response in tongue cancer cells. J Oral Pathol Med 2015.
[PMID: 25677871]

[229] Carrión-Salip D, Panosa C, Menendez JA, *et al.* Androgen-independent prostate cancer cells circumvent EGFR inhibition by overexpression of alternative HER receptors and ligands. Int J Oncol 2012; 41(3): 1128-38.
[PMID: 22684500]

[230] Ferrer-Soler L, Vazquez-Martin A, Brunet J, Menendez JA, De Llorens R, Colomer R. An update of the mechanisms of resistance to EGFR-tyrosine kinase inhibitors in breast cancer: Gefitinib (Iressa) - induced changes in the expression and nucleo-cytoplasmic trafficking of HER-ligands (Review). Int J Mol Med 2007; 20(1): 3-10. [Review].
[PMID: 17549382]

[231] Loupakis F, Cremolini C, Fioravanti A, *et al.* EGFR ligands as pharmacodynamic biomarkers in metastatic colorectal cancer patients treated with cetuximab and irinotecan. Target Oncol 2014; 9(3): 205-14.
[PMID: 23821377]

[232] Jhawer M, Goel S, Wilson AJ, *et al.* PIK3CA mutation/PTEN expression status predicts response of colon cancer cells to the epidermal growth factor receptor inhibitor cetuximab. Cancer Res 2008; 68(6): 1953-61.
[PMID: 18339877]

[233] Shahbazi M, Pravica V, Nasreen N, *et al.* Association between functional polymorphism in EGF gene and malignant melanoma. Lancet 2002; 359(9304): 397-401.
[PMID: 11844511]

[234] Hamai Y, Matsumura S, Matsusaki K, *et al.* A single nucleotide polymorphism in the 5′ untranslated region of the EGF gene is associated with occurrence and malignant progression of gastric cancer. Pathobiology 2005; 72(3): 133-8.
[PMID: 15860930]

[235] Costa BM, Ferreira P, Costa S, *et al.* Association between functional EGF+61 polymorphism and glioma risk. Clin Cancer Res 2007; 13(9): 2621-6.
[PMID: 17473192]

[236] Bhowmick DA, Zhuang Z, Wait SD, Weil RJ. A functional polymorphism in the EGF gene is found with increased frequency in glioblastoma multiforme patients and is associated with more aggressive disease. Cancer Res 2004; 64(4): 1220-3.
[PMID: 14973082]

[237] Garm Spindler KL, Pallisgaard N, Rasmussen AA, *et al.* The importance of KRAS mutations and EGF61A>G polymorphism to the effect of cetuximab and irinotecan in metastatic colorectal cancer. Ann Oncol 2009; 20(5): 879-84.
[PMID: 19179548]

[238] Graziano F, Ruzzo A, Loupakis F, *et al.* Pharmacogenetic profiling for cetuximab plus irinotecan therapy in patients with refractory advanced colorectal cancer. J Clin Oncol 2008; 26(9): 1427-34.
[PMID: 18349392]

[239] Hu-Lieskovan S, Vallbohmer D, Zhang W, *et al.* EGF61 polymorphism predicts complete pathologic response to cetuximab-based chemoradiation independent of KRAS status in locally advanced rectal cancer patients. Clin Cancer Res 2011; 17(15): 5161-9.
[PMID: 21673069]

[240] Zhang W, Gordon M, Press OA, *et al.* Cyclin D1 and epidermal growth factor polymorphisms associated with survival in patients with advanced colorectal cancer treated with Cetuximab. Pharmacogenet Genomics 2006; 16(7): 475-83.
[PMID: 16788380]

[241] Hatakeyama H, Cheng H, Wirth P, *et al.* Regulation of heparin-binding EGF-like growth factor by miR-212 and acquired cetuximab-resistance in head and neck squamous cell carcinoma. PLoS One 2010; 5(9): e12702.
[PMID: 20856931]

[242] Wheeler DL, Huang S, Kruser TJ, *et al.* Mechanisms of acquired resistance to cetuximab: role of HER (ErbB) family members. Oncogene 2008; 27(28): 3944-56.
[PMID: 18297114]

[243] Yotsumoto F, Oki E, Tokunaga E, Maehara Y, Kuroki M, Miyamoto S. HB-EGF orchestrates the complex signals involved in triple-negative and trastuzumab-resistant breast cancer. Int J Cancer 2010; 127(11): 2707-17.
[PMID: 20499311]

[244] Slamon DJ, Leyland-Jones B, Shak S, *et al.* Use of chemotherapy plus a monoclonal antibody against HER2 for metastatic breast cancer that overexpresses HER2. N Engl J Med 2001; 344(11): 783-92.
[PMID: 11248153]

[245] Vogel CL, Cobleigh MA, Tripathy D, *et al.* Efficacy and safety of trastuzumab as a single agent in first-line treatment of HER2-overexpressing metastatic breast cancer. J Clin Oncol 2002; 20(3): 719-26.
[PMID: 11821453]

[246] Wolff AC, Hammond ME, Schwartz JN, *et al.* American Society of Clinical Oncology; College of American Pathologists. American Society of Clinical Oncology/College of American Pathologists guideline recommendations for human epidermal growth factor receptor 2 testing in breast cancer. J Clin Oncol 2007; 25(1): 118-45.
[PMID: 17159189]

[247] Paik S, Kim C, Wolmark N. HER2 status and benefit from adjuvant trastuzumab in breast cancer. N Engl J Med 2008; 358(13): 1409-11.
[PMID: 18367751]

[248] Noberasco C, De Pas T, Curigliano G, *et al.* Immunohistochemical detection of HER1/HER2 can be considered a predictive marker of gefitinib activity in non-small-cell lung cancer? J Clin Oncol 2005; 23(4): 921-2.
[PMID: 15681541]

[249] Cappuzzo F, Gregorc V, Rossi E, *et al.* Gefitinib in pretreated non-small-cell lung cancer (NSCLC): analysis of efficacy and correlation with HER2 and epidermal growth factor receptor expression in locally advanced or metastatic NSCLC. J Clin Oncol 2003; 21(14): 2658-63.
[PMID: 12860941]

[250] Parra HS, Cavina R, Latteri F, *et al.* Analysis of epidermal growth factor receptor expression as a predictive factor for response to gefitinib ('Iressa', ZD1839) in non-small-cell lung cancer. Br J Cancer 2004; 91(2): 208-12.
[PMID: 15187994]

[251] Hirsch FR, Varella-Garcia M, Bunn PA Jr, *et al.* Molecular predictors of outcome with gefitinib in a phase III placebo-controlled study in advanced non-small-cell lung cancer. J Clin Oncol 2006; 24(31): 5034-42.
[PMID: 17075123]

[252] Dziadziuszko R, Witta SE, Cappuzzo F, *et al.* Epidermal growth factor receptor messenger RNA expression, gene dosage, and gefitinib sensitivity in non-small cell lung cancer. Clin Cancer Res 2006; 12(10): 3078-84.
[PMID: 16707605]

[253] Cappuzzo F, Hirsch FR, Rossi E, *et al.* Epidermal growth factor receptor gene and protein and gefitinib sensitivity in non-small-cell lung cancer. J Natl Cancer Inst 2005; 97(9): 643-55.

[PMID: 15870435]

[254] Hirsch FR, Dziadziuszko R, Thatcher N, *et al.* Epidermal growth factor receptor immunohistochemistry: comparison of antibodies and cutoff points to predict benefit from gefitinib in a phase 3 placebo-controlled study in advanced nonsmall-cell lung cancer. Cancer 2008; 112(5): 1114-21.
[PMID: 18219661]

[255] Mascaux C, Wynes MW, Kato Y, *et al.* EGFR protein expression in non-small cell lung cancer predicts response to an EGFR tyrosine kinase inhibitor--a novel antibody for immunohistochemistry or AQUA technology. Clin Cancer Res 2011; 17(24): 7796-807.
[PMID: 21994417]

[256] Wakeling AE, Guy SP, Woodburn JR, *et al.* ZD1839 (Iressa): an orally active inhibitor of epidermal growth factor signaling with potential for cancer therapy. Cancer Res 2002; 62(20): 5749-54.
[PMID: 12384534]

[257] Pirker R, Pereira JR, von Pawel J, *et al.* EGFR expression as a predictor of survival for first-line chemotherapy plus cetuximab in patients with advanced non-small-cell lung cancer: analysis of data from the phase 3 FLEX study. Lancet Oncol 2012; 13(1): 33-42.
[PMID: 22056021]

[258] Pirker R, Pereira JR, Szczesna A, *et al.* FLEX Study Team. Cetuximab plus chemotherapy in patients with advanced non-small-cell lung cancer (FLEX): an open-label randomised phase III trial. Lancet 2009; 373(9674): 1525-31.
[PMID: 19410716]

[259] Khambata-Ford S, Harbison CT, Hart LL, *et al.* Analysis of potential predictive markers of cetuximab benefit in BMS099, a phase III study of cetuximab and first-line taxane/carboplatin in advanced non-small-cell lung cancer. J Clin Oncol 2010; 28(6): 918-27.
[PMID: 20100958]

[260] Herbst RS, Prager D, Hermann R, *et al.* TRIBUTE Investigator Group. TRIBUTE: a phase III trial of erlotinib hydrochloride (OSI-774) combined with carboplatin and paclitaxel chemotherapy in advanced non-small-cell lung cancer. J Clin Oncol 2005; 23(25): 5892-9.
[PMID: 16043829]

[261] Gatzemeier U, Pluzanska A, Szczesna A, *et al.* Phase III study of erlotinib in combination with cisplatin and gemcitabine in advanced non-small-cell lung cancer: the Tarceva Lung Cancer Investigation Trial. J Clin Oncol 2007; 25(12): 1545-52.
[PMID: 17442998]

[262] Miller VA, Riely GJ, Zakowski MF, *et al.* Molecular characteristics of bronchioloalveolar carcinoma and adenocarcinoma, bronchioloalveolar carcinoma subtype, predict response to erlotinib. J Clin Oncol 2008; 26(9): 1472-8.
[PMID: 18349398]

[263] Lenz HJ, Van Cutsem E, Khambata-Ford S, *et al.* Multicenter phase II and translational study of cetuximab in metastatic colorectal carcinoma refractory to irinotecan, oxaliplatin, and fluoropyrimidines. J Clin Oncol 2006; 24(30): 4914-21.
[PMID: 17050875]

[264]   Vallböhmer D, Zhang W, Gordon M, *et al*. Molecular determinants of cetuximab efficacy. J Clin Oncol 2005; 23(15): 3536-44.
[PMID: 15908664]

[265]   Chung KY, Shia J, Kemeny NE, *et al*. Cetuximab shows activity in colorectal cancer patients with tumors that do not express the epidermal growth factor receptor by immunohistochemistry. J Clin Oncol 2005; 23(9): 1803-10.
[PMID: 15677699]

[266]   Hebbar M, Wacrenier A, Desauw C, *et al*. Lack of usefulness of epidermal growth factor receptor expression determination for cetuximab therapy in patients with colorectal cancer. Anticancer Drugs 2006; 17(7): 855-7.
[PMID: 16926635]

[267]   Fujita M, Ishida M, Tezuka N, Fujino S, Asai T, Okabe H. HER1-4 expression status correlates with the efficacy of gefitinib treatment and tumor cell proliferative activity in non-small cell lung cancer. Mol Med Rep 2008; 1(2): 225-30.
[PMID: 21479401]

[268]   Licitra L, Störkel S, Kerr KM, *et al*. Predictive value of epidermal growth factor receptor expression for first-line chemotherapy plus cetuximab in patients with head and neck and colorectal cancer: analysis of data from the EXTREME and CRYSTAL studies. Eur J Cancer 2013; 49(6): 1161-8.
[PMID: 23265711]

[269]   Neyns B, Sadones J, Joosens E, *et al*. Stratified phase II trial of cetuximab in patients with recurrent high-grade glioma. Ann Oncol 2009; 20(9): 1596-603.
[PMID: 19491283]

[270]   Taguchi T, Tsukuda M, Imagawa-Ishiguro Y, Kato Y, Sano D. Involvement of EGFR in the response of squamous cell carcinoma of the head and neck cell lines to gefitinib. Oncol Rep 2008; 19(1): 65-71.
[PMID: 18097577]

[271]   Hartmann S, Seher A, Brands RC, *et al*. Influence of epidermal growth factor receptor expression on the cetuximab and panitumumab response rates of head and neck carcinoma cells. J Craniomaxillofac Surg 2014; 42(7): 1322-8.
[PMID: 24780353]

[272]   Psyrri A, Lee JW, Pectasides E, *et al*. Prognostic biomarkers in phase II trial of cetuximab-containing induction and chemoradiation in resectable HNSCC: Eastern cooperative oncology group E2303. Clin Cancer Res 2014; 20(11): 3023-32.
[PMID: 24700741]

[273]   Wheeler S, Siwak DR, Chai R, *et al*. Tumor epidermal growth factor receptor and EGFR PY1068 are independent prognostic indicators for head and neck squamous cell carcinoma. Clin Cancer Res 2012; 18(8): 2278-89.
[PMID: 22351687]

[274]   Moehler M, Mueller A, Trarbach T, *et al*. German Arbeitsgemeinschaft Internistische Onkologie. Cetuximab with irinotecan, folinic acid and 5-fluorouracil as first-line treatment in advanced gastroesophageal cancer: a prospective multi-center biomarker-oriented phase II study. Ann Oncol 2011; 22(6): 1358-66.

[PMID: 21119032]

[275] Moroni M, Veronese S, Benvenuti S, *et al.* Gene copy number for epidermal growth factor receptor (EGFR) and clinical response to antiEGFR treatment in colorectal cancer: a cohort study. Lancet Oncol 2005; 6(5): 279-86.
[PMID: 15863375]

[276] Sartore-Bianchi A, Moroni M, Veronese S, *et al.* Epidermal growth factor receptor gene copy number and clinical outcome of metastatic colorectal cancer treated with panitumumab. J Clin Oncol 2007; 25(22): 3238-45.
[PMID: 17664472]

[277] Lièvre A, Bachet JB, Le Corre D, *et al.* KRAS mutation status is predictive of response to cetuximab therapy in colorectal cancer. Cancer Res 2006; 66(8): 3992-5.
[PMID: 16618717]

[278] Hirsch FR, Herbst RS, Olsen C, *et al.* Increased EGFR gene copy number detected by fluorescent *in situ* hybridization predicts outcome in non-small-cell lung cancer patients treated with cetuximab and chemotherapy. J Clin Oncol 2008; 26(20): 3351-7.
[PMID: 18612151]

[279] Luber B, Deplazes J, Keller G, *et al.* Biomarker analysis of cetuximab plus oxaliplatin/leucovorin/5-fluorouracil in first-line metastatic gastric and oesophago-gastric junction cancer: results from a phase II trial of the Arbeitsgemeinschaft Internistische Onkologie (AIO). BMC Cancer 2011; 11: 509.
[PMID: 22152101]

[280] Goss G, Ferry D, Wierzbicki R, *et al.* Randomized phase II study of gefitinib compared with placebo in chemotherapy-naive patients with advanced non-small-cell lung cancer and poor performance status. J Clin Oncol 2009; 27(13): 2253-60.
[PMID: 19289623]

[281] Hirsch FR, Varella-Garcia M, McCoy J, *et al.* Southwest Oncology Group. Increased epidermal growth factor receptor gene copy number detected by fluorescence *in situ* hybridization associates with increased sensitivity to gefitinib in patients with bronchioloalveolar carcinoma subtypes: a Southwest Oncology Group Study. J Clin Oncol 2005; 23(28): 6838-45.
[PMID: 15998906]

[282] Hirsch FR, Varella-Garcia M, Cappuzzo F, *et al.* Combination of EGFR gene copy number and protein expression predicts outcome for advanced non-small-cell lung cancer patients treated with gefitinib. Ann Oncol 2007; 18(4): 752-60.
[PMID: 17317677]

[283] Zhu CQ, da Cunha Santos G, Ding K, *et al.* National Cancer Institute of Canada Clinical Trials Group Study BR.21. Role of KRAS and EGFR as biomarkers of response to erlotinib in National Cancer Institute of Canada Clinical Trials Group Study BR.21. J Clin Oncol 2008; 26(26): 4268-75.
[PMID: 18626007]

[284] Lee Y, Shim HS, Park MS, *et al.* High EGFR gene copy number and skin rash as predictive markers for EGFR tyrosine kinase inhibitors in patients with advanced squamous cell lung carcinoma. Clin Cancer Res 2012; 18(6): 1760-8.
[PMID: 22271877]

[285] Dahabreh IJ, Linardou H, Kosmidis P, Bafaloukos D, Murray S. EGFR gene copy number as a predictive biomarker for patients receiving tyrosine kinase inhibitor treatment: a systematic review and meta-analysis in non-small-cell lung cancer. Ann Oncol 2011; 22(3): 545-52.
[PMID: 20826716]

[286] Yang ZY, Shen WX, Hu XF, *et al.* EGFR gene copy number as a predictive biomarker for the treatment of metastatic colorectal cancer with anti-EGFR monoclonal antibodies: a meta-analysis. J Hematol Oncol 2012; 5: 52.
[PMID: 22897982]

[287] Licitra L, Mesia R, Rivera F, *et al.* Evaluation of EGFR gene copy number as a predictive biomarker for the efficacy of cetuximab in combination with chemotherapy in the first-line treatment of recurrent and/or metastatic squamous cell carcinoma of the head and neck: EXTREME study. Ann Oncol 2011; 22(5): 1078-87.
[PMID: 21048039]

[288] Argiris A, Heron DE, Smith RP, *et al.* Induction docetaxel, cisplatin, and cetuximab followed by concurrent radiotherapy, cisplatin, and cetuximab and maintenance cetuximab in patients with locally advanced head and neck cancer. J Clin Oncol 2010; 28(36): 5294-300.
[PMID: 21079141]

[289] Kim ES, Hirsh V, Mok T, *et al.* Gefitinib *versus* docetaxel in previously treated non-small-cell lung cancer (INTEREST): a randomised phase III trial. Lancet 2008; 372(9652): 1809-18.
[PMID: 19027483]

[290] Bell DW, Lynch TJ, Haserlat SM, *et al.* Epidermal growth factor receptor mutations and gene amplification in non-small-cell lung cancer: molecular analysis of the IDEAL/INTACT gefitinib trials. J Clin Oncol 2005; 23(31): 8081-92.
[PMID: 16204011]

[291] Sone T, Kasahara K, Kimura H, *et al.* Comparative analysis of epidermal growth factor receptor mutations and gene amplification as predictors of gefitinib efficacy in Japanese patients with nonsmall cell lung cancer. Cancer 2007; 109(9): 1836-44.
[PMID: 17387741]

[292] Ichihara S, Toyooka S, Fujiwara Y, *et al.* The impact of epidermal growth factor receptor gene status on gefitinib-treated Japanese patients with non-small-cell lung cancer. Int J Cancer 2007; 120(6): 1239-47.
[PMID: 17192902]

[293] da Cunha Santos G, Dhani N, Tu D, *et al.* Molecular predictors of outcome in a phase 3 study of gemcitabine and erlotinib therapy in patients with advanced pancreatic cancer: National Cancer Institute of Canada Clinical Trials Group Study PA.3. Cancer 2010; 116(24): 5599-607.
[PMID: 20824720]

[294] Gajiwala KS, Feng J, Ferre R, *et al.* Insights into the aberrant activity of mutant EGFR kinase domain and drug recognition. Structure 2013; 21(2): 209-19.
[PMID: 23273428]

[295] Park JH, Liu Y, Lemmon MA, Radhakrishnan R. Erlotinib binds both inactive and active conformations of the EGFR tyrosine kinase domain. Biochem J 2012; 448(3): 417-23.

[PMID: 23101586]

[296] Wang Z, Longo PA, Tarrant MK, *et al.* Mechanistic insights into the activation of oncogenic forms of EGF receptor. Nat Struct Mol Biol 2011; 18(12): 1388-93.
[PMID: 22101934]

[297] Yoshikawa S, Kukimoto-Niino M, Parker L, *et al.* Structural basis for the altered drug sensitivities of non-small cell lung cancer-associated mutants of human epidermal growth factor receptor. Oncogene 2013; 32(1): 27-38.
[PMID: 22349823]

[298] Yun CH, Boggon TJ, Li Y, *et al.* Structures of lung cancer-derived EGFR mutants and inhibitor complexes: mechanism of activation and insights into differential inhibitor sensitivity. Cancer Cell 2007; 11(3): 217-27.
[PMID: 17349580]

[299] Juchum M, Günther M, Laufer SA. Fighting cancer drug resistance: Opportunities and challenges for mutation-specific EGFR inhibitors. Drug Resist Updat 2015; 20: 12-28.
[PMID: 26021435]

[300] Shigematsu H, Lin L, Takahashi T, *et al.* Clinical and biological features associated with epidermal growth factor receptor gene mutations in lung cancers. J Natl Cancer Inst 2005; 97(5): 339-46.
[PMID: 15741570]

[301] Cho J, Chen L, Sangji N, *et al.* Cetuximab response of lung cancer-derived EGF receptor mutants is associated with asymmetric dimerization. Cancer Res 2013; 73(22): 6770-9.
[PMID: 24063894]

[302] Doody JF, Wang Y, Patel SN, *et al.* Inhibitory activity of cetuximab on epidermal growth factor receptor mutations in non small cell lung cancers. Mol Cancer Ther 2007; 6(10): 2642-51.
[PMID: 17913857]

[303] Steiner P, Joynes C, Bassi R, *et al.* Tumor growth inhibition with cetuximab and chemotherapy in non-small cell lung cancer xenografts expressing wild-type and mutated epidermal growth factor receptor. Clin Cancer Res 2007; 13(5): 1540-51.
[PMID: 17332300]

[304] Perez-Torres M, Guix M, Gonzalez A, Arteaga CL. Epidermal growth factor receptor (EGFR) antibody down-regulates mutant receptors and inhibits tumors expressing EGFR mutations. J Biol Chem 2006; 281(52): 40183-92.
[PMID: 17082181]

[305] Douillard JY, Pirker R, O'Byrne KJ, *et al.* Relationship between EGFR expression, EGFR mutation status, and the efficacy of chemotherapy plus cetuximab in FLEX study patients with advanced non-small-cell lung cancer. J Thorac Oncol 2014; 9(5): 717-24.
[PMID: 24662454]

[306] Freeman DJ, Bush T, Ogbagabriel S, *et al.* Activity of panitumumab alone or with chemotherapy in non-small cell lung carcinoma cell lines expressing mutant epidermal growth factor receptor. Mol Cancer Ther 2009; 8(6): 1536-46.
[PMID: 19509246]

[307] Eichler AF, Kahle KT, Wang DL, *et al.* EGFR mutation status and survival after diagnosis of brain metastasis in nonsmall cell lung cancer. Neuro-oncol 2010; 12(11): 1193-9.
[PMID: 20627894]

[308] Gow CH, Chang YL, Hsu YC, *et al.* Comparison of epidermal growth factor receptor mutations between primary and corresponding metastatic tumors in tyrosine kinase inhibitor-naive non-small-cell lung cancer. Ann Oncol 2009; 20(4): 696-702.
[PMID: 19088172]

[309] Matsumoto S, Takahashi K, Iwakawa R, *et al.* Frequent EGFR mutations in brain metastases of lung adenocarcinoma. Int J Cancer 2006; 119(6): 1491-4.
[PMID: 16642476]

[310] Welsh JW, Komaki R, Amini A, *et al.* Phase II trial of erlotinib plus concurrent whole-brain radiation therapy for patients with brain metastases from non-small-cell lung cancer. J Clin Oncol 2013; 31(7): 895-902.
[PMID: 23341526]

[311] Daniele L, Cassoni P, Bacillo E, *et al.* Epidermal growth factor receptor gene in primary tumor and metastatic sites from non-small cell lung cancer. J Thorac Oncol 2009; 4(6): 684-8.
[PMID: 19404216]

[312] Sun M, Behrens C, Feng L, *et al.* HER family receptor abnormalities in lung cancer brain metastases and corresponding primary tumors. Clin Cancer Res 2009; 15(15): 4829-37.
[PMID: 19622585]

[313] Fan Y, Xu X, Xie C. EGFR-TKI therapy for patients with brain metastases from non-small-cell lung cancer: a pooled analysis of published data. Onco Targets Ther 2014; 7: 2075-84.
[PMID: 25419145]

[314] Kim JE, Lee DH, Choi Y, *et al.* Epidermal growth factor receptor tyrosine kinase inhibitors as a first-line therapy for never-smokers with adenocarcinoma of the lung having asymptomatic synchronous brain metastasis. Lung Cancer 2009; 65(3): 351-4.
[PMID: 19157632]

[315] Porta R, Sánchez-Torres JM, Paz-Ares L, *et al.* Brain metastases from lung cancer responding to erlotinib: the importance of EGFR mutation. Eur Respir J 2011; 37(3): 624-31.
[PMID: 20595147]

[316] Shimato S, Mitsudomi T, Kosaka T, *et al.* EGFR mutations in patients with brain metastases from lung cancer: association with the efficacy of gefitinib. Neuro-oncol 2006; 8(2): 137-44.
[PMID: 16510849]

[317] Rich JN, Reardon DA, Peery T, *et al.* Phase II trial of gefitinib in recurrent glioblastoma. J Clin Oncol 2004; 22(1): 133-42.
[PMID: 14638850]

[318] Barber TD, Vogelstein B, Kinzler KW, Velculescu VE. Somatic mutations of EGFR in colorectal cancers and glioblastomas. N Engl J Med 2004; 351(27): 2883.
[PMID: 15625347]

[319] Bhargava R, Gerald WL, Li AR, *et al.* EGFR gene amplification in breast cancer: correlation with

epidermal growth factor receptor mRNA and protein expression and HER-2 status and absence of EGFR-activating mutations. Mod Pathol 2005; 18(8): 1027-33.
[PMID: 15920544]

[320]   Stransky N, Egloff AM, Tward AD, *et al.* The mutational landscape of head and neck squamous cell carcinoma. Science 2011; 333(6046): 1157-60.
[PMID: 21798893]

[321]   Cohen EE, Lingen MW, Martin LE, *et al.* Response of some head and neck cancers to epidermal growth factor receptor tyrosine kinase inhibitors may be linked to mutation of ERBB2 rather than EGFR. Clin Cancer Res 2005; 11(22): 8105-8.
[PMID: 16299242]

[322]   Lee JW, Soung YH, Kim SY, *et al.* Somatic mutations of EGFR gene in squamous cell carcinoma of the head and neck. Clin Cancer Res 2005; 11(8): 2879-82.
[PMID: 15837736]

[323]   Nagahara H, Mimori K, Ohta M, *et al.* Somatic mutations of epidermal growth factor receptor in colorectal carcinoma. Clin Cancer Res 2005; 11(4): 1368-71.
[PMID: 15746034]

[324]   Wang Y, Jiang CQ, Guan J, *et al.* Molecular alterations of EGFR in small intestinal adenocarcinoma. Int J Colorectal Dis 2013; 28(10): 1329-35.
[PMID: 23644682]

[325]   Peraldo-Neia C, Migliardi G, Mello-Grand M, *et al.* Epidermal Growth Factor Receptor (EGFR) mutation analysis, gene expression profiling and EGFR protein expression in primary prostate cancer. BMC Cancer 2011; 11: 31.
[PMID: 21266046]

[326]   Fu M, Zhang W, Shan L, *et al.* Mutation status of somatic EGFR and KRAS genes in Chinese patients with prostate cancer (PCa). Virchows Arch 2014; 464(5): 575-81.
[PMID: 24595526]

[327]   Sudo T, Mimori K, Nagahara H, *et al.* Identification of EGFR mutations in esophageal cancer. Eur J Surg Oncol 2007; 33(1): 44-8.
[PMID: 17142003]

[328]   Zhang X, Nagahara H, Mimori K, *et al.* Mutations of epidermal growth factor receptor in colon cancer indicate susceptibility or resistance to gefitinib. Oncol Rep 2008; 19(6): 1541-4.
[PMID: 18497962]

[329]   Wheler JJ, Falchook GS, Tsimberidou AM, *et al.* Aberrations in the epidermal growth factor receptor gene in 958 patients with diverse advanced tumors: implications for therapy. Ann Oncol 2013; 24(3): 838-42.
[PMID: 23139256]

[330]   Cho J, Bass AJ, Lawrence MS, *et al.* Colon cancer-derived oncogenic EGFR G724S mutant identified by whole genome sequence analysis is dependent on asymmetric dimerization and sensitive to cetuximab. Mol Cancer 2014; 13: 141.
[PMID: 24894453]

[331] Ogino S, Meyerhardt JA, Cantor M, *et al.* Molecular alterations in tumors and response to combination chemotherapy with gefitinib for advanced colorectal cancer. Clin Cancer Res 2005; 11(18): 6650-6.
[PMID: 16166444]

[332] Sharma SV, Bell DW, Settleman J, Haber DA. Epidermal growth factor receptor mutations in lung cancer. Nat Rev Cancer 2007; 7(3): 169-81.
[PMID: 17318210]

[333] Sakurada A, Shepherd FA, Tsao MS. Epidermal growth factor receptor tyrosine kinase inhibitors in lung cancer: impact of primary or secondary mutations. Clin Lung Cancer 2006; 7 (Suppl. 4): S138-44.
[PMID: 16764754]

[334] Inoue A, Suzuki T, Fukuhara T, *et al.* Prospective phase II study of gefitinib for chemotherapy-naive patients with advanced non-small-cell lung cancer with epidermal growth factor receptor gene mutations. J Clin Oncol 2006; 24(21): 3340-6.
[PMID: 16785471]

[335] Asahina H, Yamazaki K, Kinoshita I, *et al.* A phase II trial of gefitinib as first-line therapy for advanced non-small cell lung cancer with epidermal growth factor receptor mutations. Br J Cancer 2006; 95(8): 998-1004.
[PMID: 17047648]

[336] Sutani A, Nagai Y, Udagawa K, *et al.* Gefitinib for non-small-cell lung cancer patients with epidermal growth factor receptor gene mutations screened by peptide nucleic acid-locked nucleic acid PCR clamp. Br J Cancer 2006; 95(11): 1483-9.
[PMID: 17106442]

[337] Asami K, Koizumi T, Hirai K, *et al.* Gefitinib as first-line treatment in elderly epidermal growth factor receptor-mutated patients with advanced lung adenocarcinoma: results of a Nagano Lung Cancer Research Group study. Clin Lung Cancer 2011; 12(6): 387-92.
[PMID: 21729650]

[338] Douillard JY, Ostoros G, Cobo M, *et al.* First-line gefitinib in Caucasian EGFR mutation-positive NSCLC patients: a phase-IV, open-label, single-arm study. Br J Cancer 2014; 110(1): 55-62.
[PMID: 24263064]

[339] Fujita S, Katakami N, Masago K, *et al.* Customized chemotherapy based on epidermal growth factor receptor mutation status for elderly patients with advanced non-small-cell lung cancer: a phase II trial. BMC Cancer 2012; 12: 185.
[PMID: 22613958]

[340] Inoue A, Kobayashi K, Usui K, *et al.* North East Japan Gefitinib Study Group. First-line gefitinib for patients with advanced non-small-cell lung cancer harboring epidermal growth factor receptor mutations without indication for chemotherapy. J Clin Oncol 2009; 27(9): 1394-400.
[PMID: 19224850]

[341] Maemondo M, Minegishi Y, Inoue A, *et al.* First-line gefitinib in patients aged 75 or older with advanced non-small cell lung cancer harboring epidermal growth factor receptor mutations: NEJ 003 study. J Thorac Oncol 2012; 7(9): 1417-22.
[PMID: 22895139]

[342] Morita S, Okamoto I, Kobayashi K, *et al.* Combined survival analysis of prospective clinical trials of gefitinib for non-small cell lung cancer with EGFR mutations. Clin Cancer Res 2009; 15(13): 4493-8. [PMID: 19531624]

[343] Sequist LV, Martins RG, Spigel D, *et al.* First-line gefitinib in patients with advanced non-small-cell lung cancer harboring somatic EGFR mutations. J Clin Oncol 2008; 26(15): 2442-9. [PMID: 18458038]

[344] Sugio K, Uramoto H, Onitsuka T, *et al.* Prospective phase II study of gefitinib in non-small cell lung cancer with epidermal growth factor receptor gene mutations. Lung Cancer 2009; 64(3): 314-8. [PMID: 18992959]

[345] Sunaga N, Tomizawa Y, Yanagitani N, *et al.* Phase II prospective study of the efficacy of gefitinib for the treatment of stage III/IV non-small cell lung cancer with EGFR mutations, irrespective of previous chemotherapy. Lung Cancer 2007; 56(3): 383-9. [PMID: 17368623]

[346] Takahashi K, Saito H, Hasegawa Y, *et al.* First-line gefitinib therapy for elderly patients with non-small cell lung cancer harboring EGFR mutation: Central Japan Lung Study Group 0901. Cancer Chemother Pharmacol 2014; 74(4): 721-7. [PMID: 25087097]

[347] Tamura K, Okamoto I, Kashii T, *et al.* West Japan Thoracic Oncology Group. Multicentre prospective phase II trial of gefitinib for advanced non-small cell lung cancer with epidermal growth factor receptor mutations: results of the West Japan Thoracic Oncology Group trial (WJTOG0403). Br J Cancer 2008; 98(5): 907-14. [PMID: 18283321]

[348] Rosell R, Moran T, Queralt C, *et al.* Spanish Lung Cancer Group. Screening for epidermal growth factor receptor mutations in lung cancer. N Engl J Med 2009; 361(10): 958-67. [PMID: 19692684]

[349] Park SJ, Kim HT, Lee DH, *et al.* Efficacy of epidermal growth factor receptor tyrosine kinase inhibitors for brain metastasis in non-small cell lung cancer patients harboring either exon 19 or 21 mutation. Lung Cancer 2012; 77(3): 556-60. [PMID: 22677429]

[350] Mok TS, Wu YL, Thongprasert S, *et al.* Gefitinib or carboplatin-paclitaxel in pulmonary adenocarcinoma. N Engl J Med 2009; 361(10): 947-57. [PMID: 19692680]

[351] Mitsudomi T, Kosaka T, Endoh H, *et al.* Mutations of the epidermal growth factor receptor gene predict prolonged survival after gefitinib treatment in patients with non-small-cell lung cancer with postoperative recurrence. J Clin Oncol 2005; 23(11): 2513-20. [PMID: 15738541]

[352] Chou TY, Chiu CH, Li LH, *et al.* Mutation in the tyrosine kinase domain of epidermal growth factor receptor is a predictive and prognostic factor for gefitinib treatment in patients with non-small cell lung cancer. Clin Cancer Res 2005; 11(10): 3750-7. [PMID: 15897572]

[353]   Locatelli-Sanchez M, Couraud S, Arpin D, Riou R, Bringuier PP, Souquet PJ. Routine EGFR molecular analysis in non-small-cell lung cancer patients is feasible: exons 18-21 sequencing results of 753 patients and subsequent clinical outcomes. Lung 2013; 191(5): 491-9.
[PMID: 23749122]

[354]   Wu SG, Chang YL, Hsu YC, *et al.* Good response to gefitinib in lung adenocarcinoma of complex epidermal growth factor receptor (EGFR) mutations with the classical mutation pattern. Oncologist 2008; 13(12): 1276-84.
[PMID: 19060236]

[355]   Yang CH, Yu CJ, Shih JY, *et al.* Specific EGFR mutations predict treatment outcome of stage IIIB/IV patients with chemotherapy-naive non-small-cell lung cancer receiving first-line gefitinib monotherapy. J Clin Oncol 2008; 26(16): 2745-53.
[PMID: 18509184]

[356]   Lee VH, Tin VP, Choy TS, *et al.* Association of exon 19 and 21 EGFR mutation patterns with treatment outcome after first-line tyrosine kinase inhibitor in metastatic non-small-cell lung cancer. J Thorac Oncol 2013; 8(9): 1148-55.
[PMID: 23945384]

[357]   Massarelli E, Johnson FM, Erickson HS, Wistuba II, Papadimitrakopoulou V. Uncommon epidermal growth factor receptor mutations in non-small cell lung cancer and their mechanisms of EGFR tyrosine kinase inhibitors sensitivity and resistance. Lung Cancer 2013; 80(3): 235-41.
[PMID: 23485129]

[358]   Wu JY, Yu CJ, Chang YC, Yang CH, Shih JY, Yang PC. Effectiveness of tyrosine kinase inhibitors on "uncommon" epidermal growth factor receptor mutations of unknown clinical significance in non-small cell lung cancer. Clin Cancer Res 2011; 17(11): 3812-21.
[PMID: 21531810]

[359]   Wu JY, Yu CJ, Yang CH, *et al.* First- or second-line therapy with gefitinib produces equal survival in non-small cell lung cancer. Am J Respir Crit Care Med 2008; 178(8): 847-53.
[PMID: 18583573]

[360]   Mitsudomi T, Yatabe Y. Mutations of the epidermal growth factor receptor gene and related genes as determinants of epidermal growth factor receptor tyrosine kinase inhibitors sensitivity in lung cancer. Cancer Sci 2007; 98(12): 1817-24.
[PMID: 17888036]

[361]   Shih JY, Gow CH, Yu CJ, *et al.* Epidermal growth factor receptor mutations in needle biopsy/aspiration samples predict response to gefitinib therapy and survival of patients with advanced nonsmall cell lung cancer. Int J Cancer 2006; 118(4): 963-9.
[PMID: 16152581]

[362]   Xing K, Zhou X, Zhao X, *et al.* A novel point mutation in exon 20 of EGFR showed sensitivity to erlotinib. Med Oncol 2014; 31(7): 36.
[PMID: 24908064]

[363]   Asahina H, Yamazaki K, Kinoshita I, Yokouchi H, Dosaka-Akita H, Nishimura M. Non-responsiveness to gefitinib in a patient with lung adenocarcinoma having rare EGFR mutations S768I and V769L. Lung Cancer 2006; 54(3): 419-22.

[PMID: 17045698]

[364] Murray S, Dahabreh IJ, Linardou H, Manoloukos M, Bafaloukos D, Kosmidis P. Somatic mutations of the tyrosine kinase domain of epidermal growth factor receptor and tyrosine kinase inhibitor response to TKIs in non-small cell lung cancer: an analytical database. J Thorac Oncol 2008; 3(8): 832-9.
[PMID: 18670300]

[365] He M, Capelletti M, Nafa K, *et al.* EGFR exon 19 insertions: a new family of sensitizing EGFR mutations in lung adenocarcinoma. Clin Cancer Res 2012; 18(6): 1790-7.
[PMID: 22190593]

[366] Hellmann MD, Reva B, Yu H, *et al.* Clinical and *in vivo* evidence that EGFR S768I mutant lung adenocarcinomas are sensitive to erlotinib. J Thorac Oncol 2014; 9(10): e73-4.
[PMID: 25521405]

[367] Lund-Iversen M, Kleinberg L, Fjellbirkeland L, Helland Å, Brustugun OT. Clinicopathological characteristics of 11 NSCLC patients with EGFR-exon 20 mutations. J Thorac Oncol 2012; 7(9): 1471-3.
[PMID: 22895145]

[368] Naidoo J, Sima CS, Rodriguez K, *et al.* Epidermal growth factor receptor exon 20 insertions in advanced lung adenocarcinomas: Clinical outcomes and response to erlotinib. Cancer 2015; 121(18): 3212-20.
[PMID: 26096453]

[369] Yasuda H, Park E, Yun CH, *et al.* Structural, biochemical, and clinical characterization of epidermal growth factor receptor (EGFR) exon 20 insertion mutations in lung cancer. Sci Transl Med 2013; 5(216): 216ra177.
[PMID: 24353160]

[370] Greulich H, Chen TH, Feng W, *et al.* Oncogenic transformation by inhibitor-sensitive and -resistant EGFR mutants. PLoS Med 2005; 2(11): e313.
[PMID: 16187797]

[371] Arcila ME, Nafa K, Chaft JE, *et al.* EGFR exon 20 insertion mutations in lung adenocarcinomas: prevalence, molecular heterogeneity, and clinicopathologic characteristics. Mol Cancer Ther 2013; 12(2): 220-9.
[PMID: 23371856]

[372] Gazdar AF, Minna JD. Deregulated EGFR signaling during lung cancer progression: mutations, amplicons, and autocrine loops. Cancer Prev Res (Phila) 2008; 1(3): 156-60.
[PMID: 19138950]

[373] Bahassi M, Li YQ, Wise-Draper TM, *et al.* A patient-derived somatic mutation in the epidermal growth factor receptor ligand-binding domain confers increased sensitivity to cetuximab in head and neck cancer. Eur J Cancer 2013; 49(10): 2345-55.
[PMID: 23578570]

[374] Hsieh YY, Tzeng CH, Chen MH, Chen PM, Wang WS. Epidermal growth factor receptor R521K polymorphism shows favorable outcomes in KRAS wild-type colorectal cancer patients treated with cetuximab-based chemotherapy. Cancer Sci 2012; 103(4): 791-6.
[PMID: 22321154]

[375] Arcila ME, Oxnard GR, Nafa K, *et al.* Rebiopsy of lung cancer patients with acquired resistance to EGFR inhibitors and enhanced detection of the T790M mutation using a locked nucleic acid-based assay. Clin Cancer Res 2011; 17(5): 1169-80.
[PMID: 21248300]

[376] Vikis H, Sato M, James M, *et al.* EGFR-T790M is a rare lung cancer susceptibility allele with enhanced kinase activity. Cancer Res 2007; 67(10): 4665-70.
[PMID: 17510392]

[377] Kosaka T, Yatabe Y, Endoh H, *et al.* Analysis of epidermal growth factor receptor gene mutation in patients with non-small cell lung cancer and acquired resistance to gefitinib. Clin Cancer Res 2006; 12(19): 5764-9.
[PMID: 17020982]

[378] Rosell R, Molina MA, Costa C, *et al.* Pretreatment EGFR T790M mutation and BRCA1 mRNA expression in erlotinib-treated advanced non-small-cell lung cancer patients with EGFR mutations. Clin Cancer Res 2011; 17(5): 1160-8.
[PMID: 21233402]

[379] Maheswaran S, Sequist LV, Nagrath S, *et al.* Detection of mutations in EGFR in circulating lung-cancer cells. N Engl J Med 2008; 359(4): 366-77.
[PMID: 18596266]

[380] Mack PC, Holland WS, Burich RA, *et al.* EGFR mutations detected in plasma are associated with patient outcomes in erlotinib plus docetaxel-treated non-small cell lung cancer. J Thorac Oncol 2009; 4(12): 1466-72.
[PMID: 19884861]

[381] Su KY, Chen HY, Li KC, *et al.* Pretreatment epidermal growth factor receptor (EGFR) T790M mutation predicts shorter EGFR tyrosine kinase inhibitor response duration in patients with non-smal-
-cell lung cancer. J Clin Oncol 2012; 30(4): 433-40.
[PMID: 22215752]

[382] Bell DW, Gore I, Okimoto RA, *et al.* Inherited susceptibility to lung cancer may be associated with the T790M drug resistance mutation in EGFR. Nat Genet 2005; 37(12): 1315-6.
[PMID: 16258541]

[383] Yu HA, Arcila ME, Harlan Fleischut M, *et al.* Germline EGFR T790M mutation found in multiple members of a familial cohort. J Thorac Oncol 2014; 9(4): 554-8.
[PMID: 24736080]

[384] Girard N, Lou E, Azzoli CG, *et al.* Analysis of genetic variants in never-smokers with lung cancer facilitated by an Internet-based blood collection protocol: a preliminary report. Clin Cancer Res 2010; 16(2): 755-63.
[PMID: 20068085]

[385] Sequist LV, Waltman BA, Dias-Santagata D, *et al.* Genotypic and histological evolution of lung cancers acquiring resistance to EGFR inhibitors. Sci Transl Med 2011; 3(75): 75ra26.
[PMID: 21430269]

[386] Yu HA, Arcila ME, Rekhtman N, *et al.* Analysis of tumor specimens at the time of acquired resistance

to EGFR-TKI therapy in 155 patients with EGFR-mutant lung cancers. Clin Cancer Res 2013; 19(8): 2240-7.
[PMID: 23470965]

[387]   Balak MN, Gong Y, Riely GJ, *et al.* Novel D761Y and common secondary T790M mutations in epidermal growth factor receptor-mutant lung adenocarcinomas with acquired resistance to kinase inhibitors. Clin Cancer Res 2006; 12(21): 6494-501.
[PMID: 17085664]

[388]   Yun CH, Mengwasser KE, Toms AV, *et al.* The T790M mutation in EGFR kinase causes drug resistance by increasing the affinity for ATP. Proc Natl Acad Sci USA 2008; 105(6): 2070-5.
[PMID: 18227510]

[389]   Stewart EL, Mascaux C, Pham NA, *et al.* Clinical Utility of Patient-Derived Xenografts to Determine Biomarkers of Prognosis and Map Resistance Pathways in EGFR-Mutant Lung Adenocarcinoma. J Clin Oncol 2015; 33(22): 2472-80.
[PMID: 26124487]

[390]   Erlichman C, Hidalgo M, Boni JP, *et al.* Phase I study of EKB-569, an irreversible inhibitor of the epidermal growth factor receptor, in patients with advanced solid tumors. J Clin Oncol 2006; 24(15): 2252-60.
[PMID: 16710023]

[391]   Yoshimura N, Kudoh S, Kimura T, *et al.* EKB-569, a new irreversible epidermal growth factor receptor tyrosine kinase inhibitor, with clinical activity in patients with non-small cell lung cancer with acquired resistance to gefitinib. Lung Cancer 2006; 51(3): 363-8.
[PMID: 16364494]

[392]   Sequist LV, Besse B, Lynch TJ, *et al.* Neratinib, an irreversible pan-ErbB receptor tyrosine kinase inhibitor: results of a phase II trial in patients with advanced non-small-cell lung cancer. J Clin Oncol 2010; 28(18): 3076-83.
[PMID: 20479403]

[393]   Wong KK, Fracasso PM, Bukowski RM, *et al.* A phase I study with neratinib (HKI-272), an irreversible pan ErbB receptor tyrosine kinase inhibitor, in patients with solid tumors. Clin Cancer Res 2009; 15(7): 2552-8.
[PMID: 19318484]

[394]   Chiappori AA, Ellis PM, Hamm JT, *et al.* A phase I evaluation of oral CI-1033 in combination with paclitaxel and carboplatin as first-line chemotherapy in patients with advanced non-small cell lung cancer. J Thorac Oncol 2006; 1(9): 1010-9.
[PMID: 17409987]

[395]   Jänne PA, von Pawel J, Cohen RB, *et al.* Multicenter, randomized, phase II trial of CI-1033, an irreversible pan-ERBB inhibitor, for previously treated advanced non small-cell lung cancer. J Clin Oncol 2007; 25(25): 3936-44.
[PMID: 17761977]

[396]   Ross HJ, Blumenschein GR Jr, Aisner J, *et al.* Randomized phase II multicenter trial of two schedules of lapatinib as first- or second-line monotherapy in patients with advanced or metastatic non-small cell lung cancer. Clin Cancer Res 2010; 16(6): 1938-49.

[PMID: 20215545]

[397]   Jänne PA, Boss DS, Camidge DR, *et al.* Phase I dose-escalation study of the pan-HER inhibitor, PF299804, in patients with advanced malignant solid tumors. Clin Cancer Res 2011; 17(5): 1131-9.
[PMID: 21220471]

[398]   Ramalingam SS, Blackhall F, Krzakowski M, *et al.* Randomized phase II study of dacomitinib (PF-00299804), an irreversible pan-human epidermal growth factor receptor inhibitor, *versus* erlotinib in patients with advanced non-small-cell lung cancer. J Clin Oncol 2012; 30(27): 3337-44.
[PMID: 22753918]

[399]   Liu D, Zhang L, Wu Y, *et al.* Clinical pharmacokinetics, safety, and preliminary efficacy evaluation of icotinib in patients with advanced non-small cell lung cancer. Lung Cancer 2015; 89(3): 262-7.
[PMID: 26162563]

[400]   Shi Y, Zhang L, Liu X, *et al.* Icotinib *versus* gefitinib in previously treated advanced non-small-cell lung cancer (ICOGEN): a randomised, double-blind phase 3 non-inferiority trial. Lancet Oncol 2013; 14(10): 953-61.
[PMID: 23948351]

[401]   Yap TA, Vidal L, Adam J, *et al.* Phase I trial of the irreversible EGFR and HER2 kinase inhibitor BIBW 2992 in patients with advanced solid tumors. J Clin Oncol 2010; 28(25): 3965-72.
[PMID: 20679611]

[402]   Pircher A, Manzl C, Fiegl M, Popper H, Pirker R, Hilbe W. Overcoming resistance to first generation EGFR TKIs with cetuximab in combination with chemotherapy in an EGFR mutated advanced stage NSCLC patient. Lung Cancer 2014; 83(3): 408-10.
[PMID: 24412619]

[403]   Cross DA, Ashton SE, Ghiorghiu S, *et al.* AZD9291, an irreversible EGFR TKI, overcomes T790M-mediated resistance to EGFR inhibitors in lung cancer. Cancer Discov 2014; 4(9): 1046-61.
[PMID: 24893891]

[404]   Finlay MR, Anderton M, Ashton S, *et al.* Discovery of a potent and selective EGFR inhibitor (AZD9291) of both sensitizing and T790M resistance mutations that spares the wild type form of the receptor. J Med Chem 2014; 57(20): 8249-67.
[PMID: 25271963]

[405]   Walter AO, Sjin RT, Haringsma HJ, *et al.* Discovery of a mutant-selective covalent inhibitor of EGFR that overcomes T790M-mediated resistance in NSCLC. Cancer Discov 2013; 3(12): 1404-15.
[PMID: 24065731]

[406]   Ward RA, Anderton MJ, Ashton S, *et al.* Structure- and reactivity-based development of covalent inhibitors of the activating and gatekeeper mutant forms of the epidermal growth factor receptor (EGFR). J Med Chem 2013; 56(17): 7025-48.
[PMID: 23930994]

[407]   Tartarone A, Lerose R. Clinical approaches to treat patients with non-small cell lung cancer and epidermal growth factor receptor tyrosine kinase inhibitor acquired resistance. Ther Adv Respir Dis 2015; 9(5): 242-50.
[PMID: 26016841]

[408] Jänne PA, Yang JC, Kim DW, *et al.* AZD9291 in EGFR inhibitor-resistant non-small-cell lung cancer. N Engl J Med 2015; 372(18): 1689-99.
[PMID: 25923549]

[409] Kancha RK, Peschel C, Duyster J. The epidermal growth factor receptor-L861Q mutation increases kinase activity without leading to enhanced sensitivity toward epidermal growth factor receptor kinase inhibitors. J Thorac Oncol 2011; 6(2): 387-92.
[PMID: 21252719]

[410] Tam IY, Chung LP, Suen WS, *et al.* Distinct epidermal growth factor receptor and KRAS mutation patterns in non-small cell lung cancer patients with different tobacco exposure and clinicopathologic features. Clin Cancer Res 2006; 12(5): 1647-53.
[PMID: 16533793]

[411] Costa DB, Halmos B, Kumar A, *et al.* BIM mediates EGFR tyrosine kinase inhibitor-induced apoptosis in lung cancers with oncogenic EGFR mutations. PLoS Med 2007; 4(10): 1669-79. discussion 1680
[PMID: 17973572]

[412] Engelman JA, Zejnullahu K, Gale CM, *et al.* PF00299804, an irreversible pan-ERBB inhibitor, is effective in lung cancer models with EGFR and ERBB2 mutations that are resistant to gefitinib. Cancer Res 2007; 67(24): 11924-32.
[PMID: 18089823]

[413] Harada T, Lopez-Chavez A, Xi L, Raffeld M, Wang Y, Giaccone G. Characterization of epidermal growth factor receptor mutations in non-small-cell lung cancer patients of African-American ancestry. Oncogene 2011; 30(15): 1744-52.
[PMID: 21132006]

[414] Yasuda H, Kobayashi S, Costa DB. EGFR exon 20 insertion mutations in non-small-cell lung cancer: preclinical data and clinical implications. Lancet Oncol 2012; 13(1): e23-31.
[PMID: 21764376]

[415] Yuza Y, Glatt KA, Jiang J, *et al.* Allele-dependent variation in the relative cellular potency of distinct EGFR inhibitors. Cancer Biol Ther 2007; 6(5): 661-7.
[PMID: 17495523]

[416] Bean J, Riely GJ, Balak M, *et al.* Acquired resistance to epidermal growth factor receptor kinase inhibitors associated with a novel T854A mutation in a patient with EGFR-mutant lung adenocarcinoma. Clin Cancer Res 2008; 14(22): 7519-25.
[PMID: 19010870]

[417] Avizienyte E, Ward RA, Garner AP. Comparison of the EGFR resistance mutation profiles generated by EGFR-targeted tyrosine kinase inhibitors and the impact of drug combinations. Biochem J 2008; 415(2): 197-206.
[PMID: 18588508]

[418] Godin-Heymann N, Ulkus L, Brannigan BW, *et al.* The T790M "gatekeeper" mutation in EGFR mediates resistance to low concentrations of an irreversible EGFR inhibitor. Mol Cancer Ther 2008; 7(4): 874-9.
[PMID: 18413800]

[419] Yu Z, Boggon TJ, Kobayashi S, *et al.* Resistance to an irreversible epidermal growth factor receptor (EGFR) inhibitor in EGFR-mutant lung cancer reveals novel treatment strategies. Cancer Res 2007; 67(21): 10417-27.
[PMID: 17974985]

[420] Zhou W, Ercan D, Chen L, *et al.* Novel mutant-selective EGFR kinase inhibitors against EGFR T790M. Nature 2009; 462(7276): 1070-4.
[PMID: 20033049]

[421] Ercan D, Choi HG, Yun CH, *et al.* EGFR mutations and resistance to Irreversible pyrimidine based EGFR inhibitors. Clin Cancer Res 2015; 21(17): 3913-23.
[PMID: 25948633]

[422] Thress KS, Paweletz CP, Felip E, *et al.* Acquired EGFR C797S mutation mediates resistance to AZD9291 in non-small cell lung cancer harboring EGFR T790M. Nat Med 2015; 21(6): 560-2.
[PMID: 25939061]

[423] Montagut C, Dalmases A, Bellosillo B, *et al.* Identification of a mutation in the extracellular domain of the Epidermal Growth Factor Receptor conferring cetuximab resistance in colorectal cancer. Nat Med 2012; 18(2): 221-3.
[PMID: 22270724]

[424] Arena S, Bellosillo B, Siravegna G, *et al.* Emergence of Multiple EGFR Extracellular Mutations during Cetuximab Treatment in Colorectal Cancer. Clin Cancer Res 2015; 21(9): 2157-66.
[PMID: 25623215]

[425] Bertotti A, Papp E, Jones S, *et al.* The genomic landscape of response to EGFR blockade in colorectal cancer. Nature 2015; 526(7572): 263-7.
[PMID: 26416732]

[426] Braig F, März M, Schieferdecker A, *et al.* Epidermal growth factor receptor mutation mediates cross-resistance to panitumumab and cetuximab in gastrointestinal cancer. Oncotarget 2015; 6(14): 12035-47.
[PMID: 26059438]

[427] Lu Y, Li X, Liang K, *et al.* Epidermal growth factor receptor (EGFR) ubiquitination as a mechanism of acquired resistance escaping treatment by the anti-EGFR monoclonal antibody cetuximab. Cancer Res 2007; 67(17): 8240-7.
[PMID: 17804738]

[428] Ito Y, Yamada Y, Asada K, *et al.* EGFR L2 domain mutation is not correlated with resistance to cetuximab in metastatic colorectal cancer patients. J Cancer Res Clin Oncol 2013; 139(8): 1391-6.
[PMID: 23722667]

[429] Gan HK, Kaye AH, Luwor RB. The EGFRvIII variant in glioblastoma multiforme. J Clin Neurosci 2009; 16(6): 748-54.
[PMID: 19324552]

[430] O'Rourke DM, Nute EJ, Davis JG, *et al.* Inhibition of a naturally occurring EGFR oncoprotein by the p185neu ectodomain: implications for subdomain contributions to receptor assembly. Oncogene 1998; 16(9): 1197-207.

[PMID: 9528862]

[431] Voldborg BR, Damstrup L, Spang-Thomsen M, Poulsen HS. Epidermal growth factor receptor (EGFR) and EGFR mutations, function and possible role in clinical trials. Ann Oncol 1997; 8(12): 1197-206.
[PMID: 9496384]

[432] Huang HS, Nagane M, Klingbeil CK, *et al.* The enhanced tumorigenic activity of a mutant epidermal growth factor receptor common in human cancers is mediated by threshold levels of constitutive tyrosine phosphorylation and unattenuated signaling. J Biol Chem 1997; 272(5): 2927-35.
[PMID: 9006938]

[433] Nagane M, Coufal F, Lin H, Bögler O, Cavenee WK, Huang HJ. A common mutant epidermal growth factor receptor confers enhanced tumorigenicity on human glioblastoma cells by increasing proliferation and reducing apoptosis. Cancer Res 1996; 56(21): 5079-86.
[PMID: 8895767]

[434] Wong AJ, Ruppert JM, Bigner SH, *et al.* Structural alterations of the epidermal growth factor receptor gene in human gliomas. Proc Natl Acad Sci USA 1992; 89(7): 2965-9.
[PMID: 1557402]

[435] Ge H, Gong X, Tang CK. Evidence of high incidence of EGFRvIII expression and coexpression with EGFR in human invasive breast cancer by laser capture microdissection and immunohistochemical analysis. Int J Cancer 2002; 98(3): 357-61.
[PMID: 11920586]

[436] Sok JC, Coppelli FM, Thomas SM, *et al.* Mutant epidermal growth factor receptor (EGFRvIII) contributes to head and neck cancer growth and resistance to EGFR targeting. Clin Cancer Res 2006; 12(17): 5064-73.
[PMID: 16951222]

[437] Wikstrand CJ, Hale LP, Batra SK, *et al.* Monoclonal antibodies against EGFRvIII are tumor specific and react with breast and lung carcinomas and malignant gliomas. Cancer Res 1995; 55(14): 3140-8.
[PMID: 7606735]

[438] Ji H, Zhao X, Yuza Y, *et al.* Epidermal growth factor receptor variant III mutations in lung tumorigenesis and sensitivity to tyrosine kinase inhibitors. Proc Natl Acad Sci USA 2006; 103(20): 7817-22.
[PMID: 16672372]

[439] Fukai J, Nishio K, Itakura T, Koizumi F. Antitumor activity of cetuximab against malignant glioma cells overexpressing EGFR deletion mutant variant III. Cancer Sci 2008; 99(10): 2062-9.
[PMID: 19016767]

[440] Patel D, Lahiji A, Patel S, *et al.* Monoclonal antibody cetuximab binds to and down-regulates constitutively activated epidermal growth factor receptor vIII on the cell surface. Anticancer Res 2007; 27(5A): 3355-66.
[PMID: 17970081]

[441] Wachsberger PR, Lawrence RY, Liu Y, Rice B, Daskalakis C, Dicker AP. Epidermal growth factor receptor mutation status and rad51 determine the response of glioblastoma to multimodality therapy with cetuximab, temozolomide, and radiation. Front Oncol 2013; 3: 13.

[PMID: 23383403]

[442]   Yang W, Wu G, Barth RF, *et al.* Molecular targeting and treatment of composite EGFR and EGFRvIII-positive gliomas using boronated monoclonal antibodies. Clin Cancer Res 2008; 14(3): 883-91.
[PMID: 18245552]

[443]   Reilly EB, Phillips AC, Buchanan FG, *et al.* Characterization of ABT-806, a Humanized Tumor-Specific Anti-EGFR Monoclonal Antibody. Mol Cancer Ther 2015; 14(5): 1141-51.
[PMID: 25731184]

[444]   Jutten B, Dubois L, Li Y, *et al.* Binding of cetuximab to the EGFRvIII deletion mutant and its biological consequences in malignant glioma cells. Radiother Oncol 2009; 92(3): 393-8.
[PMID: 19616334]

[445]   Luchman HA, Stechishin OD, Nguyen SA, Lun XQ, Cairncross JG, Weiss S. Dual mTORC1/2 blockade inhibits glioblastoma brain tumor initiating cells *in vitro* and *in vivo* and synergizes with temozolomide to increase orthotopic xenograft survival. Clin Cancer Res 2014; 20(22): 5756-67.
[PMID: 25316808]

[446]   Schulte A, Liffers K, Kathagen A, *et al.* Erlotinib resistance in EGFR-amplified glioblastoma cells is associated with upregulation of EGFRvIII and PI3Kp110δ. Neuro-oncol 2013; 15(10): 1289-301.
[PMID: 23877316]

[447]   Liu XJ, Wu WT, Wu WH, *et al.* A minority subpopulation of CD133(+) /EGFRvIII(+) /EGFR(-) cells acquires stemness and contributes to gefitinib resistance. CNS Neurosci Ther 2013; 19(7): 494-502.
[PMID: 23575351]

[448]   Kinsella P, Howley R, Doolan P, *et al.* Characterization and response of newly developed high-grade glioma cultures to the tyrosine kinase inhibitors, erlotinib, gefitinib and imatinib. Exp Cell Res 2012; 318(5): 641-52.
[PMID: 22285130]

[449]   Lo HW, Cao X, Zhu H, Ali-Osman F. Constitutively activated STAT3 frequently coexpresses with epidermal growth factor receptor in high-grade gliomas and targeting STAT3 sensitizes them to Iressa and alkylators. Clin Cancer Res 2008; 14(19): 6042-54.
[PMID: 18829483]

[450]   Cemeus C, Zhao TT, Barrett GM, Lorimer IA, Dimitroulakos J. Lovastatin enhances gefitinib activity in glioblastoma cells irrespective of EGFRvIII and PTEN status. J Neurooncol 2008; 90(1): 9-17.
[PMID: 18566746]

[451]   Bax DA, Gaspar N, Little SE, *et al.* EGFRvIII deletion mutations in pediatric high-grade glioma and response to targeted therapy in pediatric glioma cell lines. Clin Cancer Res 2009; 15(18): 5753-61.
[PMID: 19737945]

[452]   Greenall SA, Donoghue JF, Van Sinderen M, *et al.* EGFRvIII-mediated transactivation of receptor tyrosine kinases in glioma: mechanism and therapeutic implications. Oncogene 2015; 34(41): 5277-87.
[PMID: 25659577]

[453]   Pillay V, Allaf L, Wilding AL, *et al.* The plasticity of oncogene addiction: implications for targeted therapies directed to receptor tyrosine kinases. Neoplasia 2009; 11(5) 2 p following 458

[454] Lv S, Teugels E, Sadones J, *et al.* Correlation of EGFR, IDH1 and PTEN status with the outcome of patients with recurrent glioblastoma treated in a phase II clinical trial with the EGFR-blocking monoclonal antibody cetuximab. Int J Oncol 2012; 41(3): 1029-35.
[PMID: 22752145]

[455] Mellinghoff IK, Wang MY, Vivanco I, *et al.* Molecular determinants of the response of glioblastomas to EGFR kinase inhibitors. N Engl J Med 2005; 353(19): 2012-24.
[PMID: 16282176]

[456] Brown PD, Krishnan S, Sarkaria JN, *et al.* North Central Cancer Treatment Group Study N0177. Phase I/II trial of erlotinib and temozolomide with radiation therapy in the treatment of newly diagnosed glioblastoma multiforme: North Central Cancer Treatment Group Study N0177. J Clin Oncol 2008; 26(34): 5603-9.
[PMID: 18955445]

[457] van den Bent MJ, Brandes AA, Rampling R, *et al.* Randomized phase II trial of erlotinib *versus* temozolomide or carmustine in recurrent glioblastoma: EORTC brain tumor group study 26034. J Clin Oncol 2009; 27(8): 1268-74.
[PMID: 19204207]

[458] Prados MD, Chang SM, Butowski N, *et al.* Phase II study of erlotinib plus temozolomide during and after radiation therapy in patients with newly diagnosed glioblastoma multiforme or gliosarcoma. J Clin Oncol 2009; 27(4): 579-84.
[PMID: 19075262]

[459] Reardon DA, Desjardins A, Vredenburgh JJ, *et al.* Phase 2 trial of erlotinib plus sirolimus in adults with recurrent glioblastoma. J Neurooncol 2010; 96(2): 219-30.
[PMID: 19562254]

[460] Haas-Kogan DA, Prados MD, Tihan T, *et al.* Epidermal growth factor receptor, protein kinase B/Akt, and glioma response to erlotinib. J Natl Cancer Inst 2005; 97(12): 880-7.
[PMID: 15956649]

[461] Smilek P, Neuwirthova J, Jarkovsky J, *et al.* Epidermal growth factor receptor (EGFR) expression and mutations in the EGFR signaling pathway in correlation with anti-EGFR therapy in head and neck squamous cell carcinomas. Neoplasma 2012; 59(5): 508-15.
[PMID: 22668015]

[462] Chau NG, Perez-Ordonez B, Zhang K, *et al.* The association between EGFR variant III, HPV, p16, c-MET, EGFR gene copy number and response to EGFR inhibitors in patients with recurrent or metastatic squamous cell carcinoma of the head and neck. Head Neck Oncol 2011; 3: 11.
[PMID: 21352589]

[463] Li D, Ji H, Zaghlul S, *et al.* Therapeutic anti-EGFR antibody 806 generates responses in murine de novo EGFR mutant-dependent lung carcinomas. J Clin Invest 2007; 117(2): 346-52.
[PMID: 17256054]

[464] Bertotti A, Migliardi G, Galimi F, *et al.* A molecularly annotated platform of patient-derived xenografts ("xenopatients") identifies HER2 as an effective therapeutic target in cetuximab-resistant colorectal cancer. Cancer Discov 2011; 1(6): 508-23.
[PMID: 22586653]

[465]   Kavuri SM, Jain N, Galimi F, *et al.* HER2 activating mutations are targets for colorectal cancer treatment. Cancer Discov 2015; 5(8): 832-41.
[PMID: 26243863]

[466]   Yonesaka K, Zejnullahu K, Okamoto I, *et al.* Activation of ERBB2 signaling causes resistance to the EGFR-directed therapeutic antibody cetuximab. Sci Transl Med 2011; 3(99): 99ra86.
[PMID: 21900593]

[467]   Takezawa K, Pirazzoli V, Arcila ME, *et al.* HER2 amplification: a potential mechanism of acquired resistance to EGFR inhibition in EGFR-mutant lung cancers that lack the second-site EGFRT790M mutation. Cancer Discov 2012; 2(10): 922-33.
[PMID: 22956644]

[468]   Cappuzzo F, Varella-Garcia M, Shigematsu H, *et al.* Increased HER2 gene copy number is associated with response to gefitinib therapy in epidermal growth factor receptor-positive non-small-cell lung cancer patients. J Clin Oncol 2005; 23(22): 5007-18.
[PMID: 16051952]

[469]   Daniele L, Macrì L, Schena M, *et al.* Predicting gefitinib responsiveness in lung cancer by fluorescence *in situ* hybridization/chromogenic *in situ* hybridization analysis of EGFR and HER2 in biopsy and cytology specimens. Mol Cancer Ther 2007; 6(4): 1223-9.
[PMID: 17406029]

[470]   Martin V, Landi L, Molinari F, *et al.* HER2 gene copy number status may influence clinical efficacy to anti-EGFR monoclonal antibodies in metastatic colorectal cancer patients. Br J Cancer 2013; 108(3): 668-75.
[PMID: 23348520]

[471]   Despierre E, Vergote I, Anderson R, *et al.* European Organisation for Research and Treatment of Cancer-Gynaecological Cancer Group (EORTC-GCG), Groupe d'Investigateurs Nationaux pour les Etudes des Cancers de l'Ovaire (GINECO), Austrian Arbeitsgemeinschaft für Gynäkologische Onkologie (A-AGO), National Cancer Research Institute (NCRI), Australia New Zealand Gynaecological Oncology Group (ANZGOG), and the Mario Negri Gynecologic Oncology group (MaNGO). Epidermal Growth Factor Receptor (EGFR) Pathway Biomarkers in the Randomized Phase III Trial of Erlotinib *Versus* Observation in Ovarian Cancer Patients with No Evidence of Disease Progression after First-Line Platinum-Based Chemotherapy. Target Oncol 2015; 10(4): 583-96.
[PMID: 26004768]

[472]   Wainberg ZA, Lin LS, DiCarlo B, *et al.* Phase II trial of modified FOLFOX6 and erlotinib in patients with metastatic or advanced adenocarcinoma of the oesophagus and gastro-oesophageal junction. Br J Cancer 2011; 105(6): 760-5.
[PMID: 21811258]

[473]   Varella-Garcia M, Mitsudomi T, Yatabe Y, *et al.* EGFR and HER2 genomic gain in recurrent non-small cell lung cancer after surgery: impact on outcome to treatment with gefitinib and association with EGFR and KRAS mutations in a Japanese cohort. J Thorac Oncol 2009; 4(3): 318-25.
[PMID: 19247083]

[474]   Pugh TJ, Bebb G, Barclay L, *et al.* Correlations of EGFR mutations and increases in EGFR and HER2 copy number to gefitinib response in a retrospective analysis of lung cancer patients. BMC Cancer

2007; 7: 128.
[PMID: 17626639]

[475] Trowe T, Boukouvala S, Calkins K, *et al.* EXEL-7647 inhibits mutant forms of ErbB2 associated with lapatinib resistance and neoplastic transformation. Clin Cancer Res 2008; 14(8): 2465-75.
[PMID: 18413839]

[476] Rexer BN, Ghosh R, Narasanna A, *et al.* Human breast cancer cells harboring a gatekeeper T798M mutation in HER2 overexpress EGFR ligands and are sensitive to dual inhibition of EGFR and HER2. Clin Cancer Res 2013; 19(19): 5390-401.
[PMID: 23948973]

[477] Kancha RK, von Bubnoff N, Bartosch N, Peschel C, Engh RA, Duyster J. Differential sensitivity of ERBB2 kinase domain mutations towards lapatinib. PLoS One 2011; 6(10): e26760.
[PMID: 22046346]

[478] Stephens P, Hunter C, Bignell G, *et al.* Lung cancer: intragenic ERBB2 kinase mutations in tumours. Nature 2004; 431(7008): 525-6.
[PMID: 15457249]

[479] Buttitta F, Barassi F, Fresu G, *et al.* Mutational analysis of the HER2 gene in lung tumors from Caucasian patients: mutations are mainly present in adenocarcinomas with bronchioloalveolar features. Int J Cancer 2006; 119(11): 2586-91.
[PMID: 16988931]

[480] Lee JW, Soung YH, Seo SH, *et al.* Somatic mutations of ERBB2 kinase domain in gastric, colorectal, and breast carcinomas. Clin Cancer Res 2006; 12(1): 57-61.
[PMID: 16397024]

[481] Bekaii-Saab T, Williams N, Plass C, Calero MV, Eng C. A novel mutation in the tyrosine kinase domain of ERBB2 in hepatocellular carcinoma. BMC Cancer 2006; 6: 278.
[PMID: 17150109]

[482] Kubo T, Kuroda Y, Shimizu H, *et al.* Resequencing and copy number analysis of the human tyrosine kinase gene family in poorly differentiated gastric cancer. Carcinogenesis 2009; 30(11): 1857-64.
[PMID: 19734198]

[483] Buonanno A, Fischbach GD. Neuregulin and ErbB receptor signaling pathways in the nervous system. Curr Opin Neurobiol 2001; 11(3): 287-96.
[PMID: 11399426]

[484] Busfield SJ, Michnick DA, Chickering TW, *et al.* Characterization of a neuregulin-related gene, Don-1, that is highly expressed in restricted regions of the cerebellum and hippocampus. Mol Cell Biol 1997; 17(7): 4007-14.
[PMID: 9199335]

[485] Falls DL. Neuregulins: functions, forms, and signaling strategies. Exp Cell Res 2003; 284(1): 14-30.
[PMID: 12648463]

[486] Harari D, Tzahar E, Romano J, *et al.* Neuregulin-4: a novel growth factor that acts through the ErbB-4 receptor tyrosine kinase. Oncogene 1999; 18(17): 2681-9.
[PMID: 10348342]

[487] Zhang D, Sliwkowski MX, Mark M, *et al.* Neuregulin-3 (NRG3): a novel neural tissue-enriched protein that binds and activates ErbB4. Proc Natl Acad Sci USA 1997; 94(18): 9562-7. [PMID: 9275162]

[488] Kawakami H, Okamoto I, Yonesaka K, *et al.* The anti-HER3 antibody patritumab abrogates cetuximab resistance mediated by heregulin in colorectal cancer cells. Oncotarget 2014; 5(23): 11847-56. [PMID: 25474137]

[489] Sergina NV, Rausch M, Wang D, *et al.* Escape from HER-family tyrosine kinase inhibitor therapy by the kinase-inactive HER3. Nature 2007; 445(7126): 437-41. [PMID: 17206155]

[490] Hutcheson IR, Knowlden JM, Hiscox SE, *et al.* Heregulin beta1 drives gefitinib-resistant growth and invasion in tamoxifen-resistant MCF-7 breast cancer cells. Breast Cancer Res 2007; 9(4): R50. [PMID: 17686159]

[491] Köninki K, Barok M, Tanner M, *et al.* Multiple molecular mechanisms underlying trastuzumab and lapatinib resistance in JIMT-1 breast cancer cells. Cancer Lett 2010; 294(2): 211-9. [PMID: 20193978]

[492] Leung WY, Roxanis I, Sheldon H, *et al.* Combining lapatinib and pertuzumab to overcome lapatinib resistance due to NRG1-mediated signalling in HER2-amplified breast cancer. Oncotarget 2015; 6(8): 5678-94. [PMID: 25691057]

[493] Sato Y, Yashiro M, Takakura N. Heregulin induces resistance to lapatinib-mediated growth inhibition of HER2-amplified cancer cells. Cancer Sci 2013; 104(12): 1618-25. [PMID: 24112719]

[494] Xia W, Petricoin EF III, Zhao S, *et al.* An heregulin-EGFR-HER3 autocrine signaling axis can mediate acquired lapatinib resistance in HER2+ breast cancer models. Breast Cancer Res 2013; 15(5): R85. [PMID: 24044505]

[495] Grøvdal LM, Kim J, Holst MR, Knudsen SL, Grandal MV, van Deurs B. EGF receptor inhibitors increase ErbB3 mRNA and protein levels in breast cancer cells. Cell Signal 2012; 24(1): 296-301. [PMID: 21951604]

[496] Erjala K, Sundvall M, Junttila TT, *et al.* Signaling *via* ErbB2 and ErbB3 associates with resistance and epidermal growth factor receptor (EGFR) amplification with sensitivity to EGFR inhibitor gefitinib in head and neck squamous cell carcinoma cells. Clin Cancer Res 2006; 12(13): 4103-11. [PMID: 16818711]

[497] Iida M, Brand TM, Starr MM, *et al.* Overcoming acquired resistance to cetuximab by dual targeting HER family receptors with antibody-based therapy. Mol Cancer 2014; 13: 242. [PMID: 25344208]

[498] Engelman JA, Zejnullahu K, Mitsudomi T, *et al.* MET amplification leads to gefitinib resistance in lung cancer by activating ERBB3 signaling. Science 2007; 316(5827): 1039-43. [PMID: 17463250]

[499] Scartozzi M, Mandolesi A, Giampieri R, *et al.* The role of HER-3 expression in the prediction of clinical outcome for advanced colorectal cancer patients receiving irinotecan and cetuximab.

Oncologist 2011; 16(1): 53-60.
[PMID: 21212430]

[500] Scartozzi M, Giampieri R, Maccaroni E, *et al.* Analysis of HER-3, insulin growth factor-1, nuclear factor-kB and epidermal growth factor receptor gene copy number in the prediction of clinical outcome for K-RAS wild-type colorectal cancer patients receiving irinotecan-cetuximab. Ann Oncol 2012; 23(7): 1706-12.
[PMID: 22112971]

[501] Giampieri R, Mandolesi A, Abouelkhair KM, *et al.* Prospective study of a molecular selection profile for RAS wild type colorectal cancer patients receiving irinotecan-cetuximab. J Transl Med 2015; 13: 140.
[PMID: 25943333]

[502] Gandhi J, Zhang J, Xie Y, *et al.* Alterations in genes of the EGFR signaling pathway and their relationship to EGFR tyrosine kinase inhibitor sensitivity in lung cancer cell lines. PLoS One 2009; 4(2): e4576.
[PMID: 19238210]

[503] Witta SE, Dziadziuszko R, Yoshida K, *et al.* ErbB-3 expression is associated with E-cadherin and their coexpression restores response to gefitinib in non-small-cell lung cancer (NSCLC). Ann Oncol 2009; 20(4): 689-95.
[PMID: 19150934]

[504] Cappuzzo F, Toschi L, Domenichini I, *et al.* HER3 genomic gain and sensitivity to gefitinib in advanced non-small-cell lung cancer patients. Br J Cancer 2005; 93(12): 1334-40.
[PMID: 16288303]

[505] Black PC, Brown GA, Inamoto T, *et al.* Sensitivity to epidermal growth factor receptor inhibitor requires E-cadherin expression in urothelial carcinoma cells. Clin Cancer Res 2008; 14(5): 1478-86.
[PMID: 18316572]

[506] Jiang N, Wang D, Hu Z, *et al.* Combination of anti-HER3 antibody MM-121/SAR256212 and cetuximab inhibits tumor growth in preclinical models of head and neck squamous cell carcinoma. Mol Cancer Ther 2014; 13(7): 1826-36.
[PMID: 24748655]

[507] Wu Y, Zhang Y, Wang M, *et al.* Downregulation of HER3 by a novel antisense oligonucleotide, EZN-3920, improves the antitumor activity of EGFR and HER2 tyrosine kinase inhibitors in animal models. Mol Cancer Ther 2013; 12(4): 427-37.
[PMID: 23395887]

[508] Ju L, Zhou C, Li W, Yan L. Integrin beta1 over-expression associates with resistance to tyrosine kinase inhibitor gefitinib in non-small cell lung cancer. J Cell Biochem 2010; 111(6): 1565-74.
[PMID: 21053345]

[509] Kanda R, Kawahara A, Watari K, *et al.* Erlotinib resistance in lung cancer cells mediated by integrin β1/Src/Akt-driven bypass signaling. Cancer Res 2013; 73(20): 6243-53.
[PMID: 23872583]

[510] Aljohani H, Koncar RF, Zarzour A, Park BS, Lee SH, Bahassi M. ROS1 amplification mediates resistance to gefitinib in glioblastoma cells. Oncotarget 2015; 6(24): 20388-95.

[PMID: 25978031]

[511] Lee HJ, Zhuang G, Cao Y, Du P, Kim HJ, Settleman J. Drug resistance *via* feedback activation of Stat3 in oncogene-addicted cancer cells. Cancer Cell 2014; 26(2): 207-21. [PMID: 25065853]

[512] Argiris A, Lee SC, Feinstein T, *et al.* Serum biomarkers as potential predictors of antitumor activity of cetuximab-containing therapy for locally advanced head and neck cancer. Oral Oncol 2011; 47(10): 961-6. [PMID: 21889392]

[513] Yao Z, Fenoglio S, Gao DC, *et al.* TGF-beta IL-6 axis mediates selective and adaptive mechanisms of resistance to molecular targeted therapy in lung cancer. Proc Natl Acad Sci USA 2010; 107(35): 15535-40. [PMID: 20713723]

[514] Chen CC, Chen WC, Lu CH, *et al.* Significance of interleukin-6 signaling in the resistance of pharyngeal cancer to irradiation and the epidermal growth factor receptor inhibitor. Int J Radiat Oncol Biol Phys 2010; 76(4): 1214-24. [PMID: 20206020]

[515] Kuzumaki N, Suzuki A, Narita M, *et al.* Multiple analyses of G-protein coupled receptor (GPCR) expression in the development of gefitinib-resistance in transforming non-small-cell lung cancer. PLoS One 2012; 7(10): e44368. [PMID: 23144692]

[516] Rosa R, Melisi D, Damiano V, *et al.* Toll-like receptor 9 agonist IMO cooperates with cetuximab in K-ras mutant colorectal and pancreatic cancers. Clin Cancer Res 2011; 17(20): 6531-41. [PMID: 21890455]

[517] Cooper CS, Park M, Blair DG, *et al.* Molecular cloning of a new transforming gene from a chemically transformed human cell line. Nature 1984; 311(5981): 29-33. [PMID: 6590967]

[518] Ferracini R, Olivero M, Di Renzo MF, *et al.* Retrogenic expression of the MET proto-oncogene correlates with the invasive phenotype of human rhabdomyosarcomas. Oncogene 1996; 12(8): 1697-705. [PMID: 8622890]

[519] Ma PC, Tretiakova MS, MacKinnon AC, *et al.* Expression and mutational analysis of MET in human solid cancers. Genes Chromosomes Cancer 2008; 47(12): 1025-37. [PMID: 18709663]

[520] Olivero M, Rizzo M, Madeddu R, *et al.* Overexpression and activation of hepatocyte growth factor/scatter factor in human non-small-cell lung carcinomas. Br J Cancer 1996; 74(12): 1862-8. [PMID: 8980383]

[521] Schmidt L, Duh FM, Chen F, *et al.* Germline and somatic mutations in the tyrosine kinase domain of the MET proto-oncogene in papillary renal carcinomas. Nat Genet 1997; 16(1): 68-73. [PMID: 9140397]

[522] Bottaro DP, Rubin JS, Faletto DL, *et al.* Identification of the hepatocyte growth factor receptor as the

c-met proto-oncogene product. Science 1991; 251(4995): 802-4.
[PMID: 1846706]

[523] Inno A, Di Salvatore M, Cenci T, *et al.* Is there a role for IGF1R and c-MET pathways in resistance to cetuximab in metastatic colorectal cancer? Clin Colorectal Cancer 2011; 10(4): 325-32.
[PMID: 21729677]

[524] Kishiki T, Ohnishi H, Masaki T, *et al.* Overexpression of MET is a new predictive marker for anti-EGFR therapy in metastatic colorectal cancer with wild-type KRAS. Cancer Chemother Pharmacol 2014; 73(4): 749-57.
[PMID: 24500024]

[525] Masago K, Togashi Y, Fujita S, *et al.* Clinical significance of serum hepatocyte growth factor and epidermal growth factor gene somatic mutations in patients with non-squamous non-small cell lung cancer receiving gefitinib or erlotinib. Med Oncol 2012; 29(3): 1614-21.
[PMID: 21779929]

[526] Kasahara K, Arao T, Sakai K, *et al.* Impact of serum hepatocyte growth factor on treatment response to epidermal growth factor receptor tyrosine kinase inhibitors in patients with non-small cell lung adenocarcinoma. Clin Cancer Res 2010; 16(18): 4616-24.
[PMID: 20679350]

[527] Zucali PA, Ruiz MG, Giovannetti E, *et al.* Role of cMET expression in non-small-cell lung cancer patients treated with EGFR tyrosine kinase inhibitors. Ann Oncol 2008; 19(9): 1605-12.
[PMID: 18467317]

[528] Benedettini E, Sholl LM, Peyton M, *et al.* Met activation in non-small cell lung cancer is associated with de novo resistance to EGFR inhibitors and the development of brain metastasis. Am J Pathol 2010; 177(1): 415-23.
[PMID: 20489150]

[529] Krumbach R, Schüler J, Hofmann M, Giesemann T, Fiebig HH, Beckers T. Primary resistance to cetuximab in a panel of patient-derived tumour xenograft models: activation of MET as one mechanism for drug resistance. Eur J Cancer 2011; 47(8): 1231-43.
[PMID: 21273060]

[530] Bardelli A, Corso S, Bertotti A, *et al.* Amplification of the MET receptor drives resistance to anti-EGFR therapies in colorectal cancer. Cancer Discov 2013; 3(6): 658-73.
[PMID: 23729478]

[531] Yamada T, Takeuchi S, Kita K, *et al.* Hepatocyte growth factor induces resistance to anti-epidermal growth factor receptor antibody in lung cancer. J Thorac Oncol 2012; 7(2): 272-80.
[PMID: 22089117]

[532] Liska D, Chen CT, Bachleitner-Hofmann T, Christensen JG, Weiser MR. HGF rescues colorectal cancer cells from EGFR inhibition *via* MET activation. Clin Cancer Res 2011; 17(3): 472-82.
[PMID: 21098338]

[533] Troiani T, Martinelli E, Napolitano S, *et al.* Increased TGF-α as a mechanism of acquired resistance to the anti-EGFR inhibitor cetuximab through EGFR-MET interaction and activation of MET signaling in colon cancer cells. Clin Cancer Res 2013; 19(24): 6751-65.
[PMID: 24122793]

[534] Luraghi P, Reato G, Cipriano E, *et al.* MET signaling in colon cancer stem-like cells blunts the therapeutic response to EGFR inhibitors. Cancer Res 2014; 74(6): 1857-69.
[PMID: 24448239]

[535] Wilson TR, Fridlyand J, Yan Y, *et al.* Widespread potential for growth-factor-driven resistance to anticancer kinase inhibitors. Nature 2012; 487(7408): 505-9.
[PMID: 22763448]

[536] Gusenbauer S, Vlaicu P, Ullrich A. HGF induces novel EGFR functions involved in resistance formation to tyrosine kinase inhibitors. Oncogene 2013; 32(33): 3846-56.
[PMID: 23045285]

[537] Yano S, Wang W, Li Q, *et al.* Hepatocyte growth factor induces gefitinib resistance of lung adenocarcinoma with epidermal growth factor receptor-activating mutations. Cancer Res 2008; 68(22): 9479-87.
[PMID: 19010923]

[538] Wang W, Li Q, Yamada T, *et al.* Crosstalk to stromal fibroblasts induces resistance of lung cancer to epidermal growth factor receptor tyrosine kinase inhibitors. Clin Cancer Res 2009; 15(21): 6630-8.
[PMID: 19843665]

[539] Takeuchi S, Wang W, Li Q, *et al.* Dual inhibition of Met kinase and angiogenesis to overcome HGF-induced EGFR-TKI resistance in EGFR mutant lung cancer. Am J Pathol 2012; 181(3): 1034-43.
[PMID: 22789825]

[540] Cancer Genome Atlas Research Network. Comprehensive molecular profiling of lung adenocarcinoma. Nature 2014; 511(7511): 543-50.
[PMID: 25079552]

[541] Cappuzzo F, Jänne PA, Skokan M, *et al.* MET increased gene copy number and primary resistance to gefitinib therapy in non-small-cell lung cancer patients. Ann Oncol 2009; 20(2): 298-304.
[PMID: 18836087]

[542] Onozato R, Kosaka T, Kuwano H, Sekido Y, Yatabe Y, Mitsudomi T. Activation of MET by gene amplification or by splice mutations deleting the juxtamembrane domain in primary resected lung cancers. J Thorac Oncol 2009; 4(1): 5-11.
[PMID: 19096300]

[543] Go H, Jeon YK, Park HJ, Sung SW, Seo JW, Chung DH. High MET gene copy number leads to shorter survival in patients with non-small cell lung cancer. J Thorac Oncol 2010; 5(3): 305-13.
[PMID: 20107422]

[544] Cancer Genome Atlas Network. Comprehensive molecular characterization of human colon and rectal cancer. Nature 2012; 487(7407): 330-7.
[PMID: 22810696]

[545] Cappuzzo F, Varella-Garcia M, Finocchiaro G, *et al.* Primary resistance to cetuximab therapy in EGFR FISH-positive colorectal cancer patients. Br J Cancer 2008; 99(1): 83-9.
[PMID: 18577988]

[546] Bean J, Brennan C, Shih JY, *et al.* MET amplification occurs with or without T790M mutations in EGFR mutant lung tumors with acquired resistance to gefitinib or erlotinib. Proc Natl Acad Sci USA

2007; 104(52): 20932-7.
[PMID: 18093943]

[547] Chen HJ, Mok TS, Chen ZH, *et al.* Clinicopathologic and molecular features of epidermal growth factor receptor T790M mutation and c-MET amplification in tyrosine kinase inhibitor-resistant Chinese non-small cell lung cancer. Pathol Oncol Res 2009; 15(4): 651-8.
[PMID: 19381876]

[548] Turke AB, Zejnullahu K, Wu YL, *et al.* Preexistence and clonal selection of MET amplification in EGFR mutant NSCLC. Cancer Cell 2010; 17(1): 77-88.
[PMID: 20129249]

[549] Sohn J, Liu S, Parinyanitikul N, *et al.* cMET Activation and EGFR-Directed Therapy Resistance in Triple-Negative Breast Cancer. J Cancer 2014; 5(9): 745-53.
[PMID: 25368674]

[550] Zhang YW, Staal B, Essenburg C, *et al.* MET kinase inhibitor SGX523 synergizes with epidermal growth factor receptor inhibitor erlotinib in a hepatocyte growth factor-dependent fashion to suppress carcinoma growth. Cancer Res 2010; 70(17): 6880-90.
[PMID: 20643778]

[551] Xu H, Stabile LP, Gubish CT, Gooding WE, Grandis JR, Siegfried JM. Dual blockade of EGFR and c-Met abrogates redundant signaling and proliferation in head and neck carcinoma cells. Clin Cancer Res 2011; 17(13): 4425-38.
[PMID: 21622718]

[552] Stommel JM, Kimmelman AC, Ying H, *et al.* Coactivation of receptor tyrosine kinases affects the response of tumor cells to targeted therapies. Science 2007; 318(5848): 287-90.
[PMID: 17872411]

[553] Nanjo S, Yamada T, Nishihara H, *et al.* Ability of the Met kinase inhibitor crizotinib and new generation EGFR inhibitors to overcome resistance to EGFR inhibitors. PLoS One 2013; 8(12): e84700.
[PMID: 24386407]

[554] Van Cutsem E, Eng C, Nowara E, *et al.* Randomized phase Ib/II trial of rilotumumab or ganitumab with panitumumab *versus* panitumumab alone in patients with wild-type KRAS metastatic colorectal cancer. Clin Cancer Res 2014; 20(16): 4240-50.
[PMID: 24919569]

[555] Sequist LV, von Pawel J, Garmey EG, *et al.* Randomized phase II study of erlotinib plus tivantinib *versus* erlotinib plus placebo in previously treated non-small-cell lung cancer. J Clin Oncol 2011; 29(24): 3307-15.
[PMID: 21768463]

[556] Scagliotti G, von Pawel J, Novello S, *et al.* Phase III Multinational, Randomized, Double-Blind, Placebo-Controlled Study of Tivantinib (ARQ 197) Plus Erlotinib *Versus* Erlotinib Alone in Previously Treated Patients With Locally Advanced or Metastatic Nonsquamous Non-Small-Cell Lung Cancer. J Clin Oncol 2015; 33(24): 2667-74.
[PMID: 26169611]

[557] Spigel DR, Edelman MJ, Mok T, *et al.* MetLung Phase III Study Group. Treatment Rationale Study

Design for the MetLung Trial: A Randomized, Double-Blind Phase III Study of Onartuzumab (MetMAb) in Combination With Erlotinib *Versus* Erlotinib Alone in Patients Who Have Received Standard Chemotherapy for Stage IIIB or IV Met-Positive Non-Small-Cell Lung Cancer. Clin Lung Cancer 2012; 13(6): 500-4.
[PMID: 23063071]

[558] Adams TE, Epa VC, Garrett TP, Ward CW. Structure and function of the type 1 insulin-like growth factor receptor. Cell Mol Life Sci 2000; 57(7): 1050-93.
[PMID: 10961344]

[559] Khandwala HM, McCutcheon IE, Flyvbjerg A, Friend KE. The effects of insulin-like growth factors on tumorigenesis and neoplastic growth. Endocr Rev 2000; 21(3): 215-44.
[PMID: 10857553]

[560] LeRoith D, Roberts CT Jr. The insulin-like growth factor system and cancer. Cancer Lett 2003; 195(2): 127-37.
[PMID: 12767520]

[561] Meyer GE, Shelden E, Kim B, Feldman EL. Insulin-like growth factor I stimulates motility in human neuroblastoma cells. Oncogene 2001; 20(51): 7542-50.
[PMID: 11709726]

[562] Gilmore AP, Valentijn AJ, Wang P, *et al.* Activation of BAD by therapeutic inhibition of epidermal growth factor receptor and transactivation by insulin-like growth factor receptor. J Biol Chem 2002; 277(31): 27643-50.
[PMID: 12011069]

[563] Chakravarti A, Loeffler JS, Dyson NJ. Insulin-like growth factor receptor I mediates resistance to anti-epidermal growth factor receptor therapy in primary human glioblastoma cells through continued activation of phosphoinositide 3-kinase signaling. Cancer Res 2002; 62(1): 200-7.
[PMID: 11782378]

[564] Liu B, Fang M, Lu Y, Mendelsohn J, Fan Z. Fibroblast growth factor and insulin-like growth factor differentially modulate the apoptosis and G1 arrest induced by anti-epidermal growth factor receptor monoclonal antibody. Oncogene 2001; 20(15): 1913-22.
[PMID: 11313939]

[565] Jameson MJ, Beckler AD, Taniguchi LE, *et al.* Activation of the insulin-like growth factor-1 receptor induces resistance to epidermal growth factor receptor antagonism in head and neck squamous carcinoma cells. Mol Cancer Ther 2011; 10(11): 2124-34.
[PMID: 21878657]

[566] Masago K, Fujita S, Togashi Y, *et al.* Clinical significance of epidermal growth factor receptor mutations and insulin-like growth factor 1 and its binding protein 3 in advanced non-squamous non-small cell lung cancer. Oncol Rep 2011; 26(4): 795-803.
[PMID: 21805046]

[567] Jones HE, Goddard L, Gee JM, *et al.* Insulin-like growth factor-I receptor signalling and acquired resistance to gefitinib (ZD1839; Iressa) in human breast and prostate cancer cells. Endocr Relat Cancer 2004; 11(4): 793-814.
[PMID: 15613453]

[568] Winder T, Zhang W, Yang D, *et al.* Germline polymorphisms in genes involved in the IGF1 pathway predict efficacy of cetuximab in wild-type KRAS mCRC patients. Clin Cancer Res 2010; 16(22): 5591-602.
[PMID: 20935157]

[569] Zanella ER, Galimi F, Sassi F, *et al.* IGF2 is an actionable target that identifies a distinct subpopulation of colorectal cancer patients with marginal response to anti-EGFR therapies. Sci Transl Med 2015; 7(272): 272ra12.
[PMID: 25632036]

[570] Yang L, Li J, Ran L, *et al.* Phosphorylated insulin-like growth factor 1 receptor is implicated in resistance to the cytostatic effect of gefitinib in colorectal cancer cells. J Gastrointest Surg 2011; 15(6): 942-57.
[PMID: 21479670]

[571] Morgillo F, Woo JK, Kim ES, Hong WK, Lee HY. Heterodimerization of insulin-like growth factor receptor/epidermal growth factor receptor and induction of survivin expression counteract the antitumor action of erlotinib. Cancer Res 2006; 66(20): 10100-11.
[PMID: 17047074]

[572] Busser B, Sancey L, Josserand V, *et al.* Amphiregulin promotes BAX inhibition and resistance to gefitinib in non-small-cell lung cancers. Mol Ther 2010; 18(3): 528-35.
[PMID: 19826406]

[573] Cortot AB, Repellin CE, Shimamura T, *et al.* Resistance to irreversible EGF receptor tyrosine kinase inhibitors through a multistep mechanism involving the IGF1R pathway. Cancer Res 2013; 73(2): 834-43.
[PMID: 23172312]

[574] Ge X, Chen Q, Wu YP, *et al.* Induced IGF-1R activation contributes to gefitinib resistance following combined treatment with paclitaxel, cisplatin and gefitinib in A549 lung cancer cells. Oncol Rep 2014; 32(4): 1401-8.
[PMID: 25198583]

[575] Suda K, Mizuuchi H, Sato K, Takemoto T, Iwasaki T, Mitsudomi T. The insulin-like growth factor 1 receptor causes acquired resistance to erlotinib in lung cancer cells with the wild-type epidermal growth factor receptor. Int J Cancer 2014; 135(4): 1002-6.
[PMID: 24458568]

[576] Vazquez-Martin A, Cufí S, Oliveras-Ferraros C, *et al.* IGF-1R/epithelial-to-mesenchymal transition (EMT) crosstalk suppresses the erlotinib-sensitizing effect of EGFR exon 19 deletion mutations. Sci Rep 2013; 3: 2560.
[PMID: 23994953]

[577] Murakami A, Takahashi F, Nurwidya F, *et al.* Hypoxia increases gefitinib-resistant lung cancer stem cells through the activation of insulin-like growth factor 1 receptor. PLoS One 2014; 9(1): e86459.
[PMID: 24489728]

[578] Bodzin AS, Wei Z, Hurtt R, Gu T, Doria C. Gefitinib resistance in HCC mahlavu cells: upregulation of CD133 expression, activation of IGF-1R signaling pathway, and enhancement of IGF-1R nuclear translocation. J Cell Physiol 2012; 227(7): 2947-52.

[PMID: 21959795]

[579] Guix M, Faber AC, Wang SE, *et al.* Acquired resistance to EGFR tyrosine kinase inhibitors in cancer cells is mediated by loss of IGF-binding proteins. J Clin Invest 2008; 118(7): 2609-19.
[PMID: 18568074]

[580] Choi YJ, Park GM, Rho JK, *et al.* Role of IGF-binding protein 3 in the resistance of EGFR mutant lung cancer cells to EGFR-tyrosine kinase inhibitors. PLoS One 2013; 8(12): e81393.
[PMID: 24339922]

[581] Choi J, Kang M, Nam SH, *et al.* Bidirectional signaling between TM4SF5 and IGF1R promotes resistance to EGFR kinase inhibitors. Lung Cancer 2015; 90(1): 22-31.
[PMID: 26190015]

[582] Hurbin A, Wislez M, Busser B, *et al.* Insulin-like growth factor-1 receptor inhibition overcomes gefitinib resistance in mucinous lung adenocarcinoma. J Pathol 2011; 225(1): 83-95.
[PMID: 21598249]

[583] Hörndler C, Gallego R, García-Albeniz X, *et al.* Co-expression of matrix metalloproteinase-7 (MMP-7) and phosphorylated insulin growth factor receptor I (pIGF-1R) correlates with poor prognosis in patients with wild-type KRAS treated with cetuximab or panitumumab: a GEMCAD study. Cancer Biol Ther 2011; 11(2): 177-83.
[PMID: 21099348]

[584] Huang F, Xu LA, Khambata-Ford S. Correlation between gene expression of IGF-1R pathway markers and cetuximab benefit in metastatic colorectal cancer. Clin Cancer Res 2012; 18(4): 1156-66.
[PMID: 22294722]

[585] Fidler MJ, Basu S, Buckingham L, *et al.* Utility of insulin-like growth factor receptor-1 expression in gefitinib-treated patients with non-small cell lung cancer. Anticancer Res 2012; 32(5): 1705-10.
[PMID: 22593449]

[586] Chen B, Xiao F, Li B, *et al.* The role of epithelial-mesenchymal transition and IGF-1R expression in prediction of gefitinib activity as the second-line treatment for advanced nonsmall-cell lung cancer. Cancer Invest 2013; 31(7): 454-60.
[PMID: 23915069]

[587] Thariat J, Bensadoun RJ, Etienne-Grimaldi MC, *et al.* Contrasted outcomes to gefitinib on tumoral IGF1R expression in head and neck cancer patients receiving postoperative chemoradiation (GORTEC trial 2004-02). Clin Cancer Res 2012; 18(18): 5123-33.
[PMID: 22855581]

[588] Ramalingam SS, Spigel DR, Chen D, *et al.* Randomized phase II study of erlotinib in combination with placebo or R1507, a monoclonal antibody to insulin-like growth factor-1 receptor, for advanced-stage non-small-cell lung cancer. J Clin Oncol 2011; 29(34): 4574-80.
[PMID: 22025157]

[589] Reidy DL, Vakiani E, Fakih MG, *et al.* Randomized, phase II study of the insulin-like growth factor-1 receptor inhibitor IMC-A12, with or without cetuximab, in patients with cetuximab- or panitumumab-refractory metastatic colorectal cancer. J Clin Oncol 2010; 28(27): 4240-6.
[PMID: 20713879]

[590] Scagliotti GV, Bondarenko I, Blackhall F, *et al.* Randomized, phase III trial of figitumumab in combination with erlotinib *versus* erlotinib alone in patients with nonadenocarcinoma nonsmall-cell lung cancer. Ann Oncol 2015; 26(3): 497-504.
[PMID: 25395283]

[591] Singh D, Chan JM, Zoppoli P, *et al.* Transforming fusions of FGFR and TACC genes in human glioblastoma. Science 2012; 337(6099): 1231-5.
[PMID: 22837387]

[592] Wu YM, Su F, Kalyana-Sundaram S, *et al.* Identification of targetable FGFR gene fusions in diverse cancers. Cancer Discov 2013; 3(6): 636-47.
[PMID: 23558953]

[593] Kandoth C, Schultz N, Cherniack AD, *et al.* Cancer Genome Atlas Research Network. Integrated genomic characterization of endometrial carcinoma. Nature 2013; 497(7447): 67-73.
[PMID: 23636398]

[594] Shern JF, Chen L, Chmielecki J, *et al.* Comprehensive genomic analysis of rhabdomyosarcoma reveals a landscape of alterations affecting a common genetic axis in fusion-positive and fusion-negative tumors. Cancer Discov 2014; 4(2): 216-31.
[PMID: 24436047]

[595] Peifer M, Fernández-Cuesta L, Sos ML, *et al.* Integrative genome analyses identify key somatic driver mutations of small-cell lung cancer. Nat Genet 2012; 44(10): 1104-10.
[PMID: 22941188]

[596] Saito S, Morishima K, Ui T, *et al.* The role of HGF/MET and FGF/FGFR in fibroblast-derived growth stimulation and lapatinib-resistance of esophageal squamous cell carcinoma. BMC Cancer 2015; 15: 82.
[PMID: 25884729]

[597] Zhang Y, Pan T, Zhong X, Cheng C. Resistance to cetuximab in EGFR-overexpressing esophageal squamous cell carcinoma xenografts due to FGFR2 amplification and overexpression. J Pharmacol Sci 2014; 126(1): 77-83.
[PMID: 25242085]

[598] Huang ZQ, Buchsbaum DJ, Raisch KP, Bonner JA, Bland KI, Vickers SM. Differential responses by pancreatic carcinoma cell lines to prolonged exposure to Erbitux (IMC-C225) anti-EGFR antibody. J Surg Res 2003; 111(2): 274-83.
[PMID: 12850474]

[599] Ware KE, Marshall ME, Heasley LR, *et al.* Rapidly acquired resistance to EGFR tyrosine kinase inhibitors in NSCLC cell lines through de-repression of FGFR2 and FGFR3 expression. PLoS One 2010; 5(11): e14117.
[PMID: 21152424]

[600] Ware KE, Hinz TK, Kleczko E, *et al.* A mechanism of resistance to gefitinib mediated by cellular reprogramming and the acquisition of an FGF2-FGFR1 autocrine growth loop. Oncogenesis 2013; 2: e39.
[PMID: 23552882]

[601] Heldin CH, Johnsson A, Wennergren S, Wernstedt C, Betsholtz C, Westermark B. A human osteosarcoma cell line secretes a growth factor structurally related to a homodimer of PDGF A-chains. Nature 1986; 319(6053): 511-4.
[PMID: 3456080]

[602] Rand V, Huang J, Stockwell T, *et al*. Sequence survey of receptor tyrosine kinases reveals mutations in glioblastomas. Proc Natl Acad Sci USA 2005; 102(40): 14344-9.
[PMID: 16186508]

[603] Corless CL, Schroeder A, Griffith D, *et al*. PDGFRA mutations in gastrointestinal stromal tumors: frequency, spectrum and *in vitro* sensitivity to imatinib. J Clin Oncol 2005; 23(23): 5357-64.
[PMID: 15928335]

[604] Henriksen R, Funa K, Wilander E, Bäckström T, Ridderheim M, Oberg K. Expression and prognostic significance of platelet-derived growth factor and its receptors in epithelial ovarian neoplasms. Cancer Res 1993; 53(19): 4550-4.
[PMID: 8402626]

[605] Golub TR, Barker GF, Lovett M, Gilliland DG. Fusion of PDGF receptor beta to a novel ets-like gene, tel, in chronic myelomonocytic leukemia with t(5;12) chromosomal translocation. Cell 1994; 77(2): 307-16.
[PMID: 8168137]

[606] Kassouf W, Dinney CP, Brown G, *et al*. Uncoupling between epidermal growth factor receptor and downstream signals defines resistance to the antiproliferative effect of Gefitinib in bladder cancer cells. Cancer Res 2005; 65(22): 10524-35.
[PMID: 16288045]

[607] Thomson S, Petti F, Sujka-Kwok I, Epstein D, Haley JD. Kinase switching in mesenchymal-like non-small cell lung cancer lines contributes to EGFR inhibitor resistance through pathway redundancy. Clin Exp Metastasis 2008; 25(8): 843-54.
[PMID: 18696232]

[608] Akhavan D, Pourzia AL, Nourian AA, *et al*. De-repression of PDGFRβ transcription promotes acquired resistance to EGFR tyrosine kinase inhibitors in glioblastoma patients. Cancer Discov 2013; 3(5): 534-47.
[PMID: 23533263]

[609] Erben P, Horisberger K, Muessle B, *et al*. mRNA expression of platelet-derived growth factor receptor-beta and C-KIT: correlation with pathologic response to cetuximab-based chemoradiotherapy in patients with rectal cancer. Int J Radiat Oncol Biol Phys 2008; 72(5): 1544-50.
[PMID: 19028276]

[610] Ferrara N, Davis-Smyth T. The biology of vascular endothelial growth factor. Endocr Rev 1997; 18(1): 4-25.
[PMID: 9034784]

[611] Leung DW, Cachianes G, Kuang WJ, Goeddel DV, Ferrara N. Vascular endothelial growth factor is a secreted angiogenic mitogen. Science 1989; 246(4935): 1306-9.
[PMID: 2479986]

[612] Gerber HP, McMurtrey A, Kowalski J, *et al.* Vascular endothelial growth factor regulates endothelial cell survival through the phosphatidylinositol 3'-kinase/Akt signal transduction pathway. Requirement for Flk-1/KDR activation. J Biol Chem 1998; 273(46): 30336-43.
[PMID: 9804796]

[613] Neufeld G, Cohen T, Gengrinovitch S, Poltorak Z. Vascular endothelial growth factor (VEGF) and its receptors. FASEB J 1999; 13(1): 9-22.
[PMID: 9872925]

[614] Plate KH, Breier G, Weich HA, Risau W. Vascular endothelial growth factor is a potential tumour angiogenesis factor in human gliomas *in vivo.* Nature 1992; 359(6398): 845-8.
[PMID: 1279432]

[615] Shweiki D, Itin A, Soffer D, Keshet E. Vascular endothelial growth factor induced by hypoxia may mediate hypoxia-initiated angiogenesis. Nature 1992; 359(6398): 843-5.
[PMID: 1279431]

[616] Maity A, Pore N, Lee J, Solomon D, O'Rourke DM. Epidermal growth factor receptor transcriptionally up-regulates vascular endothelial growth factor expression in human glioblastoma cells *via* a pathway involving phosphatidylinositol 3'-kinase and distinct from that induced by hypoxia. Cancer Res 2000; 60(20): 5879-86.
[PMID: 11059786]

[617] Viloria-Petit A, Crombet T, Jothy S, *et al.* Acquired resistance to the antitumor effect of epidermal growth factor receptor-blocking antibodies *in vivo*: a role for altered tumor angiogenesis. Cancer Res 2001; 61(13): 5090-101.
[PMID: 11431346]

[618] Ciardiello F, Bianco R, Caputo R, *et al.* Antitumor activity of ZD6474, a vascular endothelial growth factor receptor tyrosine kinase inhibitor, in human cancer cells with acquired resistance to antiepidermal growth factor receptor therapy. Clin Cancer Res 2004; 10(2): 784-93.
[PMID: 14760102]

[619] Bianco R, Rosa R, Damiano V, *et al.* Vascular endothelial growth factor receptor-1 contributes to resistance to anti-epidermal growth factor receptor drugs in human cancer cells. Clin Cancer Res 2008; 14(16): 5069-80.
[PMID: 18694994]

[620] Li H, Takayama K, Wang S, *et al.* Addition of bevacizumab enhances antitumor activity of erlotinib against non-small cell lung cancer xenografts depending on VEGF expression. Cancer Chemother Pharmacol 2014; 74(6): 1297-305.
[PMID: 25344762]

[621] Chambers SK, Clouser MC, Baker AF, *et al.* Overexpression of tumor vascular endothelial growth factor A may portend an increased likelihood of progression in a phase II trial of bevacizumab and erlotinib in resistant ovarian cancer. Clin Cancer Res 2010; 16(21): 5320-8.
[PMID: 21041183]

[622] Cohen EE, Davis DW, Karrison TG, *et al.* Erlotinib and bevacizumab in patients with recurrent or metastatic squamous-cell carcinoma of the head and neck: a phase I/II study. Lancet Oncol 2009; 10(3): 247-57.

[PMID: 19201650]

[623] Byers LA, Holsinger FC, Kies MS, *et al.* Serum signature of hypoxia-regulated factors is associated with progression after induction therapy in head and neck squamous cell cancer. Mol Cancer Ther 2010; 9(6): 1755-63.
[PMID: 20530716]

[624] Vincenzi B, Santini D, Russo A, *et al.* Circulating VEGF reduction, response and outcome in advanced colorectal cancer patients treated with cetuximab plus irinotecan. Pharmacogenomics 2007; 8(4): 319-27.
[PMID: 17391070]

[625] Bukowski RM, Kabbinavar FF, Figlin RA, *et al.* Randomized phase II study of erlotinib combined with bevacizumab compared with bevacizumab alone in metastatic renal cell cancer. J Clin Oncol 2007; 25(29): 4536-41.
[PMID: 17876014]

[626] Ciuleanu T, Tsai CM, Tsao CJ, *et al.* A phase II study of erlotinib in combination with bevacizumab *versus* chemotherapy plus bevacizumab in the first-line treatment of advanced non-squamous non-small cell lung cancer. Lung Cancer 2013; 82(2): 276-81.
[PMID: 23992877]

[627] Dingemans AM, de Langen AJ, van den Boogaart V, *et al.* First-line erlotinib and bevacizumab in patients with locally advanced and/or metastatic non-small-cell lung cancer: a phase II study including molecular imaging. Ann Oncol 2011; 22(3): 559-66.
[PMID: 20702788]

[628] Herbst RS, Ansari R, Bustin F, *et al.* Efficacy of bevacizumab plus erlotinib *versus* erlotinib alone in advanced non-small-cell lung cancer after failure of standard first-line chemotherapy (BeTa): a double-blind, placebo-controlled, phase 3 trial. Lancet 2011; 377(9780): 1846-54.
[PMID: 21621716]

[629] Herbst RS, O'Neill VJ, Fehrenbacher L, *et al.* Phase II study of efficacy and safety of bevacizumab in combination with chemotherapy or erlotinib compared with chemotherapy alone for treatment of recurrent or refractory non small-cell lung cancer. J Clin Oncol 2007; 25(30): 4743-50.
[PMID: 17909199]

[630] Herbst RS, Johnson DH, Mininberg E, *et al.* Phase I/II trial evaluating the anti-vascular endothelial growth factor monoclonal antibody bevacizumab in combination with the HER-1/epidermal growth factor receptor tyrosine kinase inhibitor erlotinib for patients with recurrent non-small-cell lung cancer. J Clin Oncol 2005; 23(11): 2544-55.
[PMID: 15753462]

[631] Ichihara E, Hotta K, Nogami N, *et al.* Phase II trial of gefitinib in combination with bevacizumab as first-line therapy for advanced non-small cell lung cancer with activating EGFR gene mutations: the Okayama Lung Cancer Study Group Trial 1001. J Thorac Oncol 2015; 10(3): 486-91.
[PMID: 25695221]

[632] Tol J, Koopman M, Cats A, *et al.* Chemotherapy, bevacizumab, and cetuximab in metastatic colorectal cancer. N Engl J Med 2009; 360(6): 563-72.
[PMID: 19196673]

[633] O'Bryan JP, Frye RA, Cogswell PC, *et al.* axl, a transforming gene isolated from primary human myeloid leukemia cells, encodes a novel receptor tyrosine kinase. Mol Cell Biol 1991; 11(10): 5016-31.
[PMID: 1656220]

[634] Liu E, Hjelle B, Bishop JM. Transforming genes in chronic myelogenous leukemia. Proc Natl Acad Sci USA 1988; 85(6): 1952-6.
[PMID: 3279421]

[635] Gjerdrum C, Tiron C, Høiby T, *et al.* Axl is an essential epithelial-to-mesenchymal transition-induced regulator of breast cancer metastasis and patient survival. Proc Natl Acad Sci USA 2010; 107(3): 1124-9.
[PMID: 20080645]

[636] Byers LA, Diao L, Wang J, *et al.* An epithelial-mesenchymal transition gene signature predicts resistance to EGFR and PI3K inhibitors and identifies Axl as a therapeutic target for overcoming EGFR inhibitor resistance. Clin Cancer Res 2013; 19(1): 279-90.
[PMID: 23091115]

[637] Kim ES, Herbst RS, Wistuba II, *et al.* The BATTLE trial: personalizing therapy for lung cancer. Cancer Discov 2011; 1(1): 44-53.
[PMID: 22586319]

[638] Wilson C, Ye X, Pham T, *et al.* AXL inhibition sensitizes mesenchymal cancer cells to antimitotic drugs. Cancer Res 2014; 74(20): 5878-90.
[PMID: 25125659]

[639] Wu F, Li J, Jang C, Wang J, Xiong J. The role of Axl in drug resistance and epithelial-to-mesenchymal transition of non-small cell lung carcinoma. Int J Clin Exp Pathol 2014; 7(10): 6653-61.
[PMID: 25400744]

[640] Meyer AS, Miller MA, Gertler FB, Lauffenburger DA. The receptor AXL diversifies EGFR signaling and limits the response to EGFR-targeted inhibitors in triple-negative breast cancer cells. Sci Signal 2013; 6(287): ra66.
[PMID: 23921085]

[641] Zhang Z, Lee JC, Lin L, *et al.* Activation of the AXL kinase causes resistance to EGFR-targeted therapy in lung cancer. Nat Genet 2012; 44(8): 852-60.
[PMID: 22751098]

[642] Ji W, Choi CM, Rho JK, *et al.* Mechanisms of acquired resistance to EGFR-tyrosine kinase inhibitor in Korean patients with lung cancer. BMC Cancer 2013; 13: 606.
[PMID: 24369725]

[643] Rho JK, Choi YJ, Kim SY, *et al.* MET and AXL inhibitor NPS-1034 exerts efficacy against lung cancer cells resistant to EGFR kinase inhibitors because of MET or AXL activation. Cancer Res 2014; 74(1): 253-62.
[PMID: 24165158]

[644] Liu L, Greger J, Shi H, *et al.* Novel mechanism of lapatinib resistance in HER2-positive breast tumor cells: activation of AXL. Cancer Res 2009; 69(17): 6871-8.

[PMID: 19671800]

[645] Giles KM, Kalinowski FC, Candy PA, *et al.* Axl mediates acquired resistance of head and neck cancer cells to the epidermal growth factor receptor inhibitor erlotinib. Mol Cancer Ther 2013; 12(11): 2541-58.
[PMID: 24026012]

[646] Bae SY, Hong JY, Lee HJ, Park HJ, Lee SK. Targeting the degradation of AXL receptor tyrosine kinase to overcome resistance in gefitinib-resistant non-small cell lung cancer. Oncotarget 2015; 6(12): 10146-60.
[PMID: 25760142]

[647] Yoshida T, Zhang G, Smith MA, *et al.* Tyrosine phosphoproteomics identifies both codrivers and cotargeting strategies for T790M-related EGFR-TKI resistance in non-small cell lung cancer. Clin Cancer Res 2014; 20(15): 4059-74.
[PMID: 24919575]

[648] Wang Y, Xia H, Zhuang Z, Miao L, Chen X, Cai H. Axl-altered microRNAs regulate tumorigenicity and gefitinib resistance in lung cancer. Cell Death Dis 2014; 5: e1227.
[PMID: 24832599]

[649] Brand TM, Iida M, Stein AP, *et al.* AXL mediates resistance to cetuximab therapy. Cancer Res 2014; 74(18): 5152-64.
[PMID: 25136066]

[650] Huang SF, Liu HP, Li LH, *et al.* High frequency of epidermal growth factor receptor mutations with complex patterns in non-small cell lung cancers related to gefitinib responsiveness in Taiwan. Clin Cancer Res 2004; 10(24): 8195-203.
[PMID: 15623594]

[651] Kondo M, Yokoyama T, Fukui T, *et al.* Mutations of epidermal growth factor receptor of non-small cell lung cancer were associated with sensitivity to gefitinib in recurrence after surgery. Lung Cancer 2005; 50(3): 385-91.
[PMID: 16140420]

[652] Kim KS, Jeong JY, Kim YC, *et al.* Predictors of the response to gefitinib in refractory non-small cell lung cancer. Clin Cancer Res 2005; 11(6): 2244-51.
[PMID: 15788673]

[653] Tokumo M, Toyooka S, Kiura K, *et al.* The relationship between epidermal growth factor receptor mutations and clinicopathologic features in non-small cell lung cancers. Clin Cancer Res 2005; 11(3): 1167-73.
[PMID: 15709185]

[654] Han SW, Kim TY, Hwang PG, *et al.* Predictive and prognostic impact of epidermal growth factor receptor mutation in non-small-cell lung cancer patients treated with gefitinib. J Clin Oncol 2005; 23(11): 2493-501.
[PMID: 15710947]

[655] Cortes-Funes H, Gomez C, Rosell R, *et al.* Epidermal growth factor receptor activating mutations in Spanish gefitinib-treated non-small-cell lung cancer patients. Ann Oncol 2005; 16(7): 1081-6.
[PMID: 15851406]

[656] Tomizawa Y, Iijima H, Sunaga N, *et al.* Clinicopathologic significance of the mutations of the epidermal growth factor receptor gene in patients with non-small cell lung cancer. Clin Cancer Res 2005; 11(19 Pt 1): 6816-22.
       [PMID: 16203769]

[657] Takano T, Ohe Y, Sakamoto H, *et al.* Epidermal growth factor receptor gene mutations and increased copy numbers predict gefitinib sensitivity in patients with recurrent non-small-cell lung cancer. J Clin Oncol 2005; 23(28): 6829-37.
       [PMID: 15998907]

[658] Rosell R, Ichinose Y, Taron M, *et al.* Mutations in the tyrosine kinase domain of the EGFR gene associated with gefitinib response in non-small-cell lung cancer. Lung Cancer 2005; 50(1): 25-33.
       [PMID: 16011858]

[659] Zhang XT, Li LY, Mu XL, *et al.* The EGFR mutation and its correlation with response of gefitinib in previously treated Chinese patients with advanced non-small-cell lung cancer. Ann Oncol 2005; 16(8): 1334-42.
       [PMID: 15956035]

[660] Taron M, Ichinose Y, Rosell R, *et al.* Activating mutations in the tyrosine kinase domain of the epidermal growth factor receptor are associated with improved survival in gefitinib-treated chemorefractory lung adenocarcinomas. Clin Cancer Res 2005; 11(16): 5878-85.
       [PMID: 16115929]

[661] Uramoto H, Sugio K, Oyama T, *et al.* Epidermal growth factor receptor mutations are associated with gefitinib sensitivity in non-small cell lung cancer in Japanese. Lung Cancer 2006; 51(1): 71-7.
       [PMID: 16198442]

[662] Pan H, Liu R, Li S, *et al.* Effects of icotinib on advanced non-small cell lung cancer with different EGFR phenotypes. Cell Biochem Biophys 2014; 70(1): 553-8.
       [PMID: 24777808]

CHAPTER 2

Tumor Resistance Mechanisms to Inhibitors Targeting the Epidermal Growth Factor Receptor – Part II: Intracellular Molecules

Rodney B. Luwor[*]

Department of Surgery, The Royal Melbourne Hospital, The University of Melbourne, Parkville, Victoria 3050, Australia

Abstract: Tumor resistance to agents targeting the Epidermal Growth Factor Receptor (EGFR) is common, and well recognised as a major challenge to successful clinical outcome, because patients often present with tumors that contain pre-existing intrinsic resistance mechanisms to current EGFR inhibitors, which ultimately has no therapeutic benefit. Furthermore, patients who initially respond to these therapies commonly relapse, presenting with new tumors that have acquired resistance to the original therapy. Substantial translational and clinical research has been undertaken in order to understand, and more importantly overcome, the molecular initiators of both intrinsic and acquired tumor resistance. However, despite a multitude of cost and effort in gaining greater understanding of the molecular mechanisms that drive tumor resistance, very little has translated into clinical practice and management of patients. In these 2 back-to-back chapters, we will provide an overview of the progress made in targeting the EGFR and discuss the challenges presented by the numerous molecular mechanisms currently identified, leading to overall refractory outcomes to anti-EGFR therapeutics. In this chapter (Part II) we will specifically focus on the resistance mechanisms mediated by alterations in substrates downstream of the EGFR and review other intracellular mechanisms that mediate both sensitivity and resistance outcomes to anti-EGFR agents.

Keywords: Afatinib, Cancer, Cetuximab, Epidermal Growth Factor Receptor,

---

[*] **Corresponding author Rodney B. Luwor:** Department of Surgery, The Royal Melbourne Hospital, The University of Melbourne, Parkville, Victoria 3050, Australia; Tel: +613 8344 3027; Fax: +613 9347 6488; E-mail: rluwor@unimelb.edu.au

Atta-ur-Rahman (Ed.)

Erlotinib, Gefitinib, Lapatinib, Panitumumab, Resistance, Signaling, Therapeutics, Tumor.

1. INTRODUCTION

The HER or ErbB family consists of four members, the Epidermal Growth Factor Receptor (EGFR) (also referred to as ErbB1 or HER1) [1], HER2 (p185[Neu] or ErbB2) [2], HER3 (ErbB3) [3] and HER4 (ErbB4) [4] and is one of the most intensely studied, and targeted, receptor tyrosine kinase families. Inactive EGFR exists mainly in a "tethered" confirmation where extracellular domains II and IV associate intra-molecularly leading to an auto-inhibitory favoured state. This confirmation occludes the accessibility of the dimerization arm of the receptor (in domain II) and separates two regions in domain I and III involved in ligand binding. Upon ligand binding, the ligand binding regions of domain I and III are brought closer together and the EGFR converts into an extended confirmation resulting in a dis-association of the auto-inhibitory interaction of domain II and IV and exposure of the dimerization arm facilitating dimerization of the extracellular region [5 - 7].

In addition, the ligand induced extended confirmation of the EGFR instigates ATP binding to a lysine residue, (Lys-721), within the EGFR kinase domain [8]. This binding is a critical event required for rapid intrinsic tyrosine kinase activation and auto-phosphorylation of specific tyrosine residues in the intracellular domain of EGFR [9 - 12]. This auto-phosphorylation in turn results in a more open conformation permitting the access of cellular substrates to the tyrosine kinase domain [8, 13]. The phosphorylated tyrosines of the EGFR serve as high affinity docking sites for Src homology 2 (SH2) and phospho-tyrosine binding (PTB) domain containing signalling proteins [14, 15]. Mutational analysis has shown that the removal of the auto-phosphorylation sites has a severe effect on substrate binding if all five tyrosine sites are removed. However, when only one site is altered, the remaining auto-phosphorylated sites appear to be able to compensate for the loss of the tyrosine site [16]. Adding to the diversity of EGFR downstream signaling is the presence of other ligands including the neuregulin family that activate the EGFR indirectly by binding HER3 and HER4 and resulting in EGFR trans-phosphorylation by EGFR-HER3 or EGFR-HER4 dimerization [17, 18].

Furthermore, the EGFR can co-operate with many other non-ErbB family members receptors leading to increased diversity of signaling pathway activation downstream [19 - 30]. It is thought that each ligand within the ErbB family illicit a subtly distinct conformation between the two dimerizing receptors in the intracellular region, resulting in differential tyrosine phosphorylation profiles and unique sets of docking substrates, ultimately leading to distinct biological outcomes [31]. Proteins that directly bind the phosphorylated tyrosines of the EGFR through their SH2 domain include PLC-(, GAP, Grb2, and Crk [15, 32 - 34] whiles others such as Shc interact *via* their PTB domain [32]. HER2, HER3 and HER4 also contain areas in their intracellular region for SH2 domain containing proteins to bind [34]. However, each HER receptor displays a distinct set of C-terminal auto-phosphorylation sites resulting in the recruitment of a different set of substrates. The recruitment and activation of these molecules to the receptor in turn selectively activates downstream signaling networks which include the RAS-RAF-MAPK-ERK1/2 pathway, the PTEN regulated phosphatidylinositol 3-kinase (PI3-K)-Akt-mTOR pathway, Src-Signal transducer and activator of transcription (STAT) family members and the Phospholipase C gamma (PLCγ) signaling pathway [35] (Fig. **1**). In turn these signalling molecules interact with nuclear transcription factors and cytoskeletal proteins triggering gene transcription of many proteins involved in regulating a variety of cellular functions and changes in cell polarity and morphology [36, 37].

Furthermore, despite being originally recognised as a mechanism in which cells inactivate signalling by internalisation and degradation of activated receptors, EGFR signalling is sustained or initiated following receptor endocytosis and subsequent trafficking through early and late endosomes [38 - 40]. In addition, the EGFR (and the other HER family members) translocate into the nucleus where they are involved in direct gene transcription [41 - 47]. Finally, the presence of EGFR ligands, full length EGFR and the truncated variant EGFRvIII, that are all signaling competent have been discovered in secreted exosomes suggesting an inter-cellular role of EGFR signaling [48 - 50].

Not surprisingly, due to the EGFR's many associations at the cell membrane and the diverse network of signaling, and as outlined in our previous review (Part I of this series), EGFR activation is intimately associated with many cellular activities in both development and in the adult organism including proliferation, survival, differentiation, adhesion, migration and invasion and tumor metastasis.

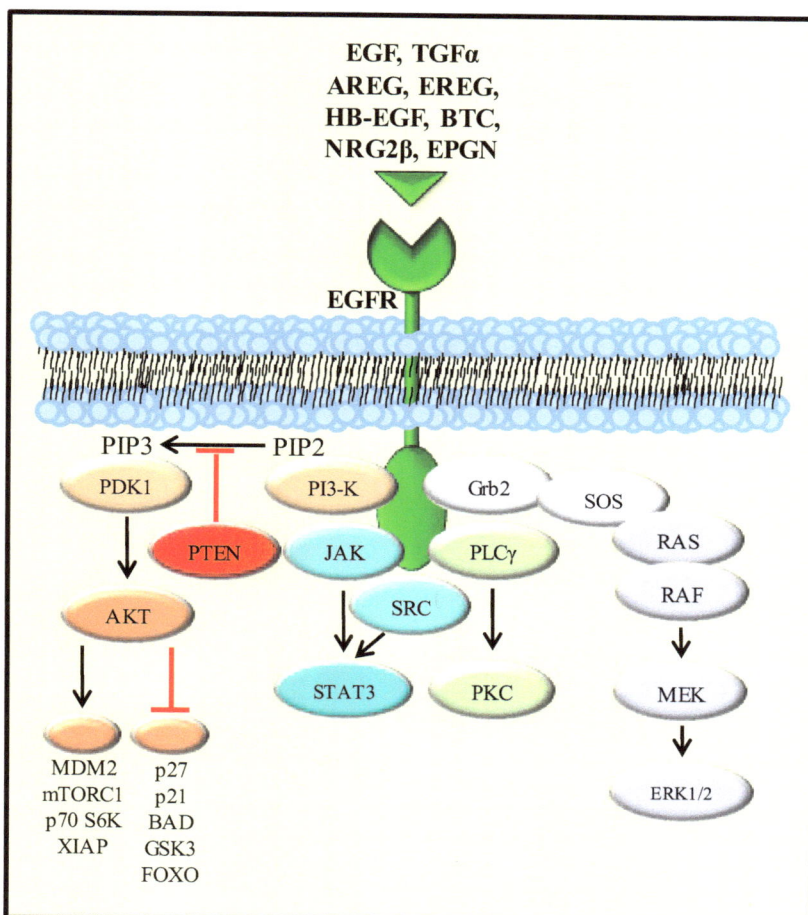

Fig. (1). Schematic of EGFR mediated signal transduction. The EGFR signals through several downstream signaling networks including the RAS/RAF, the PI3-K/AKT, PLCγ/PKC and the JAK/STAT3 pathways.

As such, several therapeutic agents directed against this receptor family have successfully entered clinical trials and have been FDA-approved for numerous cancer types (Summarised in Table **1**). Despite being commonly used clinically, therapy based around cetuximab, panitumumab, gefitinib, erlotinib, lapatinib and afatinib only results in moderate increases in overall survival of cancer patients.

The presence of pre-existing intrinsic resistance mechanisms and the ability of tumors to develop or acquire resistance to these inhibitors is common and occurs through several proposed mechanisms. Alterations in EGFR expression, copy number and mutations in both the ectodomain and the intracellular kinase domain have all been shown as potential mechanisms of resistance to anti-EGFR therapy in various cancer types. Differential expression and mutations in the other HER family members of ligands and receptors and alterative ligand and receptor signaling pathways have also been implicated in correlating with clinical response to anti-EGFR therapy. These mechanisms have all been comprehensively discussed in chapter I of this series of two reviews. In this review we will discuss the localisation of the EGFR as a potential mechanism of tumor cell resistance to anti-EGFR therapy including changes in endocytosis and nuclear localisation of the EGFR. We will also particularly highlight the current molecular mechanisms of tumor resistance to EGFR targeted therapy specifically focusing on intracellular substrates and pathways downstream of the EGFR and other alternative signaling molecules and discuss potential strategies to overcome this resistance.

Table 1. Clinically approved Anti-EGFR inhibitors.

EGFR Inhibitor	Class	Approved for treatment	Company
Cetuximab (Erbitux)	mAb	mCRC; SCCHN	Bristol-Myers Squibb and Eli Lilly and company
Panitumumab (Vectibix)	mAb	mCRC	Amgen Inc
Gefitinib (Iressa)	TKI	NSCLC	AstraZeneca
Erlotinib (Tarceva)	TKI	NSCLC	Genentech
Afatinib[a] (Gilotrif)	TKI	NSCLC	Boehringer Ingelheim Pharmaceuticals
Lapatinib[b] (Tykerb)	TKI	Breast	GlaxoSmithKline

[a]Afatinib targets EGFR, HER2 and HER4.
[b]Lapatinib is a dual EGFR, HER2 inhibitor.

2. INTRACELLULAR TRAFFICKING OF THE EGFR AND RESISTANCE TO ANTI-EGFR THERAPY

Endocytosis was widely accepted as one mechanism in which cells inactivate signalling by internalising and subsequently degrading activated receptors including the EGFR. However, internalisation of the EGFR is now regarded as an important and often essential step in progression of downstream receptor mediated signalling [39, 40, 51 - 54]. Changes in EGFR internalisation and nuclear localisation have also been implicated in the context of differential sensitivities to EGFR inhibitors.

The first pieces of evident that changes in EGFR intracellular localisation may affect the efficacy of anti-EGFR agents came from evaluating gefitinib on a series of NSCLC and epidermoid carcinoma cell lines *in vitro*. In this study by Ono and colleagues the cell sensitivity to gefitinib correlated to the speed of EGF-induced EGFR internalisation. In particular, the most sensitive cell line used in this study, PC-9 displayed rapid down-regulation of the EGFR whereas gefitinib-resistant cell lines displayed ineffective receptor internalisation [55]. A follow-up report by the same group later showed that this impaired down-regulation may involve an aberration in trafficking between the early and late endosomes [56]. More recently, it was shown that gefitinib reduced EGF-induced internalisation of the EGFR in gefitinib-sensitive NSCLC cell lines but did not in gefitinib-resistant cells suggesting that endocytosis of the EGFR is associated with reduced gefitinib efficacy [57]. Similarly, EGF-induced EGFR internalization in erlotinib-sensitive NSCLC and SCHNN cells was greater than that in erlotinib-resistant cells [58].

However, in direct contrast was the study by Kwak *et al.* who examined differences in EGFR internalisation between NSCLC cell lines with acquired resistance to gefitinib after long-term continuous exposure to gefitinib in culture with their gefitinib-sensitive parental NCI-H1650 counterparts [59]. In this study, the NCI-H1650-derived resistant cells demonstrated an enhanced EGFR internalisation compared to the gefitinib-sensitive parental cell line suggesting, as opposed to the above studies that increased EGFR internalisation may correlate with resistance to gefitinib [59]. Similarly, others have found that maintenance of EGFR at the cell surface may lead to increased gefitinib efficacy. Feng and colleagues examined the correlation of Sprouty2 expression, a protein known to increase EGFR expression on the cell membrane by regulating EGFR degradation with gefitinib efficacy in colon cancer cells. In this study, low sprouty2 expression correlated to low gefitinib efficacy while the sensitivity to gefitinib was increased after overexpression and decreased after sprouty2 knockdown [60].

Two papers from the same group also demonstrated that increased localisation of nuclear EGFR confers acquired resistance to gefitinib in other cancer cell lines. The first report, showed that acquired resistance to gefitinib following long-term culturing of A431, MDA-MB-231, BT474 and MDA-MB-468 cells in the presence of gefitinib resulted in resistant cells that displaying increased accumulation of nuclear EGFR compared to the corresponding parental gefitinib-sensitive cell lines [61]. Furthermore, the increased nuclear EGFR directly enhanced the transcriptional and protein expression of the breast cancer resistant protein (BCRP/ABCG2). Subsequently, the follow-up report found that gefitinib could only transiently inhibit EGFR activity in the gefitinib-resistant A431 cells due to a rapid efflux of gefitinib out of the cell through a BCRP dependent mechanism [62]. Interestingly, others have shown that BCRP transduced A431 cells conferred gefitinib resistance [63], while BCRP expression was detected in the recurrent tumor of a NSCLC patient who developed acquired resistance following initial response to gefitinib [64]. Thus, one may speculate that the observed nuclear EGFR dependent increase in BCRP expression results in reduced gefitinib activity by exporting gefitinib out of the cell membrane [61].

Importantly, a study by Furukawa and colleagues assessed the internalisation of the NSCLC EGFR TKI sensitizing mutation (del E746_A750) in comparison to wild type EGFR. EGF-induced endocytosis, ubiquitination and down-regulation of the exon 19 EGFR deletion mutation were all reduced compared to the wild-type EGFR [65]. This indicates that prolonged cell surface expression of the EGFR may mediate increased sensitivity to anti-EGFR therapy, although another common sensitizing EGFR mutation, L858R did not have the same impaired endocytosis profiles as the del E746_A750 mutation. Another group showed that greater association of EGFR in lipid rafts correlated with greater resistance to gefitinib in breast cancer cell lines [66], although it has been suggested that lipid rafts localisation is associated with signal transduction and not receptor internalisation or endocytosis [67]. Finally, another study directly compared a gefitinib-sensitive and a gefitinib-resistant breast cancer cell line and found that gefitinib significantly reduced nuclear NRG localisation in the gefitinib-sensitive SK-Br3 cell line but not in the gefitinib-resistant MDA-MB-468 cell line [68].

Others have identified an association of EGFR localisation with the efficacy of cetuximab. Wheeler and colleagues published a series of reports investigating the relationship of EGFR sub-cellular localisation with acquired resistance to cetuximab in H226 NSCLC cells. In their original paper, 6 stable cetuximab-resistant H226 sub-clones were generated *in vitro* following prolonged exposure to cetuximab [69]. All 6 resistant clones expressed increased EGFR levels compared to the cetuximab-sensitive H226 control. Subsequently, Wheeler and colleagues went on to find that cetuximab-resistant cells had impaired EGF-induced internalisation of the EGFR compared to the parental cell line and that this mechanism may contribute to the increased EGFR expression in the cetuximab-resistant cells. A subsequent study using these same resistant cells with impaired internalisation however showed that these resistant cells had enhanced nuclear EGFR expression compared to the parental cetuximab-sensitive cells [70]. How these cells displayed impaired EGFR internalisation yet greater nuclear localisation compared to the parental cells was not discussed and is thus open to interpretation. Nonetheless, this study went on to correlate EGFR expression in the nucleus with lack of cetuximab efficacy in not only acquired but *de novo* resistance. SCCHN cells that were sensitive to cetuximab *in vitro* contained less nuclear EGFR levels than cells that were refractory to cetuximab treatment. Furthermore, nuclear translocation of the EGFR in the H226 acquired resistant cells was dependent on src family kinase activity as blockade of this activity led to reduced nuclear accumulation and re-sensitization to cetuximab [70]. Similarly, another report by Lu and colleagues also showed that src family kinases may associate with EGFR in cetuximab-acquired resistance. In this report, cetuximab-resistant DiFi cells were generated from long-term exposure to cetuximab *in vitro*. Interestingly, however, these refractory cells displayed reduced EGFR expression through enhanced ubiquitination and EGFR down-regulation in direct contrast to that seen in H226 cells by Wheeler *et al.* [71].

The constitutively active EGFR variant, EGFRvIII has also been associated with resistance to anti-EGFR therapy in several cancer types as reviewed in part I of this series of two reviews. This variant tumor specific EGFR variant has also been shown to have impaired endocytosis and intracellular sorting to the lysosome and also translocates the nucleus [72, 73] allowing one to speculate that the EGFRvIII impaired internalisation (and enhanced signaling) may in part be one mechanism in which it mediates tumor resistance.

These laboratory studies indicate that EGFR cytoplasmic and nuclear expression may predict the efficacy of EGFR inhibitors. However, assessment of EGFR as a predictive biomarker for response to anti-EGFR therapy has been mainly performed evaluating overall staining intensity or positive *vs.* negative staining (*as discussed in Part I of this series of reviews*). Furthermore, these reports have yielded contradictory data with some studies suggesting that EGFR is a predictive biomarker of response while others have not. To date, no conclusive clinical study evaluating a possible correlation between intracellular or nuclear EGFR expression levels and tumor response and survival outcomes in patients has been performed and thus very little is known regarding the predictive value of EGFR sub-cellular localisation and response to anti-EGFR therapy. Importantly, evaluation of nuclear localisation of the EGFR should represent a surrogate biomarker of EGFR activity than overall EGFR expression and thus may be a better predictive marker for response to anti-EGFR therapy.

3. THE RAS/REF/MEK/ERK SIGNALING PATHWAY AND RESISTANCE TO ANTI-EGFR THERAPY

One of the most extensively study signaling networks in normal homeostasis, immune responses and cancer and other diseases is the RAS/RAF/MEK/ERK signaling pathway. This pathway is activated by many growth factor and cytokine receptors and aberrant signaling through either constitutively active mutations or upstream hyper-activation is very common in most cancers. In this section we specifically review the role of each of these molecules in affecting the efficacy of EGFR inhibitors across a range of cancer types.

3.1. Growth Factor Receptor-bound Protein 2 (Grb2)

Although Grb2 is the major adaptor molecule to the EGFR and a critical linking protein to the activation of RAS/RAF signaling [74], very little has been reported regarding an association of Grb2 with response to EGFR inhibitors. A recent article by Smith *et al.* used the proximity ligation assay to measure the interaction between EGFR and Grb2 [75]. In this study, intense EGFR:Grb2 association was seen in NSCLC cell lines with EGFR activating mutations but was low in cell lines with wild-type EGFR indicating that this association occurs through EGFR activation. This is important as similarly, to the evaluation of EGFR nuclear expression as reviewed above, EGFR-Grb2 association may also represent a better indication of the level of EGFR activity in a patient tumor and thus may be more predictive of response than overall EGFR expression. Smith and colleagues went on to show a correlation between EGFR:Grb2 association in 93 PDX models and cetuximab response in animal xenograft experiments. High EGFR:Grb2 association scores correlated with cetuximab response in a combined analysis of all cancer types. Finally, EGFR:Grb2 association in biopsy cores of 91 NSCLC patient treated with either gefitinib or erlotinib was assessed and correlated with improved OS, thus the level of EGFR:Grb2 signaling–associated complex may predict patients that are most likely to response to EGFR inhibitor–based therapies [75]. Supporting this hypothesis is an earlier report by Koizumi and co-workers who generated a gefitinib resistant NSCLC cell line PC9 after co-culturing parental PC9 cells with gefitinib. This resistant cell line displayed a marked reduction of both EGFR:Grb2 and EGFR:SOS association compared to the sensitive parental cell lines [76]. Similarly, differential association of Grb2 (and other adaptor molecules) with the resistance conferring EGFR T790M mutation was observed compared to the associations seen in cells expressing the EGFR TKI sensitizing EGFR mutation (delE746_A750) has been reported [77]. Thus, taken together these reports suggest in accordance to the study by Smith *et al.* that high EGFR:Grb2 (and perhaps other EGFR associations) may predict positive response to anti-EGFR treatment. Finally, the study by Hoeben and colleagues showed that SCCHN cells with reduced Grb2-associated binder 1 (GAB1) levels were more responsive to gefitinib [78].

3.2. RAS

3.2.1. The Role of K-RAS in Primary Resistance

Kirsten, Harvey and Neuroblastoma RAS are 3 members of the Ras superfamily of small guanine nucleotide-binding proteins [79 - 82]. The 3 Ras genes in humans (K-RAS, H-RAS and N-RAS) are amongst the most commonly mutated in cancer with up to 20-30% of all cancers expressing activating RAS mutations

[83, 84]. Approximately 85% of these mutations arise in the K-RAS gene with only 15% arising from N-RAS mutations and less than 1% from H-RAS mutations [84]. Just over a decade ago, an important review discussing resistance mediators to anti-EGFR therapy speculated that constitutively active downstream substrates of the EGFR could confer resistance in mCRC [85]. Shortly after, the landmark discovery that K-RAS mutations in mCRC conferred resistance to cetuximab was made. Along with the detection of EGFR sensitizing and resistance mutations in NSCLC (*discussed in our previous review*), K-RAS mutations in mCRC represents the most clinically advanced predictive biomarker in the EGFR inhibitor field and has dramatically changes the treatment rationale of mCRC patients worldwide.

Table 2. K-RAS mutations and response to EGFR inhibitors.

No of Patients[a]	Tumor type	Mutation status	Treatment[b]	Responders (%)	Study
30	mCRC	13 w mut[c]	Cetuximab	0 (0)	[86]
		17 w/o[d]	Cetuximab	11 (65)	
27	mCRC	10 w mut	Cetuximab	1 (10)	[246]
		17 w/o	Cetuximab	9 (53)	
59	mCRC	16 w mut	Cetuximab	0 (0)	[305]
		43 w/o	Cetuximab	12 (28)	
89	mCRC	24 w mut	Cetuximab	0 (0)	[306]
		65 w/o	Cetuximab	26 (40)	
80	mCRC	30 w mut	Cetuximab	0 (0)	[157]
		50 w/o	Cetuximab	5 (10)	
198	mCRC	81 w mut	Cetuximab	1 (1)	[87]
		117 w/o	Cetuximab	15 (13)	
80	mCRC	42 w mut	Cetuximab	4 (10)	[307]
		38 w/o	Cetuximab	10 (26)	
277	mCRC	105 w mut	Cetuximab	38 (36)	[308]
		172 w/o	Cetuximab	102 (59)	
113	mCRC	52 w mut	Cetuximab	17 (33)	[88]
		61 w/o	Cetuximab	37 (61)	
565	mCRC	220 w mut	Cetuximab	5 (2)	[96]
		345 w/o	Cetuximab	91 (26)	
61	mCRC	22 w mut	Cetuximab	1 (5)	[247]
		39 w/o	Cetuximab	18 (46)	
503	mCRC	299 w mut	Panitumumab	45 (15)	[93][e]
		204 w/o	Panitumumab	83 (41)	

(Table 2) contd.....

No of Patients[a]	Tumor type	Mutation status	Treatment[b]	Responders (%)	Study
21	mCRC	5 w mut	Cetuximab	0 (0)	[121]
		16 w/o	Cetuximab	6 (38)	
10	mCRC	5 w mut	Panitumumab	2 (40)	
		5 w/o	Panitumumab	2 (40)	
23	mCRC	6 w mut	Cetuximab	0 (0)	[122]
		17 w/o	Cetuximab	7 (41)	
25	mCRC	10 w mut	Panitumumab	1 (10)	
		15 w/o	Panitumumab	3 (20)	
62	mCRC	24 w mut	Panitumumab	0 (0)	[309]
		38 w/o	Panitumumab	4 (11)	
208	mCRC	84 w mut	Panitumumab	0 (0)	[310]
		124 w/o	Panitumumab	21 (17)	
62	mCRC	24 w mut	Panitumumab	0 (0)	[309]
		38 w/o	Panitumumab	4 (11)	
92	mCRC	32 w mut	Cetuximab	0 (0)	[191]
		60 w/o	Cetuximab	14 (23)	
92	mCRC	32 w mut	Cetuximab	0 (0)	[191]
		60 w/o	Cetuximab	14 (23)	
111	mCRC	55 w mut	Cetuximab[f]	2 (4)	[98][g]
		56 w/o	Cetuximab[f]	19 (34)	
98	NSCLC	13 w mut	Cetuximab	4 (31)	[103]
		85 w/o	Cetuximab	28 (33)	
199	NSCLC	38 w mut	Cetuximab	14 (37)	[104]
		161 w/o	Cetuximab	60 (37)	
39	NSCLC	17 w mut	Cetuximab	5 (29)	[105]
		22 w/o	Cetuximab	4 (18)	
24	Lung Adenocarcinoma	5 w mut	Gefitinib	0 (0)	[100]
		19 w/o	Gefitinib	12 (63)	
35	Lung Adenocarcinoma	4 w mut	Erlotinib	0 (0)	
		31 w/o	Erlotinib	9 (29)	
129	NSCLC	25 w mut	Erlotinib	2 (8)	[101]
		104 w/o	Erlotinib	27 (26)	
69	NSCLC	9 w mut	Gefitinib	0 (0)	[311]
		60 w/o	Gefitinib	16 (27)	
25	NSCLC	10 w mut	Erlotinib	0 (0)	[312]
		15 w/o	Erlotinib	4 (27)	
70	NSCLC	16 w mut	Gefitinib[h]	0 (0)	[313]
		54 w/o	Gefitinib[h]	7 (13)	
118	NSCLC	20 w mut	Erlotinib	1 (5)	[314]
		98 w/o	Erlotinib	10 (10)	

(Table 2) contd.....

No of Patients[a]	Tumor type	Mutation status	Treatment[b]	Responders (%)	Study
83	NSCLC	16 w mut 67 w/o	TKI[i] TKI[i]	0 (0) 11 (16)	[315][j]
3585[k]	-	1331 w mut 2253 w/o	-	143 (11) 687 (30)	-

[a]Number of Patients screened for K-RAS mutations, treated with EGFR inhibitor and assessed for clinical response.

[b]EGFR treatment may have also included chemotherapy

[c]w mut = with K-RAS mutation

[d]w/o = without K-RAS mutation

[e]Included mutational analysis of K-RAS and N-RAS

[f]Of the 111 patients originally included in this study, 108 were treated with cetuximab based therapy and 3 were treated with panitumumab.

[g]Mutational status based on Engineered Mutant-enriched PCR.

[h]Of the 73 patients originally included in this study, 72 were treated with gefitinib and 1 was treated with erlotinib

[i]Of the 83 patients originally included in this study, 28 were treated with gefitinib and 55 were treated with erlotinib.

[j]Mutation status based on direct sequencing data. Mutant-enriched sequencing was also performed and showed similar results.

[k]Totals of all trials (shaded in light blue).

This initial correlation of K-RAS mutation with lack of response to cetuximab in mCRC was originally discovered by Lievre and colleagues in 2006. In their study, 30 mCRC patients were treated with cetuximab monotherapy (n=1); cetuximab combined with irinotecan (n=25) or cetuximab combined with folinic acid, 5-fluorouracil and irinotecan (FOLFIRI; n=4). Retrospective analysis of K-RAS mutations revealed that patients with K-RAS mutations had a significantly poorer RR (0%; 0 out of 13 *vs.* 64.7%; 11 out of 17) and shorter OS (6.9 *vs.* 16.3 months) compared to patients with wt K-RAS expressing mCRC [86]. Following this study, a spate of retrospective studies reported similar findings to that of Lievre *et al.* observing that patients with mCRC that harboured K-RAS mutations consistently performed worst when treated with either cetuximab or panitumumab- based treatment (as summarised in Table **2**). These reports included a landmark study by Karapetis and colleagues who randomised chemo-refractory mCRC patients into cetuximab *versus* best supportive care groups and then retrospectively evaluated the association of K-RAS mutations with response and patient outcome [87]. In this study, cetuximab treated patients displayed a significantly longer median PFS (3.7 *vs.* 1.9 months) and OS (9.5 *vs.* 4.8 months) than those with best supportive care when comparing patients who expressed wt K-RAS only. However, cetuximab treatment did not provide any significant benefit compared to best supportive treatment in patients with K-RAS mutations. Furthermore, ORR in cetuximab patients with wt K-RAS was significantly better (12.8%; 15 out of 117 *vs.* 1.2%; 1 out of 81) than those treated with cetuximab with K-RAS mutations [87]. This large body of evidence clearly identifying K-RAS mutations as a consistent resistance biomarker for cetuximab and panitumumab in mCRC led the FDA in 2009 to issue guidelines for the prospective screening of mCRC patients for K-RAS status and to restrict EGFR mAb therapy to patients with mCRC expressing wt K-RAS only. The National Comprehensive Cancer Network and the European Society of Pathology also issued similar advice.

Further strengthening the advisability of these guidelines is evidence that cetuximab and panitumumab treatment is in fact detrimental to patients with K-RAS mutations. A phase II trial (OPUS) evaluating first-line therapy of cetuximab and folinic acid, fluorouracil and oxaliplatin (FOLFOX4) *vs.* FOLFOX4 alone, showed that the addition of cetuximab led to poorer median PFS (5.5 *vs.* 8.6 months) compared to patients treated with FOLFOX4 alone in the K-RAS mutated sub-population of patients [88]. Similarly, panitumumab plus FOLFOX4 produced worst PFS (7.3 *vs.* 8.7 months) and OS (15.5 *vs.* 18.7 months) compared to FOLFOX4 alone in patients with mCRC harbouring K-RAS mutations [89]. It should be noted however, that these findings presented by Douillard *et al.* included the observed additional K-RAS mutations outside of exon 2, that were not screened for in the other studies described above.

Indeed, other less common K-RAS mutations (and mutations in N-RAS) are also now routinely evaluated. The earlier studies by Lievre, Karapetis and others (Table **2**) only tested for the most common K-RAS mutations in codon 12 and 13, which are present in exon 2. In fact, the initial FDA guidelines to screen for K-RAS mutations specified the use of a K-RAS mutation kit (TheraScreen Assay) that only detected the most common mutations in codon 12 and 13. These codon 12 and 13 mutations are present in approximately 35-40% of all mCRC tumor tissue and represent approximately 98% of all K-RAS mutations in mCRC [90 - 92]. Nonetheless, the study by Douillard and colleagues highlighted the need to screen for additional K-RAS mutations. In this study, similarly to previous studies, evaluation of codon 12 and 13 K-RAS mutations in exon 2 were performed. In addition however, evaluation of mutations in K-RAS codon 61 (exon 3), codon 117 and 146 (exon 4) and N-RAS codons 12 and 13 (exon 2), codon 61 (exon 3) and codon 117 and 146 (exon 4) were also performed. Importantly, an additional 16.9% (108 out of 639) of patients with mCRC were shown to harbour RAS mutations outside of those seen in codon 12 and 13 of K-RAS and thus these patients would have been stratified into the wt K-RAS sub-group and received anti-EGFR mAb therapy if enrolled in a prospective study prior to the detection of other RAS mutations. Consistently, another recent study showed that 17.9% (107 out of 597) of mCRC patients with wt codon 12 and 13 KRAS, contained other K-RAS or N-RAS mutations [93]. Furthermore, Douillard and co-workers observed that the presence of RAS mutations overall (and not just codon 12 and 13 K-RAS mutations) predict a lack of response to panitumumab in mCRC patients. Another previous study also assessed whether additional RAS mutations were present and predictive in another large cohort of chemotherapy-refractory mCRC patients treated with cetuximab and irinotecan [94]. In this study, 747 primary tumor samples were assessed with 271 harbouring codon 12 and 13 K-RAS mutations and another 32 harbouring additional mutations. N-RAS mutations were also found in 2.6% (17 out of 644) mCRC samples. Overall, of the patients who were treated with cetuximab and chemotherapy and who were measured for response and expressed wt K-RAS displayed significantly better ORR (35.8%; 126 out of 352 *vs.* 6.7%; 17 out of 253) than those who harboured K-RAS mutations. These patients also had better median PFS (24 *vs.* 12 weeks) and OS (50 *vs.* 32 weeks) compared to patients with K-RAS mutations. Patients with the less-common codon 61 K-RAS mutation or N-RAS mutations also had poorer ORR compared to patients with wt K-RAS [94]. Another previous report has also showed that other K-RAS mutations can predict a lack of response to cetuximab based treatment [95]. Interestingly, in another report, patients with codon 13 K-RAS mutation G13D treated with cetuximab had longer median PFS (4.0 *vs.* 1.9 months) and OS (7.6 *vs.* 5.7 months) compared to patients with other K-RAS mutations which may explain why a small number of patient with K-RAS mutations respond to EGFR mAb therapy [96]. Similar findings in a subsequent study confirm these observations that not all K-RAS mutations confer refractory outcomes [97]. These findings taken together suggest greater stringency in screening for RAS mutation in order to select mCRC patients that are suitable for anti-EGFR therapy. Indeed, most recently, several associations and clinical societies worldwide have incorporated these findings into their guidelines with strong recommendations for the prospective screening of all RAS mutations prior to the commencement of anti-EGFR-based therapy. Prospective studies aimed to detect for the presence of all RAS mutations prior to the administration of cetuximab and panitumumab based treatment if suitable are ongoing. Improved and rapid screening methodology for K-RAS and N-RAS mutation detection is also vital to allow for the greatest possible accuracy in selecting patients that will respond to EGFR agents [98]. Finally, although the presence in infrequent K-RAS amplifications have also been detected in mCRC patient samples and correlate with lack of response to anti-EGFR targeted therapeutics [99].

Despite the progress made in discovering a consistent negative correlation with K-RAS mutations and response to EGFR mAbs in mCRC and the clear guidelines of use of these mAbs based on these findings, the first evaluation of K-RAS mutations as a resistance mediator was performed in the NSCLC setting focusing on EGFR TKIs (as summarised in Table **2**). The first such report was from Pao and colleagues who retrospectively evaluated 60 lung adenocarcinomas from patients with known responses to gefitinib or erlotinib either of these drugs for the presence of codon 12 and 13 K-RAS mutations. In this study, none of the 21 tumors that responded to either gefitinib or erlotinib contained K-RAS mutations, while 23.7% (9 out of 38) tumors that were refractory to gefitinib or erlotinib contained K-RAS mutations [100]. Another study published not long after the Pao report also showed similar findings [101]. In this study by Eberhard and colleagues, chemotherapy-naïve patients with locally advanced or metastatic (stage IIIB or IV) NSCLC were treated with first-line carboplatin and paclitaxel alone or in combination with erlotinib with retrospective analysis of codon 12 and 13 K-RAS mutations performed. Patients with wt K-RAS expressing tumors treated with erlotinib and chemotherapy displayed a significantly better ORR (26.0%; 27 out of 104 *vs.* 8.0%; 2 out of 25), TPP (5.3 *vs.* 3.4 months) and OS (12.1 *vs.* 4.4 months) compared to patients with K-RAS-mutant tumors treated with erlotinib and chemotherapy. In addition and as seen in mCRC patients when treated with EGFR mAbs, the addition of erlotinib to carboplatin and paclitaxel was detrimental to patients compared to carboplatin and paclitaxel alone in the K-RAS mutation sub-population of patients. Patients harbouring K-RAS mutations treated with erlotinib plus chemotherapy displayed worst median TTP (3.4 *vs.* 6.0 months) and OS (4.4 *vs.* 13.5 months) compared to those treated with chemotherapy alone [101]. Several other subsequent studies confirmed these observations (Table **2**). Based on these studies the National Comprehensive Cancer Network have also recommend (along with mCRC patients) that all NSCLC patients should be tested for K-RAS mutations prior to being considered as suitable candidates for EGFR TKI therapy [102].

However, surprisingly and unlike that seen in mCRC, K-RAS mutations did not predict response to cetuximab in NSCLC. In a study by Khambata-Ford and colleagues, advanced NSCLC patient tissue was retrospectively analysed for K-RAS mutations following cetuximab plus first-line taxane/carboplatin. There was no statistically significant difference between patients with wt K-RAS and those harbouring K-RAS mutations when assessing cetuximab-based treatment for ORR (32.9%; 28 out of 85 *vs.* 30.8%; 4 out of 13), PFS (5.1 *vs.* 5.6 months) and OS (9.7 *vs* 16.8 months) [103]. Similarly, another study found that advanced NSCLC patients with wt K-RAS treated with cetuximab combined with cisplatin and vinorelbine did not significantly differ in ORR (37.3%; 60 out of 161 *vs.* 36.8%; 14 out of 38), PFS (4.4 *vs.* 5.5 months) and OS (11.4 *vs.* 8.9 months) compared to those harbouring K-RAS mutations [104]. Finally, another study also showed no significant difference between ORR (18.2%; 4 out of 22 *vs.* 29.4%; 5 out of 17), median PFS (4 *vs.* 4 months) and OS (14 *vs.* 11 months) when comparing patients with K-RAS wt *versus* K-RAS mutations following treatment with cetuximab and taxane and carboplatin [105].

Others have shown predictive correlations between K-RAS mutations and lack of efficacy of anti-EGFR inhibitors in other tumor types including bronchioloalveolar carcinoma and oesophageal [106, 107]. However, no significant difference was seen between the disease-free or PFS and OS of wild-type or mutated K-Ras expressing pancreatic carcinoma patients treated with a combination of cetuximab and chemotherapy [108, 109]. In addition, the detection of K-RAS mutations are rare in some tumors types including SCCHN and thus offers little predictive value in selecting patients for EGFR inhibitor-based treatment [110 - 112]. Similarly, as H-RAS mutations are also rare in most cancer types, the predictive value of H-RAS mutations is limited, although some studies have identified it as a resistance marker to anti-EGFR therapy in the laboratory and in patient samples [113, 114]. Therefore, the detection of K-RAS and more recently and less commonly N-RAS mutations as a molecular biomarker for lack of response to anti-EGFR therapy currently only applies to guide the clinical treatment strategy of patients with mCRC and NSCLC.

3.2.2. The Role of K-RAS in Acquired Resistance

K-RAS mutations have also been identified as a mechanism of acquired resistance in mCRC. The role of K-RAS mutations in acquired resistance to anti-EGFR inhibitors was first reported by Bouchahda and colleagues who identified codon 12 and 13 K-RAS mutations in mCRC metachronous liver metastasis samples in one patient who had previously responded to cetuximab. The patient's primary tumor and synchronous metastases evaluated pre-treatment with cetuximab contained wt K-RAS [115]. Two ground-breaking studies published back to back in Nature in 2012 demonstrated that alterations in K-RAS were associated with acquired resistance of mCRC to cetuximab and panitumumab. The first study by Misale and colleagues initially examined differences in the DiFi and LIM1215 colon cancer cell lines with acquired resistance after long-term exposure to cetuximab compared to their EGFR inhibitor-sensitive parental cell lines. In this study, both DiFi and LIM1215 cells with acquired resistance obtain K-RAS mutations or amplification [116]. Interestingly, in depth analysis revealed that a very small percentage of parental cells contained either K-RAS amplification or point mutations suggesting that pre-existing cetuximab resistant cells may have contributed to the overall acquired resistance seen after co-culturing with cetuximab. In addition, subsequent experiments showed that resistance to cetuximab is also acquired through continued mutagenesis of K-RAS mutations under the pressure of cetuximab treatment. This acquisition of K-RAS mutations were confirmed in a subsequent study using additional colon cancer cell lines in which K-RAS and N-RAS amplification and/or mutations were seen in resistant cell lines compared to their parental counterparts [117].

Supporting these laboratory experiments were accompanying data showing that tumor biopsies taken post-cetuximab or panitumumab treatment contained K-RAS mutations and amplification which were not present in the pre-treated patient matched biopsies. Furthermore, and most importantly, K-RAS mutant alleles were detected in the plasma of patients post-treatment and were detected as early as 10 months prior to the radiological determination of disease progression [116]. Significantly, these data may represent a method of early detection of tumor recurrence superior to the current detection methods. N-RAS mutations were subsequently seen in circulating DNA from patients with acquired resistance in a subsequent report by the same authors [117]. Similar findings in the second Nature paper by Diaz and colleagues were reported, specifically examining the serum of panitumumab pre and post-treated patients for K-RAS mutations [118]. In this report circulating cell-free DNA from the serum of all 24 patients tested contained only wt K-RAS alleles. However, examination of serially acquired serum from these 24 patients post panitumumab treatment revealed that 9 patient sera contained K-RAS mutations. Furthermore, the detection of these mutations was found between 5 and 6 months following treatment. Importantly, and similarly to the study by Misale and co-workers, circulating mutant K-RAS was identified in serum samples collected prior to radiographic evidence of disease progression, again highlighting the potential use of this superior detection method in determining progression of disease [118]. Although not seen in all patients, the early detection of K-RAS amplification and mutations promises to be an important finding in potentially overcoming acquired resistance to inhibitors targeting the EGFR in the mCRC setting.

3.3. RAF

RAF kinases are a family of three (A-RAF, B-RAF and C-RAF) serine/threonine protein kinases that are downstream of RAS and play key roles in cell proliferation. B-RAF mutations are observed in approximately 50% of melanoma with the V600E mutation accounting for almost all [119]. The B-RAF V600E mutation is also reported in approximately 5-15% of mCRC [119, 120] and thus, it is logical that if activating mutations in RAS can confer resistance to anti-EGFR therapy, then similar mutations in the downstream RAF molecule should also. A series of retrospective reports have somewhat confirmed that the most prevalent

BRAF (V600E) mutation correlates with lack of response to both cetuximab and panitumumab in mCRC patients, although due to small BRAF mutation rates and small sample sizes meaningful predictive analysis was limited in some studies (Summarised in Table **3**). In an initial study by Moroni *et al.* the detection of B-RAF mutation did not correlate with patient response to panitumumab, although only one patient out of 31 was detected to harbour a B-RAF mutation [121]. Subsequently, the same group later confirmed these results observing that B-RAF mutations did not significantly associate with ORR to either cetuximab or panitumumab based therapy. However, this study by Benvenuti and colleagues observed that the presence of K-RAS and/or BRAF mutations was negatively associated with response [122]. Subsequent studies using larger sample sizes of patients such as the study by Di Nicolantonio and colleagues showed that the presence of B-RAF mutations did indeed correlate with lack of response to anti-EGFR mAbs. In this study, no mCRC patient that harboured the BRAF V600E mutation displayed response to either cetuximab or panitumumab (0%; 0 out of 11) compared to 32.4% (22 out of 68) of patients with wt B-RAF. In addition, patients harbouring B-RAF mutations had a shorter PFS and OS compared to patients with wt B-RAF [123]. Another study found similar results with B-RAF (V600E) mutations associated with poorer ORR (0%; 0 out of 5 *vs.* 47.3%; 52 out of 110), PFS (8.0 *vs.* 31.4 weeks) and OS (6.5 *vs.* 14.8 months) in patients with wt K-RAS mCRC treated with cetuximab based therapy [124]. Finally, a larger study by Tol and colleagues retrospectively analysed the presence of B-RAF mutations in mCRC patients who were treated with chemotherapy, bevacizumab and cetuximab combined therapy [125]. In this study, patients with mCRC harbouring B-RAF mutations (n=28) had a significantly shorter median PFS (6.6 *vs.* 10.4 months) and OS (15.2 *vs.* 21.5 months) compared to patients with wt B-RAF tumors (n=231) treated with chemotherapy, bevacizumab and cetuximab, although no difference in ORR was observed [125]. More recently, however, Rowland *et al.* undertook a systematic review and meta-analysis of 7 randomised controlled trials to evaluate whether B-RAF mutation was a definitive negative predictor for efficacy of anti-EGFR mAb therapy in mCRC [126]. Their data demonstrated that patients with B-RAF mutations (and wt K-RAS) did not perform significantly worst in PFS and OS when treated with cetuximab or panitumumab based regimens compared to patients with wt K-RAS and B-RAF. These findings allowed the authors to speculate that prospective analysis of B-RAF mutations to exclude patients from anti-EGFR mAb therapy remains inconclusive and should not be routinely performed in the absence of additional data [126]. Thus, based on these results one cannot conclude, based on inadequate evidence that there is a decreased benefit of EGFR based therapy for mCRC patients harbouring B-RAF mutations.

Table 3. B-RAF Mutations and response to EGFR inhibitors.

No of Patients[a]	Tumor type	Mutation status	Treatment[b]	Responders (%)	Study
15[c]	mCRC	6 w mut[d] 9 w/o[e]	Panitumumab Panitumumab	0 (0) 3 (33)	[122]
79	mCRC	4 w mut 75 w/o	Cetuximab Cetuximab	0 (0) 13 (73)	[307]
79	mCRC	11 w mut 68 w/o	Cetuximab[f] Cetuximab[f]	0 (0) 22 (32)	[123]
62	mCRC	4 w mut 58 w/o	Panitumumab Panitumumab	1 (25) 3 (5)	[309]
115	mCRC	5 w mut 110 w/o	Cetuximab Cetuximab	0 (0) 52 (47)	[124]
87	mCRC	13 w mut 74 w/o	Cetuximab Cetuximab	0 (0) 24 (32)	[95]
12	mCRC	2 w mut 10 w/o	Cetuximab Cetuximab	0 (0) 2 (20)	[316]
95	mCRC	11 w mut 84 w/o	Cetuximab[g] Cetuximab[g]	0 (0) 11 (13)	[193]
259	mCRC	28 w mut 231 w/o	Cetuximab Cetuximab	11 (39) 111 (48)	[125]
92	mCRC	9 w mut 83 w/o	Cetuximab Cetuximab	0 (0) 14 (17)	[191]
23	mCRC	2 w mut 21 w/o	Cetuximab Cetuximab	2 (100) 0 (0)	[182]
350	mCRC	24 w mut 326 w/o	Cetuximab Cetuximab	2 (8) 124 (38)	[94]
111	mCRC	9 w mut 102 w/o	Cetuximab[h] Cetuximab[h]	0 (0) 21 (21)	[98]
229	mCRC	22 w mut 207 w/o	Cetuximab Cetuximab	5 (23) 169 (82)	[127]
120	mCRC	13 w mut 107 w/o	Panitumumab Panitumumab	0 (0) 18 (17)	[129]

(Table 3) contd.....

No of Patients[a]	Tumor type	Mutation status	Treatment[b]	Responders (%)	Study
60	mCRC	3 w mut 57 w/o	Cetuximab Cetuximab	0 (0) 19 (33)	[317]
67	mCRC	12 w mut 55 w/o	Cetuximab Cetuximab	1 (8) 16 (29)	[190]
1855[i]	-	178 w mut 1677 w/o	-	22 (12) 622 (37)	-

[a]Number of Patients screened for B-RAF mutations, treated with EGFR inhibitor and assessed for clinical response.

[b]EGFR treatment may have also included chemotherapy

[c]only patients with K-RAS wt were included here

[d]w mut = with B-RAF mutation

[e]w/o = without B-RAF mutation

[f]Of the 79 patients originally included in this study, 63 were treated with cetuximab based therapy and 16 were treated with panitumumab.

[g]Of the 132 patients originally included in this study, 109 were treated with cetuximab based therapy and 23 were treated with panitumumab.

[h]Of the 111 patients originally included in this study, 108 were treated with cetuximab based therapy and 3 were treated with panitumumab.

[i]Totals of all trials (shaded in light blue).

Larger scale analysis have shown that B-RAF mutations predict poor survival rates irrespective of treatment used compared to patients with mCRC containing wt B-RAF [89, 127 - 131]. Furthermore, Douillard and colleagues found that patients with B-RAF mutations displayed similar PFS (6.1 *vs.* 5.4 months) and OS (10.5 *vs.* 9.2 months) when treated with panitumumab and FOLFOX4 *versus* FLOFOX4 alone, suggesting that the addition of panitumumab to chemotherapy did not produce any significant benefit to mCRC patients harbouring B-RAF mutations [89]. Similarly, patients with B-RAF mutations did not perform significantly better when treated with cetuximab and FOLFIRI compared to FOLFIRI alone, although a small increase in PFS (8.0 *vs.* 5.6 months) and OS (14.1 *vs.* 10.3 months) was observed [127]. Finally, Bokemeyer and colleagues evaluated B-RAF mutation status in patients from the CYSTRAL and OPUS trials combined and found in accordance to the above studies that cetuximab did not enhance survival of patients with B-RAF mutations when added to either FOLFIRI or FOLFOX4 compared to chemotherapy alone [128]. Similar results were obtained from a systematic review of meta-analysis findings evaluating B-RAF mutations in mCRC as a predictive biomarker for cetuximab or panitumumab response. In this study, Pietrantonio and colleagues assessed the benefit of first or second-line cetuximab or panitumumab treatment in a series of published phase II and III randomised trials involving a total of 463 mCRC [132]. Pietrantonio *et al.* concluded that the addition of cetuximab or panitumumab to standard therapy or best supportive care of patients with B-RAF mutations did not significantly improve ORR, PFS or OS.

The current literature examining B-RAF mutations in providing a resistance mechanism to anti-EGFR therapy in other tumor types is limited. Very few studies have evaluated B-RAF mutations outside the mCRC setting in regards to predictive value to EGFR based agents. Furthermore, the magnitude of B-RAF mutations is low in NSCLC [133 - 135], SCCHN [136] and other tumor types treated with anti-EGFR therapeutics [137], thus suggesting that B-RAF mutations may play only a limited role in generating refractory outcome to anti-EGFR agents in these clinical settings.

3.4. MAPK Extracellular Signal-regulated Kinase (MEK) and Extracellular Signal-regulated Kinase (ERK1/2)

Downstream from the intracellular substrates RAS and RAF is the mitogen activated protein kinase (MAPK) extracellular signal-regulated kinase (MEK) and extracellular signal-regulated kinase (ERK1/2). This pathway is generally activated through growth factor and cytokine receptor phosphorylation or through activating mutations of RAS or RAF. Activated MEK phosphorylates its only substrate ERK1/2 leading to dimerization, nuclear translocation and induction of target genes many of which are involved in cancer progression [138, 139]. The EGFR is well known to activate this pathway and as such inhibition of ERK1/2 is commonly evaluated as a surrogate marker for the efficacy of anti-EGFR agents [140, 141]. However, the evaluation of ERK1/2 activity as a predictive biomarker for tumor response to anti-EGFR therapy is somewhat limited compared to the body of research published on its upstream substrates RAS and RAF.

Nonetheless, several studies have identified increased ERK1/2 activation or mutations in MEK as potential mediators of resistance to EGFR targeted inhibitors. The study by Psyrri and colleagues evaluated the intratumoral expression of several potential biomarkers of response and patient outcome in a Phase II trial of operable stage II/IV SCCHN evaluating cetuximab and chemotherapy based treatment. Patients with higher ERK1/2 expression as detected by immunohistochemistry had superior PFS and OS than those with lower ERK1/2 expression [142]. Phosphorylated ERK1/2 was not evaluated in this study. However, a follow-up study by the same research team identified that activation of RAS and subsequent persistent ERK1/2 signaling led to cetuximab resistance in SCCHN cell lines [114], while another report showed similar findings in the A431 cell line [113]. Another study evaluated the level of several phosphorylated proteins with mCRC patient outcomes treated with cetuximab or panitumumab using a series of patient biopsies. In this study, increased levels of phosphorylated MEK1 were significantly associated with reduced median PFS (7.0 *vs.* 20.0 weeks) compared to patients with low MEK1 phosphorylation [143]. Others have also demonstrated that molecular alterations upstream leading to enhanced ERK1/2 activity result in reduced anti-EGFR agent efficacy [117, 144 - 149].

Amplification of ERK2 has also been identified as a possible mechanism of resistance to the third generation EGFR inhibitor, WZ4002 [150] in NSCLC [151]. A study by Ercan and colleagues generated WZ4002 resistance cells (designated WZR12) from a sub-clone of PC9 NSCLC cells which were generated previously to confer gefitinib resistance, (designated PC9GR4; that were WZ4002 sensitive). The WZ4002 resistant cells contain higher levels of both phosphorylated and total ERK2 than the PC9GR4 cells and ERK2 amplification as confirmed by FISH and qRT-PCR. Furthermore, upon examination of NSCLC tumor tissue, pre and post treatment of erlotinib developed drug resistance, Ercan *et al.* identified ERK1 amplification in one out of 21 post-treatment specimens that was not observed in the patient matched pre-treatment tumor [151]. Finally, a most recent study by Bertotti and colleagues aimed to evaluate potential mechanisms of resistance to cetuximab that had not yet been described in mCRC using patient derived xenograft models. A point mutation in the MAP2K1 gene (MEK1) was observed in one of these PDX's that had shown resistance to cetuximab [152]. However, whether these mutations or amplifications in the MAPK's is prevalent enough to warrant screening or targeted therapy are yet to be completely determined.

3.5. Dual-Specificity MAP Kinase Phosphatases (DUSPs)

Dual-specificity MAP kinase Phosphatases (DUSPs) also referred to as MKPs, are proteins that are capable of de-phosphorylating phospho-tyrosine and phospho-threonine residues on MAPKs [153, 154]. Thus not surprisingly, changes in DUSP expression and function and thereby alterations in the regulation of MEK and ERK activity have been identified as possible mechanisms for decreased cell sensitivity to EGFR inhibitors.

Baker and colleagues identified DUSP4 and DUSP6 genes associated with the disease control, ORR, and PFS of wt K-RAS mCRC patients treated with cetuximab in a large gene expression array. Increased expression of DUSP6 and subsequent reduced MAPK activity was associated with reduced likelihood of clinical benefit to cetuximab in this report [155]. Down-regulation of DUSP5 and 6 was also proposed as a mechanism of resistance to cetuximab in SCCHN cell lines [156]. Similarly, Khambata-Ford and colleagues identified high DUSP3 gene expression as a predictor for resistance to cetuximab when comparing disease control *versus* non-responding mCRC patients [157]. However in contrast, the paper by Kakiuchi *et al.* identified reduced DUSP3 levels in NSCLC patient tumor tissue that had disease progression compared to tissue from patients with response to gefitinib treatment suggesting that high MAPK activity results in reduced response to treatment. Whether the reduction of DUSP3 in these samples also resulted in enhanced MEK or ERK1/2 activity however was not performed [158]. Overall, despite a small number of articles suggesting DUSP expression as a possible biomarker for patient response, they have not been widely studied and recognised as a key resistance mediator to anti-EGFR therapy in any tumor type.

4. THE PI3-K SIGNALING PATHWAY AND RESISTANCE TO ANTI-EGFR THERAPY

Along with the RAS/RAF/ERK signaling pathway, the PI3-K/AKT pathway has been the most extensively studied signaling axis in normal cell homeostasis, cancer and other diseases. The first members of the PI3-K family were discovered in the 1980's [159, 160] and are now know to consist of 3 classes of lipid kinases that generally transduce intracellular signaling from many upstream receptors including the EGFR [161 - 164]. Class I PI3-K is further divided into 2 sub-divisions named class 1A and 1B with class 1A playing the most predominant role in cancer signaling. Class I PI3-Ks function as heterodimers consisting of one of four catalytic subunits (p110α, β, δ, γ) and a regulatory subunit (p85 or other splice variants) [165 - 167]. The regulatory subunit is responsible for recruiting the complex to phosphorylated upstream effectors at the plasma membrane where the catalytic subunit preferentially converts phosphatidylinositol-4,5-bisphosphate (PtdIns(4,5)P2 or PIP2) into phosphatidylinositol (3,4,5)-trisphosphate (PtdIns (3,4,5)P3 or PIP3) to trigger signaling transduction. PIP3 subsequently regulates the activity of many downstream molecules including PDK1, AKT, mTORC1, FOXO, BAD, GSK3 and FKHR [167 - 170] (Fig. **1**). The most studied regulatory of this pathway is the phosphatase and tensin homologue (PTEN; also named mutated in multiple advanced cancers 1 (MMAC1)) which can convert PIP3 back to PIP2 and thus directly inhibits PI3K/Akt activity [171 - 174]. Not surprisingly, mutations and dys-regulation of many of these molecules have been identified in many tumor types and have been implicated in providing resistance to anti-EGFR therapy. We will review the potential role each member of this signaling network plays in mediating resistance to EGFR inhibitors in turn below.

4.1. Phosphatidylinositol 3-kinase (PI3-K)

Although many studies have identified alterations to upstream receptor and non-receptor kinases that triggers enhanced PI3K/AKT signaling [175, 176] as discussed in Part 1 of our review series, we will not readdress this here. Instead we will focus on mutations to the PI3-K/AKT signaling axis that drive possible resistance outcomes to anti-EGFR therapies. Several studies have identified mutations in genes encoding the catalytic and regulatory subunits of PI3-K and have evaluated whether these mutations correlated with response to EGFR inhibitors (summarized in Table **4**). In particular, a mutation in the PIK3CA gene that encodes the p110α catalytic subunit has been identified in up to 10-32% of colorectal carcinoma patient tumor tissue [177 - 184]. No association was observed in two initial studies evaluating the correlation of PIK3CA mutations with anti-EGFR therapeutic response, although only a small number of samples were examined and a low level harboured PIK3CA mutations in these studies [86,

121]. Another study published by Perrone *et al.* found that 12.9% (4 out of 31) of patients contained PIK3CA mutations in there mCRC tumor. All 4 of these patients with PIK3CA mutations were non-responders to cetuximab, however the difference between partial responders and non-responders was not statistically significant. Another report also found no correlation with PIK3CA mutational status and patient outcome following cetuximab based treatments. In this study, Prenen and colleagues identified mutations in the PIK3CA gene in 11.5% (23 out of 200) of irinotecan-refractory mCRC patients who subsequently received cetuximab monotherapy or in combination with irinotecan. No correlation between the presence of a PIK3CA mutation and response to cetuximab was seen with 12.8% (5 out of 39) of patients who responded to cetuximab containing the PIK3CA mutations compared to 11.3% (18 out of 160) of patients who did not respond also containing PIK3CA mutations. Similarly, no significant difference was seen in median PFS (24 *vs.* 18 weeks) and OS (45 *vs.* 39 weeks) comparing patients with and without PIK3CA mutations [183]. Similarly, other studies also found no association between PIK3CA mutational status with PFS and OS in mCRC patients treated with cetuximab based treatment [184 - 186]. The study by Karapetis and colleagues also found that PIK3CA mutations were not predictive of benefit for cetuximab, across all patients tested or in the wt K-RAS only sub-group [187]. Finally, another study, utilising a very large number of advanced colorectal carcinomas specimens (n=1976) also found no correlation with PIK3CA mutations with ORR, PFS or OS following treatment with cetuximab-based therapy [188]. Firm conclusions for PIK3CA mutations as a potential predictive biomarker for panitumumab response could also not be made due to a small number of patients with mutations at PIK3CA in the PICCOLO study [189].

Table 4. PIK3CA mutations and response to EGFR inhibitors.

No of Patients[a]	Tumor type	Mutation status	Treatment[b]	Responders (%)	Study
21	mCRC	2 w mut[c]	Cetuximab	1 (50)	[121]
		19 w/o[d]	Cetuximab	5 (26)	
10	mCRC	1 w mut	Panitumumab	0 (0)	
		9 w/o	Panitumumab	4 (44)	
30	mCRC	2 w mut	Cetuximab	0 (0)	[86]
		28 w/o	Cetuximab	11 (39)	

(Table 4) contd.....

No of Patients[a]	Tumor type	Mutation status	Treatment[b]	Responders (%)	Study
62	mCRC	2 w mut 60 w/o	Panitumumab Panitumumab	0 (0) 4 (7)	[309]
199	mCRC	23 w mut 176 w/o	Cetuximab Cetuximab	5 (22) 33 (19)	[183]
31	mCRC	4 w mut 27 w/o	Cetuximab Cetuximab	0 (0) 10 (37)	[182]
95	mCRC	15 w mut 80 w/o	Cet or Pan[e] Cet or Pan[e]	0 (0) 22 (28)	[181]
42	mCRC	6 w mut 36 w/o	Cetuximab[f] Cetuximab[f]	0 (0) 12 (33)	[143]
111	mCRC	11 w mut 100 w/o	Cetuximab[g] Cetuximab[g]	0 (0) 21 (21)	[98]
67	mCRC	9 w mut 58 w/o	Cetuximab Cetuximab	1 (11) 16 (28)	[190]
43	mCRC	2 w mut 41 w/o	Cetuximab Cetuximab	0 (0) 10 (24)	[318]
60	mCRC	2 w mut 58 w/o	Cetuximab Cetuximab	0 (0) 19 (33)	[317]
25	NSCLC	1 w mut 24 w/o	Erlotinib Erlotinib	0 (0) 3 (13)	[312]
796[h]	-	80 w mut 716 w/o	-	7 (9) 170 (24)	-

[a]Number of Patients screened for PIK3CA mutations, treated with EGFR inhibitor and assessed for clinical response.

[b]EGFR treatment may have also included chemotherapy

[c]w mut = with PIK3CA mutation

[d]w/o = without PIK3CA mutation

[e]All 95 patients included in this study were treated with either cetuximab or panitumumab based therapy but the exact numbers of each was not clarified.

[f]Of the 42 patients originally included in this study, 41 were treated with cetuximab and 1 was treated with panitumumab.

[g]Of the 111 patients originally included in this study, 108 were treated with cetuximab based therapy and 3 were treated with panitumumab.

[h]Totals of all trials (shaded in light blue).

However, others have shown that PIK3CA mutations do correlate with mCRC patient response to cetuximab and panitumumab. The study by Sartore-Bianchi and colleagues observed that no mCRC patient with a PIK3CA mutation (0%; 0 out of 15) achieved ORR following treatment with either cetuximab or panitumumab while 27.5% (22 out of 80) of patients with wildtype PIK3CA produced OR. Furthermore, patients harbouring PIK3CA mutations had a worse PFS but not a worst OS compared to patients with tumors with wildtype PIK3CA. The study by Ulivi and colleagues also showed that PIK3CA mutations could predict mCRC patient outcomes and response to a cetuximab-based regimen. In this study, PIK3CA mutations significantly associated with poorer ORR (11.1%; 1 out of 9 *vs.* 27.6%; 16 out of 58), PFS (2.3 *vs.* 5.1 months) and OS (6.6 *vs.* 9.9 months) compared to patients with wt PIK3CA [190]. Another report also found that PIK3CA mutations in mCRC were significantly associated with shorter TTP but was not correlative with OS in a subset of K-RAS wt patients [186]. Similarly, a third study also found that PFS was significantly lower among mCRC patients whose tumors harboured PIK3CA mutations (2.5 *vs.* 3.9 months) compared to patients that contained wt PIK3CA. The presence of PIK3CA mutations did not however correlate with ORR or OS in this study [191]. Finally, a systematic review and meta-analysis also found that mutations in the PIK3CA gene significantly predicted poor ORR and shorter OS in mCRC patients [192].

The contradictory findings evaluating PIK3CA as a definitive biomarker for response to anti-EGFR mAbs in mCRC may be due to several possibilities. Firstly, analysis of PIK3CA mutations was performed in some of the studies above without assessing K-RAS and B-RAF mutations in conjunction. PIK3CA mutations can be found in the same tumor specimen as K-RAS or B-RAF mutations making evaluation of each of these molecules' specific role in EGFR agent efficacy difficult to interpret [94, 193]. In addition, De Roock and colleagues have shown that different point mutations in the PIK3CA gene lead to different response outcomes suggesting that further stratification based on these individual mutations and not overall mutations is required to better predict responders *versus* non-responders. Approximately 80% of PIK3CA mutations in CRCs are in either exon 9 or exon 20 with exon 9 mutations more common [94]. However, patients with PIK3CA exon 20 mutations are more likely to show lack of response to cetuximab compared to patients with PIK3CA exon 9 mutations, which display no significant effect on response. Furthermore, patients with PIK3CA exon 20 mutations had significantly shorter PFS and OS compared to patients with wildtype PIK3CA exon 20. However, PFS and OS of patients with PIK3CA exon 9 mutations compared to patients with wildtype or other mutations in PIK3CA were not significantly different [94, 183]. Yang and colleagues observed similar results to De Roock *et al.* In their study, they performed a systematic review with meta-analysis of a series of studies evaluating whether PIK3CA mutations could predict outcomes of patients with mCRC K-RAS wildtype tumors following treatment with cetuximab or panitumumab based therapy. In this study, PIK3CA exon 20 mutations were significantly associated with reduced ORR, shorter PFS, and worst OS compared to patients who had exon 20 wt PIK3CA. PIK3CA exon 9 mutations were not associated with any of these outcomes [194]. Another more recent meta-analysis found similar findings [195]. Finally, a most recent paper showed that PIK3CA mutations in exon 20 conferred resistance to anti-EGFR blockade in PDX models of mCRC [152]. However, other studies do not support these findings that mutations in exon 9 or 20 confer differences in anti-EGFR inhibitor efficacy [188, 196].

Furthermore, lack of response in patients expressing wt PIK3CA may still be due to over-active PI3K driven signaling due to loss of expression or function of PTEN. In this current review, we have attempted to separate individual biomarkers into separate sections, but it is clear that certain molecular mediators of resistance go hand in hand in driving the same pro-tumorigenic pathway such as PIK3CA activating mutations and loss of expression or function of PTEN. Indeed, several studies have assessed both these biomarkers together [197, 198] such as the study by Jhawer and colleagues. In this report, PIK3CA mutations were found in 8 of the 22 colon cancer cell lines examined, but PIK3CA mutation status alone did not distinguish cetuximab-sensitive from resistant cell lines. However, analysis of PTEN mutation or loss in these 22 cell lines and further classification revealed that PIK3CA mutant/PTEN null cell lines were significantly more refractory to cetuximab treatment than PIK3CA/PTEN wildtype cell lines [198]. Similar findings have revealed that combining patient sub-populations of patients with either PIK3CA mutations and PTEN loss correlated to clinical outcomes of HER2-positive metastatic breast cancer patients treated with trastuzumab and lapatinib and K-RAS mCRC patients treated with cetuximab or panitumumab [197, 199]. Nonetheless, we will assess PTEN in greater detail in the next section (section 4.2) and discuss the use of multiple markers in combination is section 5.

The PIK3CA mutations have also been evaluated as a predictive marker for tumor response to EGFR inhibitors in other tumor types with mixed conclusions. Laboratory based studies have been performed to assess the role of PIK3CA mutations in resistance to anti-EGFR therapy. In one study, two of the 8 SCCHN cell lines with PIK3CA mutations were refractory to gefitinib treatment *in vitro* [200]. Another study showed that PIK3CA mutations in breast cancer cell lines also confer resistance to lapatinib [201]. Finally, another report showed that the introduction of a PIK3CA mutation into a NSCLC cell line led to increased resistance to gefitinib [202]. A very recent report indicated that PIK3CA mutations predict poor response to cisplatin-based chemo-radiotherapy in combination with cetuximab treatment in the cervical cancer setting. This study by de la Rochefordiere and colleagues showed that no patient harbouring a PIK3CA mutation had complete responses and showed a trend toward poorer disease-free survival [203]. Another report evaluated the efficacy of panitumumab added to epirubicin, oxaliplatin and capecitabine in untreated advanced oesophagogastric adenocarcinoma. In this study, PIK3CA mutations (or K-RAS, B-RAF and loss of PTEN expression) did not predict resistance to the panitumumab based therapy, although only a small number of patients harboured a PIK3CA mutation (4.9%; 4 out of 81) [204]. Low numbers of NSCLC patients with PIK3CA mutations has also hindered the ability to truly evaluate whether this biomarker can predict response to EGFR inhibitors. In the study by Bria and colleagues next generation sequencing was used to assess the mutational status of 22 genes in poor, intermediate and good responders to first-line gefitinib treatment. Although the only PIK3CA mutation found was from a poor responder only 12 NSCLC samples were used limiting the ability to formulate definitive conclusions in this study [205]. In contrast, the two (out of 78) patients found to contain PIK3CA mutations in their NSCLC tumors had partial responses gefitinib in another study [206]. Similarly, patients with biliary tract cancers containing PIK3CA mutations did not significantly show reduced PFS or OS compared to patients with wt PIK3CA following treatment with erlotinib combined with gemcitabine and oxaliplatin [207]. The study by Jimeno *et al.* also evaluated the mutational status of PIK3CA in several PDX *in vivo* models originally surgically resected from pancreatic patients. Unexpectedly, one of the two sensitive tumors to cetuximab or erlotinib treatment contained a PIK3CA mutation indicating that this mutation did not mediate resistance in this particular tumor [208].

The role of PIK3CA mutations have also been extensively studied in the breast cancer setting when evaluating the efficacy of lapatinib and trastuzumab based treatment regimens. The expression of HER2 and PIK3CA mutations in a breast cancer animal model clearly resulted in enhanced tumor growth, metastasis and resistance to lapatinib and trastuzumab combinational therapy [209]. A phase II clinical trial also identify that HER2-positive breast cancer patients with PIK3CA mutations were less likely to benefit from dual treatment with lapatinib and trastuzumab [210]. Similarly, another group also reported that HER2-positive breast cancer patients performed better if their tumors expressed wildtype PIK3CA. In this study, Majewski and colleagues evaluated the possible correlation of PIK3CA mutational status with patient outcomes in 355 patients with HER2-positive breast cancer who were treated with neoadjuvant lapatinib and/or trastuzumab. Importantly, PIK3CA mutations, which were identified in 22.5% (80 out of 355) of these patient tumors, associated with reduced pathological complete responses in patients treated with lapatinib alone (14.8%; 4 out of 27 *vs*. 20.4%; 19 out of 93) or in combination with trastuzumab (28.6%; 8 out of 28 *vs*. 55.8%; 48 out of 86) compared to patients with wt PIK3CA. However there was no significant correlation with PIK3CA mutations and event-free survival and OS [211]. Consistently with the above reports, others have found a correlation between PIK3CA mutations and pathological complete response in HER2 positive breast cancer patients treated with the combination of lapatinib, trastuzumab and anthracycline-taxane chemotherapy. The pathological complete responses for the patients with PIK3CA mutations were (37.1% *vs*. 17.4%) compared to patients with wildtype PIK3CA. Similarly, to the study by Majewski *et al*. PIK3CA mutational status did not significantly correlate with patient disease-free survival and OS [212]. Others found that the addition of lapatinib to paclitaxel also improved the ORR and reduced the overall TTP compared to patients treated with paclitaxel alone in the subset of HER2-positive metastatic breast cancer patients who had PIK3CA wildtype expressing tumors. These differences were not seen in the patients harbouring tumors with PIK3CA mutations [213]. However, another study showed no correlation between PIK3CA mutations and pathological complete response in HER2 positive breast cancer patients treated with the combination of afatinib, trastuzumab and chemotherapy [214]. While another study found that the probability of achieving a clinical response was significantly higher in patients with hormone receptor-positive, HER2-negative operable breast cancer that expressed PIK3CA mutations compared to those who were wildtype for PIK3CA when treated with lapatinib and letrozole [215]. Another report identified that PIK3CA gene copy number did not influence PFS or OS of patients with NSCLC following gefitinib treatment. However, patients with tumors that contained increased chromosome 7 copy number, increased PIK3CA GCN and PTEN loss had significantly lower PFS (2.0 vs. 4.2 months) and OS (4.3 vs. 12.3 months) compared to patients without these combined alterations [216].

Although quite rare in occurrence, the PIK3CA gene has also been somewhat implicated in mediating acquired mCRC resistance to cetuximab. In a study by Arena *et al.* genetic mutations were assessed in pre and post cetuximab treated mCRC patient-matched biopsies. In the 37 patient-matched biopsies analysed 3 contained PIK3CA mutations in both the pre and post-treated samples while 3 others acquired PIK3CA mutations in the post cetuximab treated specimens that were not present in the patient matched pre-treated biopsy. The authors also continued to generate colon cancer cell lines with acquired resistance to cetuximab following long-term culturing in the presence of cetuximab. None of the acquired cetuximab resistant cell lines however contained newly acquired PIK3CA mutations post cetuximab treatment, although the NCIH508 acquired resistant sub-cell line retained a PIK3CA exon 9 mutation which was present in the parental cell line prior to cetuximab exposure [217]. Likewise, another study evaluated 37 NSCLC patient matched biopsies pre and post either gefitinib or erlotinib treatment. This report by Sequist detected the PIK3CA mutation in 5.4% (2 out of 37) of patient biopsies post treatment, which was not present in the pre-treated biopsy. Interestingly, both these patients were treated with erlotinib [218]. Similarly, Ji and colleagues reported the detection of an acquired PIK3CA mutation following gefitinib treatment in one NSCLC patient (out of 27 examined) [219], however Yu and co-workers did not detect any PIK3CA mutations in NSCLC patient biopsies taken post gefitinib or erlotinib treatment after the acquired resistance was observed [220]. Recently, a novel somatic mutation in the PI3K p110β isoform (PIK3Cβ^{D1067V}) was identified and was shown to promote PI3K pathway signaling and tumor formation *in vivo*. This mutation was originally identified in an erlotinib-post treated biopsy of a NSCLC patient who initially responded to erlotinib but subsequently developed resistance. The PIK3Cβ^{D1067V} mutation was not seen in the pre-treated biopsy of this patient suggesting that this novel somatic mutation may have at least in part mediated the acquired resistance to erlotinib observed clinically in this patient [221].

Despite some evidence for the causative role of PIK3CA mutations and enhanced PI3K signaling in providing resistance to anti-EGFR therapy, there are no recommended guidelines currently issued to screen for activating PI3-K signaling as a biomarker for exclusion of EGFR inhibitors in the clinical management of patients with tumors of any setting.

Mutations in AKT1 such as the activating somatic mutation E17K have been identified in several cancers including CRC [222]. A recent study subsequently indicated that mCRC patients with biopsies expressing this mutation were refractory to cetuximab treatment [223]. However, the AKT1 E17K mutation was detected in less than 1% of all mCRC patients examined [223] and thus its rarity inhibits the likelihood of any predictive value for response to anti-EGFR therapy.

4.2. PTEN

As mentioned in the previous section, several studies have reported the level of alterations in PI3-K signaling including activated PIK3CA mutations and PTEN loss in combination as a possible mechanism of resistance to EGFR targeted therapy. However, in this section we will address the role of PTEN in driving resistance to anti-EGFR therapy as a single molecule in isolation of PIK3CA mutations. The first pieces of evidence that PTEN loss may be important in the efficacy of anti-EGFR inhibitors were derived from cell line studies published over a decade ago. In two independent studies both published in 2003, Bianco and colleagues and She *et al.* both showed that the PTEN-null breast cancer cell line MDA-MB-468 was refractory to gefitinib despite the fact that gefitinib could successfully reduce EGFR phosphorylation. Both studies went on to show that the exogenous introduction of PTEN back into these cells led to a dramatic re-sensitization of gefitinib inhibition and subsequent reduced AKT phosphorylation [224, 225]. Similar results have been reported in various tumor cell models observing a key role of PTEN loss in driving resistance to other EGFR inhibitors [226 - 236]. Many studies have evaluated patient tumor tissue for PTEN loss and potential correlation with response to anti-EGFR inhibitors (as summarised in Table **5**).

Table 5. PTEN loss and response to EGFR inhibitors.

No of Patients[a]	Tumor type	Mutation status	Treatment[b]	Responders (%)	Study
59	Glioblastoma	30 neg[c] 29 pos[d]	Gef or Erl Gef or Erl	3 (10) 12 (41)	[237]
37	Glioblastoma	14 neg 23 pos	Erlotinib Erlotinib	0 (0) 3 (13)	[244]
27	mCRC	11 neg 16 pos	Cetuximab Cetuximab	0 (0) 10 (63)	[246]
66	mCRC	23 neg 43 pos	Cetuximab Cetuximab	3 (13) 18 (44)	[250]
81	mCRC	32 neg 49 pos	Cet or Pan[e] Cet or Pan[e]	1 (3) 17 (35)	[181]
85 55	mCRC (primary) mCRC (mets)	36 neg 49 pos 22 neg 33 pos	Cetuximab Cetuximab Cetuximab Cetuximab	4 (11) 11 (22) 1 (5) 12 (36)	[248]
15	mCRC	4 neg 11 pos	Cetuximab Cetuximab	0 (0) 5 (45)	[182]
111	mCRC	89 neg 22 pos	Cetuximab[f] Cetuximab[f]	41 (46) 10 (22)	[124]
61	mCRC	24 neg 37 pos	Cetuximab Cetuximab	1 (4) 18 (49)	[247]
43 24	mCRC (primary) mCRC (mets)	5 neg 38 pos 4 neg 20 pos	Cetuximab Cetuximab Cetuximab Cetuximab	1 (20) 21 (55) 0 (0) 14 (60)	[249][g]
145 139	mCRC (FISH) mCRC (IHC)	24 neg 121 pos 80 neg 59 pos	Cetuximab Cetuximab Cetuximab Cetuximab	5 (21) 25 (21) 19 (24) 9 (15)	[251]
38	Breast	29 neg 9 pos	Lapatinib Lapatinib	11 (38) 4 (44)	[262]

(Table 5) contd.....

No of Patients[a]	Tumor type	Mutation status	Treatment[b]	Responders (%)	Study
986[h]	-	427 neg 559 pos	-	90 (21) 189 (34)	-

[a]Number of Patients screened for PTEN expression, treated with EGFR inhibitor and assessed for clinical response.

[b]EGFR treatment may have also included chemotherapy

[c]neg = negative/loss or low levels of PTEN expression

[d]pos = positive or high levels of PTEN expression

[e]All 70 patients included in this study were treated with either cetuximab or panitumumab based therapy but the exact numbers of each was not clarified.

[f]Of the 111 patients originally included in this study, 108 were treated with cetuximab based therapy and 3 were treated with panitumumab.

[g]This study classified patients that showed partial response and stable disease as responders.

[h]Totals of all trials (shaded in light blue).

One of the first studies to identify PTEN loss as a potential predictor of response to EGFR targeted therapy clinically was from a trial by Mellinghoff and colleagues evaluating the efficacy of gefitinib or erlotinib in patients with recurrent glioblastoma. Of the 59 patients evaluated for response, 80.0% (12 out of 15) of responders displayed positive PTEN expression in their tumors by immunohistochemistry. In contrast only 15.9% (7 out of 44) of non-responders contained intratumoral PTEN expression. Interestingly, the predictive value of PTEN expression as a biomarker for response to gefitinib or erlotinib in glioblastoma was increased when co-expressed with the tumor specific truncated EGFR variant, EGFRvIII [237]. Untilising samples from the study by Mellinghoff described above, a subsequent study identified a novel PI3-K regulating independent mechanism of PTEN-mediated resistance to EGFR targeted therapy in glioblastoma. In this study by Fenton and colleagues, phosphorylation of PTEN on residue 240 was associated with reduced response to gefitinib and erlotinib. Furthermore, PTEN pY240 levels were found to be initially low in the tumors of two patients that originally responded to the anti-EGFR treatment but were significantly higher in levels in patient matched tumors post the acquisition of resistance to therapy [238]. However, several studies have observed contrasting findings showing that PTEN loss had no significant association with response and patient survival outcomes following anti-EGFR therapy in the glioblastoma setting [239 - 245]. Therefore, in summary, the role of PTEN expression as a predictive biomarker for glioblastoma patient responsiveness to EGFR targeted therapy is still unclear.

Evaluation of a possible correlation between PTEN expression and cetuximab efficacy in the mCRC setting has also been explored. In a study by Frattini and colleagues, PTEN protein expression was determined by immunohistochemistry in biopsies taken from 27 mCRC patients who were treated with cetuximab-based therapy. Strikingly, of the 16 patients who were positive for PTEN expression, 62.5% (10 out of 16) had an OR compared to 0% (0 out of 11) of patients who scored negative for PTEN expression [246]. The study by Sartore-Bianchi and colleagues also observed a significant association between PTEN expression and improved ORR (35.4%; 17 out of 48 *vs.* 3.1%; 1 out of 32), PFS and OS compared to patients with PTEN loss [181]. Li *et al.* also confirmed these findings in another cohort of mCRC patients [247]. Similarly, two systematic reviews with meta-analysis also established that PTEN loss or mutations significantly predicted reduced ORR, decreased PFS and poorer OS in patients with K-RAS wt mCRC compared to those with positive PTEN expression [192, 194].

The study by Loupakis assessed PTEN expression in biopsies of mCRC patients that were treated with cetuximab plus irinotecan taken from both primary and metastatic lesions. In this study, PTEN expression status in the primary tumors (n=85) as measured by immunohistochemistry did not significantly correlate with ORR, PFS and OS. However, when PTEN expression was analysed in metastatic samples, it was revealed that 36.4% (12 out of 33) of patients with PTEN positive metastatic tumors responded, while only 4.5% (1 out of 22) of patients with PTEN negative metastatic tumors responded. Furthermore, the median PFS in patients who had PTEN positive metastases was significantly longer than those who has PTEN-negative metastatic tumors (4.7 *vs.* 3.3 months), although no significant difference was seen in OS for these two patient sub-groups [248]. The study by Negri and colleagues also supports the findings by Loupakis and co-workers, suggesting that PTEN expression status in metastatic but not primary tumor lesions predicts response to cetuximab in mCRC patients. Patients with metastatic lesions containing PTEN loss as determined by immunofluorescence all showed progressive disease (100%; 4 out of 4) compared to only 30% (6 out of 20) of patients with PTEN-positive metastatic tumors. These patients with PTEN loss in their metastatic sites also showed a significantly worse ORR. However, similarly to Loupakis *et al.* no significant association was observed between PTEN loss in the primary tumor and response to cetuximab [249].

Another study however, failed to observe any significant difference in the ORR and TTP of mCRC patients with or without PTEN expression as determined by immunohistochemistry. Interestingly, FISH analysis of the same patient cohort did however identify those patients with wildtype PTEN were more likely to response and had a significantly longer TTP following cetuximab treatment compared to patients that has PTEN deletions [250]. Similarly, Perrone *et al.* evaluated PTEN expression by FISH in biopsies of 31 mCRC patients treated with cetuximab. Although they findings were not-significant, Perrone and colleagues found that patients with increased PTEN GCN were more likely to response as they observed that the 4 patients with decreased PTEN GCN were all non-responders [182]. Razis *et al.* determined PTEN expression or deletion status by immunohistochemistry and FISH and found that both detection methods showed that PTEN loss of expression and deletion did not significantly associate with ORR or TTP following treatment with cetuximab [251]. Finally, Saridaki also failed to find any significant association between PTEN expression and TTP and OS in another cohort of mCRC patients treated with cetuximab-based therapy [186]. Interestingly, patients with metastatic castration-resistant prostate cancer displayed significantly better PFS when expressing high levels of the EGFR and persistent PTEN activity [252]. Re-introduction of PTEN into PTEN-null prostate cancer cell lines also restored cetuximab or gefitinib sensitivity [253 - 255]. However, PTEN loss did not predict response to panitumumab when added to epirubicin, oxaliplatin and capecitabine in untreated advanced oesophagogastric adenocarcinoma, or undifferentiated carcinoma patients [204].

Loss of PTEN expression or function has also been proposed as a mechanism of resistance to EGR TKI treatment. Endoh and colleagues examined several potential biomarkers for survival outcomes in lung cancer patients treated with gefitinib. In this study, they found that within the subset of patients with gefitinib sensitizing EGFR mutations, those that also expressed high levels of PTEN had greater survival times compared to those that did not [206]. A more recent study evaluated the PTEN status by immunohistochemistry in 51 NSCLC patient tumor samples and found that PTEN expression negatively correlated with response to

EGFR TKIs. Higher PTEN expression also correlated with longer OS in TKI treated patients compared with patients with lower PTEN expression. Furthermore, this study by Shen and colleagues went on to show that the expression levels of miR-21, a direct regulator of PTEN expression was inversely proportional to the PTEN expression seen in these patients and thus increased miR-21 expression significantly correlated with poorer response and OS of these patients [256]. Similarly, miR-21 was shown by another group to be over-expressed in a NSCLC cell line with acquired resistance to gefitinib compared to its gefitinib-sensitive parental counterpart. In addition, miR-21 expression was significantly greater in the serum of NSCLC patients taken following gefitinib treatment and disease progression compared to the patient matched serum pre-treatment suggesting that miR-21 levels may be potentially tested for as a biomarker for acquired resistant. PTEN expression levels however, in these patients pre- and post-treatment were not reported [257]. Other studies also report that miR-214 regulates acquired resistance to gefitinib *via* a PTEN/AKT Pathway in a NSCLC cell line, while miR-217 regulates PTEN expression and breast cancer cell sensitivity to lapatinib [258, 259]. Similarly, the gefitinib-sensitive PC-9 NSCLC was shown to have significantly greater PTEN expression compared to the PC-9 gefitinib-refractory sub cell line following the acquisition of resistance after 7 months of co-culturing in the presence of gefitinib [260]. However, the study by Somlo *et al.* evaluated the combination of gefitinib, trastuzumab, and docetaxel in HER2-overexpressing metastatic breast cancer patients and found no statistically significant correlation with PTEN expression and patient response [261].

Contradictory outcomes have also been determined when assessing PTEN as a potential biomarker for lapatinib response. In a study by Dave and colleagues, PTEN expression was assessed as a possible predictive indicator of response and resistance in the pre-treatment specimens of HER2 over-expressing breast cancer patients treated with lapatinib. Distinct from the findings described in the reports above, patients with low levels of PTEN expression as detected by immunohistochemistry achieved a significantly better overall pathological complete response compared to patients with normal, suggesting that low PTEN expression predicted lapatinib sensitivity [262]. In complete contrast, PTEN expression status did not significantly predict total pathological complete response, event-free survival and OS in HER2-positive breast cancer patients treated with trastuzumab and lapatinib-based therapies in a more recent clinical study [263]. Similarly, PTEN expression status did not significantly correlate with response to lapatinib treatment in HER2 over-expressing inflammatory breast cancer patients [264]. Laboratory based research using breast cancer cell lines and HER2/neu-overexpressing PTEN homozygous loss (PTEN$^{-/-}$) NIC mice have also shown that loss of PTEN function is not associated with breast cancer cell resistance to lapatinib, although another study suggests otherwise showing that PTEN knockdown resulted in enhanced lapatinib resistance [201, 264 - 266].

Overall, clear disparities lie between the findings of many reports evaluating the possible role of PTEN as a predictive indicator of response to anti-EGFR agents across many tumor types. These inconsistencies in the predictive value of PTEN expression (and loss of function mutations) highlights the requirement of standardise methodology and the evaluation of larger prospective clinical trials utilising standardised techniques to conclusive determine whether PTEN status can guide the suitability of anti-EGFR inhibitors.

5. ANALYSIS OF SEVERAL BIOMARKERS IN COMBINATION AND RESISTANCE TO ANTI-EGFR THERAPY

As described in section 3.2 of this review, K-RAS mutations are currently the only intracellular biomarker that is used to assist in selecting patients that are less likely to benefit from anti-EGFR based cancer management. Indeed in 2013 the Evaluation of Genomic Applications in Practice and Prevention (EGAPP) Working Group (EWG) found convincing evidence for the association of K-RAS mutations with response to anti-EGFR treatment but insufficient evidence to recommend for or against BRAF V600E, N-RAS, PIK3CA mutations and/or loss of expression of PTEN or AKT testing [267].

However, over the last decade, several studies have evaluated the possibility of evaluating alterations/mutations in several intracellular molecules in combination with the aim to increase stringently of selection of patient sub-populations further improving the likelihood of accurately treating only "responders" with EGFR inhibitors. One of the first to do such was the landmark paper by De Roock and colleagues who evaluated the predictive value of the "quadruple negative" (K-RAS, N-RAS, B-RAF and PIK3CA exon 20) set of mutations expressed in mCRC *versus* tumors with wildtype expression of all 4 [94]. In this study mCRC patients were treated with cetuximab based treatment and assessed for ORR, PFS and OS. ORR was observed in 24.4% of the total population of patients prior to assessment of mutational status. However, when patients harbouring at least one of K-RAS, B-RAF, PIK3CA (exon 20) and N-RAS mutations were excluded retrospectively, the ORR was increased to 41.2%. Thus the authors concluded that patients should be screened for K-RAS mutations initially, then those with wildtype K-RAS be subsequently assessed for B-RAF, N-RAS and PIK3CA exon 20 mutations in that order and any patient with mutations in any of these 4 molecules be excluded from cetuximab or panitumumab treatment. Disappointingly however is that 58.8% of mCRC patients with wt K-RAS, B-RAF, PIK3CA and N-RAS from this study were still unresponsive to cetuximab suggesting other mechanisms of resistance [94]. Another study, observed similar findings when evaluating the correlation between the mutational status of K-RAS, B-RAF and PIK3CA and loss of PTEN with mCRC patient response to cetuximab and panitumumab. Once more, when patients were retrospectively classified to only including patients with wt K-RAS, B-RAF, PIK3CA and PTEN positive expression ORR was 51.2% as opposed to below 20% in the whole unselected patient cohort [193]. Combined mutational analysis of K-RAS, B-RAF and PIK3CA has also been shown to improve predicting cetuximab response in another mCRC patient cohort retrospectively [268]. Conversely however, when all mutations were combined, ovarian cancer patients treated with erlotinib with at least one mutation in KRAS, NRAS, BRAF, PIK3CA, or EGFR had longer PFS (33.1 *vs.* 12.3 months) compared to those with wild-type tumors [269].

Despite improving the predictive probability of patients who will respond to anti-EGFR therapy, a large percentage of patients that are still believed to be in the "responsive" sub-population similar do not response. The addition of more predictive biomarkers may be one possibility to improve these findings. In accordance with the above reports, the detection of combined N-RAS, B-RAF and PIK3CA mutation frequency in K-RAS wildtype mCRC patient tumors also significantly correlated to an anti-EGFR resistance phenotype in a more recent report. The statistical significance of these findings were enhanced when other potential predictors of resistance (FBXW7 and SMAD4) were concomitantly combined with the N-RAS, B-RAF and PIK3CA mutation positive sub-groups [270]. These results indicate that mutations at KRAS combined with N-RAS, B-RAF, PIK3CA, FBXW7 and SMAD4 have a strong combined potential for predicting response to anti-EGFR inhibitors. Others have evaluated additional putative predictive biomarkers of resistance to anti-EGFR inhibitors in a set of PDX mCRC models [271, 272]. Bertotti *et al.* particularly implicated HER2 amplification as a novel mechanism of resistance to cetuximab in PDX tumors that are wildtype for K-RAS, N-RAS, B-RAF and PIK3CA [272, 273]. Next generation sequencing has recently been shown as a possible technique to detect mutational status in a large number of genes that may significantly correlate with patient outcomes treated with cetuximab, giving hope that larger screening undertakings can be developed prospectively [270, 274].

Overall, this data highlights the fundamental importance in isolating the key predictive markers (potentially in combination) for improved EGFR-based therapy. It is clear that this has not been achieved, and evaluation of other predictive molecules is required. The next section examines another EGFR mediated signaling pathway (JAK/STAT) that seems to be consistently ignored when examining EGFR signaling and resistance mechanism to EGFR targeted therapy.

6. THE JAK/STAT SIGNALING PATHWAY AND RESISTANCE TO ANTI-EGFR THERAPY

The activation of STAT proteins, in particular STAT3, has been observed in numerous cancers, including breast, liver, prostate colorectal, head and neck, oesophageal, pancreatic, bladder, prostate and non-small cell lung cancers [275 - 281]. Up to 70% of human tumors are linked to persistent STAT3 activity leading to enhanced cellular functions, including proliferation, cell differentiation, metastasis, angiogenesis and reduced apoptosis [232, 282 - 285]. Similarly, STAT3 signaling has been implicated in mediating resistance to anti-EGFR therapy.

The most significant recent study supporting the potential role of STAT3 promoting resistance to EGFR therapeutics came from Dobi and colleagues where they evaluated STAT3 phosphorylation levels by immunohistochemistry in tumor tissue from mCRC patients treated with cetuximab [286]. Importantly, they demonstrated that only 13.0% (3 out of 23) of patients with positive phospho-STAT3 staining displayed ORR to cetuximab and chemotherapy *versus* 40.8% (29 out of 71) of patients with negative phospho-STAT3 staining. In addition, the lack of phospho-STAT3 staining correlated significantly to TTP and OS in these patients [286]. Cell culture experiments have identified STAT3-induced Akt activation as a novel mechanism for gefitinib resistance in lung cancer cells. In this study, Wu and colleagues conclude that targeting STAT3 in conjunction with EGFR inhibitors may re-sensitize tumors to EGFR blockade [287]. In fact, several reports evaluating STAT3 inhibition (or targeting upstream targets of STAT3 such as c-SRC or JAK1/2) in combination with EGFR blockade has produced encouraging outcomes in several tumor types in pre-clinical models [42, 288 - 293]. The recent report by Ung *et al.* demonstrated that the efficacy of anti-EGFR therapeutics correlates with their ability to inhibit STAT3 activation in several human colon cancer cell lines in cultures and in animal xenograft studies [294]. Similarly, STAT3 phosphorylation also strongly correlated with gefitinib sensitivity in colon cancer cell lines [295]. Likewise, human lung cancer cell lines that were largely in-sensitive to erlotinib inhibition displayed erlotinib-induced reduction in EGFR, Akt and ERK1/2 activity but maintained STAT3 activity upon erlotinib treatment, suggesting that refractory responses of these cells may be due to unabated STAT3 signaling [280]. Similar results were reported by Kim and colleagues who found that gefitinib had little effect on either STAT3 activity or *in vitro* and *in vivo* growth of the H1975 lung cancer cell line, while lapatinib could reduce STAT3 activity and cell growth in both cell culture and animal xenograft experiments. Combinational treatment of lapatinib and cetuximab further reduced STAT3 activity and tumor growth compared to single agent treatment [296]. Interestingly, combination of both cetuximab and erlotinib led to an enhanced reduction in STAT3 activity in colon cancer cells compared to single treatments [297]. The study by Lee and colleagues determined that erlotinib treated NSCLC cells secrete soluble factors including FGF16 and IL-6 which could activate STAT3 in erlotinib-naïve cells and enhance resistant. Furthermore, knockdown of STAT3 reversed this resistance which transfection of constitutively active STAT3 enhanced it [298]. Afatinib also induces IL-6 driven STAT3 activation leading to enhanced resistance in NSCLC cells [299].

STAT3 signaling has also been associated with acquired resistance to anti-EGFR inhibitors. Long-term culturing (months) of the erlotinib-sensitive human lung carcinoma cell line, HCC827 in the presence of erlotinib, resulted in an erlotinib acquired resistance sub-clone that displayed greater basal levels of phosphorylated STAT3 compared to the parental cell line [290]. Likewise, A549 NSCLC cells with acquired resistance to gefitinib also had greater STAT3 activity compared to the original parental gefitinib sensitive A549 cells [300]. Similarly, Ung and colleagues generated AG1478 (EGFR-TKI) resistant head and neck carcinoma cell line, HN5 through long-term culturing in the presence of AG1478. In this report, Ung *et al.* found that the HN5-AG resistant cells displayed more STAT3 activity after AG1478 treatment suggesting a possible alternate or compensatory pathway that maintains STAT3 activity when EGFR is de-activated in the resistant cells that was not present in the sensitive parental HN5 cell line [294]. Similarly, lapatinib could not inhibit STAT3 activity in gastric cancer cells with acquired resistant to lapatinib, but could block STAT3 activity in sensitive parental cells [301]. Another study revealed that short-term exposure (up to 9 days) to EGFR TKI's also led to enhanced STAT3 phosphorylation in residual surviving H1975 and HCC827 cells [302]. This study by Fan *et al.* also performed HCC827 xenograft studies examining the short-term effects of erlotinib treatment. They showed that erlotinib significantly reduced tumor growth compared to untreated tumors however, the residual viable tumor cells in the treated xenografts contained greater nuclear STAT3 activity *versus* the untreated xenografts [302]. Importantly, recurrent SCCHN tumor tissue taken from patient's post-cetuximab treatment displayed greater STAT3 phosphorylation compared to tumor tissue from patients pre-treatment [291]. However, this analysis was performed on non-matched pre and post-cetuximab treated patients. Another study showed that 4 SCCHN cell lines with acquired resistance to erlotinib all displayed enhanced IL-6 expression, potentially identifying a possible mechanism for the enhanced STAT3 activity often seen in post-treatment refractory cells and tumor tissue [303]. Nonetheless, collectively these cell line and ex-vivo based models for resistance and patient tumor tissue analysis indicate that enhanced or unabated STAT3 activity may protect cells from anti-EGFR therapy and may be important in driving tumor recurrence and acquired resistance. Further evidence conclusively implicating STAT3 signaling in mediating resistance to anti-EGFR inhibitors in clinical settings is required however before changes in clinical decision making is observed.

CONCLUDING REMARKS

It is clear that vast amounts of research have been published elucidating numerous possible molecular mediators of resistance to anti-EGFR based therapy. It is also clear that the research field studying the molecular mechanisms of resistance to targeted therapy is also growing and will no doubt continue to implicate novel molecules and novel mutations that may act as drivers of resistance in laboratory based research and correlate with resistance (or sensitivity) in retrospective clinical specimens. However, ultimately, most of these potential mediators will not act as suitable predictive biomarkers for patient response to EGFR targeted treatment regimens and thus one can speculate about the futility of these "non-translational" findings. This review summarises the evidence of numerous potential biomarkers including intracellular signaling molecules downstream from the EGFR signaling axes. Disappointingly, to date only K-RAS mutations (and EGFR mutations as discussed in Part 1 of this 2 set review series) can be identified quickly, cost-effectively and most importantly in high enough percentage of patient samples to be used with any confidence as a prospective predictors of response to anti-EGFR therapeutics. In addition, heterozygosity within each individual tumor represents a major limitation of all biopsy based findings as evident by a recent paper by Normanno and colleagues. This study performed quantitative assessment of K-RAS, N-RAS, B-RAF and PIK3CA mutations in neoplastic mCRC cells within the same tumor specimen. Indeed, they found that only a fraction of neoplastic cells harboured these mutant alleles [304], highlighting the need to examine not only the presence of mutations but also the level of mutational status when assessing the possible effect on response to EGFR and other targeted therapies. Another aspect of this field that is a major focus of many research laboratories is whether a detectable mutation/alteration is simply a biomarker for predicting response and overall outcome or whether this biomarker can also be targeted in potential novel combination treatment regimens. One may consider that the utility of a biomarker is dependent on whether it is "druggable" and whether a therapeutic agent directed to this target can be successfully implemented into current treatment strategies independent of and in combination with anti-EGFR agents.

As we strongly emphasized in both this review and Part I of this review series, the variation of identification and confirmation of potential mediators of resistance requires standardised methodology and state-of-the-art advanced technology to eradicate the possibility of false negatives/positives when screening for critical predictive biomarkers. Much more sophisticated techniques such as next-generation sequencing and a variety of capture approaches for the rapid detection of causative mutations in clinical samples is now widely assessable and common place allowing for the future hope of this advanced technology becoming common practice for clinical sampling prospectively. In addition coupled with precise mutational analysis, advances in detecting activated molecular predictors may allow future robust selection of the most suitable patients for anti-EGFR therapies and other targeted inhibitors. Logistically however, implementation of these methodologies universally may be extremely difficult.

It is clear that the major challenge of tumor resistance that arose when first using anti-EGFR therapy clinically many years ago remains a significant obstacle of successful cancer treatment today. However, collectively the EGFR therapeutic research field is discovering important findings rapidly and the hope that future suitable sub-populations of patients can be correctly selected and then most importantly successfully treated with anti-EGFR based therapy is still strong.

CONFLICT OF INTEREST

The author confirms that author has no conflict of interest to declare for this publication.

ACKNOWLEDGEMENTS

I acknowledge the NH&MRC for funding for Project grant #APP1080498.

ABBREVIATIONS

AREG	=	Amphiregulin
BTC	=	Betacellulin
EGF	=	Epidermal growth factor
EGFR	=	Epidermal growth factor receptor
EPGN	=	Epigen
EREG	=	Epiregulin
FISH	=	Fluorescence *in-situ* hybridization
GCN	=	Gene copy number
HB-EGF	=	Heparin-binding EGF
IL	=	Interleukin
JNK	=	c-Jun-N-terminal kinase
K-RAS	=	Kirsten rat sarcoma viral oncogene homolog
mAb	=	Monoclonal antibody
MAPK	=	Mitogen-activated protein kinase
mCRC	=	Metastatic Colorectal carcinoma
mTOR	=	mammalian target of rapamycin
NSCLC	=	Non-small cell lung carcinoma
ORR	=	Objective response rate
OS	=	Overall survival
PDX	=	Patient-derived xenografts
PFS	=	Progression-free survival
PI3-K	=	Phosphatidylinositol 3-kinase
PLCγ	=	Phospholipase-C gamma
PR	=	Partial response
RR	=	Response rate
STAT	=	Signal transducer and activator of transcription
SCCHN	=	Squamous cell carcinoma of the head and neck
SD	=	Stable disease
TGFα	=	Transforming growth factor-alpha
TKI's	=	Tyrosine kinase inhibitors
TTP	=	Time-to-progression

REFERENCES

[1]   Carpenter G, King L Jr, Cohen S. Epidermal growth factor stimulates phosphorylation in membrane preparations *in vitro*. Nature 1978; 276(5686): 409-10.
[http://dx.doi.org/10.1038/276409a0] [PMID: 309559]

[2]   Schechter AL, Stern DF, Vaidyanathan L, *et al.* The neu oncogene: An erb-B-related gene encoding a 185,000-Mr tumour antigen. Nature 1984; 312(5994): 513-6.
[http://dx.doi.org/10.1038/312513a0] [PMID: 6095109]

[3]   Plowman GD, Whitney GS, Neubauer MG, *et al.* Molecular cloning and expression of an additional epidermal growth factor receptor-related gene. Proc Natl Acad Sci USA 1990; 87(13): 4905-9.
[http://dx.doi.org/10.1073/pnas.87.13.4905] [PMID: 2164210]

[4]   Plowman GD, Culouscou JM, Whitney GS, *et al.* Ligand-specific activation of HER4/p180erbB4, a fourth member of the epidermal growth factor receptor family. Proc Natl Acad Sci USA 1993; 90(5): 1746-50.
[http://dx.doi.org/10.1073/pnas.90.5.1746] [PMID: 8383326]

[5]   Burgess AW, Cho HS, Eigenbrot C, *et al.* An open-and-shut case? Recent insights into the activation of EGF/ErbB receptors. Mol Cell 2003; 12(3): 541-52.
[http://dx.doi.org/10.1016/S1097-2765(03)00350-2] [PMID: 14527402]

[6]   Garrett TP, McKern NM, Lou M, *et al.* Crystal structure of a truncated epidermal growth factor receptor extracellular domain bound to transforming growth factor alpha. Cell 2002; 110(6): 763-73.
[http://dx.doi.org/10.1016/S0092-8674(02)00940-6] [PMID: 12297049]

[7]   Ogiso H, Ishitani R, Nureki O, *et al.* Crystal structure of the complex of human epidermal growth factor and receptor extracellular domains. Cell 2002; 110(6): 775-87.
[http://dx.doi.org/10.1016/S0092-8674(02)00963-7] [PMID: 12297050]

[8]   Moolenaar WH, Bierman AJ, Tilly BC, *et al.* A point mutation at the ATP-binding site of the EGF-receptor abolishes signal transduction. EMBO J 1988; 7(3): 707-10.
[PMID: 3260862]

[9]   Wells A, Welsh JB, Lazar CS, Wiley HS, Gill GN, Rosenfeld MG. Ligand-induced transformation by a noninternalizing epidermal growth factor receptor. Science 1990; 247(4945): 962-4.
[http://dx.doi.org/10.1126/science.2305263] [PMID: 2305263]

[10]   Cohen S, Ushiro H, Stoscheck C, Chinkers M. A native 170,000 epidermal growth factor receptor-kinase complex from shed plasma membrane vesicles. J Biol Chem 1982; 257(3): 1523-31.
[PMID: 6276390]

[11]   Ushiro H, Cohen S. Identification of phosphotyrosine as a product of epidermal growth factor-activated protein kinase in A-431 cell membranes. J Biol Chem 1980; 255(18): 8363-5.
[PMID: 6157683]

[12]   Wada T, Qian XL, Greene MI. Intermolecular association of the p185neu protein and EGF receptor modulates EGF receptor function. Cell 1990; 61(7): 1339-47.
[http://dx.doi.org/10.1016/0092-8674(90)90697-D] [PMID: 1973074]

[13]   Yarden Y, Schlessinger J. Self-phosphorylation of epidermal growth factor receptor: evidence for a model of intermolecular allosteric activation. Biochemistry 1987; 26(5): 1434-42.

[http://dx.doi.org/10.1021/bi00379a034] [PMID: 3494472]

[14]   Cantley LC, Auger KR, Carpenter C, *et al.* Oncogenes and signal transduction. Cell 1991; 64(2): 281-302.
[http://dx.doi.org/10.1016/0092-8674(91)90639-G] [PMID: 1846320]

[15]   Koch CA, Anderson D, Moran MF, Ellis C, Pawson T. SH2 and SH3 domains: elements that control interactions of cytoplasmic signaling proteins. Science 1991; 252(5006): 668-74.
[http://dx.doi.org/10.1126/science.1708916] [PMID: 1708916]

[16]   Soler C, Beguinot L, Carpenter G. Individual epidermal growth factor receptor autophosphorylation sites do not stringently define association motifs for several SH2-containing proteins. J Biol Chem 1994; 269(16): 12320-4.
[PMID: 8163537]

[17]   Holmes WE, Sliwkowski MX, Akita RW, *et al.* Identification of heregulin, a specific activator of p185erbB2. Science 1992; 256(5060): 1205-10.
[http://dx.doi.org/10.1126/science.256.5060.1205] [PMID: 1350381]

[18]   Yarden Y, Peles E. Biochemical analysis of the ligand for the neu oncogenic receptor. Biochemistry 1991; 30(14): 3543-50.
[http://dx.doi.org/10.1021/bi00228a027] [PMID: 1672825]

[19]   Daub H, Weiss FU, Wallasch C, Ullrich A. Role of transactivation of the EGF receptor in signalling by G-protein-coupled receptors. Nature 1996; 379(6565): 557-60.
[http://dx.doi.org/10.1038/379557a0] [PMID: 8596637]

[20]   Eguchi S, Numaguchi K, Iwasaki H, *et al.* Calcium-dependent epidermal growth factor receptor transactivation mediates the angiotensin II-induced mitogen-activated protein kinase activation in vascular smooth muscle cells. J Biol Chem 1998; 273(15): 8890-6.
[http://dx.doi.org/10.1074/jbc.273.15.8890] [PMID: 9535870]

[21]   Grant SL, Hammacher A, Douglas AM, *et al.* An unexpected biochemical and functional interaction between gp130 and the EGF receptor family in breast cancer cells. Oncogene 2002; 21(3): 460-74.
[http://dx.doi.org/10.1038/sj.onc.1205100] [PMID: 11821958]

[22]   Habib AA, Högnason T, Ren J, Stefánsson K, Ratan RR. The epidermal growth factor receptor associates with and recruits phosphatidylinositol 3-kinase to the platelet-derived growth factor beta receptor. J Biol Chem 1998; 273(12): 6885-91.
[http://dx.doi.org/10.1074/jbc.273.12.6885] [PMID: 9506992]

[23]   Izumi K, Zheng Y, Li Y, Zaengle J, Miyamoto H. Epidermal growth factor induces bladder cancer cell proliferation through activation of the androgen receptor. Int J Oncol 2012; 41(5): 1587-92.
[PMID: 22922989]

[24]   Jo M, Stolz DB, Esplen JE, Dorko K, Michalopoulos GK, Strom SC. Cross-talk between epidermal growth factor receptor and c-Met signal pathways in transformed cells. J Biol Chem 2000; 275(12): 8806-11.
[http://dx.doi.org/10.1074/jbc.275.12.8806] [PMID: 10722725]

[25]   Li JJ, Liu DP, Liu GT, Xie D. EphrinA5 acts as a tumor suppressor in glioma by negative regulation of epidermal growth factor receptor. Oncogene 2009; 28(15): 1759-68.

[http://dx.doi.org/10.1038/onc.2009.15] [PMID: 19270726]

[26]   Migliaccio A, Di Domenico M, Castoria G, *et al.* Steroid receptor regulation of epidermal growth factor signaling through Src in breast and prostate cancer cells: steroid antagonist action. Cancer Res 2005; 65(22): 10585-93.
[http://dx.doi.org/10.1158/0008-5472.CAN-05-0912] [PMID: 16288052]

[27]   Rodrigues S, Attoub S, Nguyen QD, *et al.* Selective abrogation of the proinvasive activity of the trefoil peptides pS2 and spasmolytic polypeptide by disruption of the EGF receptor signaling pathways in kidney and colonic cancer cells. Oncogene 2003; 22(29): 4488-97.
[http://dx.doi.org/10.1038/sj.onc.1206685] [PMID: 12881705]

[28]   Sutton P, Borgia JA, Bonomi P, Plate JM. Lyn, a Src family kinase, regulates activation of epidermal growth factor receptors in lung adenocarcinoma cells. Mol Cancer 2013; 12: 76.
[http://dx.doi.org/10.1186/1476-4598-12-76] [PMID: 23866081]

[29]   Wang Y, van Boxel-Dezaire AH, Cheon H, Yang J, Stark GR. STAT3 activation in response to IL-6 is prolonged by the binding of IL-6 receptor to EGF receptor. Proc Natl Acad Sci USA 2013; 110(42): 16975-80.
[http://dx.doi.org/10.1073/pnas.1315862110] [PMID: 24082147]

[30]   Yamashita M, Chattopadhyay S, Fensterl V, Saikia P, Wetzel JL, Sen GC. Epidermal growth factor receptor is essential for Toll-like receptor 3 signaling. Sci Signal 2012; 5(233): ra50.
[http://dx.doi.org/10.1126/scisignal.2002581] [PMID: 22810896]

[31]   Wilson KJ, Gilmore JL, Foley J, Lemmon MA, Riese DJ II. Functional selectivity of EGF family peptide growth factors: implications for cancer. Pharmacol Ther 2009; 122(1): 1-8.
[http://dx.doi.org/10.1016/j.pharmthera.2008.11.008] [PMID: 19135477]

[32]   Batzer AG, Rotin D, Ureña JM, Skolnik EY, Schlessinger J. Hierarchy of binding sites for Grb2 and Shc on the epidermal growth factor receptor. Mol Cell Biol 1994; 14(8): 5192-201.
[http://dx.doi.org/10.1128/MCB.14.8.5192] [PMID: 7518560]

[33]   Margolis B, Rhee SG, Felder S, *et al.* EGF induces tyrosine phosphorylation of phospholipase C-II: a potential mechanism for EGF receptor signaling. Cell 1989; 57(7): 1101-7.
[http://dx.doi.org/10.1016/0092-8674(89)90047-0] [PMID: 2472218]

[34]   Songyang Z, Shoelson SE, Chaudhuri M, *et al.* SH2 domains recognize specific phosphopeptide sequences. Cell 1993; 72(5): 767-78.
[http://dx.doi.org/10.1016/0092-8674(93)90404-E] [PMID: 7680959]

[35]   Burgess AW. EGFR family: structure physiology signalling and therapeutic targets. Growth Factors 2008; 26(5): 263-74.
[http://dx.doi.org/10.1080/08977190802312844] [PMID: 18800267]

[36]   Grandal MV, Madshus IH. Epidermal growth factor receptor and cancer: control of oncogenic signalling by endocytosis. J Cell Mol Med 2008; 12(5A): 1527-34.
[http://dx.doi.org/10.1111/j.1582-4934.2008.00298.x] [PMID: 18318691]

[37]   Wang Y, Du D, Fang L, *et al.* Tyrosine phosphorylated Par3 regulates epithelial tight junction assembly promoted by EGFR signaling. EMBO J 2006; 25(21): 5058-70.
[http://dx.doi.org/10.1038/sj.emboj.7601384] [PMID: 17053785]

[38]   Luwor RB, Chin X, McGeachie AB, Robinson PJ, Zhu HJ. Dynamin II function is required for EGF-mediated Stat3 activation but not Erk1/2 phosphorylation. Growth Factors 2012; 30(4): 220-9.
[http://dx.doi.org/10.3109/08977194.2012.683189] [PMID: 22574813]

[39]   Sigismund S, Argenzio E, Tosoni D, Cavallaro E, Polo S, Di Fiore PP. Clathrin-mediated internalization is essential for sustained EGFR signaling but dispensable for degradation. Dev Cell 2008; 15(2): 209-19.
[http://dx.doi.org/10.1016/j.devcel.2008.06.012] [PMID: 18694561]

[40]   Vieira AV, Lamaze C, Schmid SL. Control of EGF receptor signaling by clathrin-mediated endocytosis. Science 1996; 274(5295): 2086-9.
[http://dx.doi.org/10.1126/science.274.5295.2086] [PMID: 8953040]

[41]   Lin SY, Makino K, Xia W, et al. Nuclear localization of EGF receptor and its potential new role as a transcription factor. Nat Cell Biol 2001; 3(9): 802-8.
[http://dx.doi.org/10.1038/ncb0901-802] [PMID: 11533659]

[42]   Lo HW, Hsu SC, Ali-Seyed M, et al. Nuclear interaction of EGFR and STAT3 in the activation of the iNOS/NO pathway. Cancer Cell 2005; 7(6): 575-89.
[http://dx.doi.org/10.1016/j.ccr.2005.05.007] [PMID: 15950906]

[43]   Marti U, Burwen SJ, Wells A, et al. Localization of epidermal growth factor receptor in hepatocyte nuclei. Hepatology 1991; 13(1): 15-20.
[http://dx.doi.org/10.1002/hep.1840130104] [PMID: 1988335]

[44]   Ni CY, Murphy MP, Golde TE, Carpenter G. gamma -Secretase cleavage and nuclear localization of ErbB-4 receptor tyrosine kinase. Science 2001; 294(5549): 2179-81.
[http://dx.doi.org/10.1126/science.1065412] [PMID: 11679632]

[45]   Offterdinger M, Schöfer C, Weipoltshammer K, Grunt TW. c-erbB-3: A nuclear protein in mammary epithelial cells. J Cell Biol 2002; 157(6): 929-39.
[http://dx.doi.org/10.1083/jcb.200109033] [PMID: 12045181]

[46]   Wang SC, Lien HC, Xia W, et al. Binding at and transactivation of the COX-2 promoter by nuclear tyrosine kinase receptor ErbB-2. Cancer Cell 2004; 6(3): 251-61.
[http://dx.doi.org/10.1016/j.ccr.2004.07.012] [PMID: 15380516]

[47]   Xie Y, Hung MC. Nuclear localization of p185neu tyrosine kinase and its association with transcriptional transactivation. Biochem Biophys Res Commun 1994; 203(3): 1589-98.
[http://dx.doi.org/10.1006/bbrc.1994.2368] [PMID: 7945309]

[48]   Graner MW, Alzate O, Dechkovskaia AM, et al. Proteomic and immunologic analyses of brain tumor exosomes. FASEB J 2009; 23(5): 1541-57.
[http://dx.doi.org/10.1096/fj.08-122184] [PMID: 19109410]

[49]   Higginbotham JN, Demory Beckler M, Gephart JD, et al. Amphiregulin exosomes increase cancer cell invasion. Curr Biol 2011; 21(9): 779-86.
[http://dx.doi.org/10.1016/j.cub.2011.03.043] [PMID: 21514161]

[50]   Sanderson MP, Keller S, Alonso A, Riedle S, Dempsey PJ, Altevogt P. Generation of novel, secreted epidermal growth factor receptor (EGFR/ErbB1) isoforms via metalloprotease-dependent ectodomain shedding and exosome secretion. J Cell Biochem 2008; 103(6): 1783-97.

[http://dx.doi.org/10.1002/jcb.21569] [PMID: 17910038]

[51]   Barbieri MA, Fernandez-Pol S, Hunker C, Horazdovsky BH, Stahl PD. Role of rab5 in EGF receptor-mediated signal transduction. Eur J Cell Biol 2004; 83(6): 305-14.
[http://dx.doi.org/10.1078/0171-9335-00381] [PMID: 15511088]

[52]   Kranenburg O, Verlaan I, Moolenaar WH. Dynamin is required for the activation of mitogen-activated protein (MAP) kinase by MAP kinase kinase. J Biol Chem 1999; 274(50): 35301-4.
[http://dx.doi.org/10.1074/jbc.274.50.35301] [PMID: 10585393]

[53]   Ringerike T, Stang E, Johannessen LE, Sandnes D, Levy FO, Madshus IH. High-affinity binding of epidermal growth factor (EGF) to EGF receptor is disrupted by overexpression of mutant dynamin (K44A). J Biol Chem 1998; 273(27): 16639-42.
[http://dx.doi.org/10.1074/jbc.273.27.16639] [PMID: 9642213]

[54]   Tosoni D, Cestra G. CAP (Cbl associated protein) regulates receptor-mediated endocytosis. FEBS Lett 2009; 583(2): 293-300.
[http://dx.doi.org/10.1016/j.febslet.2008.12.047] [PMID: 19116150]

[55]   Ono M, Hirata A, Kometani T, *et al.* Sensitivity to gefitinib (Iressa, ZD1839) in non-small cell lung cancer cell lines correlates with dependence on the epidermal growth factor (EGF) receptor/extracellular signal-regulated kinase 1/2 and EGF receptor/Akt pathway for proliferation. Mol Cancer Ther 2004; 3(4): 465-72.
[PMID: 15078990]

[56]   Nishimura Y, Bereczky B, Ono M. The EGFR inhibitor gefitinib suppresses ligand-stimulated endocytosis of EGFR *via* the early/late endocytic pathway in non-small cell lung cancer cell lines. Histochem Cell Biol 2007; 127(5): 541-53.
[http://dx.doi.org/10.1007/s00418-007-0281-y] [PMID: 17361439]

[57]   Jo U, Park KH, Whang YM, *et al.* EGFR endocytosis is a novel therapeutic target in lung cancer with wild-type EGFR. Oncotarget 2014; 5(5): 1265-78.
[http://dx.doi.org/10.18632/oncotarget.1711] [PMID: 24658031]

[58]   Huang DH, Su L, Peng XH, *et al.* Quantum dot-based quantification revealed differences in subcellular localization of EGFR and E-cadherin between EGFR-TKI sensitive and insensitive cancer cells. Nanotechnology 2009; 20(22): 225102.
[http://dx.doi.org/10.1088/0957-4484/20/22/225102] [PMID: 19433879]

[59]   Kwak EL, Sordella R, Bell DW, *et al.* Irreversible inhibitors of the EGF receptor may circumvent acquired resistance to gefitinib. Proc Natl Acad Sci USA 2005; 102(21): 7665-70.
[http://dx.doi.org/10.1073/pnas.0502860102] [PMID: 15897464]

[60]   Feng YH, Tsao CJ, Wu CL, *et al.* Sprouty2 protein enhances the response to gefitinib through epidermal growth factor receptor in colon cancer cells. Cancer Sci 2010; 101(9): 2033-8.
[http://dx.doi.org/10.1111/j.1349-7006.2010.01637.x] [PMID: 20624167]

[61]   Huang WC, Chen YJ, Li LY, *et al.* Nuclear translocation of epidermal growth factor receptor by Akt-dependent phosphorylation enhances breast cancer-resistant protein expression in gefitinib-resistant cells. J Biol Chem 2011; 286(23): 20558-68.
[http://dx.doi.org/10.1074/jbc.M111.240796] [PMID: 21487020]

[62]   Chen YJ, Huang WC, Wei YL, *et al.* Elevated BCRP/ABCG2 expression confers acquired resistance to gefitinib in wild-type EGFR-expressing cells. PLoS One 2011; 6(6): e21428.
[http://dx.doi.org/10.1371/journal.pone.0021428] [PMID: 21731744]

[63]   Sugimoto Y, Tsukahara S, Ishikawa E, Mitsuhashi J. Breast cancer resistance protein: molecular target for anticancer drug resistance and pharmacokinetics/pharmacodynamics. Cancer Sci 2005; 96(8): 457-65.
[http://dx.doi.org/10.1111/j.1349-7006.2005.00081.x] [PMID: 16108826]

[64]   Usuda J, Ohira T, Suga Y, *et al.* Breast cancer resistance protein (BCRP) affected acquired resistance to gefitinib in a "never-smoked" female patient with advanced non-small cell lung cancer. Lung Cancer 2007; 58(2): 296-9.
[http://dx.doi.org/10.1016/j.lungcan.2007.05.019] [PMID: 17618705]

[65]   Furukawa M, Nagatomo I, Kumagai T, *et al.* Gefitinib-sensitive EGFR lacking residues 746-750 exhibits hypophosphorylation at tyrosine residue 1045, hypoubiquitination, and impaired endocytosis. DNA Cell Biol 2007; 26(3): 178-85.
[http://dx.doi.org/10.1089/dna.2006.0573] [PMID: 17417946]

[66]   Irwin ME, Mueller KL, Bohin N, Ge Y, Boerner JL. Lipid raft localization of EGFR alters the response of cancer cells to the EGFR tyrosine kinase inhibitor gefitinib. J Cell Physiol 2011; 226(9): 2316-28.
[http://dx.doi.org/10.1002/jcp.22570] [PMID: 21660955]

[67]   Thomsen P, Roepstorff K, Stahlhut M, van Deurs B. Caveolae are highly immobile plasma membrane microdomains, which are not involved in constitutive endocytic trafficking. Mol Biol Cell 2002; 13(1): 238-50.
[http://dx.doi.org/10.1091/mbc.01-06-0317] [PMID: 11809836]

[68]   Ferrer-Soler L, Vazquez-Martin A, Brunet J, Menendez JA, De Llorens R, Colomer R. An update of the mechanisms of resistance to EGFR-tyrosine kinase inhibitors in breast cancer: Gefitinib (Iressa) - induced changes in the expression and nucleo-cytoplasmic trafficking of HER-ligands (Review). Int J Mol Med 2007; 20(1): 3-10. [Review].
[PMID: 17549382]

[69]   Wheeler DL, Huang S, Kruser TJ, *et al.* Mechanisms of acquired resistance to cetuximab: role of HER (ErbB) family members. Oncogene 2008; 27(28): 3944-56.
[http://dx.doi.org/10.1038/onc.2008.19] [PMID: 18297114]

[70]   Li C, Iida M, Dunn EF, Ghia AJ, Wheeler DL. Nuclear EGFR contributes to acquired resistance to cetuximab. Oncogene 2009; 28(43): 3801-13.
[http://dx.doi.org/10.1038/onc.2009.234] [PMID: 19684613]

[71]   Lu Y, Li X, Liang K, *et al.* Epidermal growth factor receptor (EGFR) ubiquitination as a mechanism of acquired resistance escaping treatment by the anti-EGFR monoclonal antibody cetuximab. Cancer Res 2007; 67(17): 8240-7.
[http://dx.doi.org/10.1158/0008-5472.CAN-07-0589] [PMID: 17804738]

[72]   Lo HW, Cao X, Zhu H, Ali-Osman F. Constitutively activated STAT3 frequently coexpresses with epidermal growth factor receptor in high-grade gliomas and targeting STAT3 sensitizes them to Iressa and alkylators. Clin Cancer Res 2008; 14(19): 6042-54.

[http://dx.doi.org/10.1158/1078-0432.CCR-07-4923] [PMID: 18829483]

[73] Grandal MV, Zandi R, Pedersen MW, Willumsen BM, van Deurs B, Poulsen HS. EGFRvIII escapes down-regulation due to impaired internalization and sorting to lysosomes. Carcinogenesis 2007; 28(7): 1408-17.
[http://dx.doi.org/10.1093/carcin/bgm058] [PMID: 17372273]

[74] Lowenstein EJ, Daly RJ, Batzer AG, *et al.* The SH2 and SH3 domain-containing protein GRB2 links receptor tyrosine kinases to ras signaling. Cell 1992; 70(3): 431-42.
[http://dx.doi.org/10.1016/0092-8674(92)90167-B] [PMID: 1322798]

[75] Smith MA, Hall R, Fisher K, *et al.* Annotation of human cancers with EGFR signaling-associated protein complexes using proximity ligation assays. Sci Signal 2015; 8(359): ra4.
[http://dx.doi.org/10.1126/scisignal.2005906] [PMID: 25587191]

[76] Koizumi F, Shimoyama T, Taguchi F, Saijo N, Nishio K. Establishment of a human non-small cell lung cancer cell line resistant to gefitinib. Int J Cancer 2005; 116(1): 36-44.
[http://dx.doi.org/10.1002/ijc.20985] [PMID: 15761868]

[77] Li J, Bennett K, Stukalov A, *et al.* Perturbation of the mutated EGFR interactome identifies vulnerabilities and resistance mechanisms. Mol Syst Biol 2013; 9: 705.
[http://dx.doi.org/10.1038/msb.2013.61] [PMID: 24189400]

[78] Hoeben A, Martin D, Clement PM, Cools J, Gutkind JS. Role of GRB2-associated binder 1 in epidermal growth factor receptor-induced signaling in head and neck squamous cell carcinoma. Int J Cancer 2013; 132(5): 1042-50.
[http://dx.doi.org/10.1002/ijc.27763] [PMID: 22865653]

[79] Chang EH, Gonda MA, Ellis RW, Scolnick EM, Lowy DR. Human genome contains four genes homologous to transforming genes of Harvey and Kirsten murine sarcoma viruses. Proc Natl Acad Sci USA 1982; 79(16): 4848-52.
[http://dx.doi.org/10.1073/pnas.79.16.4848] [PMID: 6289320]

[80] Parada LF, Tabin CJ, Shih C, Weinberg RA. Human EJ bladder carcinoma oncogene is homologue of Harvey sarcoma virus ras gene. Nature 1982; 297(5866): 474-8.
[http://dx.doi.org/10.1038/297474a0] [PMID: 6283357]

[81] Marshall CJ, Hall A, Weiss RA. A transforming gene present in human sarcoma cell lines. Nature 1982; 299(5879): 171-3.
[http://dx.doi.org/10.1038/299171a0] [PMID: 6287287]

[82] Hall A, Marshall CJ, Spurr NK, Weiss RA. Identification of transforming gene in two human sarcoma cell lines as a new member of the ras gene family located on chromosome 1. Nature 1983; 303(5916): 396-400.
[http://dx.doi.org/10.1038/303396a0] [PMID: 6304521]

[83] Bos JL. ras oncogenes in human cancer: A review. Cancer Res 1989; 49(17): 4682-9.
[PMID: 2547513]

[84] Downward J. Targeting RAS signalling pathways in cancer therapy. Nat Rev Cancer 2003; 3(1): 11-22.
[http://dx.doi.org/10.1038/nrc969] [PMID: 12509763]

[85]   Camp ER, Summy J, Bauer TW, Liu W, Gallick GE, Ellis LM. Molecular mechanisms of resistance to therapies targeting the epidermal growth factor receptor. Clin Cancer Res 2005; 11(1): 397-405.
[PMID: 15671571]

[86]   Lièvre A, Bachet JB, Le Corre D, *et al.* KRAS mutation status is predictive of response to cetuximab therapy in colorectal cancer. Cancer Res 2006; 66(8): 3992-5.
[http://dx.doi.org/10.1158/0008-5472.CAN-06-0191] [PMID: 16618717]

[87]   Karapetis CS, Khambata-Ford S, Jonker DJ, *et al.* K-ras mutations and benefit from cetuximab in advanced colorectal cancer. N Engl J Med 2008; 359(17): 1757-65.
[http://dx.doi.org/10.1056/NEJMoa0804385] [PMID: 18946061]

[88]   Bokemeyer C, Bondarenko I, Makhson A, *et al.* Fluorouracil, leucovorin, and oxaliplatin with and without cetuximab in the first-line treatment of metastatic colorectal cancer. J Clin Oncol 2009; 27(5): 663-71.
[http://dx.doi.org/10.1200/JCO.2008.20.8397] [PMID: 19114683]

[89]   Douillard JY, Oliner KS, Siena S, *et al.* Panitumumab-FOLFOX4 treatment and RAS mutations in colorectal cancer. N Engl J Med 2013; 369(11): 1023-34.
[http://dx.doi.org/10.1056/NEJMoa1305275] [PMID: 24024839]

[90]   Andreyev HJ, Norman AR, Cunningham D, *et al.* Kirsten ras mutations in patients with colorectal cancer: the 'RASCAL II' study. Br J Cancer 2001; 85(5): 692-6.
[http://dx.doi.org/10.1054/bjoc.2001.1964] [PMID: 11531254]

[91]   Andreyev HJ, Norman AR, Cunningham D, Oates JR, Clarke PA. Kirsten ras mutations in patients with colorectal cancer: the multicenter "RASCAL" study. J Natl Cancer Inst 1998; 90(9): 675-84.
[http://dx.doi.org/10.1093/jnci/90.9.675] [PMID: 9586664]

[92]   Wang HL, Lopategui J, Amin MB, Patterson SD. KRAS mutation testing in human cancers: The pathologist's role in the era of personalized medicine. Adv Anat Pathol 2010; 17(1): 23-32.
[PMID: 20032635]

[93]   Peeters M, Oliner K, Price TJ, *et al.* Analysis of KRAS/NRAS Mutations in a Phase 3 Study of Panitumumab With FOLFIRI Compared With FOLFIRI Alone as Second-Line Treatment for Metastatic Colorectal Cancer. Clin Cancer Res 2015; 21(24): 5469-79.
[http://dx.doi.org/10.1158/1078-0432.CCR-15-0526] [PMID: 26341920]

[94]   De Roock W, Claes B, Bernasconi D, *et al.* Effects of KRAS, BRAF, NRAS, and PIK3CA mutations on the efficacy of cetuximab plus chemotherapy in chemotherapy-refractory metastatic colorectal cancer: a retrospective consortium analysis. Lancet Oncol 2010; 11(8): 753-62.
[http://dx.doi.org/10.1016/S1470-2045(10)70130-3] [PMID: 20619739]

[95]   Loupakis F, Ruzzo A, Cremolini C, *et al.* KRAS codon 61, 146 and BRAF mutations predict resistance to cetuximab plus irinotecan in KRAS codon 12 and 13 wild-type metastatic colorectal cancer. Br J Cancer 2009; 101(4): 715-21.
[http://dx.doi.org/10.1038/sj.bjc.6605177] [PMID: 19603018]

[96]   De Roock W, Jonker DJ, Di Nicolantonio F, *et al.* Association of KRAS p.G13D mutation with outcome in patients with chemotherapy-refractory metastatic colorectal cancer treated with cetuximab. JAMA 2010; 304(16): 1812-20.

[http://dx.doi.org/10.1001/jama.2010.1535] [PMID: 20978259]

[97]   Tejpar S, Celik I, Schlichting M, Sartorius U, Bokemeyer C, Van Cutsem E. Association of KRAS
       G13D tumor mutations with outcome in patients with metastatic colorectal cancer treated with first-
       line chemotherapy with or without cetuximab. J Clin Oncol 2012; 30(29): 3570-7.
       [http://dx.doi.org/10.1200/JCO.2012.42.2592] [PMID: 22734028]

[98]   Molinari F, Felicioni L, Buscarino M, *et al.* Increased detection sensitivity for KRAS mutations
       enhances the prediction of anti-EGFR monoclonal antibody resistance in metastatic colorectal cancer.
       Clin Cancer Res 2011; 17(14): 4901-14.
       [http://dx.doi.org/10.1158/1078-0432.CCR-10-3137] [PMID: 21632860]

[99]   Valtorta E, Misale S, Sartore-Bianchi A, *et al.* KRAS gene amplification in colorectal cancer and
       impact on response to EGFR-targeted therapy. Int J Cancer 2013; 133(5): 1259-65.
       [http://dx.doi.org/10.1002/ijc.28106] [PMID: 23404247]

[100] Pao W, Wang TY, Riely GJ, *et al.* KRAS mutations and primary resistance of lung adenocarcinomas
       to gefitinib or erlotinib. PLoS Med 2005; 2(1): e17.
       [http://dx.doi.org/10.1371/journal.pmed.0020017] [PMID: 15696205]

[101] Eberhard DA, Johnson BE, Amler LC, *et al.* Mutations in the epidermal growth factor receptor and in
       KRAS are predictive and prognostic indicators in patients with non-small-cell lung cancer treated with
       chemotherapy alone and in combination with erlotinib. J Clin Oncol 2005; 23(25): 5900-9.
       [http://dx.doi.org/10.1200/JCO.2005.02.857] [PMID: 16043828]

[102] Shackelford RE, Whitling NA, McNab P, Japa S, Coppola D. KRAS Testing: A Tool for the
       Implementation of Personalized Medicine. Genes Cancer 2012; 3(7-8): 459-66.
       [http://dx.doi.org/10.1177/1947601912460547] [PMID: 23264846]

[103] Khambata-Ford S, Harbison CT, Hart LL, *et al.* Analysis of potential predictive markers of cetuximab
       benefit in BMS099, a phase III study of cetuximab and first-line taxane/carboplatin in advanced non-
       small-cell lung cancer. J Clin Oncol 2010; 28(6): 918-27.
       [http://dx.doi.org/10.1200/JCO.2009.25.2890] [PMID: 20100958]

[104] O'Byrne KJ, Gatzemeier U, Bondarenko I, *et al.* Molecular biomarkers in non-small-cell lung cancer:
       a retrospective analysis of data from the phase 3 FLEX study. Lancet Oncol 2011; 12(8): 795-805.
       [http://dx.doi.org/10.1016/S1470-2045(11)70189-9] [PMID: 21782507]

[105] Herbst RS, Kelly K, Chansky K, *et al.* Phase II selection design trial of concurrent chemotherapy and
       cetuximab *versus* chemotherapy followed by cetuximab in advanced-stage non-small-cell lung cancer:
       Southwest Oncology Group study S0342. J Clin Oncol 2010; 28(31): 4747-54.
       [http://dx.doi.org/10.1200/JCO.2009.27.9356] [PMID: 20921467]

[106] Janmaat ML, Gallegos-Ruiz MI, Rodriguez JA, *et al.* Predictive factors for outcome in a phase II study
       of gefitinib in second-line treatment of advanced esophageal cancer patients. J Clin Oncol 2006;
       24(10): 1612-9.
       [http://dx.doi.org/10.1200/JCO.2005.03.4900] [PMID: 16575012]

[107] Miller VA, Riely GJ, Zakowski MF, *et al.* Molecular characteristics of bronchioloalveolar carcinoma
       and adenocarcinoma, bronchioloalveolar carcinoma subtype, predict response to erlotinib. J Clin
       Oncol 2008; 26(9): 1472-8.
       [http://dx.doi.org/10.1200/JCO.2007.13.0062] [PMID: 18349398]

[108] Fensterer H, Schade-Brittinger C, Müller HH, *et al.* Arbeitsgemeinschaft Internistische Onkologie. Multicenter phase II trial to investigate safety and efficacy of gemcitabine combined with cetuximab as adjuvant therapy in pancreatic cancer (ATIP). Ann Oncol 2013; 24(10): 2576-81. [http://dx.doi.org/10.1093/annonc/mdt270] [PMID: 23897705]

[109] Kullmann F, Hartmann A, Stöhr R, *et al.* KRAS mutation in metastatic pancreatic ductal adenocarcinoma: results of a multicenter phase II study evaluating efficacy of cetuximab plus gemcitabine/oxaliplatin (GEMOXCET) in first-line therapy. Oncology 2011; 81(1): 3-8. [http://dx.doi.org/10.1159/000330194] [PMID: 21894049]

[110] Boeckx C, Weyn C, Vanden Bempt I, *et al.* Mutation analysis of genes in the EGFR pathway in Head and Neck cancer patients: implications for anti-EGFR treatment response. BMC Res Notes 2014; 7: 337. [http://dx.doi.org/10.1186/1756-0500-7-337] [PMID: 24899223]

[111] Van Damme N, Deron P, Van Roy N, *et al.* Epidermal growth factor receptor and K-RAS status in two cohorts of squamous cell carcinomas. BMC Cancer 2010; 10: 189. [http://dx.doi.org/10.1186/1471-2407-10-189] [PMID: 20459770]

[112] Szabó B, Nelhubel GA, Kárpáti A, *et al.* Clinical significance of genetic alterations and expression of epidermal growth factor receptor (EGFR) in head and neck squamous cell carcinomas. Oral Oncol 2011; 47(6): 487-96. [http://dx.doi.org/10.1016/j.oraloncology.2011.03.020] [PMID: 21498106]

[113] Luwor RB, Lu Y, Li X, Liang K, Fan Z. Constitutively active Harvey Ras confers resistance to epidermal growth factor receptor-targeted therapy with cetuximab and gefitinib. Cancer Lett 2011; 306(1): 85-91. [http://dx.doi.org/10.1016/j.canlet.2011.02.035] [PMID: 21411223]

[114] Rampias T, Giagini A, Siolos S, *et al.* RAS/PI3K crosstalk and cetuximab resistance in head and neck squamous cell carcinoma. Clin Cancer Res 2014; 20(11): 2933-46. [http://dx.doi.org/10.1158/1078-0432.CCR-13-2721] [PMID: 24696319]

[115] Bouchahda M, Karaboué A, Saffroy R, *et al.* Acquired KRAS mutations during progression of colorectal cancer metastases: possible implications for therapy and prognosis. Cancer Chemother Pharmacol 2010; 66(3): 605-9. [http://dx.doi.org/10.1007/s00280-010-1298-9] [PMID: 20361188]

[116] Misale S, Yaeger R, Hobor S, *et al.* Emergence of KRAS mutations and acquired resistance to anti-EGFR therapy in colorectal cancer. Nature 2012; 486(7404): 532-6. [PMID: 22722830]

[117] Misale S, Arena S, Lamba S, *et al.* Blockade of EGFR and MEK intercepts heterogeneous mechanisms of acquired resistance to anti-EGFR therapies in colorectal cancer. Sci Transl Med 2014; 6(224): 224ra26. [http://dx.doi.org/10.1126/scitranslmed.3007947] [PMID: 24553387]

[118] Diaz LA Jr, Williams RT, Wu J, *et al.* The molecular evolution of acquired resistance to targeted EGFR blockade in colorectal cancers. Nature 2012; 486(7404): 537-40. [PMID: 22722843]

[119] Davies H, Bignell GR, Cox C, *et al.* Mutations of the BRAF gene in human cancer. Nature 2002; 417(6892): 949-54.
[http://dx.doi.org/10.1038/nature00766] [PMID: 12068308]

[120] Rajagopalan H, Bardelli A, Lengauer C, Kinzler KW, Vogelstein B, Velculescu VE. Tumorigenesis: RAF/RAS oncogenes and mismatch-repair status. Nature 2002; 418(6901): 934.
[http://dx.doi.org/10.1038/418934a] [PMID: 12198537]

[121] Moroni M, Veronese S, Benvenuti S, *et al.* Gene copy number for epidermal growth factor receptor (EGFR) and clinical response to antiEGFR treatment in colorectal cancer: a cohort study. Lancet Oncol 2005; 6(5): 279-86.
[http://dx.doi.org/10.1016/S1470-2045(05)70102-9] [PMID: 15863375]

[122] Benvenuti S, Sartore-Bianchi A, Di Nicolantonio F, *et al.* Oncogenic activation of the RAS/RAF signaling pathway impairs the response of metastatic colorectal cancers to anti-epidermal growth factor receptor antibody therapies. Cancer Res 2007; 67(6): 2643-8.
[http://dx.doi.org/10.1158/0008-5472.CAN-06-4158] [PMID: 17363584]

[123] Di Nicolantonio F, Martini M, Molinari F, *et al.* Wild-type BRAF is required for response to panitumumab or cetuximab in metastatic colorectal cancer. J Clin Oncol 2008; 26(35): 5705-12.
[http://dx.doi.org/10.1200/JCO.2008.18.0786] [PMID: 19001320]

[124] Laurent-Puig P, Cayre A, Manceau G, *et al.* Analysis of PTEN, BRAF, and EGFR status in determining benefit from cetuximab therapy in wild-type KRAS metastatic colon cancer. J Clin Oncol 2009; 27(35): 5924-30.
[http://dx.doi.org/10.1200/JCO.2008.21.6796] [PMID: 19884556]

[125] Tol J, Nagtegaal ID, Punt CJ. BRAF mutation in metastatic colorectal cancer. N Engl J Med 2009; 361(1): 98-9.
[http://dx.doi.org/10.1056/NEJMc0904160] [PMID: 19571295]

[126] Rowland A, Dias MM, Wiese MD, *et al.* Meta-analysis of BRAF mutation as a predictive biomarker of benefit from anti-EGFR monoclonal antibody therapy for RAS wild-type metastatic colorectal cancer. Br J Cancer 2015; 112(12): 1888-94.
[http://dx.doi.org/10.1038/bjc.2015.173] [PMID: 25989278]

[127] Van Cutsem E, Köhne CH, Láng I, *et al.* Cetuximab plus irinotecan, fluorouracil, and leucovorin as first-line treatment for metastatic colorectal cancer: updated analysis of overall survival according to tumor KRAS and BRAF mutation status. J Clin Oncol 2011; 29(15): 2011-9.
[http://dx.doi.org/10.1200/JCO.2010.33.5091] [PMID: 21502544]

[128] Bokemeyer C, Van Cutsem E, Rougier P, *et al.* Addition of cetuximab to chemotherapy as first-line treatment for KRAS wild-type metastatic colorectal cancer: pooled analysis of the CRYSTAL and OPUS randomised clinical trials. Eur J Cancer 2012; 48(10): 1466-75.
[http://dx.doi.org/10.1016/j.ejca.2012.02.057] [PMID: 22446022]

[129] Peeters M, Oliner KS, Parker A, *et al.* Massively parallel tumor multigene sequencing to evaluate response to panitumumab in a randomized phase III study of metastatic colorectal cancer. Clin Cancer Res 2013; 19(7): 1902-12.
[http://dx.doi.org/10.1158/1078-0432.CCR-12-1913] [PMID: 23325582]

[130] Maughan TS, Adams RA, Smith CG, *et al.* MRC COIN Trial Investigators. Addition of cetuximab to oxaliplatin-based first-line combination chemotherapy for treatment of advanced colorectal cancer: results of the randomised phase 3 MRC COIN trial. Lancet 2011; 377(9783): 2103-14.
[http://dx.doi.org/10.1016/S0140-6736(11)60613-2] [PMID: 21641636]

[131] Tveit KM, Guren T, Glimelius B, *et al.* Phase III trial of cetuximab with continuous or intermittent fluorouracil, leucovorin, and oxaliplatin (Nordic FLOX) *versus* FLOX alone in first-line treatment of metastatic colorectal cancer: the NORDIC-VII study. J Clin Oncol 2012; 30(15): 1755-62.
[http://dx.doi.org/10.1200/JCO.2011.38.0915] [PMID: 22473155]

[132] Pietrantonio F, Petrelli F, Coinu A, *et al.* Predictive role of BRAF mutations in patients with advanced colorectal cancer receiving cetuximab and panitumumab: a meta-analysis. Eur J Cancer 2015; 51(5): 587-94.
[http://dx.doi.org/10.1016/j.ejca.2015.01.054] [PMID: 25673558]

[133] Li S, Li L, Zhu Y, *et al.* Coexistence of EGFR with KRAS, or BRAF, or PIK3CA somatic mutations in lung cancer: a comprehensive mutation profiling from 5125 Chinese cohorts. Br J Cancer 2014; 110(11): 2812-20.
[http://dx.doi.org/10.1038/bjc.2014.210] [PMID: 24743704]

[134] Han JY, Kim SH, Lee YS, *et al.* Comparison of targeted next-generation sequencing with conventional sequencing for predicting the responsiveness to epidermal growth factor receptor-tyrosine kinase inhibitor (EGFR-TKI) therapy in never-smokers with lung adenocarcinoma. Lung Cancer 2014; 85(2): 161-7.
[http://dx.doi.org/10.1016/j.lungcan.2014.04.009] [PMID: 24857785]

[135] Brustugun OT, Khattak AM, Trømborg AK, *et al.* BRAF-mutations in non-small cell lung cancer. Lung Cancer 2014; 84(1): 36-8.
[http://dx.doi.org/10.1016/j.lungcan.2014.01.023] [PMID: 24552757]

[136] Weber A, Langhanki L, Sommerer F, Markwarth A, Wittekind C, Tannapfel A. Mutations of the BRAF gene in squamous cell carcinoma of the head and neck. Oncogene 2003; 22(30): 4757-9.
[http://dx.doi.org/10.1038/sj.onc.1206705] [PMID: 12879021]

[137] Vakiani E, Solit DB. KRAS and BRAF: drug targets and predictive biomarkers. J Pathol 2011; 223(2): 219-29.
[http://dx.doi.org/10.1002/path.2796] [PMID: 21125676]

[138] Chang L, Karin M. Mammalian MAP kinase signalling cascades. Nature 2001; 410(6824): 37-40.
[http://dx.doi.org/10.1038/35065000] [PMID: 11242034]

[139] Khokhlatchev AV, Canagarajah B, Wilsbacher J, *et al.* Phosphorylation of the MAP kinase ERK2 promotes its homodimerization and nuclear translocation. Cell 1998; 93(4): 605-15.
[http://dx.doi.org/10.1016/S0092-8674(00)81189-7] [PMID: 9604935]

[140] Albanell J, Rojo F, Averbuch S, *et al.* Pharmacodynamic studies of the epidermal growth factor receptor inhibitor ZD1839 in skin from cancer patients: histopathologic and molecular consequences of receptor inhibition. J Clin Oncol 2002; 20(1): 110-24.
[http://dx.doi.org/10.1200/JCO.20.1.110] [PMID: 11773160]

[141] Luwor RB, Lu Y, Li X, Mendelsohn J, Fan Z. The antiepidermal growth factor receptor monoclonal

antibody cetuximab/C225 reduces hypoxia-inducible factor-1 alpha, leading to transcriptional inhibition of vascular endothelial growth factor expression. Oncogene 2005; 24(27): 4433-41.
[http://dx.doi.org/10.1038/sj.onc.1208625] [PMID: 15806152]

[142]　Psyrri A, Lee JW, Pectasides E, *et al.* Prognostic biomarkers in phase II trial of cetuximab-containing induction and chemoradiation in resectable HNSCC: Eastern cooperative oncology group E2303. Clin Cancer Res 2014; 20(11): 3023-32.
[http://dx.doi.org/10.1158/1078-0432.CCR-14-0113] [PMID: 24700741]

[143]　Perkins G, Lièvre A, Ramacci C, *et al.* Additional value of EGFR downstream signaling phosphoprotein expression to KRAS status for response to anti-EGFR antibodies in colorectal cancer. Int J Cancer 2010; 127(6): 1321-31.
[http://dx.doi.org/10.1002/ijc.25152] [PMID: 20049837]

[144]　Clark PA, Iida M, Treisman DM, *et al.* Activation of multiple ERBB family receptors mediates glioblastoma cancer stem-like cell resistance to EGFR-targeted inhibition. Neoplasia 2012; 14(5): 420-8.
[http://dx.doi.org/10.1596/neo.12432] [PMID: 22745588]

[145]　Buonato JM, Lazzara MJ. ERK1/2 blockade prevents epithelial-mesenchymal transition in lung cancer cells and promotes their sensitivity to EGFR inhibition. Cancer Res 2014; 74(1): 309-19.
[http://dx.doi.org/10.1158/0008-5472.CAN-12-4721] [PMID: 24108744]

[146]　Furcht CM, Buonato JM, Skuli N, *et al.* Multivariate signaling regulation by SHP2 differentially controls proliferation and therapeutic response in glioma cells. J Cell Sci 2014; 127(Pt 16): 3555-67.
[http://dx.doi.org/10.1242/jcs.150862] [PMID: 24951116]

[147]　Uchida A, Hirano S, Kitao H, *et al.* Activation of downstream epidermal growth factor receptor (EGFR) signaling provides gefitinib-resistance in cells carrying EGFR mutation. Cancer Sci 2007; 98(3): 357-63.
[http://dx.doi.org/10.1111/j.1349-7006.2007.00387.x] [PMID: 17270025]

[148]　Wykosky J, Hu J, Gomez GG, *et al.* A urokinase receptor-Bim signaling axis emerges during EGFR inhibitor resistance in mutant EGFR glioblastoma. Cancer Res 2015; 75(2): 394-404.
[http://dx.doi.org/10.1158/0008-5472.CAN-14-2004] [PMID: 25432173]

[149]　Xu J, Zeng LF, Shen W, Turchi JJ, Zhang ZY. Targeting SHP2 for EGFR inhibitor resistant non-small cell lung carcinoma. Biochem Biophys Res Commun 2013; 439(4): 586-90.
[http://dx.doi.org/10.1016/j.bbrc.2013.09.028] [PMID: 24041688]

[150]　Zhou W, Ercan D, Chen L, *et al.* Novel mutant-selective EGFR kinase inhibitors against EGFR T790M. Nature 2009; 462(7276): 1070-4.
[http://dx.doi.org/10.1038/nature08622] [PMID: 20033049]

[151]　Ercan D, Xu C, Yanagita M, *et al.* Reactivation of ERK signaling causes resistance to EGFR kinase inhibitors. Cancer Discov 2012; 2(10): 934-47.
[http://dx.doi.org/10.1158/2159-8290.CD-12-0103] [PMID: 22961667]

[152]　Bertotti A, Papp E, Jones S, *et al.* The genomic landscape of response to EGFR blockade in colorectal cancer. Nature 2015; 526(7572): 263-7.
[http://dx.doi.org/10.1038/nature14969] [PMID: 26416732]

[153] Guan KL, Broyles SS, Dixon JE. A Tyr/Ser protein phosphatase encoded by vaccinia virus. Nature 1991; 350(6316): 359-62.
[http://dx.doi.org/10.1038/350359a0] [PMID: 1848923]

[154] Farooq A, Zhou MM. Structure and regulation of MAPK phosphatases. Cell Signal 2004; 16(7): 769-79.
[http://dx.doi.org/10.1016/j.cellsig.2003.12.008] [PMID: 15115656]

[155] Baker JB, Dutta D, Watson D, *et al.* Tumour gene expression predicts response to cetuximab in patients with KRAS wild-type metastatic colorectal cancer. Br J Cancer 2011; 104(3): 488-95.
[http://dx.doi.org/10.1038/sj.bjc.6606054] [PMID: 21206494]

[156] Boeckx C, Op de Beeck K, Wouters A, *et al.* Overcoming cetuximab resistance in HNSCC: the role of AURKB and DUSP proteins. Cancer Lett 2014; 354(2): 365-77.
[http://dx.doi.org/10.1016/j.canlet.2014.08.039] [PMID: 25192874]

[157] Khambata-Ford S, Garrett CR, Meropol NJ, *et al.* Expression of epiregulin and amphiregulin and K-ras mutation status predict disease control in metastatic colorectal cancer patients treated with cetuximab. J Clin Oncol 2007; 25(22): 3230-7.
[http://dx.doi.org/10.1200/JCO.2006.10.5437] [PMID: 17664471]

[158] Kakiuchi S, Daigo Y, Ishikawa N, *et al.* Prediction of sensitivity of advanced non-small cell lung cancers to gefitinib (Iressa, ZD1839). Hum Mol Genet 2004; 13(24): 3029-43.
[http://dx.doi.org/10.1093/hmg/ddh331] [PMID: 15496427]

[159] Berridge MJ, Irvine RF. Inositol trisphosphate, a novel second messenger in cellular signal transduction. Nature 1984; 312(5992): 315-21.
[http://dx.doi.org/10.1038/312315a0] [PMID: 6095092]

[160] Whitman M, Kaplan DR, Schaffhausen B, Cantley L, Roberts TM. Association of phosphatidylinositol kinase activity with polyoma middle-T competent for transformation. Nature 1985; 315(6016): 239-42.
[http://dx.doi.org/10.1038/315239a0] [PMID: 2987699]

[161] Whitman M, Downes CP, Keeler M, Keller T, Cantley L. Type I phosphatidylinositol kinase makes a novel inositol phospholipid, phosphatidylinositol-3-phosphate. Nature 1988; 332(6165): 644-6.
[http://dx.doi.org/10.1038/332644a0] [PMID: 2833705]

[162] MacDougall LK, Domin J, Waterfield MD. A family of phosphoinositide 3-kinases in Drosophila identifies a new mediator of signal transduction. Curr Biol 1995; 5(12): 1404-15.
[http://dx.doi.org/10.1016/S0960-9822(95)00278-8] [PMID: 8749393]

[163] Schu PV, Takegawa K, Fry MJ, Stack JH, Waterfield MD, Emr SD. Phosphatidylinositol 3-kinase encoded by yeast VPS34 gene essential for protein sorting. Science 1993; 260(5104): 88-91.
[http://dx.doi.org/10.1126/science.8385367] [PMID: 8385367]

[164] Burgering BM, Coffer PJ. Protein kinase B (c-Akt) in phosphatidylinositol-3-OH kinase signal transduction. Nature 1995; 376(6541): 599-602.
[http://dx.doi.org/10.1038/376599a0] [PMID: 7637810]

[165] Vanhaesebroeck B, Guillermet-Guibert J, Graupera M, Bilanges B. The emerging mechanisms of isoform-specific PI3K signalling. Nat Rev Mol Cell Biol 2010; 11(5): 329-41.
[http://dx.doi.org/10.1038/nrm2882] [PMID: 20379207]

[166] Hooshmand-Rad R, Hájková L, Klint P, *et al.* The PI 3-kinase isoforms p110(alpha) and p110(beta) have differential roles in PDGF- and insulin-mediated signaling. J Cell Sci 2000; 113(Pt 2): 207-14. [PMID: 10633072]

[167] Vanhaesebroeck B, Alessi DR. The PI3K-PDK1 connection: more than just a road to PKB. Biochem J 2000; 346(Pt 3): 561-76. [PMID: 10698680]

[168] Stephens L, Anderson K, Stokoe D, *et al.* Protein kinase B kinases that mediate phosphatidylinositol 3,4,5-trisphosphate-dependent activation of protein kinase B. Science 1998; 279(5351): 710-4. [http://dx.doi.org/10.1126/science.279.5351.710] [PMID: 9445477]

[169] James SR, Downes CP, Gigg R, Grove SJ, Holmes AB, Alessi DR. Specific binding of the Akt-1 protein kinase to phosphatidylinositol 3,4,5-trisphosphate without subsequent activation. Biochem J 1996; 315(Pt 3): 709-13. [http://dx.doi.org/10.1042/bj3150709] [PMID: 8645147]

[170] Alessi DR, James SR, Downes CP, *et al.* Characterization of a 3-phosphoinositide-dependent protein kinase which phosphorylates and activates protein kinase Balpha. Curr Biol 1997; 7(4): 261-9. [http://dx.doi.org/10.1016/S0960-9822(06)00122-9] [PMID: 9094314]

[171] Steck PA, Pershouse MA, Jasser SA, *et al.* Identification of a candidate tumour suppressor gene, MMAC1, at chromosome 10q23.3 that is mutated in multiple advanced cancers. Nat Genet 1997; 15(4): 356-62. [http://dx.doi.org/10.1038/ng0497-356] [PMID: 9090379]

[172] Li J, Yen C, Liaw D, *et al.* PTEN, a putative protein tyrosine phosphatase gene mutated in human brain, breast, and prostate cancer. Science 1997; 275(5308): 1943-7. [http://dx.doi.org/10.1126/science.275.5308.1943] [PMID: 9072974]

[173] Li DM, Sun H. TEP1, encoded by a candidate tumor suppressor locus, is a novel protein tyrosine phosphatase regulated by transforming growth factor beta. Cancer Res 1997; 57(11): 2124-9. [PMID: 9187108]

[174] Maehama T, Dixon JE. The tumor suppressor, PTEN/MMAC1, dephosphorylates the lipid second messenger, phosphatidylinositol 3,4,5-trisphosphate. J Biol Chem 1998; 273(22): 13375-8. [http://dx.doi.org/10.1074/jbc.273.22.13375] [PMID: 9593664]

[175] Engelman JA, Jänne PA, Mermel C, *et al.* ErbB-3 mediates phosphoinositide 3-kinase activity in gefitinib-sensitive non-small cell lung cancer cell lines. Proc Natl Acad Sci USA 2005; 102(10): 3788-93. [http://dx.doi.org/10.1073/pnas.0409773102] [PMID: 15731348]

[176] Guix M, Faber AC, Wang SE, *et al.* Acquired resistance to EGFR tyrosine kinase inhibitors in cancer cells is mediated by loss of IGF-binding proteins. J Clin Invest 2008; 118(7): 2609-19. [PMID: 18568074]

[177] Samuels Y, Velculescu VE. Oncogenic mutations of PIK3CA in human cancers. Cell Cycle 2004; 3(10): 1221-4. [http://dx.doi.org/10.4161/cc.3.10.1164] [PMID: 15467468]

[178] Samuels Y, Wang Z, Bardelli A, *et al.* High frequency of mutations of the PIK3CA gene in human

cancers. Science 2004; 304(5670): 554.
[http://dx.doi.org/10.1126/science.1096502] [PMID: 15016963]

[179]   Barault L, Veyrie N, Jooste V, *et al.* Mutations in the RAS-MAPK, PI(3)K (phosphatidylinositol--
        -OH kinase) signaling network correlate with poor survival in a population-based series of colon
        cancers. Int J Cancer 2008; 122(10): 2255-9.
        [http://dx.doi.org/10.1002/ijc.23388] [PMID: 18224685]

[180]   Nosho K, Kawasaki T, Ohnishi M, *et al.* PIK3CA mutation in colorectal cancer: relationship with
        genetic and epigenetic alterations. Neoplasia 2008; 10(6): 534-41.
        [http://dx.doi.org/10.1593/neo.08336] [PMID: 18516290]

[181]   Sartore-Bianchi A, Martini M, Molinari F, *et al.* PIK3CA mutations in colorectal cancer are associated
        with clinical resistance to EGFR-targeted monoclonal antibodies. Cancer Res 2009; 69(5): 1851-7.
        [http://dx.doi.org/10.1158/0008-5472.CAN-08-2466] [PMID: 19223544]

[182]   Perrone F, Lampis A, Orsenigo M, *et al.* PI3KCA/PTEN deregulation contributes to impaired
        responses to cetuximab in metastatic colorectal cancer patients. Ann Oncol 2009; 20(1): 84-90.
        [http://dx.doi.org/10.1093/annonc/mdn541] [PMID: 18669866]

[183]   Prenen H, De Schutter J, Jacobs B, *et al.* PIK3CA mutations are not a major determinant of resistance
        to the epidermal growth factor receptor inhibitor cetuximab in metastatic colorectal cancer. Clin
        Cancer Res 2009; 15(9): 3184-8.
        [http://dx.doi.org/10.1158/1078-0432.CCR-08-2961] [PMID: 19366826]

[184]   Wong NS, Fernando NH, Nixon AB, *et al.* A phase II study of capecitabine, oxaliplatin, bevacizumab
        and cetuximab in the treatment of metastatic colorectal cancer. Anticancer Res 2011; 31(1): 255-61.
        [PMID: 21273607]

[185]   Tol J, Dijkstra JR, Klomp M, *et al.* Markers for EGFR pathway activation as predictor of outcome in
        metastatic colorectal cancer patients treated with or without cetuximab. Eur J Cancer 2010; 46(11):
        1997-2009.
        [http://dx.doi.org/10.1016/j.ejca.2010.03.036] [PMID: 20413299]

[186]   Saridaki Z, Tzardi M, Papadaki C, *et al.* Impact of KRAS, BRAF, PIK3CA mutations, PTEN, AREG,
        EREG expression and skin rash in ≥ 2 line cetuximab-based therapy of colorectal cancer patients.
        PLoS One 2011; 6(1): e15980.
        [http://dx.doi.org/10.1371/journal.pone.0015980] [PMID: 21283802]

[187]   Karapetis CS, Jonker D, Daneshmand M, *et al.* NCIC Clinical Trials Group and the Australasian
        Gastro-Intestinal Trials Group. PIK3CA, BRAF, and PTEN status and benefit from cetuximab in the
        treatment of advanced colorectal cancer--results from NCIC CTG/AGITG CO.17. Clin Cancer Res
        2014; 20(3): 744-53.
        [http://dx.doi.org/10.1158/1078-0432.CCR-13-0606] [PMID: 24218517]

[188]   Smith CG, Fisher D, Claes B, *et al.* Somatic profiling of the epidermal growth factor receptor pathway
        in tumors from patients with advanced colorectal cancer treated with chemotherapy ± cetuximab. Clin
        Cancer Res 2013; 19(15): 4104-13.
        [http://dx.doi.org/10.1158/1078-0432.CCR-12-2581] [PMID: 23741067]

[189]   Seymour MT, Brown SR, Middleton G, *et al.* Panitumumab and irinotecan *versus* irinotecan alone for
        patients with KRAS wild-type, fluorouracil-resistant advanced colorectal cancer (PICCOLO): a

prospectively stratified randomised trial. Lancet Oncol 2013; 14(8): 749-59.
[http://dx.doi.org/10.1016/S1470-2045(13)70163-3] [PMID: 23725851]

[190] Ulivi P, Capelli L, Valgiusti M, *et al.* Predictive role of multiple gene alterations in response to cetuximab in metastatic colorectal cancer: a single center study. J Transl Med 2012; 10: 87.
[http://dx.doi.org/10.1186/1479-5876-10-87] [PMID: 22569004]

[191] Souglakos J, Philips J, Wang R, *et al.* Prognostic and predictive value of common mutations for treatment response and survival in patients with metastatic colorectal cancer. Br J Cancer 2009; 101(3): 465-72.
[http://dx.doi.org/10.1038/sj.bjc.6605164] [PMID: 19603024]

[192] Therkildsen C, Bergmann TK, Henrichsen-Schnack T, Ladelund S, Nilbert M. The predictive value of KRAS, NRAS, BRAF, PIK3CA and PTEN for anti-EGFR treatment in metastatic colorectal cancer: A systematic review and meta-analysis. Acta Oncol 2014; 53(7): 852-64.
[http://dx.doi.org/10.3109/0284186X.2014.895036] [PMID: 24666267]

[193] Sartore-Bianchi A, Di Nicolantonio F, Nichelatti M, *et al.* Multi-determinants analysis of molecular alterations for predicting clinical benefit to EGFR-targeted monoclonal antibodies in colorectal cancer. PLoS One 2009; 4(10): e7287.
[http://dx.doi.org/10.1371/journal.pone.0007287] [PMID: 19806185]

[194] Yang ZY, Wu XY, Huang YF, *et al.* Promising biomarkers for predicting the outcomes of patients with KRAS wild-type metastatic colorectal cancer treated with anti-epidermal growth factor receptor monoclonal antibodies: a systematic review with meta-analysis. Int J Cancer 2013; 133(8): 1914-25.
[http://dx.doi.org/10.1002/ijc.28153] [PMID: 23494461]

[195] Huang L, Liu Z, Deng D, *et al.* Anti-epidermal growth factor receptor monoclonal antibody-based therapy for metastatic colorectal cancer: a meta-analysis of the effect of PIK3CA mutations in KRAS wild-type patients. Arch Med Sci 2014; 10(1): 1-9.
[http://dx.doi.org/10.5114/aoms.2014.40728] [PMID: 24701207]

[196] Pentheroudakis G, Kotoula V, De Roock W, *et al.* Biomarkers of benefit from cetuximab-based therapy in metastatic colorectal cancer: interaction of EGFR ligand expression with RAS/RAF, PIK3CA genotypes. BMC Cancer 2013; 13: 49.
[http://dx.doi.org/10.1186/1471-2407-13-49] [PMID: 23374602]

[197] Sood A, McClain D, Maitra R, *et al.* PTEN gene expression and mutations in the PIK3CA gene as predictors of clinical benefit to anti-epidermal growth factor receptor antibody therapy in patients with KRAS wild-type metastatic colorectal cancer. Clin Colorectal Cancer 2012; 11(2): 143-50.
[http://dx.doi.org/10.1016/j.clcc.2011.12.001] [PMID: 22285706]

[198] Jhawer M, Goel S, Wilson AJ, *et al.* PIK3CA mutation/PTEN expression status predicts response of colon cancer cells to the epidermal growth factor receptor inhibitor cetuximab. Cancer Res 2008; 68(6): 1953-61.
[http://dx.doi.org/10.1158/0008-5472.CAN-07-5659] [PMID: 18339877]

[199] Wang L, Zhang Q, Zhang J, *et al.* PI3K pathway activation results in low efficacy of both trastuzumab and lapatinib. BMC Cancer 2011; 11: 248.
[http://dx.doi.org/10.1186/1471-2407-11-248] [PMID: 21676217]

[200] Young NR, Liu J, Pierce C, *et al.* Molecular phenotype predicts sensitivity of squamous cell carcinoma

of the head and neck to epidermal growth factor receptor inhibition. Mol Oncol 2013; 7(3): 359-68.
[http://dx.doi.org/10.1016/j.molonc.2012.11.001] [PMID: 23200321]

[201] Eichhorn PJ, Gili M, Scaltriti M, *et al.* Phosphatidylinositol 3-kinase hyperactivation results in lapatinib resistance that is reversed by the mTOR/phosphatidylinositol 3-kinase inhibitor NVP-BEZ235. Cancer Res 2008; 68(22): 9221-30.
[http://dx.doi.org/10.1158/0008-5472.CAN-08-1740] [PMID: 19010894]

[202] Engelman JA, Mukohara T, Zejnullahu K, *et al.* Allelic dilution obscures detection of a biologically significant resistance mutation in EGFR-amplified lung cancer. J Clin Invest 2006; 116(10): 2695-706.
[http://dx.doi.org/10.1172/JCI28656] [PMID: 16906227]

[203] de la Rochefordiere A, Kamal M, Floquet A, *et al.* PIK3CA Pathway Mutations Predictive of Poor Response Following Standard Radiochemotherapy ± Cetuximab in Cervical Cancer Patients. Clin Cancer Res 2015; 21(11): 2530-7.
[http://dx.doi.org/10.1158/1078-0432.CCR-14-2368] [PMID: 25724520]

[204] Okines AF, Gonzalez de Castro D, Cunningham D, *et al.* Biomarker analysis in oesophagogastric cancer: Results from the REAL3 and TransMAGIC trials. Eur J Cancer 2013; 49(9): 2116-25.
[http://dx.doi.org/10.1016/j.ejca.2013.02.007] [PMID: 23481512]

[205] Bria E, Pilotto S, Amato E, *et al.* Molecular heterogeneity assessment by next-generation sequencing and response to gefitinib of EGFR mutant advanced lung adenocarcinoma. Oncotarget 2015; 6(14): 12783-95.
[http://dx.doi.org/10.18632/oncotarget.3727] [PMID: 25904052]

[206] Endoh H, Yatabe Y, Kosaka T, Kuwano H, Mitsudomi T. PTEN and PIK3CA expression is associated with prolonged survival after gefitinib treatment in EGFR-mutated lung cancer patients. J Thorac Oncol 2006; 1(7): 629-34.
[PMID: 17409929]

[207] Kim ST, Jang KT, Lee J, *et al.* Molecular subgroup analysis of clinical outcomes in a phase 3 study of gemcitabine and oxaliplatin with or without erlotinib in advanced biliary tract cancer. Transl Oncol 2015; 8(1): 40-6.
[http://dx.doi.org/10.1016/j.tranon.2014.12.003] [PMID: 25749176]

[208] Jimeno A, Tan AC, Coffa J, *et al.* Coordinated epidermal growth factor receptor pathway gene overexpression predicts epidermal growth factor receptor inhibitor sensitivity in pancreatic cancer. Cancer Res 2008; 68(8): 2841-9.
[http://dx.doi.org/10.1158/0008-5472.CAN-07-5200] [PMID: 18413752]

[209] Hanker AB, Pfefferle AD, Balko JM, *et al.* Mutant PIK3CA accelerates HER2-driven transgenic mammary tumors and induces resistance to combinations of anti-HER2 therapies. Proc Natl Acad Sci USA 2013; 110(35): 14372-7.
[http://dx.doi.org/10.1073/pnas.1303204110] [PMID: 23940356]

[210] Guarneri V, Dieci MV, Frassoldati A, *et al.* Prospective biomarker analysis of the randomized CHER-LOB study evaluating the dual anti-HER2 treatment with trastuzumab and lapatinib plus chemotherapy as neoadjuvant therapy for HER2-positive breast cancer. Oncologist 2015; 20(9): 1001-10.
[http://dx.doi.org/10.1634/theoncologist.2015-0138] [PMID: 26245675]

[211] Majewski IJ, Nuciforo P, Mittempergher L, *et al.* PIK3CA mutations are associated with decreased benefit to neoadjuvant human epidermal growth factor receptor 2-targeted therapies in breast cancer. J Clin Oncol 2015; 33(12): 1334-9.
[http://dx.doi.org/10.1200/JCO.2014.55.2158] [PMID: 25559818]

[212] Loibl S, von Minckwitz G, Schneeweiss A, *et al.* PIK3CA mutations are associated with lower rates of pathologic complete response to anti-human epidermal growth factor receptor 2 (her2) therapy in primary HER2-overexpressing breast cancer. J Clin Oncol 2014; 32(29): 3212-20.
[http://dx.doi.org/10.1200/JCO.2014.55.7876] [PMID: 25199759]

[213] Xu B, Guan Z, Shen Z, *et al.* Association of phosphatase and tensin homolog low and phosphatidylinositol 3-kinase catalytic subunit alpha gene mutations on outcome in human epidermal growth factor receptor 2-positive metastatic breast cancer patients treated with first-line lapatinib plus paclitaxel or paclitaxel alone. Breast Cancer Res 2014; 16(4): 405.
[http://dx.doi.org/10.1186/s13058-014-0405-y] [PMID: 25056500]

[214] Hanusch C, Schneeweiss A, Loibl S, *et al.* Dual Blockade with AFatinib and Trastuzumab as NEoadjuvant Treatment for Patients with Locally Advanced or Operable Breast Cancer Receiving Taxane-Anthracycline Containing Chemotherapy-DAFNE (GBG-70). Clin Cancer Res 2015; 21(13): 2924-31.
[http://dx.doi.org/10.1158/1078-0432.CCR-14-2774] [PMID: 25825476]

[215] Guarneri V, Generali DG, Frassoldati A, *et al.* Double-blind, placebo-controlled, multicenter, randomized, phase IIb neoadjuvant study of letrozole-lapatinib in postmenopausal hormone receptor-positive, human epidermal growth factor receptor 2-negative, operable breast cancer. J Clin Oncol 2014; 32(10): 1050-7.
[http://dx.doi.org/10.1200/JCO.2013.51.4737] [PMID: 24590635]

[216] Fidler MJ, Morrison LE, Basu S, *et al.* PTEN and PIK3CA gene copy numbers and poor outcomes in non-small cell lung cancer patients with gefitinib therapy. Br J Cancer 2011; 105(12): 1920-6.
[http://dx.doi.org/10.1038/bjc.2011.494] [PMID: 22095222]

[217] Arena S, Bellosillo B, Siravegna G, *et al.* Emergence of multiple EGFR extracellular mutations during cetuximab treatment in colorectal cancer. Clin Cancer Res 2015; 21(9): 2157-66.
[http://dx.doi.org/10.1158/1078-0432.CCR-14-2821] [PMID: 25623215]

[218] Sequist LV, Waltman BA, Dias-Santagata D, *et al.* Genotypic and histological evolution of lung cancers acquiring resistance to EGFR inhibitors. Sci Transl Med 2011; 3(75): 75ra26.
[http://dx.doi.org/10.1126/scitranslmed.3002003] [PMID: 21430269]

[219] Ji W, Choi CM, Rho JK, *et al.* Mechanisms of acquired resistance to EGFR-tyrosine kinase inhibitor in Korean patients with lung cancer. BMC Cancer 2013; 13: 606.
[http://dx.doi.org/10.1186/1471-2407-13-606] [PMID: 24369725]

[220] Yu HA, Arcila ME, Rekhtman N, *et al.* Analysis of tumor specimens at the time of acquired resistance to EGFR-TKI therapy in 155 patients with EGFR-mutant lung cancers. Clin Cancer Res 2013; 19(8): 2240-7.
[http://dx.doi.org/10.1158/1078-0432.CCR-12-2246] [PMID: 23470965]

[221] Pazarentzos E, Giannikopoulos P, Hrustanovic G, *et al.* Oncogenic activation of the PI3-kinase p110beta isoform *via* the tumor-derived PIK3Cbeta kinase domain mutation. Oncogene 2015.

[PMID: 25982275]

[222] Carpten JD, Faber AL, Horn C, *et al.* A transforming mutation in the pleckstrin homology domain of AKT1 in cancer. Nature 2007; 448(7152): 439-44.
[http://dx.doi.org/10.1038/nature05933] [PMID: 17611497]

[223] Hechtman JF, Sadowska J, Huse JT, *et al.* AKT1 E17K in Colorectal Carcinoma Is Associated with BRAF V600E but Not MSI-H Status: A Clinicopathologic Comparison to PIK3CA Helical and Kinase Domain Mutants. Mol Cancer Res 2015; 13(6): 1003-8.
[http://dx.doi.org/10.1158/1541-7786.MCR-15-0062-T] [PMID: 25714871]

[224] She QB, Solit D, Basso A, Moasser MM. Resistance to gefitinib in PTEN-null HER-overexpressing tumor cells can be overcome through restoration of PTEN function or pharmacologic modulation of constitutive phosphatidylinositol 3'-kinase/Akt pathway signaling. Clin Cancer Res 2003; 9(12): 4340-6.
[PMID: 14555504]

[225] Bianco R, Shin I, Ritter CA, *et al.* Loss of PTEN/MMAC1/TEP in EGF receptor-expressing tumor cells counteracts the antitumor action of EGFR tyrosine kinase inhibitors. Oncogene 2003; 22(18): 2812-22.
[http://dx.doi.org/10.1038/sj.onc.1206388] [PMID: 12743604]

[226] Sos ML, Koker M, Weir BA, *et al.* PTEN loss contributes to erlotinib resistance in EGFR-mutant lung cancer by activation of Akt and EGFR. Cancer Res 2009; 69(8): 3256-61.
[http://dx.doi.org/10.1158/0008-5472.CAN-08-4055] [PMID: 19351834]

[227] Yamasaki F, Johansen MJ, Zhang D, *et al.* Acquired resistance to erlotinib in A-431 epidermoid cancer cells requires down-regulation of MMAC1/PTEN and up-regulation of phosphorylated Akt. Cancer Res 2007; 67(12): 5779-88.
[http://dx.doi.org/10.1158/0008-5472.CAN-06-3020] [PMID: 17575145]

[228] Sarkaria JN, Yang L, Grogan PT, *et al.* Identification of molecular characteristics correlated with glioblastoma sensitivity to EGFR kinase inhibition through use of an intracranial xenograft test panel. Mol Cancer Ther 2007; 6(3): 1167-74.
[http://dx.doi.org/10.1158/1535-7163.MCT-06-0691] [PMID: 17363510]

[229] Messner I, Cadeddu G, Huckenbeck W, *et al.* KRAS p.G13D mutations are associated with sensitivity to anti-EGFR antibody treatment in colorectal cancer cell lines. J Cancer Res Clin Oncol 2013; 139(2): 201-9.
[http://dx.doi.org/10.1007/s00432-012-1319-7] [PMID: 23015072]

[230] Maeda M, Murakami Y, Watari K, Kuwano M, Izumi H, Ono M. CpG hypermethylation contributes to decreased expression of PTEN during acquired resistance to gefitinib in human lung cancer cell lines. Lung Cancer 2015; 87(3): 265-71.
[http://dx.doi.org/10.1016/j.lungcan.2015.01.009] [PMID: 25638724]

[231] Kokubo Y, Gemma A, Noro R, *et al.* Reduction of PTEN protein and loss of epidermal growth factor receptor gene mutation in lung cancer with natural resistance to gefitinib (IRESSA). Br J Cancer 2005; 92(9): 1711-9.
[http://dx.doi.org/10.1038/sj.bjc.6602559] [PMID: 15870831]

[232] Albitar L, Carter MB, Davies S, Leslie KK. Consequences of the loss of p53, RB1, and PTEN:

relationship to gefitinib resistance in endometrial cancer. Gynecol Oncol 2007; 106(1): 94-104.
[http://dx.doi.org/10.1016/j.ygyno.2007.03.006] [PMID: 17490733]

[233] Noro R, Gemma A, Miyanaga A, *et al.* PTEN inactivation in lung cancer cells and the effect of its recovery on treatment with epidermal growth factor receptor tyrosine kinase inhibitors. Int J Oncol 2007; 31(5): 1157-63.
[PMID: 17912443]

[234] Guillamo JS, de Boüard S, Valable S, *et al.* Molecular mechanisms underlying effects of epidermal growth factor receptor inhibition on invasion, proliferation, and angiogenesis in experimental glioma. Clin Cancer Res 2009; 15(11): 3697-704.
[http://dx.doi.org/10.1158/1078-0432.CCR-08-2042] [PMID: 19435839]

[235] Bidkhori G, Moeini A, Masoudi-Nejad A. Modeling of tumor progression in NSCLC and intrinsic resistance to TKI in loss of PTEN expression. PLoS One 2012; 7(10): e48004.
[http://dx.doi.org/10.1371/journal.pone.0048004] [PMID: 23133538]

[236] Okamoto K, Okamoto I, Hatashita E, *et al.* Overcoming erlotinib resistance in EGFR mutation-positive non-small cell lung cancer cells by targeting survivin. Mol Cancer Ther 2012; 11(1): 204-13.
[http://dx.doi.org/10.1158/1535-7163.MCT-11-0638] [PMID: 22075159]

[237] Mellinghoff IK, Wang MY, Vivanco I, *et al.* Molecular determinants of the response of glioblastomas to EGFR kinase inhibitors. N Engl J Med 2005; 353(19): 2012-24.
[http://dx.doi.org/10.1056/NEJMoa051918] [PMID: 16282176]

[238] Fenton TR, Nathanson D, Ponte de Albuquerque C, *et al.* Resistance to EGF receptor inhibitors in glioblastoma mediated by phosphorylation of the PTEN tumor suppressor at tyrosine 240. Proc Natl Acad Sci USA 2012; 109(35): 14164-9.
[http://dx.doi.org/10.1073/pnas.1211962109] [PMID: 22891331]

[239] Brown PD, Krishnan S, Sarkaria JN, *et al.* North Central Cancer Treatment Group Study N0177. Phase I/II trial of erlotinib and temozolomide with radiation therapy in the treatment of newly diagnosed glioblastoma multiforme: North Central Cancer Treatment Group Study N0177. J Clin Oncol 2008; 26(34): 5603-9.
[http://dx.doi.org/10.1200/JCO.2008.18.0612] [PMID: 18955445]

[240] van den Bent MJ, Brandes AA, Rampling R, *et al.* Randomized phase II trial of erlotinib *versus* temozolomide or carmustine in recurrent glioblastoma: EORTC brain tumor group study 26034. J Clin Oncol 2009; 27(8): 1268-74.
[http://dx.doi.org/10.1200/JCO.2008.17.5984] [PMID: 19204207]

[241] Thiessen B, Stewart C, Tsao M, *et al.* A phase I/II trial of GW572016 (lapatinib) in recurrent glioblastoma multiforme: clinical outcomes, pharmacokinetics and molecular correlation. Cancer Chemother Pharmacol 2010; 65(2): 353-61.
[http://dx.doi.org/10.1007/s00280-009-1041-6] [PMID: 19499221]

[242] Reardon DA, Desjardins A, Vredenburgh JJ, *et al.* Phase 2 trial of erlotinib plus sirolimus in adults with recurrent glioblastoma. J Neurooncol 2010; 96(2): 219-30.
[http://dx.doi.org/10.1007/s11060-009-9950-0] [PMID: 19562254]

[243] Reardon DA, Groves MD, Wen PY, *et al.* A phase I/II trial of pazopanib in combination with lapatinib in adult patients with relapsed malignant glioma. Clin Cancer Res 2013; 19(4): 900-8.

[http://dx.doi.org/10.1158/1078-0432.CCR-12-1707] [PMID: 23363814]

[244] Yung WK, Vredenburgh JJ, Cloughesy TF, *et al.* Safety and efficacy of erlotinib in first-relapse glioblastoma: a phase II open-label study. Neuro-oncol 2010; 12(10): 1061-70.
[http://dx.doi.org/10.1093/neuonc/noq072] [PMID: 20615922]

[245] de Groot JF, Gilbert MR, Aldape K, *et al.* Phase II study of carboplatin and erlotinib (Tarceva, OSI-774) in patients with recurrent glioblastoma. J Neurooncol 2008; 90(1): 89-97.
[http://dx.doi.org/10.1007/s11060-008-9637-y] [PMID: 18581057]

[246] Frattini M, Saletti P, Romagnani E, *et al.* PTEN loss of expression predicts cetuximab efficacy in metastatic colorectal cancer patients. Br J Cancer 2007; 97(8): 1139-45.
[http://dx.doi.org/10.1038/sj.bjc.6604009] [PMID: 17940504]

[247] Li FH, Shen L, Li ZH, *et al.* Impact of KRAS mutation and PTEN expression on cetuximab-treated colorectal cancer. World J Gastroenterol 2010; 16(46): 5881-8.
[http://dx.doi.org/10.3748/wjg.v16.i46.5881] [PMID: 21155011]

[248] Loupakis F, Pollina L, Stasi I, *et al.* PTEN expression and KRAS mutations on primary tumors and metastases in the prediction of benefit from cetuximab plus irinotecan for patients with metastatic colorectal cancer. J Clin Oncol 2009; 27(16): 2622-9.
[http://dx.doi.org/10.1200/JCO.2008.20.2796] [PMID: 19398573]

[249] Negri FV, Bozzetti C, Lagrasta CA, *et al.* PTEN status in advanced colorectal cancer treated with cetuximab. Br J Cancer 2010; 102(1): 162-4.
[http://dx.doi.org/10.1038/sj.bjc.6605471] [PMID: 19953097]

[250] Razis E, Briasoulis E, Vrettou E, *et al.* Potential value of PTEN in predicting cetuximab response in colorectal cancer: an exploratory study. BMC Cancer 2008; 8: 234.
[http://dx.doi.org/10.1186/1471-2407-8-234] [PMID: 18700047]

[251] Razis E, Pentheroudakis G, Rigakos G, *et al.* EGFR gene gain and PTEN protein expression are favorable prognostic factors in patients with KRAS wild-type metastatic colorectal cancer treated with cetuximab. J Cancer Res Clin Oncol 2014; 140(5): 737-48.
[http://dx.doi.org/10.1007/s00432-014-1626-2] [PMID: 24595598]

[252] Cathomas R, Rothermundt C, Klingbiel D, *et al.* Swiss Group for Clinical Cancer Research SAKK. Efficacy of cetuximab in metastatic castration-resistant prostate cancer might depend on EGFR and PTEN expression: results from a phase II trial (SAKK 08/07). Clin Cancer Res 2012; 18(21): 6049-57.
[http://dx.doi.org/10.1158/1078-0432.CCR-12-2219] [PMID: 22977195]

[253] Bouali S, Chrétien AS, Ramacci C, Rouyer M, Becuwe P, Merlin JL. PTEN expression controls cellular response to cetuximab by mediating PI3K/AKT and RAS/RAF/MAPK downstream signaling in KRAS wild-type, hormone refractory prostate cancer cells. Oncol Rep 2009; 21(3): 731-5.
[PMID: 19212633]

[254] Festuccia C, Muzi P, Millimaggi D, *et al.* Molecular aspects of gefitinib antiproliferative and pro-apoptotic effects in PTEN-positive and PTEN-negative prostate cancer cell lines. Endocr Relat Cancer 2005; 12(4): 983-98.
[http://dx.doi.org/10.1677/erc.1.00986] [PMID: 16322337]

[255] Wu Z, Gioeli D, Conaway M, Weber MJ, Theodorescu D. Restoration of PTEN expression alters the

sensitivity of prostate cancer cells to EGFR inhibitors. Prostate 2008; 68(9): 935-44.
[http://dx.doi.org/10.1002/pros.20745] [PMID: 18386291]

[256] Shen H, Zhu F, Liu J, *et al.* Alteration in Mir-21/PTEN expression modulates gefitinib resistance in non-small cell lung cancer. PLoS One 2014; 9(7): e103305.
[http://dx.doi.org/10.1371/journal.pone.0103305] [PMID: 25058005]

[257] Li B, Ren S, Li X, *et al.* MiR-21 overexpression is associated with acquired resistance of EGFR-TKI in non-small cell lung cancer. Lung Cancer 2014; 83(2): 146-53.
[http://dx.doi.org/10.1016/j.lungcan.2013.11.003] [PMID: 24331411]

[258] Wang YS, Wang YH, Xia HP, Zhou SW, Schmid-Bindert G, Zhou CC. MicroRNA-214 regulates the acquired resistance to gefitinib *via* the PTEN/AKT pathway in EGFR-mutant cell lines. Asian Pac J Cancer Prev 2012; 13(1): 255-60.
[http://dx.doi.org/10.7314/APJCP.2012.13.1.255] [PMID: 22502680]

[259] Zhang AX, Lu FQ, Yang YP, Ren XY, Li ZF, Zhang W. MicroRNA-217 overexpression induces drug resistance and invasion of breast cancer cells by targeting PTEN signaling. Cell Biol Int 2015. [Epub ahead of print]
[http://dx.doi.org/10.1002/cbin.10506] [PMID: 26109338]

[260] Yamamoto C, Basaki Y, Kawahara A, *et al.* Loss of PTEN expression by blocking nuclear translocation of EGR1 in gefitinib-resistant lung cancer cells harboring epidermal growth factor receptor-activating mutations. Cancer Res 2010; 70(21): 8715-25.
[http://dx.doi.org/10.1158/0008-5472.CAN-10-0043] [PMID: 20959484]

[261] Somlo G, Martel CL, Lau SK, *et al.* A phase I/II prospective, single arm trial of gefitinib, trastuzumab, and docetaxel in patients with stage IV HER-2 positive metastatic breast cancer. Breast Cancer Res Treat 2012; 131(3): 899-906.
[http://dx.doi.org/10.1007/s10549-011-1850-2] [PMID: 22042372]

[262] Dave B, Migliaccio I, Gutierrez MC, *et al.* Loss of phosphatase and tensin homolog or phosphoinositol-3 kinase activation and response to trastuzumab or lapatinib in human epidermal growth factor receptor 2-overexpressing locally advanced breast cancers. J Clin Oncol 2011; 29(2): 166-73.
[http://dx.doi.org/10.1200/JCO.2009.27.7814] [PMID: 21135276]

[263] Nuciforo PG, Aura C, Holmes E, *et al.* Benefit to neoadjuvant anti-human epidermal growth factor receptor 2 (HER2)-targeted therapies in HER2-positive primary breast cancer is independent of phosphatase and tensin homolog deleted from chromosome 10 (PTEN) status. Ann Oncol 2015; 26(7): 1494-500.
[PMID: 25851628]

[264] Xia W, Husain I, Liu L, *et al.* Lapatinib antitumor activity is not dependent upon phosphatase and tensin homologue deleted on chromosome 10 in ErbB2-overexpressing breast cancers. Cancer Res 2007; 67(3): 1170-5.
[http://dx.doi.org/10.1158/0008-5472.CAN-06-2101] [PMID: 17283152]

[265] O'Brien NA, Browne BC, Chow L, *et al.* Activated phosphoinositide 3-kinase/AKT signaling confers resistance to trastuzumab but not lapatinib. Mol Cancer Ther 2010; 9(6): 1489-502.
[http://dx.doi.org/10.1158/1535-7163.MCT-09-1171] [PMID: 20501798]

[266] Sahin O, Wang Q, Brady SW, *et al.* Biomarker-guided sequential targeted therapies to overcome therapy resistance in rapidly evolving highly aggressive mammary tumors. Cell Res 2014; 24(5): 542-59.
[http://dx.doi.org/10.1038/cr.2014.37] [PMID: 24675532]

[267] Evaluation of Genomic Applications in Practice and Prevention (EGAPP) Working Group. Recommendations from the EGAPP Working Group: can testing of tumor tissue for mutations in EGFR pathway downstream effector genes in patients with metastatic colorectal cancer improve health outcomes by guiding decisions regarding anti-EGFR therapy? Genet Med 2013; 15(7): 517-27.
[http://dx.doi.org/10.1038/gim.2012.184] [PMID: 23429431]

[268] Tian S, Simon I, Moreno V, *et al.* A combined oncogenic pathway signature of BRAF, KRAS and PI3KCA mutation improves colorectal cancer classification and cetuximab treatment prediction. Gut 2013; 62(4): 540-9.
[http://dx.doi.org/10.1136/gutjnl-2012-302423] [PMID: 22798500]

[269] Despierre E, Vergote I, Anderson R, *et al.* European Organisation for Research and Treatment of Cancer-Gynaecological Cancer Group (EORTC-GCG), Groupe d'Investigateurs Nationaux pour les Etudes des Cancers de l'Ovaire (GINECO), Austrian Arbeitsgemeinschaft für Gynäkologische Onkologie (A-AGO), National Cancer Research Institute (NCRI), Australia New Zealand Gynaecological Oncology Group (ANZGOG), and the Mario Negri Gynecologic Oncology group (MaNGO). Epidermal Growth Factor Receptor (EGFR) Pathway Biomarkers in the Randomized Phase III Trial of Erlotinib *Versus* Observation in Ovarian Cancer Patients with No Evidence of Disease Progression after First-Line Platinum-Based Chemotherapy. Target Oncol 2015; 10(4): 583-96.
[http://dx.doi.org/10.1007/s11523-015-0369-6] [PMID: 26004768]

[270] Lupini L, Bassi C, Mlcochova J, *et al.* Prediction of response to anti-EGFR antibody-based therapies by multigene sequencing in colorectal cancer patients. BMC Cancer 2015; 15: 808.
[http://dx.doi.org/10.1186/s12885-015-1752-5] [PMID: 26508446]

[271] Nunes M, Vrignaud P, Vacher S, *et al.* Evaluating patient-derived colorectal cancer xenografts as preclinical models by comparison with patient clinical data. Cancer Res 2015; 75(8): 1560-6.
[http://dx.doi.org/10.1158/0008-5472.CAN-14-1590] [PMID: 25712343]

[272] Bertotti A, Migliardi G, Galimi F, *et al.* A molecularly annotated platform of patient-derived xenografts ("xenopatients") identifies HER2 as an effective therapeutic target in cetuximab-resistant colorectal cancer. Cancer Discov 2011; 1(6): 508-23.
[http://dx.doi.org/10.1158/2159-8290.CD-11-0109] [PMID: 22586653]

[273] Kavuri SM, Jain N, Galimi F, *et al.* HER2 activating mutations are targets for colorectal cancer treatment. Cancer Discov 2015; 5(8): 832-41.
[http://dx.doi.org/10.1158/2159-8290.CD-14-1211] [PMID: 26243863]

[274] Ciardiello F, Normanno N, Maiello E, *et al.* Clinical activity of FOLFIRI plus cetuximab according to extended gene mutation status by next-generation sequencing: findings from the CAPRI-GOIM trial. Ann Oncol 2014; 25(9): 1756-61.
[http://dx.doi.org/10.1093/annonc/mdu230] [PMID: 24942275]

[275] Barton BE, Karras JG, Murphy TF, Barton A, Huang HF. Signal transducer and activator of transcription 3 (STAT3) activation in prostate cancer: Direct STAT3 inhibition induces apoptosis in

prostate cancer lines. Mol Cancer Ther 2004; 3(1): 11-20.
[http://dx.doi.org/10.1186/1476-4598-3-11] [PMID: 14749471]

[276]　Campbell CL, Jiang Z, Savarese DM, Savarese TM. Increased expression of the interleukin-11 receptor and evidence of STAT3 activation in prostate carcinoma. Am J Pathol 2001; 158(1): 25-32.
[http://dx.doi.org/10.1016/S0002-9440(10)63940-5] [PMID: 11141475]

[277]　Chen RJ, Ho YS, Guo HR, Wang YJ. Rapid activation of Stat3 and ERK1/2 by nicotine modulates cell proliferation in human bladder cancer cells. Toxicological sciences : an official journal of the Society of Toxicology 2008; 104(2): 283-93.
[http://dx.doi.org/10.1093/toxsci/kfn086] [PMID: 18448488]

[278]　Chung SS, Giehl N, Wu Y, Vadgama JV. STAT3 activation in HER2-overexpressing breast cancer promotes epithelial-mesenchymal transition and cancer stem cell traits. Int J Oncol 2014; 44(2): 403-11.
[PMID: 24297508]

[279]　Lin L, Fuchs J, Li C, Olson V, Bekaii-Saab T, Lin J. STAT3 signaling pathway is necessary for cell survival and tumorsphere forming capacity in ALDH(+)/CD133(+) stem cell-like human colon cancer cells. Biochem Biophys Res Commun 2011; 416(3-4): 246-51.
[http://dx.doi.org/10.1016/j.bbrc.2011.10.112] [PMID: 22074823]

[280]　Looyenga BD, Hutchings D, Cherni I, Kingsley C, Weiss GJ, Mackeigan JP. STAT3 is activated by JAK2 independent of key oncogenic driver mutations in non-small cell lung carcinoma. PLoS One 2012; 7(2): e30820.
[http://dx.doi.org/10.1371/journal.pone.0030820] [PMID: 22319590]

[281]　Zhang Y, Du XL, Wang CJ, *et al.* Reciprocal activation between PLK1 and Stat3 contributes to survival and proliferation of esophageal cancer cells. Gastroenterology 2012; 142(3): 521-30 e3.
[http://dx.doi.org/10.1053/j.gastro.2011.11.023]

[282]　Graf U, Casanova EA, Cinelli P. The Role of the Leukemia Inhibitory Factor (LIF) - Pathway in Derivation and Maintenance of Murine Pluripotent Stem Cells. Genes (Basel) 2011; 2(1): 280-97.
[http://dx.doi.org/10.3390/genes2010280] [PMID: 24710148]

[283]　Luwor RB, Stylli SS, Kaye AH. The role of Stat3 in glioblastoma multiforme. J Clin Neurosci 2013; 20(7): 907-11.
[http://dx.doi.org/10.1016/j.jocn.2013.03.006] [PMID: 23688441]

[284]　Organ SL, Tsao MS. An overview of the c-MET signaling pathway. Ther Adv Med Oncol 2011; 3(1) (Suppl.): S7-S19.
[http://dx.doi.org/10.1177/1758834011422556] [PMID: 22128289]

[285]　Ren Z, Schaefer TS. ErbB-2 activates Stat3 alpha in a Src- and JAK2-dependent manner. J Biol Chem 2002; 277(41): 38486-93.
[http://dx.doi.org/10.1074/jbc.M112438200] [PMID: 11940572]

[286]　Dobi E, Monnien F, Kim S, *et al.* Impact of STAT3 phosphorylation on the clinical effectiveness of anti-EGFR-based therapy in patients with metastatic colorectal cancer. Clin Colorectal Cancer 2013; 12(1): 28-36.
[http://dx.doi.org/10.1016/j.clcc.2012.09.002] [PMID: 23083634]

[287] Wu K, Chang Q, Lu Y, *et al.* Gefitinib resistance resulted from STAT3-mediated Akt activation in lung cancer cells. Oncotarget 2013; 4(12): 2430-8.
[http://dx.doi.org/10.18632/oncotarget.1431] [PMID: 24280348]

[288] Bonner JA, Yang ES, Trummell HQ, Nowsheen S, Willey CD, Raisch KP. Inhibition of STAT-3 results in greater cetuximab sensitivity in head and neck squamous cell carcinoma. Radiother Oncol 2011; 99(3): 339-43.
[http://dx.doi.org/10.1016/j.radonc.2011.05.070] [PMID: 21704410]

[289] Li L, Han R, Xiao H, *et al.* Metformin sensitizes EGFR-TKI-resistant human lung cancer cells *in vitro* and *in vivo* through inhibition of IL-6 signaling and EMT reversal. Clin Cancer Res 2014; 20(10): 2714-26.
[http://dx.doi.org/10.1158/1078-0432.CCR-13-2613] [PMID: 24644001]

[290] Li R, Hu Z, Sun SY, *et al.* Niclosamide overcomes acquired resistance to erlotinib through suppression of STAT3 in non-small cell lung cancer. Mol Cancer Ther 2013; 12(10): 2200-12.
[http://dx.doi.org/10.1158/1535-7163.MCT-13-0095] [PMID: 23894143]

[291] Sen M, Joyce S, Panahandeh M, *et al.* Targeting Stat3 abrogates EGFR inhibitor resistance in cancer. Clin Cancer Res 2012; 18(18): 4986-96.
[http://dx.doi.org/10.1158/1078-0432.CCR-12-0792] [PMID: 22825581]

[292] Zhang FQ, Yang WT, Duan SZ, Xia YC, Zhu RY, Chen YB. JAK2 inhibitor TG101348 overcomes erlotinib-resistance in non-small cell lung carcinoma cells with mutated EGF receptor. Oncotarget 2015; 6(16): 14329-43.
[http://dx.doi.org/10.18632/oncotarget.3685] [PMID: 25869210]

[293] Cao W, Liu Y, Zhang R, *et al.* Homoharringtonine induces apoptosis and inhibits STAT3 *via* IL-6/JAK1/STAT3 signal pathway in Gefitinib-resistant lung cancer cells. Sci Rep 2015; 5: 8477.
[http://dx.doi.org/10.1038/srep08477] [PMID: 26166037]

[294] Ung N, Putoczki TL, Stylli SS, *et al.* Anti-EGFR therapeutic efficacy correlates directly with inhibition of STAT3 activity. Cancer Biol Ther 2014; 15(5): 623-32.
[http://dx.doi.org/10.4161/cbt.28179] [PMID: 24556630]

[295] Li Q, Zhang D, Chen X, *et al.* Nuclear PKM2 contributes to gefitinib resistance *via* upregulation of STAT3 activation in colorectal cancer. Sci Rep 2015; 5: 16082.
[http://dx.doi.org/10.1038/srep16082] [PMID: 26542452]

[296] Kim HP, Han SW, Kim SH, *et al.* Combined lapatinib and cetuximab enhance cytotoxicity against gefitinib-resistant lung cancer cells. Mol Cancer Ther 2008; 7(3): 607-15.
[http://dx.doi.org/10.1158/1535-7163.MCT-07-2068] [PMID: 18347147]

[297] Weickhardt AJ, Price TJ, Chong G, *et al.* Dual targeting of the epidermal growth factor receptor using the combination of cetuximab and erlotinib: preclinical evaluation and results of the phase II DUX study in chemotherapy-refractory, advanced colorectal cancer. J Clin Oncol 2012; 30(13): 1505-12.
[http://dx.doi.org/10.1200/JCO.2011.38.6599] [PMID: 22412142]

[298] Lee HJ, Zhuang G, Cao Y, Du P, Kim HJ, Settleman J. Drug resistance *via* feedback activation of Stat3 in oncogene-addicted cancer cells. Cancer Cell 2014; 26(2): 207-21.
[http://dx.doi.org/10.1016/j.ccr.2014.05.019] [PMID: 25065853]

[299] Kim SM, Kwon OJ, Hong YK, *et al.* Activation of IL-6R/JAK1/STAT3 signaling induces de novo resistance to irreversible EGFR inhibitors in non-small cell lung cancer with T790M resistance mutation. Mol Cancer Ther 2012; 11(10): 2254-64.
[http://dx.doi.org/10.1158/1535-7163.MCT-12-0311] [PMID: 22891040]

[300] Jung MJ, Rho JK, Kim YM, *et al.* Upregulation of CXCR4 is functionally crucial for maintenance of stemness in drug-resistant non-small cell lung cancer cells. Oncogene 2013; 32(2): 209-21.
[http://dx.doi.org/10.1038/onc.2012.37] [PMID: 22370645]

[301] Kim HP, Han SW, Song SH, *et al.* Testican-1-mediated epithelial-mesenchymal transition signaling confers acquired resistance to lapatinib in HER2-positive gastric cancer. Oncogene 2014; 33(25): 3334-41.
[http://dx.doi.org/10.1038/onc.2013.285] [PMID: 23873022]

[302] Fan W, Tang Z, Yin L, *et al.* MET-independent lung cancer cells evading EGFR kinase inhibitors are therapeutically susceptible to BH3 mimetic agents. Cancer Res 2011; 71(13): 4494-505.
[http://dx.doi.org/10.1158/0008-5472.CAN-10-2668] [PMID: 21555370]

[303] Stanam A, Love-Homan L, Joseph TS, Espinosa-Cotton M, Simons AL. Upregulated interleukin-6 expression contributes to erlotinib resistance in head and neck squamous cell carcinoma. Mol Oncol 2015; 9(7): 1371-83.
[http://dx.doi.org/10.1016/j.molonc.2015.03.008] [PMID: 25888065]

[304] Normanno N, Rachiglio AM, Lambiase M, *et al.* CAPRI-GOIM investigators. Heterogeneity of KRAS, NRAS, BRAF and PIK3CA mutations in metastatic colorectal cancer and potential effects on therapy in the CAPRI GOIM trial. Ann Oncol 2015; 26(8): 1710-4.
[http://dx.doi.org/10.1093/annonc/mdv176] [PMID: 25851630]

[305] Di Fiore F, Blanchard F, Charbonnier F, *et al.* Clinical relevance of KRAS mutation detection in metastatic colorectal cancer treated by Cetuximab plus chemotherapy. Br J Cancer 2007; 96(8): 1166-9.
[http://dx.doi.org/10.1038/sj.bjc.6603685] [PMID: 17375050]

[306] Lièvre A, Bachet JB, Boige V, *et al.* KRAS mutations as an independent prognostic factor in patients with advanced colorectal cancer treated with cetuximab. J Clin Oncol 2008; 26(3): 374-9.
[http://dx.doi.org/10.1200/JCO.2007.12.5906] [PMID: 18202412]

[307] Cappuzzo F, Varella-Garcia M, Finocchiaro G, *et al.* Primary resistance to cetuximab therapy in EGFR FISH-positive colorectal cancer patients. Br J Cancer 2008; 99(1): 83-9.
[http://dx.doi.org/10.1038/sj.bjc.6604439] [PMID: 18577988]

[308] Van Cutsem E, Köhne CH, Hitre E, *et al.* Cetuximab and chemotherapy as initial treatment for metastatic colorectal cancer. N Engl J Med 2009; 360(14): 1408-17.
[http://dx.doi.org/10.1056/NEJMoa0805019] [PMID: 19339720]

[309] Freeman DJ, Juan T, Reiner M, *et al.* Association of K-ras mutational status and clinical outcomes in patients with metastatic colorectal cancer receiving panitumumab alone. Clin Colorectal Cancer 2008; 7(3): 184-90.
[http://dx.doi.org/10.3816/CCC.2008.n.024] [PMID: 18621636]

[310] Amado RG, Wolf M, Peeters M, *et al.* Wild-type KRAS is required for panitumumab efficacy in

patients with metastatic colorectal cancer. J Clin Oncol 2008; 26(10): 1626-34.
[http://dx.doi.org/10.1200/JCO.2007.14.7116] [PMID: 18316791]

[311] Han SW, Kim TY, Jeon YK, *et al.* Optimization of patient selection for gefitinib in non-small cell lung cancer by combined analysis of epidermal growth factor receptor mutation, K-ras mutation, and Akt phosphorylation. Clin Cancer Res 2006; 12(8): 2538-44.
[http://dx.doi.org/10.1158/1078-0432.CCR-05-2845] [PMID: 16638863]

[312] Giaccone G, Gallegos Ruiz M, Le Chevalier T, *et al.* Erlotinib for frontline treatment of advanced non-small cell lung cancer: a phase II study. Clin Cancer Res 2006; 12(20 Pt 1): 6049-55.
[http://dx.doi.org/10.1158/1078-0432.CCR-06-0260] [PMID: 17062680]

[313] Massarelli E, Varella-Garcia M, Tang X, *et al.* KRAS mutation is an important predictor of resistance to therapy with epidermal growth factor receptor tyrosine kinase inhibitors in non-small-cell lung cancer. Clin Cancer Res 2007; 13(10): 2890-6.
[http://dx.doi.org/10.1158/1078-0432.CCR-06-3043] [PMID: 17504988]

[314] Zhu CQ, da Cunha Santos G, Ding K, *et al.* National Cancer Institute of Canada Clinical Trials Group Study BR.21. Role of KRAS and EGFR as biomarkers of response to erlotinib in National Cancer Institute of Canada Clinical Trials Group Study BR.21. J Clin Oncol 2008; 26(26): 4268-75.
[http://dx.doi.org/10.1200/JCO.2007.14.8924] [PMID: 18626007]

[315] Marchetti A, Milella M, Felicioni L, *et al.* Clinical implications of KRAS mutations in lung cancer patients treated with tyrosine kinase inhibitors: an important role for mutations in minor clones. Neoplasia 2009; 11(10): 1084-92.
[http://dx.doi.org/10.1593/neo.09814] [PMID: 19794967]

[316] Molinari F, Martin V, Saletti P, *et al.* Differing deregulation of EGFR and downstream proteins in primary colorectal cancer and related metastatic sites may be clinically relevant. Br J Cancer 2009; 100(7): 1087-94.
[http://dx.doi.org/10.1038/sj.bjc.6604848] [PMID: 19293803]

[317] Iwamoto S, Hazama S, Kato T, *et al.* Multicenter phase II study of second-line cetuximab plus folinic acid/5-fluorouracil/irinotecan (FOLFIRI) in KRAS wild-type metastatic colorectal cancer: the FLIER study. Anticancer Res 2014; 34(4): 1967-73.
[PMID: 24692733]

[318] Soeda H, Shimodaira H, Watanabe M, *et al.* Clinical usefulness of KRAS, BRAF, and PIK3CA mutations as predictive markers of cetuximab efficacy in irinotecan- and oxaliplatin-refractory Japanese patients with metastatic colorectal cancer. Int J Clin Oncol 2013; 18(4): 670-7.
[http://dx.doi.org/10.1007/s10147-012-0422-8] [PMID: 22638623]

CHAPTER 3

Chemotherapeutic, Immunologic, and Molecularly Targeted Therapy for the Treatment of Advanced Melanoma

Saïd C. Azoury[1], David M. Straughan[2], Robert D. Bennett[2], Vivek Shukla[3,*]

[1] *Department of Surgery, The Johns Hopkins Hospital, Baltimore, MD, USA*

[2] *Department of Surgery, University of South Florida, Morsani College of Medicine, Tampa, FL, USA*

[3] *Thoracic and GI Oncology Branch, National Cancer Institute, National Institutes of Health, Bethesda, MD, USA*

Abstract: Over the past several decades, the incidence of melanoma has increased. Although surgery remains the primary treatment modality for localized early-stage lesions, melanoma is often diagnosed following locoregional and distant disease spread. Prognosis for advanced stage disease is dismal as one would expect; however, nowadays, the myriad of systemic therapies have allowed for improvements in disease free and overall survival. Such systemic treatment approaches include chemotherapy, immunotherapy, and molecularly targeted agents. Since the time of the approval of dacarbazine by the Food and Drug Administration for the treatment of metastatic melanoma in 1975, other agents have gained approval including interleukin-2, immune checkpoint inhibitors such as ipilimumab (anti-CTLA-4), and others. More recently, studies suggest that combination regimens of the aforementioned approaches may further improve outcomes when compared to monotherapy. Herein, the authors provide an up-to-date comprehensive review on the chemotherapeutic, immunologic, and molecularly targeted therapy approaches to the treatment of advanced melanoma.

Keywords: Advanced Stage, Anti-PD-1, Anti-CTLA-4, Anti-PD-L1, Chemotherapy, Dacarbazine, Immune Checkpoint, Immunotherapy, Interleukin-2,

* **Corresponding author Vivek Shukla:** 10 Center Drive, Room 3W5848, Thoracic and GI Oncology Branch, Clinical Center, National Cancer Center, National Institutes of Health, Bethesda, MD-20892, USA; Tel: 301-594-8961; E-mails: shuklav@mail.nih.gov, vivek.shukla@nih.gov

Atta-ur-Rahman (Ed.)

Melanoma, Metastatic, Systemic, Targeted Therapy, Vaccine.

INTRODUCTION

Over the past several decades, the incidence of melanoma has markedly increased [1 - 3]. Worldwide, approximately 50,000 deaths can be attributed to melanoma each year [4]. Melanomas originate from melanocytes, which reside in the basal layer of the epidermis and produce melanin. Several mechanisms are thought to underlie the malignant transformation of normal melanocytes in melanoma development. Perhaps one of the most well studied risk factors for melanoma development is ultraviolet radiation [5]. Under normal circumstances, melanin helps protect the skin from ultraviolet light. Overtime, excessive sun exposure, results in excessive DNA damage to proliferating melanocytes, thereby over-whelming the normal DNA repair mechanisms. Occasionally in the process, a cell will undergo malignant transformation [5]. Furthermore, several genes, such as *BRAF*, *PTEN,c-Kit*, *p53*, *CDKN2A/p16* are implicated in the development by mutation, deletion, or amplification. Mutations in these genes may be induced by UV radiation or are inherited and ultimately result in the dysregulation of the normal cell cycle checkpoints. Understanding the complex interplay of genetic and environmental factors in melanoma pathogenesis is an ongoing area of investigation.

Surgery is the primary treatment modality for localized early stage lesions, with estimated 5 and 10-year survival rates approximating 97% and 93% for patients with Stage 1a, T1aN0M0 melanomas ($\leq$ 1mm, without ulceration and mitosis $\leq$ 1/mm^2) [6]. Metastatic melanoma carries an overall median survival of 4-12 months, depending on the site of distant disease [7]. The current melanoma TNM staging system was recently updated using data from an expanded American Joint Committee on Cancer (AJCC) Melanoma Staging Database [4]. For metastatic melanoma (stage IV), elevated serum levels of LDH and site(s) of metastases define the M1 stage into three categories: M1a - only distant skin, subcutaneous or nodal metastases and normal LDH, M1b - lung metastases is present with a normal LDH, or M1c - metastases to any other visceral site and elevated LDH [4]. As one would expect, prognosis worsens as disease progresses from M1a to M1c disease.

While the prognosis after surgical resection in patients with early stage disease is favorable, the median overall survival for patients with distant metastases (stage IV) treated with chemotherapy is less than a year, and 5-year survival approximates 10% [3]. When considering metastatic disease, surgery may improve outcomes, and complete resection has been shown to improve survival when compared to incomplete resection [8, 9]. Melanoma is generally considered to be a relatively radio-resistant tumor; however, radiation therapy (*e.g.*, whole brain irradiation or stereotactic radiosurgery) has been used in adjuvant and palliative settings, such as in cases of metastasis to the brain [10 - 12].

Table 1. Select agents approved by the US Food and Drug Administration (FDA) for the treatment of advanced melanoma.

Class	Agent	Year FDA Approved	Indication
Chemotherapy	Dacarbazine	1975	Stage IV melanoma
Immunotherapy	High-Dose Interferon alfa-2b (IFN-α)	1996	Adjuvant treatment of intermediate and high-risk melanoma (Stage IIB/C, Stage III)
	High-Dose Interleukin-2 (IL-2)	1998	Stage IV melanoma
	Ipilimumab	2011	Unresectable Stage III or Stage IV melanoma
	Nivolumab	2014	Unresectable Stage III or Stage IV melanoma
	Pembrolizumab	2014	Unresectable Stage III or Stage IV melanoma
Molecularly Targeted Therapy	Vemurafenib	2011	Patients with BRAF V600E mutation with unresectable Stage III or Stage IV melanoma
	Trametinib	2013	Patients with BRAF V600E/V600K mutation who have unresectable Stage III or Stage IV melanoma
	Dabrafenib	2013	Patients with BRAF V600E mutation with unresectable Stage III or Stage IV melanoma
	Trametinib/ Dabrafenib Combination	2014	Patients with BRAF V600E/V600K mutation who have unresectable Stage III or Stage IV melanoma

Systemic therapy remains the primary treatment modality for stage IV disease [13]. Prior to 2011, high dose interleukin-2 (IL-2) and an alkylating agent, dacarbazine (5-3,3-dimethyl-1-triazenyl-imidazole-4-carboxamide, or DTIC), were the only FDA approved drugs for the treatment of metastatic melanoma [14]. Dacarbazine, based on its demonstrated successes in pre-clinical studies and clinical trials, was FDA approved for the treatment of metastatic melanoma in 1975 [15 - 17]. Unfortunately, when used as a single agent, majority of responses are partial and often not durable, with fewer than 2% of patients alive at 6 years [18]. High dose bolus interleukin-2 was first shown to mediate complete cancer regression in patients with metastatic melanoma, and was therefore approved by the US Food and Drug Administration (FDA) for this use in 1998 [19 - 21]. In addition to these treatment options, the management of advanced-stage disease has evolved more recently [1]. Options for systemic therapy now include new cytotoxic chemotherapy regimens, targeted agents (*e.g.*, BRAF Inhibitors) and immunotherapeutics (*e.g.*, IL-2, anti-PD-1). With immunotherapy as a treatment option for instance, median 5-year survival for patients with stage IV melanoma has nearly doubled, approximating 20% [22]. Furthermore, recent studies suggest the combination regimens that include conventional treatment options (*e.g.* surgery, radiosurgery) and systemic therapy (*e.g.* BRAF inhibitor, anti-CTLA-4) may produce better outcomes than either option alone [23, 24]. Herein, the authors provide an update on major breakthroughs in chemotherapeutic, immunologic, and molecularly target agents used in the treatment of advanced melanoma (Table 1).

CHEMOTHERAPEUTIC AGENTS

An evolving knowledge regarding the complex pathophysiology of melanoma on a molecular level has led to an increase in the number of options for systemic therapy in malignant melanoma. Currently, only one cytotoxic chemotherapeutic agent has been approved for use in metastatic melanoma. While not yet FDA approved, several other cytotoxic chemotherapeutic agents are available for use, including temozolamide, platinum compounds, taxanes, and nitrosoureas.

Alkylating Agents

Dacarbazine

Dacarbazine (di-methyl triazeno imidazole carboxamide, DTIC) is a cell-cycle non-specific aklylating agent. It is a prodrug requiring hepatic metabolism to yield the active metabolite 5-(3-methyl-1-triazeno) imidazole 4-carboxamide (MTIC), thus potentially limiting its use in the setting of liver dysfunction or liver metastases. Common adverse effects include nausea, vomiting, thrombocytopenia, leukopenia, and others. A potential limitation to its use is the presence of brain metastasis, as dacarbazine is unable to cross the blood-brain barrier. Since its FDA approval in 1975, it has remained the only cytotoxic chemotherapeutic drug approved for treatment of advanced melanoma. As such, it has long served as the standard by which other interventions for systemic disease are compared.

In recent randomized controlled trials, dacarbazine monotherapy has demonstrated response rates of 5-15% [25 - 27]. A single institution experience spanning several decades with dacarbazine monotherapy demonstrated similar results, with an approximately 20% objective response rate, 5% complete response rate and 5-6 month median duration of response [14]. A 6.4 month median overall survival (OS) was seen in a randomized phase III trial comparing dacarbazine and temozolamide monotherapy, another oral chemotherapeutic alkylating agent [28, 29]. Despite these phase I and II trial results, to our knowledge, there is no phase III trial to date that has shown a survival benefit of dacarbazine over placebo. The fact that it is still considered the gold standard for cytotoxic chemotherapeutic treatment of advanced melanoma underscores the difficulty in management of these patients and need for continued development of other treatment modalities.

Temozolomide

Temozolomide is an oral active congener of dacarbazine that is converted to the active metabolite MTIC at physiologic pH, thereby overcoming the need for hepatic metabolism. It is also able to cross the blood-brain barrier with documented activity in the central nervous system [30]. While temozolomide has yet to gain FDA approval for the treatment of metastatic melanoma, it is widely used in clinical practice as a substitute for dacarbazine, especially for patients with brain metastases. The most common side effects of temozolomide therapy are nausea, vomiting, constipation, hair loss, lymphopenia, headache, and fatigue.

In a randomized phase III trial involving 305 patients comparing temozolomide to dacarbazine treatment in chemotherapy naïve patients, temozolomide was noted to result in a trend towards improved median overall survival (OS) (7.7 *vs.* 6.4 months), although this finding was not statistically significant [28]. Median progression free survival (PFS) was significantly longer in the temozolomide group than the dacarbazine group (1.9 *vs.* 1.4 months), leading the study authors to conclude that temozolomide was at least as effective as dacarbazine monotherapy [28]. Considering the potential side effects of therapy, whether this represents a clinically significant difference is debatable. Both *in vitro* and *in vivo* work has demonstrated that the effect of temozolomide is dose schedule dependent, with a low dose extended schedule resulting in increased drug activity [31].

Platinum Compounds

Platinum containing compounds, including cisplatin and carboplatin, are cytotoxic, non–cell cycle–specific agents. The most common side-effects reported are ototoxicity, nephrotoxicity, neuropathy, myelotoxicity, and electrolyte abnormalities. Trials investigating cisplatin have shown overall objective response rates ranging from 11–50%, with median response duration of 4-7 months and median survival of 7.5 months [32, 33]. While no studies have compared cisplatin or other platinum compounds directly to the alkylating agents dacarbazine or temozolomide, the results from phase I and II trials are similar. Unfortunately, the clinical benefits of platinum containing compounds and alkylating agents do not appear to be synergistic.

Taxanes

The most extensively studied taxanes for the treatment of metastatic melanoma include paclitaxel and docetaxel. Taxanes are cell-cycle specific cytotoxic agents, acting in the M phase by promoting assembly and stabilization of microtubules, thus preventing further cell cycle progression [34].

Paclitaxel and docetaxel monotherapy for metastatic melanoma have been evaluated and found to have response rates of approximately 11% across multiple studies [35 - 37]. Paclitaxel has also been bound to various vehicle molecules, including fatty acids and albumin, in an attempt to limit toxicity and improve efficacy. In comparison to dacarbazine, when bound to a fatty acid vehicle, paclitaxel demonstrates an improved side effect profile, but no improvement in response rate, duration of response, time to progression, time to treatment or overall survival [38]. Phase I trials of abraxane, paclitaxel bound to albumin, have shown response rates of 38-49%, progression-free survival of 4 months, and median overall survival of 9.6 to 12.1 months [39]. Despite the similar survival statistics, improved side effect profile makes paclitaxel potentially clinically useful in the setting of adverse response to first line dacarbazine or temozolomide.

Nitrosureas

Nitrosoureas are DNA alkylating agents and include carmustine, lomustine and fotemustine. Overall objective response rates in metastatic melanoma treated with this class of drug range from 13 to 18%, with fotemustine appearing to be the most active amongst the group with response rates of 20-25% [40 - 43]. These agents are potentially useful in patients with brain metastases, as they are able to cross the blood brain barrier.

Chemotherapy in Combination

While it remains the "gold standard" for chemotherapy, dacarbazine monotherapy has had disappointing overall results. This has led to it being combined with other chemotherapeutic drugs in an attempt to prolong response and increase survival. The two most commonly studied combinations include cisplatin/vinblastine/ dacarbazine (CVD) and cisplatin/carmustine/ dacarbazine/tamoxifen (CBDT), also known as the Dartmouth Regimen. Similar to monotherapy, phase I and II trials have yielded promising results for combination therapy, but confirmatory phase III trials have been disappointing. Combination therapy with CVD has resulted in increased response rates, but response was partial, and median overall survival was similar to that for monotherapy [44]. When CBDT is compared to monotherapy with dacarbazine, neither response rates nor median overall survival are significantly different [44]. Also of note, toxicity is increased with both combination regimens, making them less appealing than monotherapy. A combination of bleomycin, vincristine, lomustine and dacarbazine (BOLD) was shown in a small case series to induce complete remission of brain metastases in a proportion of patients while providing 12.5 month median survival [45]. Both BOLD and CVD regimens have been shown to induce responses in metastases commonly unresponsive to dacarbazine alone, but to our knowledge, there are no studies demonstrating an impact on overall patient survival with these combination regimens [14].

Temozolomide monotherapy has been compared to combination therapy with several other agents. A phase II trial comparing monotherapy to temozolomide plus interferon-alpha 2b showed no differences in overall survival, response rate, or time to progression [46]. A subsequent phase III trial showed a statistically significant increase in response rate with combination therapy (24% *vs.* 13%), but no statistically significant difference was seen in median overall survival (9.7 *vs.* 8.4 months). Additionally, combination with interferon-alpha resulted in increased rates of thrombocytopenia and leukopenia [47]. A randomized phase II trial comparing monotherapy to temozolomide plus cisplatin also had disappointing results, showing no statistically significant differences in the overall median survival, time to disease progression, or objective response rate between the two treatment groups [30]. Combination with thalidomide in a randomized phase II trial produced a 6-month progression free survival of 15%, a 1-year overall survival of 35% and a response rate of 13%.[48]. As seen with dacarbazine combination therapy, despite encouraging data from phase I and II trials, no evidence exists from well designed phase III trials to support an improvement in patient survival with temozolomide combination therapy compared to mono-therapy.

Several combinations of chemotherapeutic agents have been studied as second line therapy for failed treatment with dacarbazine or temozolomide with median progression free survival between 1.3 and 4.1 months and overall survival between 3.5 and 9.8 months [49 - 52]. In this setting, taxanes in combination with platinum containing compounds have produced the best survival statistics [51, 52]. This setting may be where taxanes are the most useful. Combination carboplatin/ paclitaxel (CP) with or without sorafenib (CPS) was investigated as first-line therapy in a phase III randomized trial [53]. There was no significant difference in the median overall survival for the CP (11.3 months) and CPS (11.1

months) groups (P=0.878). The median progression free survival was also similar between groups (CP - 4.2 months, CPS - 4.9 months, *P*=0.092) and there was no significant difference in overall response rate (CP- 18%, CPS-20%, *P*=0.427). The addition of sorafenib to the combination chemotherapy arm resulted in more grade 3 or higher toxicities (CPS- 84%, CP – 78%, *P* = 0.027). This study established the benchmark end points for the use of combination carboplatin and paclitaxel [53].

Evidence exists from phase II trials to support the use of anti-angiogenic agents in combination with chemotherapy. The rationale for use of angiogenesis inhibitors in the treatment of melanoma comes from studies suggesting that vascular endothelial growth factor (VEGF) is highly expressed in melanoma and seems to play an important role in disease progression [54]. When patients without *c-kit* or *BRAF* mutations were assigned randomly to receive dacarbazine plus recombinant human endostatin (rhES) or dacarbazine plus placebo, the group receiving rhES showed a statistically improved progression free survival (4.5 *vs.* 1.5 months) and overall survival (12 *vs.* 8 months) [55]. Furthermore, a recently published phase II trial showed favorable results for dacarbazine in combination with the selective anti-VEGF monoclonal antibody bevacizumab (Avastin). In comparison to the historical 5-6 month median response duration for dacarbazine, combination therapy with bevacizumab yielded a median response duration of 16.9 months [56]. While this was not a randomized trial, preliminary results for dacarbazine with bevacizumab are promising. Kim and colleagues further sought to investigate the use of carboplatin and paclitaxel (CP) in combination with bevacizumab (CPB) in a randomized phase II study of patients with treatment naïve advanced melanoma [57]. Overall response rates in the CP and CPB groups were similar at 16.4% and 25.5%, respectively (*P*=0.1577). Furthermore, there was no significant improvement in progression free survival for the CPB arm (5.6 months) compared with the CP arm (4.5 months) (HR, 0.78; log-rank *P* = 0.1414) [57].

IMMUNOTHERAPY

Although cytotoxic chemotherapy has a palliative role in patients with metastatic melanoma, as mentioned previously, treatment results are rarely durable, and such a therapy offers little survival benefit [16]. Immunotherapeutics have recently demonstrated promising results for treatment of patients with metastatic melanoma, and may offer a chance for cure [58 - 60]. Such options include interleukin-2, vaccine therapy, adoptive cell transfer, and agents that target inhibitory receptors on T-cells (*i.e.* immune checkpoint inhibitors) [60].

Interferon Alpha

Interferon alfa-2b (IFN- α; Intron A; Merck, White House Station, NJ) is expressed by multiple cell types in response to various stimuli (*e.g.* pathogens and malignant cells) and is thought to enhance activity of host immune cells [61 - 63]. In a randomized controlled study in 287 patients with deep primary (T4, Stage IIB) or regionally metastatic melanoma (N1, Stage III), IFN alfa-2b was compared to observation alone [64]. This agent was the first to show a significant benefit in disease-free survival (from 1 to 1.7 years, $P = 0.0023$) and overall survival (OS) (from 2.8 to 3.8 years, $P=0.0237$) when compared to no intervention for the treatment of advanced melanoma. IFN-α was FDA approved for adjuvant treatment of intermediate and high-risk melanoma in 1996. A follow-up, three-arm intergroup trial, evaluated the efficacy of low and high-dose interferon alfa-2b when compared to observation for the same high-risk melanoma patients (Stage IIB and III) [65]. The data supported that interferon alfa-2b improved relapse-free survival, not OS, compared to observation alone, with high-dose producing better results than low-dose [65]. A similar finding with regards to improved relapse-free survival and not OS was seen in a pooled analysis of ECOG and intergroup trials [66]. Subsequent studies on the impact of dose and maintenance therapy have reported variable results.

Pegylated IFN-α-2b (PEG-IFN, PEG-Intron, Sylatron; Merck) was evaluated in 1,256 patients with stage III melanoma following lymphadenectomy who received the agent or observation alone [67, 68]. There was a significant increase in recurrence-free survival (18%) in the treatment compared to the observation group, and this improvement was sustained [67, 68]. Pegylated alfa-2b was initially approved "for the treatment hepatitis C" in 2001, and received FDA approval for the treatment of Stage III melanoma after surgical resection in 2011. Pegylation is thought to enhance the pharmacokinetics of the agent.

Interleukin-2 (IL-2)

Interleukin-2 (IL-2) initially referred to as T cell growth factor, was one of the earliest milestones in immunotherapy for human cancer [69]. It has been estimated that high-dose IL-2 induces responses in 15-20% of patients with advanced melanoma and 5-8% of these responses are durable CRs [70]. IL-2 is a cytokine predominantly secreted by Ag-stimulated CD4+ T cells, but also CD8+ cells, activated dendritic and natural killer (NK) cells [69]. It stimulates the immune system by way of T- and NK-cell activation and proliferation, and causes a release of various cytokines including tumor necrosis factor and interferon-γ from activated lymphocytes [71]. More specifically, IL-2 maintains CD4+ regulatory T cells and mediates their differentiation to subsets with many different functions; for CD8+ cells, IL-2 stimulates their growth as well as differentiation to memory and more terminally differentiated lymphocytes.

In 1984, a 33 year-old female with metastatic melanoma was treated with recombinant IL-2, with subsequent regression of disease burden on follow-up evaluations, and she has remained disease free for nearly thirty years [69]. This was the first time that IL-2 demonstrated durable and curative regression of metastatic melanoma by way of manipulating an individual's immune response to eradicate cancer [69]. IL-2 has also helped advance the field of adoptive cell transfer (ACT), or the expansion of natural or genetically modified autologous human antitumor T cells (lymphokine-activated killer cells, or LAK cells) *in vitro* for the treatment of advanced human disease *in vivo* [72]. Subsequent experiments of IL-2 treatment alone in a murine model for pulmonary sarcoma and melanoma metastasis demonstrated inhibition of tumor growth at 3-days and regression of grossly visible tumor metastases at 10-days [73]. When an initial in-human study failed to demonstrate anti-tumor responses following administration of recombinant IL-2 alone [74] investigations began to focus on co-administration of IL-2 with LAK cells [20, 74]. The first successful report of systemic administration of autologous lymphokine-activated killer (LAK) cells and increasing doses of the recombinant-derived lymphokine interleukin-2 in humans was by Rosenberg and colleagues in 1985 at the National Cancer Institute, Bethesda Maryland [20]. This study included 25 patients with advanced cancer including metastatic melanoma who had failed prior systemic therapies. Objective tumor response was observed in 11 of the 25 patients (44%) overall, 4 of 7 partial responses were noted in patients with hepatic and pulmonary melanoma metastases, and one patient with metastatic melanoma had complete tumor regression sustained for 10 years after therapy [20]. The main adverse event associated with treatment was severe fluid retention, which resolved following treatment [20]. A subsequent study, also at the National Cancer Institute, evaluated 157 patients with advanced disease including renal cell cancer (RCC) and melanoma, who received either LAK cells and IL-2 (n=108) or high-dose IL-2 alone (n=49) [75]. Overall, objective tumor regression was noted in 30 patients, and this included 12 of 42 patients (29%) with melanoma [75]. A randomized control trial expanded on these findings, and sought to evaluate whether the administration of LAK cells in combination with high-dose IL-2 improved anti-tumor response and survival compared with the same IL-2 dose alone [76]. This study included a total of 181 patients (97 with RCC and 54 with melanoma) who failed to respond to other conventional therapies or for whom no other treatment option existed. Overall, in the combination arm, there were 10 complete responses and 14 partial responses, whereas in the IL-2 alone group, there were 4 complete and 12 partial responses [76]. There was no significant difference in the 3-year actuarial survival in the IL-2/LAK and IL-2 alone groups (IL-2/LAK: 31%, IL-2 alone: 17%; $P = 0.089$). Of the patients with metastatic melanoma, 5 of 28 who received IL-2/LAK were alive at the time of data analysis, but none were alive in the IL-2 alone group. Overall, there were 6 treatment deaths in the study, 3 of which were due to myocardial infarction [76]. A later study was conducted on 283 consecutive patients treated with high-dose bolus interleukin-2 for metastatic RCC or melanoma from September 1985 to December 1992 [19]. Of the patients treated with metastatic melanoma, 14 (10%) and 9 (7%) achieved partial and complete regression, respectively [19]. A follow-up study of 409 patients treated with high-dose bolus interleukin-2 conducted several years later (September 1985 to November 1996) showed an objective response in 28 of 187 patients (15%) and complete regression in 12 of 187 (6.6%) in patients with metastatic melanoma [19]. Similarly, the National Biotherapy Study Group evaluated the use of IL-2 in 788 patients with cancer, in various combinations including with LAK cells, cyclophosphamide, tumor-infiltrating lymphocytes, tumor necrosis factor (TNF), alpha-interferon, and LAK alternating with combination chemotherapy [77].

Objective responses were observed in 13 of 188 patients (18%) with melanoma, with a overall median survival of 9.6 months for patients with melanoma [77].

Even more persuasive evidence highlighting the benefit of high-dose recombinant IL-2 for patients with metastatic melanoma comes from a multi-institutional collaborative conducted between 1985 and 1993, which included 270 patients [21]. In this study, there were 6 mortalities, all due to sepsis. There were 43 objective responses (16%), 17 complete responses (6%) and 26 partial responses (10%), all independent of tumor burden or disease site [21]. The median survival for the 43 responders was at least 1 year, and 12 of these patients remained without disease progression for ≥ 70 months [78]. At the time of data analysis, the median response duration for those achieving a complete response had not been achieved, and was 5.9 months for those who achieved a partial response. In the patients who responded, tumor regression was seen at all tumor sites. Impressively, disease did not progress in any patient responding for more than 30 months. This further emphasized the observation that if a patient were to have significant anti-tumor response to IL-2, by way of a complete response, that the effects would also be durable. Based on these findings and other data from the aforementioned studies, the FDA approved IL-2 for the treatment of metastatic melanoma in 1998 [69].

Toxicities resulting from the administration of IL-2 are due to capillary permeability and resultant extravasation of fluid into tissues and organs through out the body [69]. This manifests clinically as cardiac arrhythmias, volume overload, pulmonary edema, and hypotension. Other drug related symptoms and toxicities include fevers, chills, diarrhea, and neuropsychiatric changes (*e.g.* delirium) [79]. Furthermore, central line sepsis, perhaps due in part to the neutrophil chemotactic defects, complicates the clinical efficacy and safety of IL-2 administration and prophylactic antibiotics administration has been shown to reduce the rate of this complication [69, 80]. However, with growing experience in the administration of IL-2, treatment-related toxicities have been reduced significantly with attributable mortalities estimated at <1% [79].

Vaccine Therapy

Therapeutic cancer vaccines were one of the first immunotherapies investigated for the treatment of metastatic melanoma [81]. Tumor-associated antigens (TAAs) are uniquely expressed or up-regulated on tumors and include cancer-testis antigens (CTAs), differentiation antigens, mutated antigens, and viral antigens [58]. These antigens are delivered as whole proteins/peptides, recombinant viruses, or loaded onto dendritic antigen-presenting cells. Various attempts have been made to co-administer such vaccines with other treatments such as IL-2, immune-checkpoint inhibitors, and GM-CSF as a method to boost their immunogenicity [58]. Although some approaches have been able to elicit an immune regulated response to TAAs, the response has not been definitively linked to clinical benefit and improved overall survival, and therefore discussion in this text will be limited [82]. Nevertheless, given their minimal toxicity and ease of administration, vaccines remain a popular area of research interest for the treatment of metastatic melanoma and prevention of disease spread in patients at a high risk of recurrence [81].

Antigen MZ2-E, also known as melanoma-associated antigen (MAGE-1, and later MAGE-A1), was the first of such TAAs on melanoma recognized by CD8(+) T cells in the context of HLA-A1 [83]. In this initial observation, it was noted that the antigens such as MAGE-A1, referred to as cancer-testis antigens (CTA), were expressed on tumor but not normal tissues (other than testicular tissue), making them ideal candidates for immune-targeted therapy. Subsequent studies demonstrated that *in vivo* administration of peptide vaccines derived from TAAs as MAGE-A1, MAGE-A3, NY-ESO-1, and melan-A/MART-1 enhance cytotoxic T cell reactivity with a well-tolerated safety profile; however, tumor regression was not achieved [84 - 88].

Peptide Vaccines

Differentiation and Cancer-Testis Antigens (CTAs)

Differentiation antigens include gp100, Melan-A/MART-1, tyrosinase, and tyrosinase related protein 1 and 2 [89, 90]. Granulocyte macrophage colony stimulating-factor (GMCSF), a cytokine, in part facilitates the interaction between the antigen-presenting dendritic cell and naïve T cells [58]. In a randomized phase II trial, twenty-six patients with advanced melanoma were assigned randomly to vaccination with a mixture of four melanoma peptides co-administered in GM-CSF in adjuvant or pulsed on monocyte-derived dendritic cells melanoma [91]. The immunogens included a mixture of four gp100 and tyrosinase peptides restricted by HLA-A1, HLA-A2, and HLA-A3, plus a tetanus helper peptide. The overall immune response was greater in the GM-CSF group (P <0.02): objective clinical responses were observed in one patient in the DC arm and in two patients in the GM-CSF arm. Furthermore, stable disease was noted in one patient in the dendritic cell arm and two patients in the GM-CSF group [91]. A separate pilot study sought to evaluate the efficacy of immune adjuvants, IL-2 and GM-CSF, in potentiating an immune response when co-administered with a multi-peptide gp100(207-217), MART-1a, and survivin melanoma vaccine in patients with completely resected stage II-IV melanoma [92]. This study failed to show significant improvements in the immunologic response with the addition of GM-CSF and IL-2 compared with GM-CSF alone, although IL-2 treatment did increase T regulatory and NK cells compared with no IL-2 treatment [92]. The addition of IL-2 or increase in GM-CSF did not result in an increased frequency of vaccine-specific cytotoxic T lymphocytes [92]. A subsequent multicenter trial vaccinated patients with resected stage IIB-IV melanoma with 12 class I MHC-restricted melanoma peptides (12MP) to stimulate CD8(+) T cells and randomly assigned them to receive either a mixture of six melanoma-associated helper peptides (6MHP) to stimulate CD4(+) T cells or a tetanus helper peptide [93]. Patients were further randomly assigned to receive cyclophosphamide pre-treatment. At the time of data analysis, there was no significant difference in OS in either treatment arm (overall 3-year survival was 79%), and contrary to what one would expect, melanoma-associated helper peptides decreased CD8(+) T-cell responses to the melanoma vaccine (P < 0.001) [93].

Another differentiation peptide, gp100, has been extensively studied and compared to other immunotherapeutics in patients with advanced melanoma. Three separate phase II trials of gp100 (210M) peptide plus high-dose IL-2 in patients with HLA-A2-positive advanced melanoma showed an overall response rate of 16% for 121 evaluable patients: 11 (9%) were CRs, and 9 (7%) were partial responses. When compared to historical data, the addition of the vaccine did not offer a clinical advantage when compared to IL-2 alone [70]. Schwartzentruber *et al.* conducted a randomized, phase 3 trial that included 185 patients from 21 institutions [94]. These patients had locally advanced stage III or IV melanoma, expressed HLA*A0201, and did not have brain metastases. The two randomly assigned arms were patients who received IL-2 alone or gp100:209-217(210M) plus incomplete Freund's adjuvant (Montanide ISA-51) once per cycle, followed by IL-2 [94]. The median overall survival was longer in the vaccine-IL-2 group (17.8 months) compared to the IL-2 group alone (11.1 months), though not of statistical significance ($P = 0.06$). Furthermore, there was a significant improvement in the overall objective response (vaccine-IL-2 group: 16% *vs.* IL-2 group: 6%, $P = 0.03$) and longer PFS in the vaccine-IL-2-group (vaccine-IL-2 group: 2.2 months *vs.* IL-2 alone: 1.6 months, $P = 0.008$) [94]. However, this study failed to demonstrate a correlation between immune response elicited by the vaccine and clinical response.

As mentioned previously, cancer-testis antigens are expressed on normal testicular tissue but also tumor cells, and include the MAGE family, PRAME and NYESO-1 [89, 95]. NYESO-1 and MAGE-A3 are overexpressed in approximately 45% and 70% of melanomas, respectively [95, 96]. A phase I study, LUD99-008, conducted by Davis *et al.* demonstrated that administration of NYESO-1 vaccine and saponin-based adjuvant ISCOMATRIX was safe and capable of eliciting an immune response [97]. A later study further showed a significant association between the stage of disease, the amount of T regulatory cells in the blood, and the efficacy of the NYESO-1/ISCOMATRIX vaccine [98]. When considering MAGE-A3, a Phase I/II study of recombinant MAGE-A3 subcutaneous and intradermal administration to patients with metastatic melanoma demonstrated a partial response in 1 patient and mixed response in 4 patients out of 26 [99]. Time to progression for these 5 responders varied from 3 to 51+ months (continued response at the time of data analysis) [99]. Based on data from phase II studies, ongoing investigations are seeking to evaluate whether the addition of various immunostimulants (AS02B or AS15) increase immunogenicity or extend disease free survival when coupled with recombinant MAGE-A3 vaccine [100].

Rosenberg and colleagues conducted a study on 440 individuals with metastatic cancer, of whom 422 had metastatic melanoma, treated with 541 various cancer vaccines at the NCI/NIH Surgery Branch between 1995 and 2004 [101]. Peptide vaccines were given to 323 individuals alone and were derived from melanoma-differentiated antigens including MART-1, tyrosinase/TRP-2, gp100 and CTAs such as NY-ESO-1 or MAGE-12. The overall objective response rate for all vaccine treatments was 2.6%: 11 partial and 3 complete. The majority of these objective responders (79%) had disease confined to cutaneous or lymph node sites, and the remainder (n=3, 21%) had visceral disease. This may perhaps suggest that vaccines may be more successful in patients with locoregional (cutaneous, lymph node) disease [101].

Cell Surface Glycolipids

GD2, GD3 and GM2 are cell surface glycolipids and these form another class of melanoma tumor antigens [102]. Livingston *et al.* conducted a study with 122 patients with stage III melanoma, disease-free after surgery, and randomized patients to receive treatment with GM2/bacilli Calmette-Guèrin (BCG) vaccine or BCG alone [103]. This trial demonstrated an induction of IgM antibodies in the majority (86%) of patients who received GM2/BCG and a prolonged DFS for patients who had GM2 antibody production; however, there was no difference in overall survival or disease-free survival in both treatment arms [103]. Further-more, the Eastern Cooperative Oncology Group (ECOG) conducted a study in collaboration with the North American cooperative groups that compared GM2 vaccine with high-dose interferon-α2b in patients with resected stage IIB/III melanoma [104]. This trial was closed after interim analysis, as the high dose interferon group demonstrated significant treatment benefit in terms of improved relapse-free survival and OS when compared to GM2 vaccine [104]. Similarly, the EORTC 18961 phase III trial showed no difference in outcomes for patients who received GM-2KLH/Qs-21 vaccination *versus* observation for stage II melanoma, and therefore was closed at the second interim analysis [105].

Recombinant Viral Vector Vaccines

Viruses can be engineered to express tumor antigens. Once they are taken up by

APCs, these tumor antigens are expressed to the immune system, thereby enhancing the anti-tumor T-cell directed response. A phase II trial evaluated 56 patients with unresectable metastatic melanoma who received GM-CSF-encoding, second-generation oncolytic herpesvirus [106]. This study demonstrated an overall 26% response rate (8 CRs, 5 PRs), with an OS of 58% and 52% at 1 and 2 years, respectively [106]. A newly published study from Andtbacka and colleagues randomized 436 patients with advanced melanoma (stage IIIB-IV) to Talimogene laherparepvec (T-VEC), a herpes simplex virus type 1-derived oncolytic immunotherapy, or GM-CSF alone [107]. T-VEC was designed to selectively replicate within tumors and produce GM-CSF, which then enhances the antitumor T-cell response. T-VEC was well tolerated and when compared to GM-CSF alone, its administration resulted in a higher durable response rate ($P < 0.001$) and longer median OS ($P = 0.051$).

Tumor Cell-Derived Antigens

Autologous Melanoma Vaccines

The use of the patient's own tumor as the antigen source refers to an autologous vaccine approach. This method offers a personalized approach, as the antigens that are unique to the patient are incorporated into the vaccine. Heat shock proteins (HSPs) are soluble intracellular proteins that bind peptides, such as TAAs, and are believed to play an important role in chaperoning these antigens for presentation [108]. Heat shock protein peptide complex (HSPPC)-96-based vaccine vitespen (formerly Oncophage ®) was the first autologous cancer vaccine and has shown considerable benefit in advanced melanoma studies with an excellent safety profile [109]. One open-label trial conducted at 71 centers worldwide, randomized 322 patients 2:1 to receive vitespan or a provider's choice of alternative including dacarbazine, interleukin-2, temozolomide, or complete tumor resection [110]. There was no difference in overall survival (OS) in patients who received autologous vaccine *versus* physicians' choice; however, patients who received more than 10 doses of vaccine and had M1a/b disease had a longer OS compared to those receiving fewer vaccines [110]. Another autologous vaccine, M-VaxTM (AVAX Technologies, MO, USA) consists of multiple intradermal injections of a mixture comprised of dnitrophenyl (DNP)-modified autologous tumor cells and bacilli Calmette-Guerin (BCG) [111]. Following pretreatment with cyclophosphamide, 97 patients with surgically incurable metastatic melanoma were treated with DNP vaccine [112]. Of the 83 evaluable patients, there were 11 patients with antitumor responses: 4 partial, 5 mixed, and 2 complete [112] Overall, it was observed that DNP-modified melanoma vaccine was able to induce meaningful regression of melanoma metastases, particularly small pulmonary nodules. The median overall survival for non-responders was 8.7 months, compared to 21.4 months in responders, and this finding was found to be statistically significant ($P = 0.01$) [112]. A phase III trial comparing M-Vax or placebo to low-dose IL-2 was suspended in 2009 and to our knowledge, the results have not been reported [113].

Allogeneic Melanoma Vaccines

Allogenic whole-cell vaccines are composed of tumor cells isolated from cell lines or individual tumors from other patients. Canvaxin is one such example that expresses 20 tumor antigens *via* three different melanoma cell lines [113]. Morton *et al.* conducted a phase II trial of patients who underwent complete resection of metastatic melanoma to regional lymph nodes (stage III), and compared patients who received the Canvaxin polyvalent vaccine to those who did not [114]. Median OS and 5-year OS were higher in the vaccinated patients compared to the non-vaccinated group. A Phase II adjuvant trial compared patients with completely resected stage IV melanoma who received Canvaxin to those who did not [115]. There was a significant overall survival advantage in the vaccine group, with 5-year OS approximating 39% for vaccine patients compared to 20% in the non-vaccine group (P < 0.001) [115]. Interestingly, in the adjuvant vaccine group, a significant delayed-type hypersensitivity reaction was observed and this correlated with OS [115]. However, OS did not correlate with delayed-type hypersensitivity reaction to a control antigen, purified protein derivative. In contrast to what would be expected based on these early phase studies, two large randomized double-blinded placebo-controlled phase III trials evaluating Canvaxin plus BCG *versus* placebo plus BCG in resected stage III and IV melanoma were discontinued, as both studies demonstrated poorer overall survival in the Canvaxin groups [58].

Additional examples of allogeneic vaccines include vaccinia melanoma oncolysate (VMO), vaccinia melanoma cell lysate (VMCL), and Melacine [113]. A follow-up analysis of a randomized phase III double-blind trial assessed the long-term effectiveness of the VMO vaccine in patients with stage III melanoma [116]. The two groups compared included patients receiving vaccinia alone to those receiving the VMO vaccine. There was no difference in the median OS between the groups (VMO: 7.71 years, vaccinia: 7.95 years, $P = 0.70$) and the median disease free interval for the VMO group was 6 years whereas that for the vaccinia group had not been reached by the time of data analysis [116]. Simply, this study did not demonstrate a benefit in the use of VMO for patients with advanced melanoma when compared to a control group.

Vaccinia melanoma cell lysate (VMCL) vaccine incorporates a single melanoma cell line combined with vaccinia cell lysate *in vitro* [117]. One prospective, multicenter phase III trial included 700 patients with melanoma stage IIB and III, randomized 1:1 to receive the VMCL vaccine or to no treatment [118]. This study demonstrated a longer 5-year OS in the vaccine group (60.6%) compared to control (54.8%), although not statistically significant ($P = 0.068$).

Melacine consists of a detoxified Freund adjuvant (DETOX) combined with a lysate of two melanoma cell lines [119]. In one of the largest randomized, phase III studies of adjuvant vaccine therapy in human cancer to date, the Southwest Oncology Group compared patients who received the allogeneic Melacine vaccine for two years *versus* observation for intermediate thickness (1.5 to 4.0 mm), node negative melanoma (T3N0M0) [120]. This study demonstrated no improvement in disease-free survival in the treated *versus* observation groups [120].

Two recent single arm, phase II trials evaluated the efficacy and toxicity of an adjuvant treatment using Hyper-IL-6 gene modified whole-cell allogeneic melanoma vaccine in patients with resected stage IIIB-IV disease [121]. When compared to historical non-treated controls, an extension of DFS and OS were observed, with no grade 3 or 4 toxicities.

Dendritic Cell-Based Vaccines

Dendritic cells are antigen-presenting cells (APCs) that have been used as immune adjuvants to induce *in vivo* anti-tumor responses [122]. One key pilot study used autologous dendritic cells cultured in IL-4 and GM-CSF and then pulsed with tumor lysate or peptides prior to infusion in 16 patients with advanced melanoma [123]. Objective responses, with disease regression at multiple visceral sites, were noted in 5 of 16 patients (31%): two complete and three partial responses [123].

Schadendorf and colleagues evaluated a dendritic cell vaccine in a phase III randomized trial of 108 patients with metastatic melanoma [124]. Dendritic cell vaccines were loaded with MHC class I and II-restricted peptides and was compared to conventional dacarbazine (DTIC). The Data Safety & Monitoring Board recommended closure of the study, as the dendritic cell vaccine failed to prove more effective than conventional DTIC [124]. More recently, a pilot study generated dendritic cells by culturing monocytes with GM-CSF, IL-2, TNF, and CD40 ligand [125]. The autologous monocyte-derived dendritic cells were then loaded with killed allogeneic Colo829 melanoma cell line that was then used to vaccinate 20 patients with stage IV metastatic melanoma [125]. The estimated median overall survival was 22.5 months (range, 2-35.5 months), and the vaccines were considered to be safe and tolerable. Durable objective clinical responses were achieved in two patients, 1 with a complete regression lasting 18 months and the other with a partial regression lasting 23 months [125]. A later study treated 22 high-risk stage III melanoma patients following lymph node dissection with adjuvant dendritic cell vaccine loaded with MHC-class-1-restricted melanoma peptides respective to the patient's haplotype and these patients were matched to an unvaccinated control group [126]. The 3-year OS was higher in the vaccinated group (vaccinated: 68.2%, *versus* unvaccinated: 25.7%, $P = 0.0290$) and the 3-year DFS rate longer in the vaccinated (40.9%) compared to the control group (14.5%), although not statistically significant ($P = 0.1083$) [126].

Many clinicians and researchers continue to question the true clinical effectiveness and practicality of vaccine therapy; however, some of the newer strategies and combination approaches may overcome some of the presented shortcomings.

Adoptive Cell Therapy

Unfortunately, one of the challenges of the various aforementioned vaccine approaches is the inability to generate large numbers of anti-tumor T-cells with high reactivity/affinity to a particular antigen target [127]. A solution to this problem, Adoptive Cell Therapy (ACT), or the transfer of autologous tumor-infiltrating lymphocytes (TILs) as a therapeutic modality for patients with cancer, has led to objective disease regression in 49-72% of patients with metastatic melanoma [127]. More specifically, lymphocytes are collected from a patient, followed by *in vitro* selection, expansion and activation and are then infused back into the patient. One of the first reports of the adoptive transfer of tumor-reactive cells that overexpressed self-derived differentiation antigens to patients with metastatic melanoma was out of the Surgery Branch at the National Cancer Institute [128]. This transfer not only led to complete regression of the patient's disease, but also resulted in autoimmune destruction of melanocytes. It was also observed that there was a persistent repopulation of T cells, with proliferation of highly functioning T cells *in vivo* and migration to tumor sites [128]. Hunder *et al.* developed an *in vitro* method by which CD4(+) T-cell clones with specificity for NY-ESO-1 were isolated, expanded, and then infused into a patient with refractory metastatic melanoma [129]. Impressively, a durable clinical remission was achieved as well as immunogenic responses to other melanoma antigens [129]. Furthermore, it was noticed early on that such antitumor responses were potentiated with co-administration of IL-2. A study by Dudley *et al.* evaluated increasing intensities of myeloablative chemoradiation using fludarabine plus cyclophosphamide with 2 or 12 Gy of total-body irradiation followed by ACT and HD IL-2 [130]. An objective response rate of 52 and 72% was observed in the 2 and 12 Gy TBI groups, and responses were seen at all sites including the brain. Ten patients achieved a CR and remained disease free with a median follow-up of 31 months [130]. Rosenberg and colleagues also investigated the use of autologous TILs in conjunction with IL-2 across three clinical trials following lymphodepletion in 93 patients with measurable metastatic melanoma, the majority of whom (95%) had progressive disease on prior treatments. Examples of prior treatments included chemotherapy, immune checkpoint blockade (*i.e.* anti-CTLA-4), IFN, and IL-2 coupled with the aforementioned therapies. The lymphodepleting preparative regimens included chemotherapy alone, and 2 or 12 Gy irradiation and the objective response rates were 49%, 52%, and 72%, respectively [131]. Impressively, twenty of the patients (22%) achieved CR, 19 of who had an extension of this response beyond 3 years. The actuarial survival for the entire group at 3 and 5 years was 36% and 29%, respectively [131]. Those who achieved a complete response had a 3- and 5-year survival of 100% and 93%.

Immune Checkpoint Inhibitors

Immune checkpoints include those regulatory pathways that allow for the maintenance of self-tolerance and modulate normal physiologic immune responses in order to protect the host from collateral damage [132]. The discovery of immune checkpoint inhibitory proteins led to major breakthroughs in the immunotherapeutic approach to cancer treatment [133]. These immune check-points include cytotoxic T-lymphocyte Associated Protein 4 (CTLA-4), Programmed Death-1 (PD-1), and Programmed Death- Ligand 1 (PD-L1) (Fig. **1**) [134 - 138].

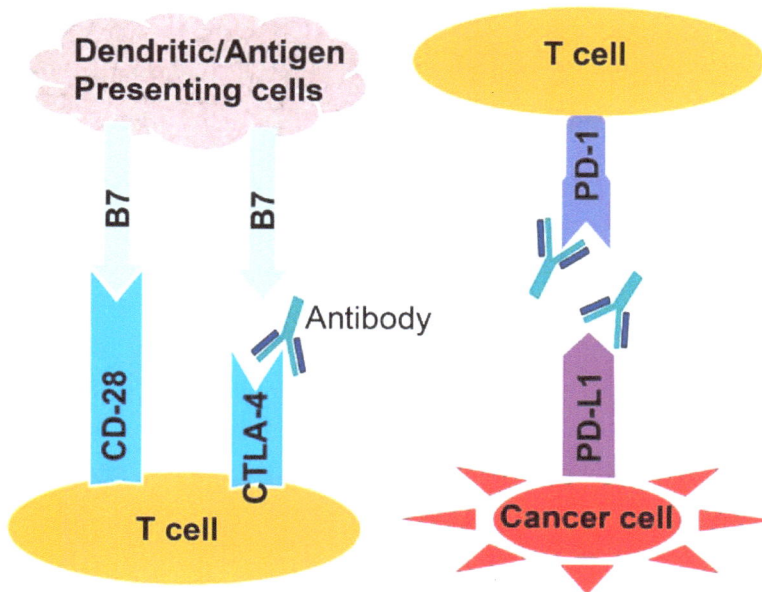

Fig. (1). Antibody blockade of Cytotoxic T-Lymphocyte Associated Protein-4, Programmed Death-1, and Programmed-Death Ligand 1 Immune Checkpoints as therapy for metastatic melanoma.

Early investigations demonstrated that blocking such inhibitory pathways allows for activation of dormant T-cells, with downstream processes that ultimately result in an anti-tumor immune response.

Anti-CTLA-4

Anti-CTLA-4 therapy was the first immune checkpoint inhibitor to be approved by FDA for metastatic melanoma. In some of the first investigations, Hodi *et al.* studied the efficacy of CTLA-4 blockade (MDX-010) in previously vaccinated ovarian cancer and melanoma patients.[139]. Interestingly, MDX-010 resulted in granulocyte/lymphocyte infiltration and extensive tumor necrosis in 3 metastatic melanoma patients previously vaccinated with irradiated, autologous GM-CS--secreting tumor cells [139]. Around the same time, Phan *et al.* reported on 14 patients who received MDX-010 and vaccination with two modified HLA-A*0201-restricted peptides from the gp100 melanosomal differentiation antigen [140]. Objective cancer regression was observed in 3 patients (21%) [140]. Other studies of anti-CTLA-4 in patients with metastatic melanoma have demonstrated objective response rates of 11-13%, with durable responses as far out as 31 months, which marked the time of data analysis [141, 142]. When anti-CTLA-4 is coupled with IL-2 treatment, observed response rates have been reported to be around 22%, with similar grade III/IV immune-related events when compared to either therapy alone [143].

Hodi *et al.* evaluated ipilimumab with or without gp100 peptide vaccine and gp100 vaccine alone for the treatment of patients with metastatic melanoma (stage III or IV) in a phase III study [136]. The best overall response rate in the ipilimumab, ipilimumab/gp100, and gp100 alone groups were 10.9%, 5.7%, and 1.5%, respectively, and the difference observed between the ipilimumab groups and the gp100 alone group was statistically significant ($P<0.05$). The adverse events related to the treatment with ipilimumab were mostly immune related as a result of its mechanism of action, with the most common being diarrhea. Grade 3 or 4 immune-related adverse events occurred in 10-15% of patients in the ipilimumab groups compared to 3% with gp100 alone. Patients treated with ipilimumab with or without gp100 peptide vaccine had improved median overall survival (10-10.1 months) when compared to gp100 alone (6.4 months). This was the first phase III study that demonstrated a survival benefit with anti-CTLA-4 therapy, yet there was no survival benefit with the addition of gp100 to the ipilimumab group.

Other studies similarly demonstrated a survival benefit in patients receiving ipilimumab (anti-CTLA-4 monoclonal antibody, trade name Yervoy®; Bristol Myers Squibb, New York, NY) compared to prior conventional treatments for advanced melanoma [144]. A phase III study by Robert *et al.* randomly assigned treatment naïve patients with metastatic melanoma to receiving ipilimumab plus dacarbazine or dacarbazine plus placebo [144]. Ipilimumab in combination with dacarbazine was found to have a longer median duration of response (19.3 *vs.* 8.1 months) and longer median OS (11.2 *vs.* 9.1 months) compared to dacarbazine/ placebo [144]. Given the presented evidence as well as data from other studies, ipilimumab was approved by the FDA for the treatment of unresectable Stage III or IV melanoma in 2011.

These findings were recently confirmed in a separate controlled phase III trial that randomized treatment-naïve patients with metastatic melanoma 1:1 to receiving ipilimumab plus dacarbazine or placebo plus dacarbazine [145]. The five-year survival for patients in the combination treatment arm was 18.2% compared to 8% for patients treated with placebo plus dacarbazine [145]. While the aforementioned results seem convincing, dacarbazine plus ipilimumab has not yet replaced dacarbazine monotherapy as the standard regimen used in the setting of metastatic melanoma.

Anti-PD-1

Since the break through investigations that supported the clinical use of anti-CTLA-4 for the treatment for advanced melanoma, evidence supporting the safety and clinical efficacy of anti-PD-1 has continued to surface [134, 146, 147]. In a pilot dose-escalation study, MDX-1106 (also known as BMS-936558), an antibody to PD-1, was evaluated for the treatment of advanced solid malignancies (*e.g.* colorectal cancer, renal cell carcinoma), including melanoma [146]. One of the patients with melanoma achieved a partial response and another had significant lesional tumor regression that did not achieve PR criteria [146]. This study further suggested that that immune-related toxicities following treatment with anti-PD-1 therapy may be less severe and better tolerated than those following anti-CTLA-4 therapy. Similarly, Topalian *et al.* evaluated the use of BMS-936558, another antibody that blocks PD-1, in patients with various malignancies including advanced melanoma [134]. Overall, the objective response rate was 19-41% depending on the dose administered, with an overall object response rate of 28% across all doses. This study provided additional valuable findings, in that no tumor responses were observed in patients with PD-L1 (ligand for PD-1) negative tumors, whereas over a third of the patients with PD-L1 positive tumors had an objective response [134].

Nivolumab, another antibody to PD-1 (previously known as BMS-936558, MDX-1106, ONO-4538, trade name Opdivo®), was evaluated for survival benefits and long-term safety in patients with advanced melanoma and other cancers.[148]. The 1- and 2- year survival rates were 62% and 43%, respectively; median OS and PFS were 16.8 months and 3.7 months, respectively.[148]. Impressively, the median response duration was 2 years in 33 of the patients (31%) who achieved an objective response [148]. In December 2014, nivolumab was FDA-approved for use in stage III or stage IV melanoma. Additionally, nivolumab results in longer PFS and improved survival rate when compared to dacarbazine alone in previously untreated melanoma patients without BRAF mutation [25]. Response rates for those receiving anti-CTLA-4 therapy have been estimated to be 12%, while those for anti-PD-1 are about 40% [133]. Furthermore, toxicity with PD-1 antibodies has been observed to be less than that following treatment with other immunotherapeutics (*e.g.* anti-CTLA-4, IL-2) [149].

In a study by Hamid and colleagues, another anti-PD-1 agent, MK-3475, was administered to 135 patients with advanced [137]. This study included both patients who had prior treatment with ipilimumab and those who did not. Across all dosages, the overall confirmed response rate was 38% (44 of 117 patients), the majority of which were durable; the highest confirmed response rate was seen in patients who received the higher dose of MK-3475.[137]. The most common adverse events were low grade, which is similar to what was seen with BMS-936558 [137]. It was also observed that prior treatment with other immuno-therapeutics (*e.g.* IL-2 and anti-CTLA-4) did not alter outcomes [137].

Pembrolizumab (formerly MK-3475) has also proven efficacious for the treatment of advanced melanoma in ipilimumab-refractory patients [150]. Based on the proven clinical efficacy of this anti-PD-1 therapy, pembrolizumab (trade name Keytruda®), gained FDA approval in September 2014 for use in Stage III or Stage IV melanoma [151, 152].

Recently, a phase 3 study enrolled 834 patients with advanced melanoma and randomly assigned them in a 1:1:1 ratio to receive pembrolizumab (10 mg/kg) every 2 weeks or every 3 weeks or four doses of ipilimumab (3 mg/kg) every 3 weeks [153]. There was a higher incidence of treatment-related adverse events ≥ grade 3 in the ipilimumab group (19.9%) compared with the pembrolizumab groups (2 week group - 13.3%; 3 week group- 10.1%). Fatigue was the most common treatment-related event of any grade in the pembrolizumab groups, while pruritus and diarrhea were the two most common events in the ipilimumab group. The efficacy of both pembrolizumab regimens was found to be similar. The pembrolizumab regimens had improved overall response rates (2 week group - 33.7%; 3 week group - 32.9%) compared with ipilimumab (11.9%) ($P<0.001$). The estimated 6-month progression-free survival rates were 47.3% and 46.4% for those receiving pembrolizumab every 2 and 3 weeks, respectively, *versus* 26.5% for ipilimumab ($P < 0.001$). One-year estimates of survival for both pembro-lizumab groups (2 week group- 74.1%, 3 week group- 68.4%) were significantly superior to the ipilimumab group (58.2%); therefore, the study was stopped early to allow patients in the ipilimumab group the option of receiving pembrolizumab [153]. As seen in prior studies, responses appeared to be durable in all groups, with ongoing responses in 87.8% of patients in the ipilimumab group and 93% in the combined pembrolizumab groups. Overall, this study was key in that it demonstrated improved overall and progression free survival following pembrolizumab treatment with fewer high-grade toxic events when compared with ipilimumab for advanced melanoma.

Anti-PD-L1

PD-L1, the ligand for the PD-1 protein, has also been the subject of investigations over the past several years. Brahmer *et al.* conducted a multicenter phase 1 trial that included 207 patients with advanced malignancies (*e.g.* colorectal cancer, renal-cell cancer, ovarian cancer) in addition to 55 patients with advanced melanoma [135]. High-grade (3 or 4) treatment related effects occurred in 9% of patients, overall. Of the patients with melanoma, 9 (17%) experienced an objective response [135]. Additional investigations are underway currently to determine benefits of anti-PD-L1 therapy compared with anti-PD-1 and anti-CTLA-4 [154].

More recently, the safety, activity and biomarkers of yet another high affinity antibody targeting PD-L1 (MPDL-3280A) was evaluated across multiple cancer types (eg NSCLC, melanoma, renal cell carcinoma, colorectal cancer, gastric cancer, and head and neck squamous cell cancer) [155]. Out of 175 efficacy-evaluable patients, confirmed responses were observed in 32 of 175 patients (18%) overall. When analyzed according to tumor type, 11 of 43 (26%), 11 of 53 (21%), 7 of 56 (13%), and 3 of 23 (13%) of patients with melanoma, NSCLC, renal cell carcinoma, and other cancers (including colorectal cancer, gastric cancer, and head and neck squamous cell carcinoma) [155]. Treatment-related grade 3-4 adverse events were observed in 35 patients overall (13%) and immune-relate grade 3-4 AEs were observed in 3 patients (1%); however, most adverse events did not require medical treatment. Also, responses were observed in tumors expressing high levels of PD-L1. Specific to the melanoma, pre-treatment tumors in responding patients exhibited upregulation of IFN-(as well as IFN-(-inducible genes such as *CXCL9*. This anti-PD-L1 agent and others continue to be developed and additional investigations are underway.

Immune Checkpoint Inhibitors in Combination

The clinical utility of combining immune checkpoint and other immuno-therapeutic approaches was further elaborated in a study that provided follow-up data on 177 patients with stage IV melanoma from the National Cancer Institute comparing gp100, ipilimumab with IL-2, and ipilimumab with intrapatient dose-escalation [156]. Objective response rates were 13%, 25%, and 23% in the gp100, ipilimumab with IL-2 and ipilimumab with intrapatient dose escalation groups, respectively [156]. A recent phase 2 clinical trial by Hodi and colleagues randomized patients with advanced melanoma to receive ipilimumab plus sargramostim (granulocyte-macrophage colony-stimulating factor) or ipilimumab alone [157]. This study noted a lower toxicity and longer overall survival in the combination arm [157]. Median overall survival for the ipilimumab plus sargramostim group was 17.5 months compared to 12.7 months for the ipilimumab alone group; however, there was no difference in progression free survival. One-year survival rate for the ipilimumab group was 52.9%, compared to 68.9% for the combination group [157].

Recent interest has been devoted to elucidating the benefits of combination immune checkpoint blockade. A study by Wolchok *et al.* evaluated the efficacy of combining checkpoint blockade in a phase-I study dose escalation of concurrent treatment with nivolumab (anti-PD-1) and ipilimumab (anti-CTLA-4) in patients with advanced melanoma.[158]. This study demonstrated an overall objective-response rate of 40%, exceeding prior experience with either check-point antibody alone, and the observed anti-tumor effects were rapid [158]. Subsequent investigations demonstrated that nivolumab (anti-PD-1) and ipilimumab (anti-CTLA-4) dual therapy is better than nivolumab or ipilimumab monotherapy for untreated melanoma [159, 160]. In a double-blind study that included 142 patients with metastatic melanoma who had not received prior treatment, patients were randomly assigned in a 2:1 ratio to receive ipilimumab (3 mg/kg) combined with nivolumab (1 mg/kg) or placebo every 2 weeks [159]. The confirmed objective response rate among patients with BRAF wild-type tumors in the combination group (61%) was significantly higher than the ipilimumab plus placebo group (11%) ($P<0.001$). Of those in the combination arm, 22% achieved complete responses while no complete responses were observed in the monotherapy group. Similar response rates and progression free survival were demonstrated in patients with BRAF mutation-positive tumors [159]. While the median PFS was not reached in the ipilimumab/nivolumab combination arm, a PFS of 4.4 months was observed with ipilimumab monotherapy [159]. Not surprising, there was a higher incidence of grade 3 or 4 drug-related adverse events in the combination therapy group (54%) compared with ipilimumab monotherapy (24%). A phase 3 study randomized 945 previously untreated patients with unresectable stage III or IV melanoma in a 1:1:1 ratio to treatment with nivolumab alone, nivolumab plus ipilimumab, or ipilimumab alone [160]. Again, a higher percentage of treatment-related adverse events of grade 3 or 4 occurred in the combination group (55%)

compared with nivolumab (16.3%) and ipilimumab (27.3%) groups. The median progression-free survival was significantly improved in the combination group (11.5 months) when compared with ipilimumab (2.9 months) and nivolumab (6.9 months) groups ($P < 0.001$). In patients with PD-L1 negative tumors, combining ipilimumab and nivolumab proved more effective than either agent alone [160]. Based on these studies comparing combined immune checkpoint blockade with single agent therapy, findings suggest that combination PD-1 and CTLA-4 is more efficacious in the treatment of advanced melanoma but at the cost of more treatment-related adverse events.

MOLECULARLY TARGETED THERAPY

Increasing evidence over the past decades has shed light on the fact that cancers are a disease caused by genetic mutations that are responsible for both the silencing of tumor suppressor genes as well as the unopposed activation of oncogenes [161]. Studies have demonstrated that of all cancer types, melanoma is associated with the highest prevalence of somatic mutations, most likely secondary to its link with ultraviolet radiation [162]. Numerous studies elucidating the genetic aberrations leading to melanoma carcinogenesis have allowed scientists to design specific small molecules to block the genetic drivers of this disease.

MAPK Signaling Pathway

One cell signaling pathway that is altered in many different cancer histologies is that of the mitogen activated protein kinase (MAPK) pathway, also known as the RAS-RAF-MEK-ERK pathway (Fig. **2**) [163].

This signaling pathway is initiated when an extracellular ligand such as epidermal growth factor (EGF) binds to a transmembrane receptor kinase. After binding, the receptor kinase dimerizes and becomes activated. This in turn leads to downstream activation of another protein called RAS. RAS subsequently phosphorylates and activates a family of 3 kinases known as the RAF kinases, ARAF, BRAF, and CRAF. These activated proteins can then phosphorylate and activate their downstream targets of MEK1 and MEK2. These in turn activate ERK1 and ERK2. ERK1/2 activate transcription factors of the AP-1 family, which after activation can traverse the nuclear membrane and directly bind to the DNA of the nucleus leading to cellular proliferation and survival (Fig. **1**) [164].

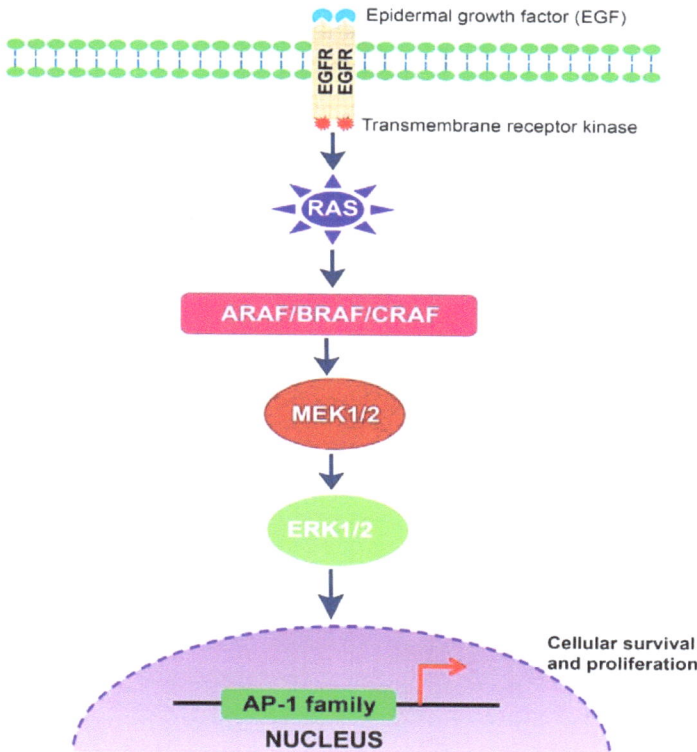

Fig. (2). MAPK pathway: The transmembrane receptor kinase is activated by binding to a ligand such as EGF. This leads to downstream phosphorylation and activation of a series of kinases including RAS, RAF, MEK, and ERK causing subsequent activation of transcription factors in the AP-1 family. Ultimately, this results in cellular poliferation and survival.

While this signaling pathway plays a key role in cell survival, mutations of the different kinases that contribute to the pathway can lead to constant activation and subsequent unopposed cellular proliferation and cancer formation. Furthermore, these mutations have been shown to lead to angiogenesis as well as invasion of cancers [165]. Specifically, mutations of BRAF have been identified in 50-70% of melanomas [166, 167], and up to 80% of these BRAF mutations are of the V600E variety representing a substitution of valine for glutamic acid at position 600 of the protein. Furthermore, although to a lesser degree, mutations of the different RAS proteins (NRAS, KRAS, and HRAS) have also been identified in up to 30% of melanomas.

BRAF Inhibitors

Vemurafenib

Vemurafenib (PLX4032, trade name Zelboraf®) is an oral, competitive and reversible selective inhibitor of BRAF V600E [168]. The clinical efficacy of vemurafenib was first demonstrated in a phase I study (BRIM-1) [169]. Two arms were included in this trial. First, a dose escalation cohort was amassed which included patients with different cancer types but 89% of whom had melanoma. Thirty-two of the patients had metastatic melanoma harboring a V600E mutation and were included in an extension phase arm so that data regarding response could be obtained. The maximum tolerated dose (MTD) was established at 960mg bid. Within the extension phase arm, 24 of the 32 (75%) patients had a partial response, and 2 (6%) had a complete response. The authors were able to conclude that vemurafenib was a well-tolerated drug and seemingly had activity in patients with V600E mutated melanoma.

Because of this, a phase II study was undertaken (BRIM-2) [170]. This cohort of 132 patients included heavily pre-treated advanced melanoma patients with V600E mutations. The overall response rate was found to be 53% with 6% having a CR. The median duration of response, however, was found to be 6.7 months. The median OS was 15.9 months. Of note, one interesting finding was that 26% of patients developed cutaneous squamous cell carcinoma or keratocanthoma while being treated with vemurafenib.

A phase III multi-center randomized control trial (BRIM-3) comparing vemurafenib to dacarbazine standard treatment was published in 2011 [26]. This study had an interim analysis, which concluded that overall and progression-free survival favored the vemurafenib arm, so patients within the dacarbazine arm were allowed to cross over. The estimated progression-free survival in the vemurafenib arm was 5.3 months compared to 1.6 months in the dacarbazine arm. The objective response rates were 48% *vs.* 5% in the vemurafenib and dacarbazine arms, respectively (p<0.001). The most common grade 2+ adverse events seen with vemurafenib in BRIM-3 were arthralgias, rash, fatigue, and cutaneous squamous cell carcinoma. These studies led to the FDA-approval of vemurafenib as a treatment for unresectable stage III or stage IV melanoma with a V600E BRAF mutation in 2011 [26].

While these results were promising, resistance to vemurafenib has been emerging as most patients relapse within 6-7 months. Different mechanisms explaining this resistance have been identified. Upstream bypass mechanisms including activation of NRAS have been identified [171]. Other alternative pathways have also been identified including "RAF switching" *via* activation of either ARAF or CRAF and dysregulation of tyrosine kinase signaling *via* insulin-like growth factor 1 [172, 173].

Dabrafenib (GSK2118436)

Dabrafenib (trade name Tafinlar) is another FDA-approved drug that acts as an inhibitor of the BRAF V600E mutation in non-resectable melanoma. The phase I study including dabrafenib as a treatment option for non-resectable melanoma was the BREAK trial [174]. One hundred eighty-four patients were enrolled, of whom 156 had metastatic melanoma. The most common adverse events grade 2+ was cutaneous squamous-cell carcinoma. An MTD of 150mg bid was selected, and of the 36 patients with a V600E BRAF mutation who received that dose, 56% of patients had a response with a median duration of response of 6.2 months.

The phase 2 study (BREAK-2) was carried out and published in 2013 [175]. An overall response rate of 59% was seen in patients with metastatic melanoma harboring a V600E BRAF mutation with a progression-free survival of 6.3 months. The median overall survival was 13.1 months. Again, cutaneous malignancies including basal cell and squamous cell carcinomas were seen in patients treated with dabrafenib [175].

A phase 3 randomized control trial (BREAK-3) compared dabrafenib to dacarbazine in patients with unresectable malonoma with a V600E BRAF mutation [176]. Progression-free survival was superior in the dabrafenib arm as were response rates. The FDA approved this drug as a single agent for patients with

BRAF V600E mutation with unresectable Stage III or Stage IV melanoma in 2013.

MEK Inhibitors

Trametinib

Trametinib (trade name Mekinist) was granted approval by the FDA in 2013, for the treatment of unresectable stage III or stage IV melanoma with either a V600E or V600K BRAF mutation. The approval was based on a phase 3 randomized control trial comparing patients treated with trametinib or chemotherapy (dacarbazine or paclitaxel) [177]. Patients who were previously treated with BRAF or other MEK inhibitors were excluded from the study. A significantly improved progression-free survival of 4.8 months was seen in the trametinib arm compared to that of 1.5 months in the chemotherapy arm. Furthermore, there was a 22% objective response rate seen in the trametinib arm compared to 8% for the chemotherapy arm [177].

Other MEK Inhibitors

Based on the promising results of trametinib in the treatment of unresectable melanoma, other MEK inhibitors are currently in clinical trials including selumetinib, MEK162, pimasertib, and GDC-0973. Selumetinib, a selective MEK1/2 inhibitor, has been studied in combination with dacarbazine compared to dacarbazine alone in the treatment of patients with unresectable melanoma. While no difference was seen in overall survival between the 2 groups, a trend of longer progression-free survival was appreciated in the combination arm compared to the dacarbazine-alone arm [178].

Ascierto and colleagues aimed to assess the use of small-molecule MEK1/2 inhibitor, MEK162, in patients with NRAS-mutated or Val600 BRAF-mutated advanced melanoma [179]. Eight of 41 patients (20%) with BRAF-mutated melanoma had a partial response as did six of 30 patients (20%) with NRAS-mutated melanoma. There were no complete responses observed. Adverse events occurring in the treatment groups included acneiform dermatitis, rash, peripheral and facial edema, diarrhea and elevation in creatine phosphokinase. There were no deaths observed as a result of treatment. At the time, this was the first study that demonstrated activity of MEK162 in patients with NRAS-mutated melanoma [179].

C-KIT Inhibitors

C-Kit (CD117) is a receptor kinase whose activation has been linked to many cancers including gastrointestinal stromal tumors and leukemias [180]. KIT receptor tyrosine kinase activation ultimately results in evasion of apoptosis, cell survival, dysregulation of normal cell cycle pathways, angiogenesis, and ultimately carcinogenesis. The role of this receptor kinase in melanoma has also been elucidated and investigations into the efficacy of c-Kit inhibitor in melanoma are currently underway [181].

Molecularly Targeted Therapies in Combination

As yet another area for combining treatment approaches, understanding the MAPK signaling pathway led to the development of the blockade of its different components including *MEK* and *BRAF*. Early on, attempts at simultaneously blocking these different steps in the pathway proved beneficial. A study combining cobimetinib, a noncompetitive inhibitor of MEK1/2, with vemurafenib demonstrated an improved progression-free survival and overall survival in the combination group when compared to vemurafenib alone [182]. In 2014, the FDA approved the combination treatment of dabrafenib and trametinib with unresectable Stage III or Stage IV melanoma with *BRAF* V600E or V600K mutations. This approval was based on a randomized control trial comparing the combination treatment of dabrafenib and trametinib to dabrafenib alone [183]. Both objective response rates and response duration time were superior in the combination arm with 2mg trametinib compared to the dabrafenib-alone arm [183]. Serious adverse drug events seen in the combination arm included hemorrhage, venous thromboembolism, and new primary lung malignancy.

Several phase 3 trials have investigated the combination of *BRAF* and *MEK* small molecule inhibition. A study by Long and colleagues randomized 423 treatment naïve patients with unresectable stage IIIC or stage IV melanoma with BRAF V600E or V600K mutation to combination dabrafenib and trametinib or dabrafenib and placebo alone [184]. The overall response rate was 67% in the dabrafenib-trametinib group compared to 51% in the dabrafenib-placebo group (P=0.002), and the rate of progression-free survival was improved (P=0.03) in the combined treatment group (9.3 months) compared to the dabrafenib-only group (8.8 months) [184]. A follow-up double-blind phase 3 study evaluated dabrafenib and trametinib *versus* dabrafenib and placebo for BRAF Val600 mutation-positive stage IIIC or stage IV melanoma [185]. Median overall survival was significantly improved (P=0.0107) in the dabrafenib-trametinib group (25.1 months) compared to dabrafenib-only group (18.7 months). Another phase 3 trial by Robert *et al.* randomly assigned 704 patients with metastatic melanoma with a BRAF V600 mutation to received either a combination of dabrafenib and trametinib or vemurafenib orally as first line therapy [186]. When compared to vemurafenib monotherapy, dabrafenib plus trametinib significantly improved overall survival without increased overall toxicity [186]. Additional studies assessing the efficacy and safety of BRAF and MEK inhibition with immunotherapies are underway.

Given the success of BRAF inhibition monotherapy and immune checkpoint blockade when used alone, there has been considerable interest in targeting both pathways in combination. A phase 1 study conducted by Ribas and colleagues indeed investigated the concurrent administration of vemurafenib and ipilimumab in patients with BRAF V600 mutated metastatic melanoma who had not received prior treatment with BRAF or MEK inhibition or with CTLA-4/PD-1 blocking antibodies [187]. Hepatic adverse events were noted in both treatment cohorts (the first cohort that included full approved doses of both agents, and the second with a lower dose of vemurafenib but with the full dose of ipilimumab). Given the liver toxic events, the study was closed to further patient accrual. This study highlights the importance of investigating the safety of various combination regimens, even if the agents, when given alone, have obtained regulatory approval and proven efficacious.

The utility of combination MEK and cyclin-dependent kinase inhibitors is the subject of ongoing investigations. CDKs are often overexpressed/amplified in cancer as a result of various genetic and epigenetic alterations. CDK inhibitors are small molecules and their use with hormonal therapy in breast cancer has recently gained FDA approval. Early results from the use of combination MEK1/2 inhibitor binimetinib (MEK162) and and Ribociclib (LEE011), an orally available cyclin-dependent kinase (CDK) 4/6 inhibitor, in NRAS-mutant melanoma are promising [188]. Out of 14 enrolled patients in a phase 1b/2 study, six (43%) achieved a partial response, 6 (43%) had stable disease (4 with tumor shrinkage >20%), and several patients experienced symptomatic improvement associated with tumor shrinkage [188]. Optimal dose, schedule and combination strategies of CDK and MEK inhibitors continue to be investigated.

CONCLUSION

Metastatic melanoma has a dismal prognosis. Cytotoxic chemotherapeutic drugs have been studied extensively in the setting of metastatic melanoma in an effort to improve its dire prognosis. Overall, chemotherapy alone and in combination regimens have produced underwhelming results, highlighting the devastating nature of this disease. Dacarbazine, an intravenous alkylating agent approved by the FDA in 1975 for the treatment of advanced melanoma, remains the "gold standard" of traditional chemotherapy. The poor results obtained with dacarbazine underscore the need for further research into targeted molecular and immunomodulatory therapies, discussed elsewhere in this chapter. Advances in the immunotherapeutic approach to targeting advanced melanoma has led to the FDA approval of IL-2, ipilimumab, nivolumab, and other immune-modulating agents for the treatment of metastatic disease. Such approval was granted based off of data that demonstrated improved survival and tolerable safety profile when compared to other conventional treatment options such as chemotherapy or previously studied vaccine treatments. Furthermore, understanding the genetic mutations that cause melanoma carcinogenesis has given scientists and physicians new targets to combat the disease. Promising results have been seen in studies as presented in this chapter, but unfortunately, issues with acquired resistance have been seen as a hurdle that will need to be overcome in the future development of these targeted therapies. Nevertheless, the advances made in the management of advanced stage melanoma are impressive and many believe that the ultimate benefit will be achieved by combining different treatments and agents. Additional prospective studies are necessary to ensure that the added benefit of such combination regimens does not come with additional toxicity risk and to ensure that the treatments remain safe.

CONFLICT OF INTEREST

The authors confirm that they have no conflict of interest to declare for this publication.

ACKNOWLEDGEMENTS

SCA, DMS, RDB, and VS are listed as authors and have contributed substantially to the design of the chapter and accompanying figures/tables, as well as writing and editing of the text.

REFERENCES

[1]   Azoury SC, Lange JR. Epidemiology, risk factors, prevention, and early detection of melanoma. Surg Clin North Am 2014; 94(5): 945-962, vii.
        [http://dx.doi.org/10.1016/j.suc.2014.07.013] [PMID: 25245960]

[2]   Siegel R, Ma J, Zou Z, Jemal A. Cancer statistics, 2014. CA Cancer J Clin 2014; 64(1): 9-29.
        [http://dx.doi.org/10.3322/caac.21208] [PMID: 24399786]

[3]   Howlader N, Ries LA, Mariotto AB, Reichman ME, Ruhl J, Cronin KA. Improved estimates of cancer-specific survival rates from population-based data. J Natl Cancer Inst 2010; 102(20): 1584-98.
        [http://dx.doi.org/10.1093/jnci/djq366] [PMID: 20937991]

[4]   Ferlay J, Shin H-R, Bray F, Forman D, Mathers C, Parkin DM. Estimates of worldwide burden of cancer in 2008: GLOBOCAN 2008. Int J Cancer 2010; 127(12): 2893-917.
        [http://dx.doi.org/10.1002/ijc.25516] [PMID: 21351269]

[5]   Rass K, Reichrath J. UV damage and DNA repair in malignant melanoma and nonmelanoma skin cancer. Adv Exp Med Biol 2008; 624: 162-78.
        [http://dx.doi.org/10.1007/978-0-387-77574-6_13] [PMID: 18348455]

[6]   Balch CM, Gershenwald JE, Soong S-J, *et al.* Final version of 2009 AJCC melanoma staging and classification. J Clin Oncol 2009; 27(36): 6199-206.
        [http://dx.doi.org/10.1200/JCO.2009.23.4799] [PMID: 19917835]

[7]   Barth A, Wanek LA, Morton DL. Prognostic factors in 1,521 melanoma patients with distant metastases. J Am Coll Surg 1995; 181(3): 193-201.
        [PMID: 7670677]

[8]   Wong JH, Skinner KA, Kim KA, Foshag LJ, Morton DL. The role of surgery in the treatment of nonregionally recurrent melanoma. Surgery 1993; 113(4): 389-94.
        [PMID: 8456394]

[9]   Fletcher WS, Pommier RF, Lum S, Wilmarth TJ. Surgical treatment of metastatic melanoma. Am J Surg 1998; 175(5): 413-7.
        [http://dx.doi.org/10.1016/S0002-9610(98)00041-5] [PMID: 9600290]

[10]   Shi W. Role for radiation therapy in melanoma. Surg Oncol Clin N Am 2015; 24(2): 323-35.

[http://dx.doi.org/10.1016/j.soc.2014.12.009] [PMID: 25769715]

[11]   Huttenlocher S, Sehmisch L, Schild SE, Blank O, Hornung D, Rades D. Identifying melanoma patients with 1-3 brain metastases who may benefit from whole-brain irradiation in addition to radiosurgery. Anticancer Res 2014; 34(10): 5589-92.
[PMID: 25275060]

[12]   Burmeister BH, Henderson MA, Ainslie J, *et al.* Adjuvant radiotherapy *versus* observation alone for patients at risk of lymph-node field relapse after therapeutic lymphadenectomy for melanoma: a randomised trial. Lancet Oncol 2012; 13(6): 589-97.
[http://dx.doi.org/10.1016/S1470-2045(12)70138-9] [PMID: 22575589]

[13]   Bhatia S, Tykodi SS, Thompson JA. Treatment of metastatic melanoma: an overview. Oncology (Huntingt) 2009; 23(6): 488-96.
[PMID: 19544689]

[14]   Serrone L, Zeuli M, Sega FM, Cognetti F. Dacarbazine-based chemotherapy for metastatic melanoma: thirty-year experience overview. J Exp Clin Cancer Res 2000; 19(1): 21-34.
[PMID: 10840932]

[15]   Luce JK, Thurman WG, Isaacs BL, Talley RW. Clinical trials with the antitumor agent 5-(3,-dimethyl-1-triazeno)imidazole-4-carboxamide(NSC-45388). Cancer Chemother Rep 1970; 54(2): 119-24.
[PMID: 4334086]

[16]   Wagner DE, Ramirez G, Weiss AJ, Hill G Jr. Combination phase 1-II study of imidazole carboxamide (NCS45388). Oncology 1972; 26(2): 310-6.
[http://dx.doi.org/10.1159/000224680] [PMID: 5049924]

[17]   Skibba JL, Ertürk E, Bryan GT. Induction of thymic lymphosarcoma and mammary adenocarcinomas in rats by oral administration of the antitumor agent, 4 (5)-(3,3-dimethyl-1-triazeno) imidazole-5 (4)-carboxamide. Cancer 1970; 26(5): 1000-5.
[http://dx.doi.org/10.1002/1097-0142(197011)26:5<1000::AID-CNCR2820260506>3.0.CO;2-2]
[PMID: 4320033]

[18]   Hill GJ II, Krementz ET, Hill HZ. Dimethyl triazeno imidazole carboxamide and combination therapy for melanoma. IV. Late results after complete response to chemotherapy (Central Oncology Group protocols 7130, 7131, and 7131A). Cancer 1984; 53(6): 1299-305.
[http://dx.doi.org/10.1002/1097-0142(19840315)53:6<1299::AID-CNCR2820530613>3.0.CO;2-4]
[PMID: 6362841]

[19]   Rosenberg SA, Yang JC, Topalian SL, *et al.* Treatment of 283 consecutive patients with metastatic melanoma or renal cell cancer using high-dose bolus interleukin 2. JAMA 1994; 271(12): 907-13.
[http://dx.doi.org/10.1001/jama.1994.03510360033032] [PMID: 8120958]

[20]   Rosenberg SA, Lotze MT, Muul LM, *et al.* Observations on the systemic administration of autologous lymphokine-activated killer cells and recombinant interleukin-2 to patients with metastatic cancer. N Engl J Med 1985; 313(23): 1485-92.
[http://dx.doi.org/10.1056/NEJM198512053132327] [PMID: 3903508]

[21]   Atkins MB, Lotze MT, Dutcher JP, *et al.* High-dose recombinant interleukin 2 therapy for patients with metastatic melanoma: analysis of 270 patients treated between 1985 and 1993. J Clin Oncol 1999;

17(7): 2105-16.
[PMID: 10561265]

[22]   Wolchok J. How recent advances in immunotherapy are changing the standard of care for patients with metastatic melanoma. Ann Oncol 2012; 23 (Suppl. 8): viii15-21.
[http://dx.doi.org/10.1093/annonc/mds258] [PMID: 22918923]

[23]   Patel KR, Shoukat S, Oliver DE, *et al.* Ipilimumab and stereotactic radiosurgery *versus* stereotactic radiosurgery alone for newly diagnosed melanoma brain metastases. Am J Clin Oncol 2015.
[http://dx.doi.org/10.1097/COC.0000000000000199] [PMID: 26017484]

[24]   Kiess AP, Wolchok JD, Barker CA, *et al.* Stereotactic radiosurgery for melanoma brain metastases in patients receiving ipilimumab: safety profile and efficacy of combined treatment. Int J Radiat Oncol Biol Phys 2015; 92(2): 368-75.
[http://dx.doi.org/10.1016/j.ijrobp.2015.01.004] [PMID: 25754629]

[25]   Robert C, Long GV, Brady B, *et al.* Nivolumab in previously untreated melanoma without BRAF mutation. N Engl J Med 2015; 372(4): 320-30.
[http://dx.doi.org/10.1056/NEJMoa1412082] [PMID: 25399552]

[26]   Chapman PB, Hauschild A, Robert C, *et al.* BRIM-3 Study Group. Improved survival with vemurafenib in melanoma with BRAF V600E mutation. N Engl J Med 2011; 364(26): 2507-16.
[http://dx.doi.org/10.1056/NEJMoa1103782] [PMID: 21639808]

[27]   McArthur GA, Chapman PB, Robert C, *et al.* Safety and efficacy of vemurafenib in BRAF(V600E) and BRAF(V600K) mutation-positive melanoma (BRIM-3): extended follow-up of a phase 3, randomised, open-label study. Lancet Oncol 2014; 15(3): 323-32.
[http://dx.doi.org/10.1016/S1470-2045(14)70012-9] [PMID: 24508103]

[28]   Middleton MR, Grob JJ, Aaronson N, *et al.* Randomized phase III study of temozolomide *versus* dacarbazine in the treatment of patients with advanced metastatic malignant melanoma. J Clin Oncol 2000; 18(1): 158-66.
[PMID: 10623706]

[29]   Coates AS, Segelov E. Long term response to chemotherapy in patients with visceral metastatic melanoma. Ann Oncol 1994; 5(3): 249-51.
[PMID: 8186173]

[30]   Bafaloukos D, Tsoutsos D, Kalofonos H, *et al.* Temozolomide and cisplatin *versus* temozolomide in patients with advanced melanoma: a randomized phase II study of the Hellenic Cooperative Oncology Group. Ann Oncol 2005; 16(6): 950-7.
[http://dx.doi.org/10.1093/annonc/mdi190] [PMID: 15829494]

[31]   Brock CS, Newlands ES, Wedge SR, *et al.* Phase I trial of temozolomide using an extended continuous oral schedule. Cancer Res 1998; 58(19): 4363-7.
[PMID: 9766665]

[32]   Glover D, Glick JH, Weiler C, Fox K, Guerry D. WR-2721 and high-dose cisplatin: an active combination in the treatment of metastatic melanoma. J Clin Oncol 1987; 5(4): 574-8.
[PMID: 3031224]

[33]   Glover D, Ibrahim J, Kirkwood J, *et al.* Eastern Cooperative Oncology Group. Phase II randomized

trial of cisplatin and WR-2721 *versus* cisplatin alone for metastatic melanoma: an Eastern Cooperative Oncology Group Study (E1686). Melanoma Res 2003; 13(6): 619-26.
[http://dx.doi.org/10.1097/00008390-200312000-00012] [PMID: 14646626]

[34]   Huizing MT, Misser VH, Pieters RC, *et al.* Taxanes: A new class of antitumor agents. Cancer Invest 1995; 13(4): 381-404.
[http://dx.doi.org/10.3109/07357909509031919] [PMID: 7627725]

[35]   Legha SS, Ring S, Papadopoulos N, Raber M, Benjamin RS. A phase II trial of taxol in metastatic melanoma. Cancer 1990; 65(11): 2478-81.
[http://dx.doi.org/10.1002/1097-0142(19900601)65:11<2478::AID-CNCR2820651114>3.0.CO;2-S] [PMID: 1970948]

[36]   Einzig AI, Hochster H, Wiernik PH, *et al.* A phase II study of taxol in patients with malignant melanoma. Invest New Drugs 1991; 9(1): 59-64.
[http://dx.doi.org/10.1007/BF00194546] [PMID: 1673965]

[37]   Einzig AI, Wiernik PH, Wadler S, *et al.* Phase I study of paclitaxel (taxol) and granulocyte colony stimulating factor (G-CSF) in patients with unresectable malignancy. Invest New Drugs 1998; 16(1): 29-36.
[http://dx.doi.org/10.1023/A:1006004809169] [PMID: 9740541]

[38]   Bedikian AY, DeConti RC, Conry R, *et al.* Phase 3 study of docosahexaenoic acid-paclitaxel *versus* dacarbazine in patients with metastatic malignant melanoma. Ann Oncol 2011; 22(4): 787-93.
[http://dx.doi.org/10.1093/annonc/mdq438] [PMID: 20855467]

[39]   Hersh EM, O'Day SJ, Ribas A, *et al.* A phase 2 clinical trial of nab-paclitaxel in previously treated and chemotherapy-naive patients with metastatic melanoma. Cancer 2010; 116(1): 155-63.
[PMID: 19877111]

[40]   Gasent Blesa JM, Grande Pulido E, Alberola Candel V, Provencio Pulla M. Melanoma: from darkness to promise. Am J Clin Oncol 2011; 34(2): 179-87.
[PMID: 20498590]

[41]   Kleeberg UR, Engel E, Israels P, *et al.* Palliative therapy of melanoma patients with fotemustine. Inverse relationship between tumour load and treatment effectiveness. A multicentre phase II trial of the EORTC-Melanoma Cooperative Group (MCG). Melanoma Res 1995; 5(3): 195-200.
[http://dx.doi.org/10.1097/00008390-199506000-00009] [PMID: 7543785]

[42]   Jacquillat C, Khayat D, Banzet P, *et al.* Final report of the French multicenter phase II study of the nitrosourea fotemustine in 153 evaluable patients with disseminated malignant melanoma including patients with cerebral metastases. Cancer 1990; 66(9): 1873-8.
[http://dx.doi.org/10.1002/1097-0142(19901101)66:9<1873::AID-CNCR2820660904>3.0.CO;2-5] [PMID: 2224783]

[43]   Calabresi F, Aapro M, Becquart D, *et al.* Multicenter phase II trial of the single agent fotemustine in patients with advanced malignant melanoma. Ann Oncol 1991; 2(5): 377-8.
[PMID: 1954183]

[44]   Chapman PB, Einhorn LH, Meyers ML, *et al.* Phase III multicenter randomized trial of the Dartmouth regimen *versus* dacarbazine in patients with metastatic melanoma. J Clin Oncol 1999; 17(9): 2745-51.
[PMID: 10561349]

[45]   Bottoni U, Bonaccorsi P, Devirgiliis V, *et al*. Complete remission of brain metastases in three patients with stage IV melanoma treated with BOLD and G-CSF. Jpn J Clin Oncol 2005; 35(9): 507-13.
[http://dx.doi.org/10.1093/jjco/hyi141] [PMID: 16120623]

[46]   Richtig E, Hofmann-Wellenhof R, Pehamberger H, *et al*. Temozolomide and interferon alpha 2b in metastatic melanoma stage IV. Br J Dermatol 2004; 151(1): 91-8.
[http://dx.doi.org/10.1111/j.1365-2133.2004.06019.x] [PMID: 15270876]

[47]   Kaufmann R, Spieth K, Leiter U, *et al*. Dermatologic Cooperative Oncology Group. Temozolomide in combination with interferon-alfa *versus* temozolomide alone in patients with advanced metastatic melanoma: a randomized, phase III, multicenter study from the Dermatologic Cooperative Oncology Group. J Clin Oncol 2005; 23(35): 9001-7.
[http://dx.doi.org/10.1200/JCO.2005.01.1551] [PMID: 16260697]

[48]   Clark JI, Moon J, Hutchins LF, *et al*. Phase 2 trial of combination thalidomide plus temozolomide in patients with metastatic malignant melanoma: Southwest Oncology Group S0508. Cancer 2010; 116(2): 424-31.
[http://dx.doi.org/10.1002/cncr.24739] [PMID: 19918923]

[49]   Rao RD, Holtan SG, Ingle JN, *et al*. Combination of paclitaxel and carboplatin as second-line therapy for patients with metastatic melanoma. Cancer 2006; 106(2): 375-82.
[http://dx.doi.org/10.1002/cncr.21611] [PMID: 16342250]

[50]   Eisen T, Trefzer U, Hamilton A, *et al*. Results of a multicenter, randomized, double-blind phase 2/3 study of lenalidomide in the treatment of pretreated relapsed or refractory metastatic malignant melanoma. Cancer 2010; 116(1): 146-54.
[PMID: 19862820]

[51]   Hauschild A, Agarwala SS, Trefzer U, *et al*. Results of a phase III, randomized, placebo-controlled study of sorafenib in combination with carboplatin and paclitaxel as second-line treatment in patients with unresectable stage III or stage IV melanoma. J Clin Oncol 2009; 27(17): 2823-30.
[http://dx.doi.org/10.1200/JCO.2007.15.7636] [PMID: 19349552]

[52]   Lee C-K, Jung M, Choi HJ, Kim HR, Kim HS, Roh MR, *et al*. Results of a phase II study to evaluate the efficacy of docetaxel and carboplatin in metastatic malignant melanoma patients who failed first-line therapy containing darcabazine. Cancer Res Treat 2015; 47(4): 781-9.
[http://dx.doi.org/10.4143/crt.2014.261] [PMID: 25687848]

[53]   Flaherty KT, Lee SJ, Zhao F, *et al*. Phase III trial of carboplatin and paclitaxel with or without sorafenib in metastatic melanoma. J Clin Oncol 2013; 31(3): 373-9.
[http://dx.doi.org/10.1200/JCO.2012.42.1529] [PMID: 23248256]

[54]   Ugurel S, Rappl G, Tilgen W, Reinhold U. Increased serum concentration of angiogenic factors in malignant melanoma patients correlates with tumor progression and survival. J Clin Oncol 2001; 19(2): 577-83.
[PMID: 11208853]

[55]   Cui C, Mao L, Chi Z, *et al*. A phase II, randomized, double-blind, placebo-controlled multicenter trial of Endostar in patients with metastatic melanoma. Mol Ther 2013; 21(7): 1456-63.
[http://dx.doi.org/10.1038/mt.2013.79] [PMID: 23670576]

[56] Ferrucci PF, Minchella I, Mosconi M, *et al.* Dacarbazine in combination with bevacizumab for the treatment of unresectable/metastatic melanoma: a phase II study. Melanoma Res 2015; 25(3): 239-45. [http://dx.doi.org/10.1097/CMR.0000000000000146] [PMID: 25746039]

[57] Kim KB, Sosman JA, Fruehauf JP, *et al.* BEAM: A randomized phase II study evaluating the activity of bevacizumab in combination with carboplatin plus paclitaxel in patients with previously untreated advanced melanoma. J Clin Oncol 2012; 30(1): 34-41. [http://dx.doi.org/10.1200/JCO.2011.34.6270] [PMID: 22124101]

[58] Weiss SA, Chandra S, Pavlick AC. Update on vaccines for high-risk melanoma. Curr Treat Options Oncol 2014; 15(2): 269-80. [http://dx.doi.org/10.1007/s11864-014-0283-7] [PMID: 24788575]

[59] Topalian SL, Wolchok JD, Chan TA, *et al.* Immunotherapy: The path to win the war on cancer? Cell 2015; 161(2): 185-6. [http://dx.doi.org/10.1016/j.cell.2015.03.045] [PMID: 26042237]

[60] Turcotte S, Rosenberg SA. Immunotherapy for metastatic solid cancers. Adv Surg 2011; 45: 341-60. [http://dx.doi.org/10.1016/j.yasu.2011.04.003] [PMID: 21954698]

[61] Conta BS, Powell MB, Ruddle NH. Production of lymphotoxin, IFN-gamma and IFN-alpha, beta by murine T cell lines and clones. J Immunol 1983; 130(5): 2231-5. [PMID: 6403618]

[62] Lesinski GB, Anghelina M, Zimmerer J, *et al.* The antitumor effects of IFN-alpha are abrogated in a STAT1-deficient mouse. J Clin Invest 2003; 112(2): 170-80. [http://dx.doi.org/10.1172/JCI16603] [PMID: 12865406]

[63] Palathinkal DM, Sharma TR, Koon HB, Bordeaux JS. Current systemic therapies for melanoma. Dermatol Surg 2014; 40(9): 948-63. [http://dx.doi.org/10.1097/01.DSS.0000452626.09513.55] [PMID: 25072125]

[64] Kirkwood JM, Strawderman MH, Ernstoff MS, Smith TJ, Borden EC, Blum RH. Interferon alfa-2b adjuvant therapy of high-risk resected cutaneous melanoma: the Eastern Cooperative Oncology Group Trial EST 1684. J Clin Oncol 1996; 14(1): 7-17. [PMID: 8558223]

[65] Kirkwood JM, Ibrahim JG, Sondak VK, *et al.* High- and low-dose interferon alfa-2b in high-risk melanoma: first analysis of intergroup trial E1690/S9111/C9190. J Clin Oncol 2000; 18(12): 2444-58. [PMID: 10856105]

[66] Kirkwood JM, Manola J, Ibrahim J, Sondak V, Ernstoff MS, Rao U. Eastern Cooperative Oncology Group. A pooled analysis of eastern cooperative oncology group and intergroup trials of adjuvant high-dose interferon for melanoma. Clin Cancer Res 2004; 10(5): 1670-7. [http://dx.doi.org/10.1158/1078-0432.CCR-1103-3] [PMID: 15014018]

[67] Bottomley A, Coens C, Suciu S, *et al.* Adjuvant therapy with pegylated interferon alfa-2b *versus* observation in resected stage III melanoma: a phase III randomized controlled trial of health-related quality of life and symptoms by the European Organisation for Research and Treatment of Cancer Melanoma Group. J Clin Oncol 2009; 27(18): 2916-23. [http://dx.doi.org/10.1200/JCO.2008.20.2069] [PMID: 19433686]

[68] Eggermont AM, Suciu S, Santinami M, *et al.* EORTC Melanoma Group. Adjuvant therapy with pegylated interferon alfa-2b *versus* observation alone in resected stage III melanoma: final results of EORTC 18991, a randomised phase III trial. Lancet 2008; 372(9633): 117-26.
[http://dx.doi.org/10.1016/S0140-6736(08)61033-8] [PMID: 18620949]

[69] Rosenberg SA. IL-2: the first effective immunotherapy for human cancer. J Immunol 2014; 192(12): 5451-8.
[http://dx.doi.org/10.4049/jimmunol.1490019] [PMID: 24907378]

[70] Sosman JA, Carrillo C, Urba WJ, *et al.* Three phase II cytokine working group trials of gp100 (210M) peptide plus high-dose interleukin-2 in patients with HLA-A2-positive advanced melanoma. J Clin Oncol 2008; 26(14): 2292-8.
[http://dx.doi.org/10.1200/JCO.2007.13.3165] [PMID: 18467720]

[71] Sim GC, Radvanyi L. The IL-2 cytokine family in cancer immunotherapy. Cytokine Growth Factor Rev 2014; 25(4): 377-90.
[http://dx.doi.org/10.1016/j.cytogfr.2014.07.018] [PMID: 25200249]

[72] Rosenberg SA, Lotze MT, Muul LM, *et al.* A new approach to the therapy of cancer based on the systemic administration of autologous lymphokine-activated killer cells and recombinant interleukin-2. Surgery 1986; 100(2): 262-72.
[PMID: 3526604]

[73] Rosenberg SA, Mulé JJ, Spiess PJ, Reichert CM, Schwarz SL. Regression of established pulmonary metastases and subcutaneous tumor mediated by the systemic administration of high-dose recombinant interleukin 2. J Exp Med 1985; 161(5): 1169-88.
[http://dx.doi.org/10.1084/jem.161.5.1169] [PMID: 3886826]

[74] Lotze MT, Matory YL, Ettinghausen SE, *et al. In vivo* administration of purified human interleukin 2. II. Half life, immunologic effects, and expansion of peripheral lymphoid cells *in vivo* with recombinant IL 2. J Immunol 1985; 135(4): 2865-75.
[PMID: 2993418]

[75] Rosenberg SA, Lotze MT, Muul LM, *et al.* A progress report on the treatment of 157 patients with advanced cancer using lymphokine-activated killer cells and interleukin-2 or high-dose interleukin-2 alone. N Engl J Med 1987; 316(15): 889-97.
[http://dx.doi.org/10.1056/NEJM198704093161501] [PMID: 3493432]

[76] Rosenberg SA, Lotze MT, Yang JC, *et al.* Prospective randomized trial of high-dose interleukin-2 alone or in conjunction with lymphokine-activated killer cells for the treatment of patients with advanced cancer. J Natl Cancer Inst 1993; 85(8): 622-32.
[http://dx.doi.org/10.1093/jnci/85.8.622] [PMID: 8468720]

[77] Dillman RO, Church C, Oldham RK, West WH, Schwartzberg L, Birch R. Inpatient continuous-infusion interleukin-2 in 788 patients with cancer. The National Biotherapy Study Group experience. Cancer 1993; 71(7): 2358-70.
[http://dx.doi.org/10.1002/1097-0142(19930401)71:7<2358::AID-CNCR2820710730>3.0.CO;2-M]
[PMID: 8453558]

[78] Atkins MB, Kunkel L, Sznol M, Rosenberg SA. High-dose recombinant interleukin-2 therapy in patients with metastatic melanoma: long-term survival update. Cancer J Sci Am 2000; 6 (Suppl. 1):

S11-4.
[PMID: 10685652]

[79]   Kammula US, White DE, Rosenberg SA. Trends in the safety of high dose bolus interleukin-2 administration in patients with metastatic cancer. Cancer 1998; 83(4): 797-805.
[http://dx.doi.org/10.1002/(SICI)1097-0142(19980815)83:4<797::AID-CNCR25>3.0.CO;2-M]
[PMID: 9708948]

[80]   Bock SN, Lee RE, Fisher B, *et al.* A prospective randomized trial evaluating prophylactic antibiotics to prevent triple-lumen catheter-related sepsis in patients treated with immunotherapy. J Clin Oncol 1990; 8(1): 161-9.
[PMID: 2404087]

[81]   Ott PA, Fritsch EF, Wu CJ, Dranoff G. Vaccines and melanoma. Hematol Oncol Clin North Am 2014; 28(3): 559-69.
[http://dx.doi.org/10.1016/j.hoc.2014.02.008] [PMID: 24880947]

[82]   Dillman RO. Cancer vaccines: can they improve survival? Cancer Biother Radiopharm 2015; 30(4): 147-51.
[http://dx.doi.org/10.1089/cbr.2014.1805] [PMID: 25747158]

[83]   van der Bruggen P, Traversari C, Chomez P, *et al.* A gene encoding an antigen recognized by cytolytic T lymphocytes on a human melanoma. Science 1991; 254(5038): 1643-7.
[http://dx.doi.org/10.1126/science.1840703] [PMID: 1840703]

[84]   Chaux P, Vantomme V, Stroobant V, *et al.* Identification of MAGE-3 epitopes presented by HLA-DR molecules to CD4(+) T lymphocytes. J Exp Med 1999; 189(5): 767-78.
[http://dx.doi.org/10.1084/jem.189.5.767] [PMID: 10049940]

[85]   Cormier JN, Salgaller ML, Prevette T, *et al.* Enhancement of cellular immunity in melanoma patients immunized with a peptide from MART-1/Melan A. Cancer J Sci Am 1997; 3(1): 37-44.
[PMID: 9072306]

[86]   Marchand M, van Baren N, Weynants P, *et al.* Tumor regressions observed in patients with metastatic melanoma treated with an antigenic peptide encoded by gene MAGE-3 and presented by HLA-A1. Int J Cancer 1999; 80(2): 219-30.
[http://dx.doi.org/10.1002/(SICI)1097-0215(19990118)80:2<219::AID-IJC10>3.0.CO;2-S]   [PMID: 9935203]

[87]   Kawakami Y, Eliyahu S, Delgado CH, *et al.* Identification of a human melanoma antigen recognized by tumor-infiltrating lymphocytes associated with *in vivo* tumor rejection. Proc Natl Acad Sci USA 1994; 91(14): 6458-62.
[http://dx.doi.org/10.1073/pnas.91.14.6458] [PMID: 8022805]

[88]   Kawakami Y, Eliyahu S, Delgado CH, *et al.* Cloning of the gene coding for a shared human melanoma antigen recognized by autologous T cells infiltrating into tumor. Proc Natl Acad Sci USA 1994; 91(9): 3515-9.
[http://dx.doi.org/10.1073/pnas.91.9.3515] [PMID: 8170938]

[89]   Kawakami Y, Robbins PF, Wang RF, Parkhurst M, Kang X, Rosenberg SA. The use of melanosomal proteins in the immunotherapy of melanoma. J Immunother 1998; 21(4): 237-46.
[http://dx.doi.org/10.1097/00002371-199807000-00001] [PMID: 9672845]

[90]   Kawakami Y, Rosenberg SA. Immunobiology of human melanoma antigens MART-1 and gp100 and their use for immuno-gene therapy. Int Rev Immunol 1997; 14(2-3): 173-92.
[http://dx.doi.org/10.3109/08830189709116851] [PMID: 9131386]

[91]   Slingluff CL Jr, Petroni GR, Yamshchikov GV, *et al.* Clinical and immunologic results of a randomized phase II trial of vaccination using four melanoma peptides either administered in granulocyte-macrophage colony-stimulating factor in adjuvant or pulsed on dendritic cells. J Clin Oncol 2003; 21(21): 4016-26.
[http://dx.doi.org/10.1200/JCO.2003.10.005] [PMID: 14581425]

[92]   Block MS, Suman VJ, Nevala WK, *et al.* Pilot study of granulocyte-macrophage colony-stimulating factor and interleukin-2 as immune adjuvants for a melanoma peptide vaccine. Melanoma Res 2011; 21(5): 438-45.
[http://dx.doi.org/10.1097/CMR.0b013e32834640c0] [PMID: 21697748]

[93]   Slingluff CL Jr, Petroni GR, Chianese-Bullock KA, *et al.* Randomized multicenter trial of the effects of melanoma-associated helper peptides and cyclophosphamide on the immunogenicity of a multipeptide melanoma vaccine. J Clin Oncol 2011; 29(21): 2924-32.
[http://dx.doi.org/10.1200/JCO.2010.33.8053] [PMID: 21690475]

[94]   Schwartzentruber DJ, Lawson DH, Richards JM, *et al.* gp100 peptide vaccine and interleukin-2 in patients with advanced melanoma. N Engl J Med 2011; 364(22): 2119-27.
[http://dx.doi.org/10.1056/NEJMoa1012863] [PMID: 21631324]

[95]   Ferrucci PF, Tosti G, di Pietro A, *et al.* Newly identified tumor antigens as promising cancer vaccine targets for malignant melanoma treatment. Curr Top Med Chem 2012; 12(1): 11-31.
[http://dx.doi.org/10.2174/156802612798919213] [PMID: 22196269]

[96]   Barrow C, Browning J, MacGregor D, *et al.* Tumor antigen expression in melanoma varies according to antigen and stage. Clin Cancer Res 2006; 12(3 Pt 1): 764-71.
[http://dx.doi.org/10.1158/1078-0432.CCR-05-1544] [PMID: 16467087]

[97]   Davis ID, Chen W, Jackson H, *et al.* Recombinant NY-ESO-1 protein with ISCOMATRIX adjuvant induces broad integrated antibody and CD4(+) and CD8(+) T cell responses in humans. Proc Natl Acad Sci USA 2004; 101(29): 10697-702.
[http://dx.doi.org/10.1073/pnas.0403572101] [PMID: 15252201]

[98]   Nicholaou T, Ebert LM, Davis ID, *et al.* Regulatory T-cell-mediated attenuation of T-cell responses to the NY-ESO-1 ISCOMATRIX vaccine in patients with advanced malignant melanoma. Clin Cancer Res 2009; 15(6): 2166-73.
[http://dx.doi.org/10.1158/1078-0432.CCR-08-2484] [PMID: 19276262]

[99]   Kruit WH, van Ojik HH, Brichard VG, *et al.* Phase 1/2 study of subcutaneous and intradermal immunization with a recombinant MAGE-3 protein in patients with detectable metastatic melanoma. Int J Cancer 2005; 117(4): 596-604.
[http://dx.doi.org/10.1002/ijc.21264] [PMID: 15945101]

[100]   Kruit WH, Suciu S, Dreno B, *et al.* Selection of immunostimulant AS15 for active immunization with MAGE-A3 protein: results of a randomized phase II study of the European Organisation for Research and Treatment of Cancer Melanoma Group in Metastatic Melanoma. J Clin Oncol 2013; 31(19): 2413-20.

[http://dx.doi.org/10.1200/JCO.2012.43.7111] [PMID: 23715572]

[101]   Rosenberg SA, Yang JC, Restifo NP. Cancer immunotherapy: moving beyond current vaccines. Nat Med 2004; 10(9): 909-15.
[http://dx.doi.org/10.1038/nm1100] [PMID: 15340416]

[102]   Livingston P. The unfulfilled promise of melanoma vaccines. Clin Cancer Res 2001; 7(7): 1837-8.
[PMID: 11448892]

[103]   Livingston PO, Wong GY, Adluri S, *et al.* Improved survival in stage III melanoma patients with GM2 antibodies: a randomized trial of adjuvant vaccination with GM2 ganglioside. J Clin Oncol 1994; 12(5): 1036-44.
[PMID: 8164027]

[104]   Kirkwood JM, Ibrahim JG, Sosman JA, *et al.* High-dose interferon alfa-2b significantly prolongs relapse-free and overall survival compared with the GM2-KLH/QS-21 vaccine in patients with resected stage IIB-III melanoma: results of intergroup trial E1694/S9512/C509801. J Clin Oncol 2001; 19(9): 2370-80.
[PMID: 11331315]

[105]   Eggermont AM, Suciu S, Rutkowski P, *et al.* Adjuvant ganglioside GM2-KLH/QS-21 vaccination *versus* observation after resection of primary tumor > 1.5 mm in patients with stage II melanoma: results of the EORTC 18961 randomized phase III trial. J Clin Oncol 2013; 31(30): 3831-7.
[http://dx.doi.org/10.1200/JCO.2012.47.9303] [PMID: 24019551]

[106]   Senzer NN, Kaufman HL, Amatruda T, *et al.* Phase II clinical trial of a granulocyte-macrophage colony-stimulating factor-encoding, second-generation oncolytic herpesvirus in patients with unresectable metastatic melanoma. J Clin Oncol 2009; 27(34): 5763-71.
[http://dx.doi.org/10.1200/JCO.2009.24.3675] [PMID: 19884534]

[107]   Andtbacka RH, Kaufman HL, Collichio F, *et al.* Talimogene Laherparepvec Improves Durable Response Rate in Patients With Advanced Melanoma. J Clin Oncol 2015; 33(25): 2780-8.
[http://dx.doi.org/10.1200/JCO.2014.58.3377] [PMID: 26014293]

[108]   Murshid A, Gong J, Calderwood SK. The role of heat shock proteins in antigen cross presentation. Front Immunol 2012; 3: 63.
[http://dx.doi.org/10.3389/fimmu.2012.00063] [PMID: 22566944]

[109]   Tosti G, di Pietro A, Ferrucci PF, Testori A. HSPPC-96 vaccine in metastatic melanoma patients: from the state of the art to a possible future. Expert Rev Vaccines 2009; 8(11): 1513-26.
[http://dx.doi.org/10.1586/erv.09.108] [PMID: 19863242]

[110]   Testori A, Richards J, Whitman E, *et al.* C-100-21 Study Group. Phase III comparison of vitespen, an autologous tumor-derived heat shock protein gp96 peptide complex vaccine, with physician's choice of treatment for stage IV melanoma: the C-100-21 Study Group. J Clin Oncol 2008; 26(6): 955-62.
[http://dx.doi.org/10.1200/JCO.2007.11.9941] [PMID: 18281670]

[111]   Berd D. M-Vax: an autologous, hapten-modified vaccine for human cancer. Expert Rev Vaccines 2004; 3(5): 521-7.
[http://dx.doi.org/10.1586/14760584.3.5.521] [PMID: 15485331]

[112]   Berd D, Sato T, Cohn H, Maguire HC Jr, Mastrangelo MJ. Treatment of metastatic melanoma with

autologous, hapten-modified melanoma vaccine: regression of pulmonary metastases. Int J Cancer 2001; 94(4): 531-9.
[http://dx.doi.org/10.1002/ijc.1506.abs] [PMID: 11745440]

[113]   Ozao-Choy J, Lee DJ, Faries MB. Melanoma vaccines: mixed past, promising future. Surg Clin North Am 2014; 94(5): 1017-1030, viii. [–viii.].
[http://dx.doi.org/10.1016/j.suc.2014.07.005] [PMID: 25245965]

[114]   Morton DL, Hsueh EC, Essner R, *et al.* Prolonged survival of patients receiving active immunotherapy with Canvaxin therapeutic polyvalent vaccine after complete resection of melanoma metastatic to regional lymph nodes. Annals of Surgery 2002; 236(4): 438-8. discussion 448-9
[http://dx.doi.org/10.1097/00000658-200210000-00006]

[115]   Hsueh EC, Essner R, Foshag LJ, *et al.* Prolonged survival after complete resection of disseminated melanoma and active immunotherapy with a therapeutic cancer vaccine. J Clin Oncol 2002; 20(23): 4549-54.
[http://dx.doi.org/10.1200/JCO.2002.01.151] [PMID: 12454111]

[116]   Suriano R, Rajoria S, George AL, Geliebter J, Tiwari RK, Wallack M. Follow-up analysis of a randomized phase III immunotherapeutic clinical trial on melanoma. Mol Clin Oncol 2013; 1(3): 466-72.
[PMID: 24649193]

[117]   Hersey P, Edwards A, Coates A, Shaw H, McCarthy W, Milton G. Evidence that treatment with vaccinia melanoma cell lysates (VMCL) may improve survival of patients with stage II melanoma. Treatment of stage II melanoma with viral lysates. Cancer Immunol Immunother 1987; 25(3): 257-65.
[http://dx.doi.org/10.1007/BF00199156] [PMID: 3677126]

[118]   Hersey P, Coates AS, McCarthy WH, *et al.* Adjuvant immunotherapy of patients with high-risk melanoma using vaccinia viral lysates of melanoma: results of a randomized trial. J Clin Oncol 2002; 20(20): 4181-90.
[http://dx.doi.org/10.1200/JCO.2002.12.094] [PMID: 12377961]

[119]   Sosman JA, Sondak VK. Melacine: an allogeneic melanoma tumor cell lysate vaccine. Expert Rev Vaccines 2003; 2(3): 353-68.
[http://dx.doi.org/10.1586/14760584.2.3.353] [PMID: 12903801]

[120]   Sondak VK, Liu P-Y, Tuthill RJ, *et al.* Adjuvant immunotherapy of resected, intermediate-thickness, node-negative melanoma with an allogeneic tumor vaccine: overall results of a randomized trial of the Southwest Oncology Group. J Clin Oncol 2002; 20(8): 2058-66.
[http://dx.doi.org/10.1200/JCO.2002.08.071] [PMID: 11956266]

[121]   Mackiewicz A, Mackiewicz J, Wysocki PJ, *et al.* Long-term survival of high-risk melanoma patients immunized with a Hyper-IL-6-modified allogeneic whole-cell vaccine after complete resection. Expert Opin Investig Drugs 2012; 21(6): 773-83.
[http://dx.doi.org/10.1517/13543784.2012.684753] [PMID: 22577889]

[122]   Butterfield LH. Dendritic cells in cancer immunotherapy clinical trials: are we making progress? Front Immunol 2013; 4: 454.
[http://dx.doi.org/10.3389/fimmu.2013.00454] [PMID: 24379816]

[123]   Nestle FO, Alijagic S, Gilliet M, *et al.* Vaccination of melanoma patients with peptide- or tumor

lysate-pulsed dendritic cells. Nat Med 1998; 4(3): 328-32.
[http://dx.doi.org/10.1038/nm0398-328] [PMID: 9500607]

[124] Schadendorf D, Ugurel S, Schuler-Thurner B, *et al.* DC study group of the DeCOG. Dacarbazine (DTIC) *versus* vaccination with autologous peptide-pulsed dendritic cells (DC) in first-line treatment of patients with metastatic melanoma: a randomized phase III trial of the DC study group of the DeCOG. Ann Oncol 2006; 17(4): 563-70.
[http://dx.doi.org/10.1093/annonc/mdj138] [PMID: 16418308]

[125] Palucka AK, Ueno H, Connolly J, *et al.* Dendritic cells loaded with killed allogeneic melanoma cells can induce objective clinical responses and MART-1 specific CD8+ T-cell immunity. J Immunother 2006; 29(5): 545-57.
[http://dx.doi.org/10.1097/01.cji.0000211309.90621.8b] [PMID: 16971810]

[126] Markowicz S, Nowecki ZI, Rutkowski P, *et al.* Adjuvant vaccination with melanoma antigen-pulsed dendritic cells in stage III melanoma patients. Med Oncol 2012; 29(4): 2966-77.
[http://dx.doi.org/10.1007/s12032-012-0168-1] [PMID: 22302285]

[127] Rosenberg SA. Cell transfer immunotherapy for metastatic solid cancer--what clinicians need to know. Nat Rev Clin Oncol 2011; 8(10): 577-85.
[http://dx.doi.org/10.1038/nrclinonc.2011.116] [PMID: 21808266]

[128] Dudley ME, Wunderlich JR, Robbins PF, *et al.* Cancer regression and autoimmunity in patients after clonal repopulation with antitumor lymphocytes. Science 2002; 298(5594): 850-4.
[http://dx.doi.org/10.1126/science.1076514] [PMID: 12242449]

[129] Hunder NN, Wallen H, Cao J, *et al.* Treatment of metastatic melanoma with autologous CD4+ T cells against NY-ESO-1. N Engl J Med 2008; 358(25): 2698-703.
[http://dx.doi.org/10.1056/NEJMoa0800251] [PMID: 18565862]

[130] Dudley ME, Yang JC, Sherry R, *et al.* Adoptive cell therapy for patients with metastatic melanoma: evaluation of intensive myeloablative chemoradiation preparative regimens. J Clin Oncol 2008; 26(32): 5233-9.
[http://dx.doi.org/10.1200/JCO.2008.16.5449] [PMID: 18809613]

[131] Rosenberg SA, Yang JC, Sherry RM, *et al.* Durable complete responses in heavily pretreated patients with metastatic melanoma using T-cell transfer immunotherapy. Clin Cancer Res 2011; 17(13): 4550-7.
[http://dx.doi.org/10.1158/1078-0432.CCR-11-0116] [PMID: 21498393]

[132] Pardoll DM. The blockade of immune checkpoints in cancer immunotherapy. Nat Rev Cancer 2012; 12(4): 252-64.
[http://dx.doi.org/10.1038/nrc3239] [PMID: 22437870]

[133] Eggermont AM, Maio M, Robert C. Immune checkpoint inhibitors in melanoma provide the cornerstones for curative therapies. Semin Oncol 2015; 42(3): 429-35.
[http://dx.doi.org/10.1053/j.seminoncol.2015.02.010] [PMID: 25965361]

[134] Topalian SL, Hodi FS, Brahmer JR, *et al.* Safety, activity, and immune correlates of anti-PD-1 antibody in cancer. N Engl J Med 2012; 366(26): 2443-54.
[http://dx.doi.org/10.1056/NEJMoa1200690] [PMID: 22658127]

[135] Brahmer JR, Tykodi SS, Chow LQ, *et al.* Safety and activity of anti-PD-L1 antibody in patients with advanced cancer. N Engl J Med 2012; 366(26): 2455-65.
[http://dx.doi.org/10.1056/NEJMoa1200694] [PMID: 22658128]

[136] Hodi FS, O'Day SJ, McDermott DF, *et al.* Improved survival with ipilimumab in patients with metastatic melanoma. N Engl J Med 2010; 363(8): 711-23.
[http://dx.doi.org/10.1056/NEJMoa1003466] [PMID: 20525992]

[137] Hamid O, Robert C, Daud A, *et al.* Safety and tumor responses with lambrolizumab (anti-PD-1) in melanoma. N Engl J Med 2013; 369(2): 134-44.
[http://dx.doi.org/10.1056/NEJMoa1305133] [PMID: 23724846]

[138] Postow MA, Callahan MK, Wolchok JD. Immune Checkpoint Blockade in Cancer Therapy. J Clin Oncol 2015; 33(17): 1974-82.
[http://dx.doi.org/10.1200/JCO.2014.59.4358] [PMID: 25605845]

[139] Hodi FS, Mihm MC, Soiffer RJ, *et al.* Biologic activity of cytotoxic T lymphocyte-associated antigen 4 antibody blockade in previously vaccinated metastatic melanoma and ovarian carcinoma patients. Proc Natl Acad Sci USA 2003; 100(8): 4712-7.
[http://dx.doi.org/10.1073/pnas.0830997100] [PMID: 12682289]

[140] Phan GQ, Yang JC, Sherry RM, *et al.* Cancer regression and autoimmunity induced by cytotoxic T lymphocyte-associated antigen 4 blockade in patients with metastatic melanoma. Proc Natl Acad Sci USA 2003; 100(14): 8372-7.
[http://dx.doi.org/10.1073/pnas.1533209100] [PMID: 12826605]

[141] Attia P, Phan GQ, Maker AV, *et al.* Autoimmunity correlates with tumor regression in patients with metastatic melanoma treated with anti-cytotoxic T-lymphocyte antigen-4. J Clin Oncol 2005; 23(25): 6043-53.
[http://dx.doi.org/10.1200/JCO.2005.06.205] [PMID: 16087944]

[142] Maker AV, Yang JC, Sherry RM, *et al.* Intrapatient dose escalation of anti-CTLA-4 antibody in patients with metastatic melanoma. J Immunother 2006; 29(4): 455-63.
[http://dx.doi.org/10.1097/01.cji.0000208259.73167.58] [PMID: 16799341]

[143] Maker AV, Phan GQ, Attia P, *et al.* Tumor regression and autoimmunity in patients treated with cytotoxic T lymphocyte-associated antigen 4 blockade and interleukin 2: a phase I/II study. Ann Surg Oncol 2005; 12(12): 1005-16.
[http://dx.doi.org/10.1245/ASO.2005.03.536] [PMID: 16283570]

[144] Robert C, Thomas L, Bondarenko I, *et al.* Ipilimumab plus dacarbazine for previously untreated metastatic melanoma. N Engl J Med 2011; 364(26): 2517-26.
[http://dx.doi.org/10.1056/NEJMoa1104621] [PMID: 21639810]

[145] Maio M, Grob J-J, Aamdal S, *et al.* Five-year survival rates for treatment-naive patients with advanced melanoma who received ipilimumab plus dacarbazine in a phase III trial. J Clin Oncol 2015; 33(10): 1191-6.
[http://dx.doi.org/10.1200/JCO.2014.56.6018] [PMID: 25713437]

[146] Brahmer JR, Drake CG, Wollner I, *et al.* Phase I study of single-agent anti-programmed death-1 (MDX-1106) in refractory solid tumors: safety, clinical activity, pharmacodynamics, and immunologic

correlates. J Clin Oncol 2010; 28(19): 3167-75.
[http://dx.doi.org/10.1200/JCO.2009.26.7609] [PMID: 20516446]

[147]   Ribas A. Tumor immunotherapy directed at PD-1. N Engl J Med 2012; 366(26): 2517-9.
[http://dx.doi.org/10.1056/NEJMe1205943] [PMID: 22658126]

[148]   Topalian SL, Sznol M, McDermott DF, *et al.* Survival, durable tumor remission, and long-term safety
in patients with advanced melanoma receiving nivolumab. J Clin Oncol 2014; 32(10): 1020-30.
[http://dx.doi.org/10.1200/JCO.2013.53.0105] [PMID: 24590637]

[149]   Mahoney KM, Freeman GJ, McDermott DF. The Next Immune-Checkpoint Inhibitors: PD-1/PD-L1
Blockade in Melanoma. Clin Ther 2015; 37(4): 764-82.
[http://dx.doi.org/10.1016/j.clinthera.2015.02.018] [PMID: 25823918]

[150]   Robert C, Ribas A, Wolchok JD, *et al.* Anti-programmed-death-receptor-1 treatment with
pembrolizumab in ipilimumab-refractory advanced melanoma: a randomised dose-comparison cohort
of a phase 1 trial. Lancet 2014; 384(9948): 1109-17.
[http://dx.doi.org/10.1016/S0140-6736(14)60958-2] [PMID: 25034862]

[151]   Rajakulendran T, Adam DN. Spotlight on pembrolizumab in the treatment of advanced melanoma.
Drug Des Devel Ther 2015; 9: 2883-6.
[PMID: 26082618]

[152]   Shin DS, Ribas A. The evolution of checkpoint blockade as a cancer therapy: what's here, what's
next? Curr Opin Immunol 2015; 33: 23-35.
[http://dx.doi.org/10.1016/j.coi.2015.01.006] [PMID: 25621841]

[153]   Robert C, Schachter J, Long GV, *et al.* KEYNOTE-006 investigators. Pembrolizumab *versus*
Ipilimumab in Advanced Melanoma. N Engl J Med 2015; 372(26): 2521-32.
[http://dx.doi.org/10.1056/NEJMoa1503093] [PMID: 25891173]

[154]   Sunshine J, Taube JM. PD-1/PD-L1 inhibitors. Curr Opin Pharmacol 2015; 23: 32-8.
[http://dx.doi.org/10.1016/j.coph.2015.05.011] [PMID: 26047524]

[155]   Herbst RS, Soria J-C, Kowanetz M, *et al.* Predictive correlates of response to the anti-PD-L1 antibody
MPDL3280A in cancer patients. Nature 2014; 515(7528): 563-7.
[http://dx.doi.org/10.1038/nature14011] [PMID: 25428504]

[156]   Prieto PA, Yang JC, Sherry RM, *et al.* CTLA-4 blockade with ipilimumab: long-term follow-up of 177
patients with metastatic melanoma. Clin Cancer Res 2012; 18(7): 2039-47.
[http://dx.doi.org/10.1158/1078-0432.CCR-11-1823] [PMID: 22271879]

[157]   Hodi FS, Lee S, McDermott DF, *et al.* Ipilimumab plus sargramostim *vs.* ipilimumab alone for
treatment of metastatic melanoma: a randomized clinical trial. JAMA 2014; 312(17): 1744-53.
[http://dx.doi.org/10.1001/jama.2014.13943] [PMID: 25369488]

[158]   Wolchok JD, Kluger H, Callahan MK, *et al.* Nivolumab plus ipilimumab in advanced melanoma. N
Engl J Med 2013; 369(2): 122-33.
[http://dx.doi.org/10.1056/NEJMoa1302369] [PMID: 23724867]

[159]   Postow MA, Chesney J, Pavlick AC, *et al.* Nivolumab and ipilimumab *versus* ipilimumab in untreated
melanoma. N Engl J Med 2015; 372(21): 2006-17.
[http://dx.doi.org/10.1056/NEJMoa1414428] [PMID: 25891304]

[160]   Larkin J, Chiarion-Sileni V, Gonzalez R, *et al.* Combined Nivolumab and Ipilimumab or Monotherapy in Untreated Melanoma. N Engl J Med 2015; 373(1): 23-34.
[http://dx.doi.org/10.1056/NEJMoa1504030] [PMID: 26027431]

[161]   Curtin JA, Fridlyand J, Kageshita T, *et al.* Distinct sets of genetic alterations in melanoma. N Engl J Med 2005; 353(20): 2135-47.
[http://dx.doi.org/10.1056/NEJMoa050092] [PMID: 16291983]

[162]   Alexandrov LB, Nik-Zainal S, Wedge DC, *et al.* Australian Pancreatic Cancer Genome Initiative; ICGC Breast Cancer Consortium; ICGC MMML-Seq Consortium; ICGC PedBrain. Signatures of mutational processes in human cancer. Nature 2013; 500(7463): 415-21.
[http://dx.doi.org/10.1038/nature12477] [PMID: 23945592]

[163]   Santarpia L, Lippman SM, El-Naggar AK. Targeting the MAPK-RAS-RAF signaling pathway in cancer therapy. Expert Opin Ther Targets 2012; 16(1): 103-19.
[http://dx.doi.org/10.1517/14728222.2011.645805] [PMID: 22239440]

[164]   Sun Y, Liu W-Z, Liu T, Feng X, Yang N, Zhou H-F. Signaling pathway of MAPK/ERK in cell proliferation, differentiation, migration, senescence and apoptosis. J Recept Signal Transduct Res 2015; 35(6): 600-4.
[http://dx.doi.org/10.3109/10799893.2015.1030412] [PMID: 26096166]

[165]   Sharma A, Trivedi NR, Zimmerman MA, Tuveson DA, Smith CD, Robertson GP. Mutant V599EB-Raf regulates growth and vascular development of malignant melanoma tumors. Cancer Res 2005; 65(6): 2412-21.
[http://dx.doi.org/10.1158/0008-5472.CAN-04-2423] [PMID: 15781657]

[166]   Davies H, Bignell GR, Cox C, *et al.* Mutations of the BRAF gene in human cancer. Nature 2002; 417(6892): 949-54.
[http://dx.doi.org/10.1038/nature00766] [PMID: 12068308]

[167]   Mercer KE, Pritchard CA. Raf proteins and cancer: B-Raf is identified as a mutational target. Biochim Biophys Acta 2003; 1653(1): 25-40.
[PMID: 12781369]

[168]   Bollag G, Hirth P, Tsai J, *et al.* Clinical efficacy of a RAF inhibitor needs broad target blockade in BRAF-mutant melanoma. Nature 2010; 467(7315): 596-9.
[http://dx.doi.org/10.1038/nature09454] [PMID: 20823850]

[169]   Flaherty KT, Puzanov I, Kim KB, *et al.* Inhibition of mutated, activated BRAF in metastatic melanoma. N Engl J Med 2010; 363(9): 809-19.
[http://dx.doi.org/10.1056/NEJMoa1002011] [PMID: 20818844]

[170]   Sosman JA, Kim KB, Schuchter L, *et al.* Survival in BRAF V600-mutant advanced melanoma treated with vemurafenib. N Engl J Med 2012; 366(8): 707-14.
[http://dx.doi.org/10.1056/NEJMoa1112302] [PMID: 22356324]

[171]   Su F, Bradley WD, Wang Q, *et al.* Resistance to selective BRAF inhibition can be mediated by modest upstream pathway activation. Cancer Res 2012; 72(4): 969-78.
[http://dx.doi.org/10.1158/0008-5472.CAN-11-1875] [PMID: 22205714]

[172]   Fedorenko IV, Paraiso KH, Smalley KS. Acquired and intrinsic BRAF inhibitor resistance in BRAF

V600E mutant melanoma. Biochem Pharmacol 2011; 82(3): 201-9.
[http://dx.doi.org/10.1016/j.bcp.2011.05.015] [PMID: 21635872]

[173] Solit DB, Rosen N. Resistance to BRAF inhibition in melanomas. N Engl J Med 2011; 364(8): 772-4.
[http://dx.doi.org/10.1056/NEJMcibr1013704] [PMID: 21345109]

[174] Falchook GS, Long GV, Kurzrock R, *et al.* Dabrafenib in patients with melanoma, untreated brain
metastases, and other solid tumours: a phase 1 dose-escalation trial. Lancet 2012; 379(9829): 1893-
901.
[http://dx.doi.org/10.1016/S0140-6736(12)60398-5] [PMID: 22608338]

[175] Ascierto PA, Minor D, Ribas A, *et al.* Phase II trial (BREAK-2) of the BRAF inhibitor dabrafenib
(GSK2118436) in patients with metastatic melanoma. J Clin Oncol 2013; 31(26): 3205-11.
[http://dx.doi.org/10.1200/JCO.2013.49.8691] [PMID: 23918947]

[176] Hauschild A, Grob J-J, Demidov LV, *et al.* Dabrafenib in BRAF-mutated metastatic melanoma: a
multicentre, open-label, phase 3 randomised controlled trial. Lancet 2012; 380(9839): 358-65.
[http://dx.doi.org/10.1016/S0140-6736(12)60868-X] [PMID: 22735384]

[177] Flaherty KT, Robert C, Hersey P, *et al.* METRIC Study Group. Improved survival with MEK
inhibition in BRAF-mutated melanoma. N Engl J Med 2012; 367(2): 107-14.
[http://dx.doi.org/10.1056/NEJMoa1203421] [PMID: 22663011]

[178] Robert C, Dummer R, Gutzmer R, *et al.* Selumetinib plus dacarbazine *versus* placebo plus dacarbazine
as first-line treatment for BRAF-mutant metastatic melanoma: a phase 2 double-blind randomised
study. Lancet Oncol 2013; 14(8): 733-40.
[http://dx.doi.org/10.1016/S1470-2045(13)70237-7] [PMID: 23735514]

[179] Ascierto PA, Schadendorf D, Berking C, *et al.* MEK162 for patients with advanced melanoma
harbouring NRAS or Val600 BRAF mutations: a non-randomised, open-label phase 2 study. Lancet
Oncol 2013; 14(3): 249-56.
[http://dx.doi.org/10.1016/S1470-2045(13)70024-X] [PMID: 23414587]

[180] Roberts R, Govender D. Gene of the month: KIT. J Clin Pathol 2015; 68(9): 671-4.
[http://dx.doi.org/10.1136/jclinpath-2015-203207] [PMID: 26135312]

[181] Curtin JA, Busam K, Pinkel D, Bastian BC. Somatic activation of KIT in distinct subtypes of
melanoma. J Clin Oncol 2006; 24(26): 4340-6.
[http://dx.doi.org/10.1200/JCO.2006.06.2984] [PMID: 16908931]

[182] Larkin J, Ascierto PA, Dréno B, *et al.* Combined vemurafenib and cobimetinib in BRAF-mutated
melanoma. N Engl J Med 2014; 371(20): 1867-76.
[http://dx.doi.org/10.1056/NEJMoa1408868] [PMID: 25265494]

[183] Flaherty KT, Infante JR, Daud A, *et al.* Combined BRAF and MEK inhibition in melanoma with
BRAF V600 mutations. N Engl J Med 2012; 367(18): 1694-703.
[http://dx.doi.org/10.1056/NEJMoa1210093] [PMID: 23020132]

[184] Long GV, Stroyakovskiy D, Gogas H, *et al.* Combined BRAF and MEK inhibition *versus* BRAF
inhibition alone in melanoma. N Engl J Med 2014; 371(20): 1877-88.
[http://dx.doi.org/10.1056/NEJMoa1406037] [PMID: 25265492]

[185] Long GV, Stroyakovskiy D, Gogas H, *et al.* Dabrafenib and trametinib *versus* dabrafenib and placebo

for Val600 BRAF-mutant melanoma: a multicentre, double-blind, phase 3 randomised controlled trial. Lancet 2015; 386(9992): 444-51.
[http://dx.doi.org/10.1016/S0140-6736(15)60898-4] [PMID: 26037941]

[186]   Robert C, Karaszewska B, Schachter J, *et al.* Improved overall survival in melanoma with combined dabrafenib and trametinib. N Engl J Med 2015; 372(1): 30-9.
[http://dx.doi.org/10.1056/NEJMoa1412690] [PMID: 25399551]

[187]   Ribas A, Hodi FS, Callahan M, Konto C, Wolchok J. Hepatotoxicity with combination of vemurafenib and ipilimumab. N Engl J Med 2013; 368(14): 1365-6.
[http://dx.doi.org/10.1056/NEJMc1302338] [PMID: 23550685]

[188]   Sosman JA, Kittaneh M, Lolkema MP, Postow MA, Schwartz G, Franklin C, *et al.* A phase 1b/2 study of LEE011 in combination with binimetinib (MEK162) in patients with NRAS-mutant melanoma: Early encouraging clinical activity. ASCO Meeting Abstracts. 32 (15 Suppl): 2009. Available at: http://meetinglibrary.asco.org/content/130034-144

Frontiers in Clinical Drug Research - Anti-Cancer Agents, 2016, *Vol. 3*, 271-324

CHAPTER 4

Targeting the Warburg Effect for Cancer Therapy: A Long and Winding Road

Patrícia L. Abreu*, **Ana M. Urbano***,#

Unidade de Química-Física Molecular and Departamento de Ciências da Vida, Faculdade de Ciências e Tecnologia, Universidade de Coimbra, Coimbra, Portugal

Abstract: In the 1920s, Otto Warburg, one of the leading biochemists of the 20th century, uncovered a striking phenotype of cancer cells: their increased dependence on lactic acid fermentation for energy production compared to that of the normal cells from which they derived. Warburg viewed this metabolic particularity of cancer cells, which came to be known as the Warburg effect, as a driving force in carcinogenesis. This perception suggested a novel path for cancer therapy, a strategy that Warburg himself proposed and defended with passion to his death. However, for many decades, both his metabolic theory of cancer and suggested therapeutic approach were essentially ignored by cancer researchers, who were mostly focused on the genetic basis of the disease and on the intricacies of the pathways known to promote cellular proliferation, differentiation and death. Still, thanks to the combined efforts of those who chose to pursue Warburg's line of research, experimental evidence supporting and extending Warburg's findings on the metabolism of cancer cells accumulated. In the 1980s, ^{18}F-deoxyglucose positron emission tomography (^{18}FDG–PET) was implemented in the clinic. This metabolic imaging technique, which is based on the avidity of cancer cells for glucose, represents, to this day, the only successful exploitation of the Warburg effect for medical purposes. The wide success of ^{18}FDG–PET in the diagnosis and staging of tumors is among the factors most responsible for renewing interest in the central carbon metabolism of cancer cells. This renewed interest was further boosted by the discovery of multiple links between central carbon metabolism and cellular proliferation, differentiation and death and culminated

* **Corresponding authors Ana M. Urbano and Patrícia L. Abreu:** Department of Life Sciences and Molecular Physical Chemistry Research Unit, University of Coimbra, Coimbra, Portugal; Tel/Fax: +351-239-826541; E-mails: amurbano@ci.uc.pt & patricia.lonaabreu@gmail.com
# Centro de Investigação em Meio Ambiente, Genética e Oncobiologia (CIMAGO), Faculdade de Medicina, Universidade de Coimbra, Coimbra, Portugal.

Atta-ur-Rahman (Ed.)

in the recent classification, by Weinberg and Hanahan, of tumor metabolism as an emerging cancer hallmark. Tremendous research effort is now being devoted into a more detailed and comprehensive elucidation of the metabolic rewiring that accompanies neoplastic transformation and, unsurprisingly, targeting the metabolic peculiarities of tumors has become a hot topic in drug discovery. This chapter summarizes past and current efforts at targeting the Warburg effect for selective cancer therapies.

Keywords: Aerobic glycolysis, Central carbon metabolism, Clinical trials, Diabetes, Emerging cancer hallmark, ^{18}F-Deoxyglucose positron emission tomography (^{18}FDG–PET), Hypoxia, Ketogenic diet, Metabolic cancer therapies, Metformin, Pasteur effect, Targeted cancer therapies, Warburg effect.

1.   THERAPEUTICAL   APPROACHES   TO   CANCER: FROM CHEMOTHERAPY TO TARGETED THERAPIES

The oldest written description of cancer known to exist can be found in the Edwin Smith Papyrus, which is based on what was known in surgery and medicine up to 3000 BC [1, 2]. But humans must have, in all likelihood, been fighting against cancer throughout their existence. Although this papyrus describes the treatment of tumors with cauterization, it also acknowledges the absence of a cure for the disease. By 400 BC, Hippocrates, the "Father of Medicine", advised against the treatment of deep-seated tumors, as this would shorten the lives of patients [2]. Fortunately, this perception of cancer as an incurable disease did not prevent significant advances in cancer therapy, mostly during the last century. Some milestones in cancer therapy will be briefly discussed in this section.

The first successful inductions of tumor regression *via* systemic administration of chemical substances can be traced back to the 1940s. At that time, our understanding of human cancer biology was very limited and the discovery of the anticancer activity of the first cancer drugs stemmed from chance observations. Namely, from the post-mortem observation of severe myelosuppression and lymphoid hypoplasia in First World War soldiers dying of mustard gas exposure, which suggested the use of nitrogen mustards for the treatment of lymphomas [3, 4], and the observation of increased proliferation of acute lymphoblastic leukemia (ALL) cells upon administration of folic acid to children with ALL [5], which suggested the use of two folate analogues (aminopterin and amethopterin (methotrexate; brand names Abitrexate™ and Brimexate™)[1]) to treat this neoplasy [6]. Although brief, due to development of tumor resistance to the drugs, these remissions stimulated further research on cancer therapy [7].

By this time, attempts were also being made at the rational design of compounds capable of interrupting cell proliferation. These early attempts led to the development of several purine analogs, designed to interfere with the natural production of DNA. The two most promising analogs, 6-mercaptopurine (Purinethol™, Alti-Mercaptopurine™) and thioguanine (Tabloid™, Lanvis™), were introduced in the clinic in the 1950s, establishing a novel class of cancer drugs [8, 9]. Notwithstanding these attempts at rational drug design, serendipity continued to play a role in the discovery of novel classes of cancer drugs. That was the case with vinca alkaloids, whose anticancer potential emerged in a screen for antidiabetic activity [10]. Other discoveries were the result of systematic screenings, most notably that conducted on thousands of natural products by the National Cancer Institute, which led to the discovery of the anticancer activity of taxanes and camptothecins [11].

Once the mechanisms of action of these cancer drugs became known, new compounds with similar actions, but with refined structures, could be synthesized. It was hoped that these novel structures would improve their pharmacological properties, namely in terms of stability and efficacy. However, gains achieved using this approach were rather modest [7]. Those achieved through further systematic screenings were, likewise, modest, as most of the new cancer drugs thus discovered belonged to the classes already in clinical use [12].

It is worth noting that, in spite of exhibiting distinct mechanisms of action, all cancer drug classes used in the clinic up to the mid 1970s acted by directly interfering with cellular proliferation: nitrogen mustards are non-specific DNA alkylating agents [13]; the antimetabolite methotrexate inhibits the enzyme dihydrofolate reductase (DHFR), thereby compromising the synthesis of thymidine and purines and, ultimately, DNA synthesis [14]; vinca alkaloids and taxanes are both antimitotic agents [15]; camptothecin is an inhibitor of topoisomerase I [16], an enzyme essential for DNA unwinding during replication and transcription [17]. As such, rather than acting specifically against cancer cells, these traditional cytotoxics act against all actively dividing cells, often producing severe side effects. It soon became apparent that significant improvements in drug efficacy and safety could only be achieved through novel drugs targeting molecules specifically associated with cancer [18]. Research carried out over the last few decades allowed a clear definition of some of the unique properties and requirements of malignant cells, now commonly described as cancer hallmarks [19, 20], unraveling several potential targets for cancer therapy. Advances in genomic screening were particularly invaluable in the identification of genes that are frequently altered in tumors. Unsurprisingly, it was found that many of them are associated with growth signaling pathways. Amongst the identified "druggable" targets are growth factors, signaling molecules, cell-cycle proteins, apoptosis modulators and angiogenesis promoting molecules [21]. Nowadays, targeting is achieved both pharmacologically, with antibodies and small molecule inhibitors, and through genetic inhibition, using RNA interference (RNAi)-mediated depletion and microRNAs [22, 23].

Hormone therapy was one of the first examples of targeted cancer therapies. The beneficial effects of removing the ovaries in women with breast cancer had been known since the 19th century [12]. By the middle of the 20th century, it was found that the removal of their adrenal glands and hypophysis had similar effects [24, 25]. Once it became apparent that this therapeutic effect was related to the stimulatory effect that estrogens have on the growth of tumors derived from tissues associated with the reproductive system, namely breast tissue, efforts began at the development of drugs that prevent the production of those hormones or their use by cancer cells. Tamoxifen (Nolvadex™, Apo-Tamox™), an estrogen receptor modulator, is the most successful drug in this category. It has been in the clinic since 1977, when the Food and Drug Administration (FDA) approved its use for the treatment of metastatic breast cancer [26]. Tamoxifen also targets other specialized tissues, such as breast epithelium, thereby inhibiting their proliferation, but this inhibition does not compromise the survival of the organism.

Meanwhile, the discovery that interferon, a pleiotropic cytokine primarily produced by lymphoid-type cells, could activate immune cells and improve their ability to attack cancer cells prompted investigations into its potential in cancer therapy. Its approval by the FDA, in 1995, established immunotherapy as a new targeted approach in cancer therapy. Interferon (Alferon N™, Intron A™) is still the most used cytokine in immunotherapy [27].

A more specific cancer immunotherapy approach uses monoclonal antibodies against selected tumor antigens known to play an active role in the development or progression of human cancers [28]. Rituximab (Rituxan™, Mabthera™) was the first antibody to receive FDA approval (for the treatment of follicular lymphomas). This antibody, introduced in the clinic in 1997, targets the protein CD20, present in the surface of B cells, whose numbers are frequently increased in hematological malignancies [29]. However, the truly first great success in this new era of targeted therapies was trastuzumab (Herceptin™), a monoclonal antibody against the extracellular domain of the HER2 receptor, a tyrosine kinase receptor frequently overexpressed in breast cancers [30]. The HER proteins stimulate cell proliferation and their overexpression in cancer cells promotes their uncontrolled proliferation [31]. Trastuzumab binds a non-essential protein with restricted expression in adult tissues, which contributed to its success in the clinic [21].

Since trastuzumab's FDA approval in 1998, ten other antibodies have been approved for cancer treatment: gemtuzumab ozogamicin (Mylotarg™) (2000), alemtuzumab (Campath™) (2001), ibritumomab tiuxetan (Zevalin™) (2002), tositumomab (Bexxar™) (2003), cetuximab (Erbitux™) (2004), bevacizumab (Avastin™) (2004), panitumumab (Vectibix™) (2006), ofatumumab (Arzerra™, HuMax-CD20™) (2009), ipilimumab (Yervoy™) (2011) and brentuximab vedotin (Adcetris™) (2011) [32, 33].

Meanwhile, great efforts have been made towards the development of active specific immunotherapies, commonly known as "cancer vaccines". In 2010, the FDA approved the first of these vaccines, Sipuleucel-T (Provenge™), which is used for the treatment of advanced prostate cancer [34].

The message that emerges from clinical outcomes is that ideal cancer drug targets must have a function that is essential in cancer cells, but not in normal cells, so that the intentional inhibition of this specific function does not result in toxicity to normal cells. In other words, these ideal targets are both essential and unique to the cancer cells.

The Abelson kinase is a paradigm of an ideal target, and the success obtained with its inhibitor, imatinib (Gleevec™, Glivec™), in the treatment of certain cancers amply justifies continued efforts towards the identification of other ideal targets. The Abelson kinase is an abnormal tyrosine kinase and is encoded by a fusion gene, resulting from the juxtaposing of the v-abl Abelson murine leukemia viral oncogene homolog (ABL) to a part of the breakpoint cluster region (BCR) [35, 36]. These two genes are located in chromosomes 9 and 22, respectively, and the fusion gene results from a reciprocal translocation between the long arms of the two chromosomes. The chromosome containing the fusion gene, known as the Philadelphia chromosome [37], is consistently found in chronic myelogenous leukemia (CML) cells, but not in the normal cells of the same patients. It is the absolute and unique dependence of CML cells on the Abelson kinase that explains the selectivity of imatinib, which, in 2001, received FDA approval for the treatment of patients with advanced, Philadelphia chromosome positive CML. In the earlier chronic phase of the disease, the success rate of imatinib is impressive, with over ninety percent of CML patients achieving complete hematological remission [38]. It is worth noting that almost three decades elapsed between the discovery of the fusion gene by John Groffen in 1984 [35] and the introduction of imatinib in the clinic, clearly showing how lengthy the development of new therapies can be.

Theories to explain neoplasia, as well as all other pathologies, have always been much influenced by the existing knowledge and technology. For instance, the Philadelphia chromosome could not have been identified before major advances in the cytogenetic techniques of banding, particularly Giemsa banding, took place. In fact, cancer could not even have been perceived as a cellular disease before the discovery of the cell. Neither could it have been perceived as a disease of the genes before the discovery of the chromosomes. By the time of the development of the chromosomal theory of inheritance and the proposal, by Boveri, that certain chromosome combinations lead to abnormal development [39], major discoveries were also taking place in other areas of the biosciences.

The beginning of the 20th century was the golden age of central carbon metabolism, with a large number of scientists focusing their research efforts on a detailed elucidation of its major pathways. Prominent among them was Otto Warburg, a German scientist who, in 1931, was awarded the Nobel Prize in Physiology or Medicine for his discoveries on the nature and mode of action of the respiratory enzyme (cytochrome c oxidase, in current nomenclature). As described in more detail in section 3, his seminal studies, conducted in the early 1920s, unveiled the first cancer-specific metabolic phenotype, *i.e.*, a significantly increased reliance of well-aerated cancer cells on lactic acid fermentation ("aerobic glycolysis") for the generation of metabolic energy. This phenotype, which was later dubbed the Warburg effect, was largely ignored for many decades, but there is now a growing interest in exploring the possibilities that this and other, meanwhile discovered, metabolic traits of cancer cells might open in terms of targeted cancer therapies. Section 4 summarizes past and current efforts at targeting the Warburg effect for targeted cancer therapies.

2. BIOENERGETICS: A VERY BRIEF OVERVIEW

All living cells depend on a constant supply of metabolic energy to survive, grow and proliferate. Humans, just like all other heterotrophs, obtain this energy from the oxidation of organic fuel molecules present in the diet. These molecules are characterized by a high free energy content, which is used to generate other forms of energy that can be readily used by the cells, most notably adenosine triphosphate (ATP). There are basically two types of cellular processes for the generation of ATP, both composed of a long series of reactions: fermentations, in which the electrons extracted from the fuel molecules are ultimately transferred to an endogenous electron acceptor, and cellular respirations, which are characterized by exogenous terminal electron acceptors, namely molecular oxygen (in the case of aerobic respiration). With endogenous acceptors, the oxidation of fuel molecules is inevitably partial, whereas exogenous acceptors allow their complete oxidation. As a consequence, the energy yield of fermentations is much lower than that of respirations (starting from the same fuel molecule).

For most human cells, glucose is the substrate of choice for energy generation (as well as for the generation of reducing power and as a precursor for biosynthesis). To this end, glucose is either partially oxidized *via* lactic acid fermentation or fully oxidized *via* aerobic respiration (Fig. **1**). Both processes are initiated in the cytosol and share the first ten reactions, known globally as glycolysis. In lactic acid fermentation, pyruvate, the final product of glycolysis, acts as the terminal electron acceptor and is directly converted to lactate. Aerobic respiration is much more complex and intricate. In addition to glycolysis, it includes three other processes: the oxidative decarboxylation of pyruvate to acetyl coenzyme A (acetyl CoA),   the tricarboxylic   acid   (TCA)   cycle and   oxidative phosphorylation (OXPHOS), all occurring, in the case of eukaryotic cells, in the mitochondria.

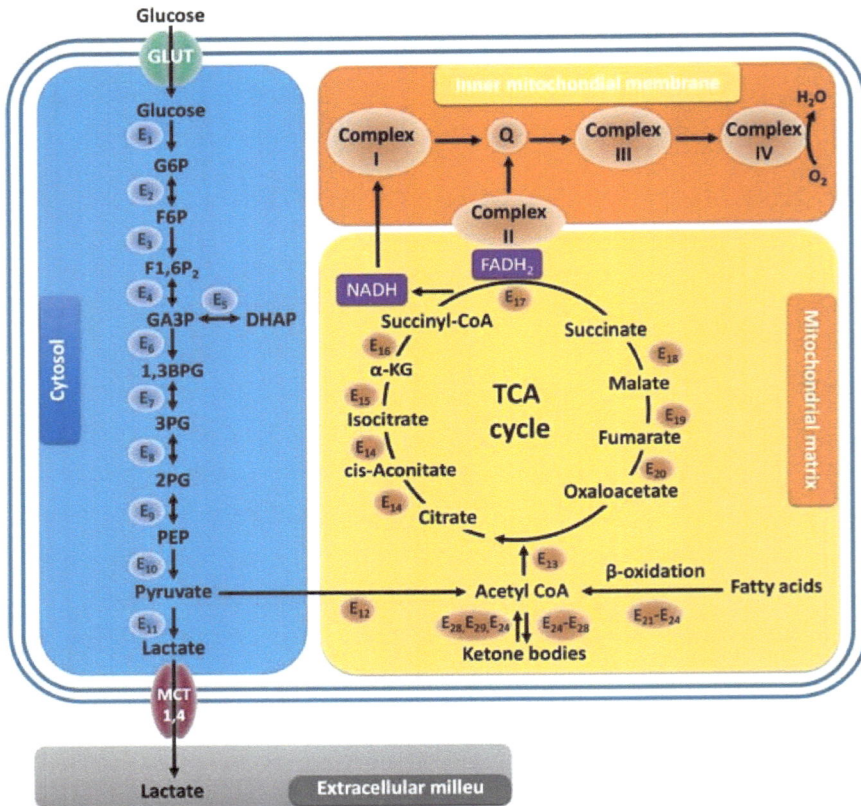

Fig. (1). Overview of the metabolic processes used by human cells to generate ATP through the oxidation of glucose, fatty acids or ketone bodies. Glucose is the substrate of choice for most human cells, whereas certain cell types, such as heart and liver cells, rely mostly on fatty acids. When glucose is scarce, the brain can adapt to use ketone bodies as a source of energy. In the presence of oxygen, these fuel molecules can be completely oxidized to CO_2 and H_2O, generating large amounts of ATP (essentially during OXPHOS, which is depicted in the orange box; the actual ATP generation is not depicted). The initial oxidation steps are fuel specific, but they all generate acetyl CoA, which then enters the TCA cycle to be fully oxidized. The initial oxidation of glucose takes place in the cytosol. It produces pyruvate through a series of 10 steps collectively known as glycolysis. Two molecules of ATP are generated per molecule of glucose (not depicted in the figure). The fate of pyruvate varies according to oxygen availability (and also cell type; see main manuscript for more details). In the absence of oxygen, pyruvate is converted to lactate. The overall metabolic process, *i.e.*, from glucose to lactate, is called lactic acid fermentation. In the presence of an adequate oxygen supply, pyruvate is first converted to acetyl CoA and then enters the TCA cycle. The conversion of pyruvate to acetyl CoA is catalized by the enzyme PDH, which is generally perceived as the gate-keeper of the TCA cycle. In the case of fatty acids, their initial oxidation takes place in the mitochondrial matrix through a recurring sequence of four steps known as β-oxidation. This process generates acetyl CoA which normally enters the TCA cycle. Under certain metabolic conditions, namely glucose scarcity, acetyl CoA is also used by the liver to produce ketone bodies. Ketone bodies are then transported in the blood to several extra-hepatic tissues, most notably brain tissue, which convert them back to acetyl CoA to use as an energy source. The catabolism of fatty acids and ketone bodies is strictly aerobic. The reduced coenzymes (NADH and $FADH_2$) produced during the oxidation of fuel molecules transfer their electrons to the mitochondrial electron transport chain (depicted in the orange box) and the energy released during the flow of electrons from these coenzymes to oxygen is used to produce large amounts of ATP through OXPHOS. Acetyl CoA, acetyl coenzyme A; α-KG, alpha-ketoglutarate; 1,3BPG, 1,3-bisphosphoglycerate; DHAP, dihydroxyacetone phosphate; $F1,6P_2$, fructose 1,6-bisphosphate; F6P, fructose 6-phosphate; GAP3P, glyceraldehyde 3-phosphate; G6P, glucose 6-phosphate; GLUT, glucose transporter; MCT, monocarboxylate transporter; OXPHOS, oxidative phosphorylation; PDH, pyruvate dehydrogenase; PEP, phosphoenolpyruvate; 2-PG, 2-phosphoglycerate; 3PG, 3-phosphoglycerate; Succinyl CoA, succinyl coenzyme A; TCA, tricarboxylic acid; Q, ubiquinone, E_1, hexokinase; E_2, phosphoglucose isomerase; E_3, 6-phosphofructo-1-kinase; E_4, aldolase; E_5, triose phosphate isomerase; E_6, glyceraldehyde 3-phosphate dehydrogenase; E_7, phosphoglycerate kinase; E_8, phosphoglucomutase; E_9, enolase; E_{10}, pyruvate kinase; E_{11}, lactate dehydrogenase; E_{12}, pyruvate dehydrogenase; E_{13}, citrate synthase; E_{14}, aconitase; E_{15}, isocitrate dehydrogenase; E_{16}, α-ketoglutarate dehydrogenase; E_{17}, succinyl-CoA synthase; E_{18}, succinate dehydrogenase; E_{19}, fumarase; E_{20}, malate dehydrogenase; E_{21}, acyl-CoA dehydrogenase; E_{22}, enoyl-CoA hydratase, E_{23}, β-hydroxyacyl-CoA dehydrogenase; E_{24}, acyl-CoA acetyltransferase (thiolase); E_{25}, β-hydroxy-β-methylglutaryl-CoA (HMG-CoA) synthase; E_{26}, HMG-CoA lyase; E_{27}, acetoacetate decarboxylase; E_{28}, D-β-hydroxybutyrate dehydrogenase; E_{29}, β-ketoacyl-CoA transferase.

The TCA cycle completes the oxidation of acetyl CoA, generating carbon dioxide (CO_2). All electrons extracted from the fuel molecules during the overall process are ultimately accepted by molecular oxygen (O_2), which is reduced to water. This electron flux involves a chain of electron transporters, known collectively as the mitochondrial electron transport chain (ETC), located in the inner mitochondrial membrane. Three of the protein complexes of the ETC couple the electron flux to the transfer of protons across the inner mitochondrial membrane, generating an electrochemical gradient that is ultimately used by the mitochondrial ATP synthase to synthesize ATP from adenosine diphosphate (ADP) and inorganic phosphate (P_i).

Contrary to CO_2, lactate is still a relatively energy-rich molecule, which explains the very low yield of lactic acid fermentation (2 ATP molecules per molecule of glucose) compared to that of aerobic respiration (30 ATP molecules per molecule of glucose). Not surprisingly, aerobic respiration is the process of choice for energy production for most human cells, as well as for those of other aerobic organisms. In fact, already in the 1860s, Louis Pasteur observed the abolishment of fermentation by oxygen in yeast cells [40], a phenomenon that later became known as the Pasteur effect. Nonetheless, it must be stressed that, despite their much lower energy yields, fermentations can be advantageous in certain circumstances. For instance, during strenuous exercise, muscle cells rely strongly on lactic acid fermentation, an extremely rapid process, because the inflow of oxygen to these cells is insufficient to generate enough ATP solely *via* respiration. However, this shift to lactic acid fermentation can only take place during brief periods of time, as muscle cells would not cope with the acidification of the milieu resulting from an excessive accumulation of lactate. In fact, the acidification produced by this accumulation could, ultimately, result in necrosis or p53- and caspase-3-dependent apoptosis [41, 42]. In the case of human mature red blood cells, the reliance on lactic acid fermentation for ATP generation is absolute.

The molecular basis of the Pasteur effect has not been completely elucidated. For a long time, it was essentially perceived as resulting from the feedback inhibition of the glycolytic enzyme 6-phosphofructo-1-kinase (PFK-1) by citrate and ATP [43]. This enzyme, which catalyzes the phosphorylation of fructose 6-phosphate by ATP, is controlled by a large number of intracellular metabolites and proteins and mediates the actions of various drugs [44]. This extensive regulation of its activity contributed to the still generalized, but controversial [45], perception of this enzyme as the pacemaker of glycolysis and, ultimately, of both lactic acid fermentation and aerobic respiration.

In fact, two other metabolic enzymes, lactate dehydrogenase (LDH) and pyruvate dehydrogenase (PDH) or, more precisely, the pyruvate dehydrogenase complex, are probably more suited to promote the Pasteur effect, as each is unique to only one of the energy-generating processes. LDH catalyzes the last step of lactic acid fermentation, whereas PDH catalyzes the conversion of pyruvate to acetyl CoA. By establishing a link between glycolysis and the TCA cycle, PDH controls the flux of acetyl CoA to this cycle. Importantly, it has been shown that pyruvate dehydrogenase kinase 1 (PDK1) [46], an enzyme that phosphorylates PDH, leading to its inactivation [47], is a direct target of the hypoxia-inducible transcription factor 1 (HIF-1). This transcription factor is stabilized by hypoxia and is inactivated in the presence of an adequate oxygen supply. Thus, the presence of oxygen favors the mitochondrial oxidation of pyruvate, whereas hypoxia results in the inactivation of PDH, shifting the energy metabolism to lactic acid fermentation.

Another aspect worth mentioning is that some types of human cells not only can, but actually prefer to use alternative fuels for energy generation, namely fatty acids. For instance, fatty acids provide up to 80% of the energetic needs of heart and liver cells. In the presence of oxygen, fatty acids can be completely oxidized to CO_2 and H_2O, just like glucose and all other organic fuel molecules. In eukaryotic cells, the complete oxidation of fatty acids occurs entirely in the mitochondrial matrix. These molecules are initially oxidized to acetyl CoA through a recurring sequence of four steps named β-oxidation (Fig. 1). As is the case for the aerobic oxidation of glucose, the TCA cycle concludes the oxidation of acetyl CoA and (most) ATP molecules are synthesized *via* OXPHOS. Since fatty acids are initially in a much more reduced state than glucose, the final ATP yield per gram of fuel molecule is, correspondingly, much higher.

The TCA cycle is not the only fate of the acetyl CoA molecules obtained from the initial oxidation of fatty acids. Under some conditions, namely glucose scarcity, the liver uses the TCA cycle intermediate oxaloacetate to produce glucose by the gluconeogenic pathway. This reaction depletes the pool of oxaloacetate available for condensation with acetyl CoA (the first step of the TCA cycle), slowing down the flux through this cycle. Under these conditions, acetyl CoA is used to produce the ketone bodies acetoacetate, D-β-hydroxybutyrate and acetone. Acetone is produced in minimal quantities and is generally exhaled, but acetoacetate and D-β -hydroxybutyrate are transported in the blood to several extra-hepatic tissues that can use them as energy sources. Heart muscle and the renal cortex actually prefer to use acetoacetate over glucose. Even brain cells can adapt their metabolism to use ketone bodies under starvation conditions.

As can be appreciated, most human cells have a certain metabolic plasticity, making it possible to modulate metabolism only by adjusting the dietary composition. This perception is the rationale behind several types of diets, as further discussed in section 4.

3. THE WARBURG EFFECT: CURRENT PERSPECTIVE

In the 1920s, Warburg uncovered a striking phenotype of cancer cells: contrary to the tissues from which they derived, well-aerated cancer cells exhibited high rates of lactic acid fermentation, or high rates of aerobic glycolysis, as this phenomenon was then named [48]. Thus, cancer cells failed to efficiently suppress fermentation in the presence of oxygen.

Contrary to many important biomedical findings, the discovery of what came to be known as the Warburg effect [49] was not due to chance. One of Warburg's major early ambitions, even before graduating, was to find a cure for cancer [50]. His comprehensive research into the energetics of growth, conducted in the early 1900s, had shown that the respiration of the sea urchin egg was raised after fertilization, presumably to sustain the active cell growth and division that was taking place in the developing embryo. As cancer cells are characterized by uncontrolled growth, Warburg reasoned that they should, likewise, exhibit respiratory rates higher than those of the normal tissues from which they derived. Therefore, he set out to determine the respiration rates of the Flexner-Jobling rat carcinoma, a transplantable cancer. To his surprise, the oxygen consumption rate of tumor tissue was identical to those of normal tissues. Equally unexpected was the finding that, despite the presence of oxygen, cancer cells exhibited important fermentation rates [48, 51]. These findings were soon confirmed by Warburg and others [48, 52 - 54], not only for other types of experimental cancers, but also for human cancers.

Considering that the energy yield of fermentation is significantly lower than that of respiration (see preceding section), the increased reliance of cancer cells on fermentation seemed paradoxical. Based on his extensive knowledge of energy metabolism, Warburg postulated that it could only be explained by permanent respiratory defects, firmly stating that there was no other way to upregulate fermentation in the presence of oxygen. Furthermore, having observed that the fermentation to respiration ratio increased as the cells became more malignant, Warburg also proposed that malignant progression was associated with cumulative respiratory defects. Warburg speculated that, to compensate for the lower energy yield of fermentation, cells needed to consume more glucose, which demanded an increased glucose uptake. This increase was soon confirmed, albeit indirectly, by Warburg and some of his contemporaries [48, 52 - 54].

Although Warburg had, by this time, already established himself as an outstanding scientist, his proposal that a metabolic shift played a fundamental role in carcinogenesis was received with skepticism. In fact, it was difficult to understand, in the light of contemporary knowledge, how alterations in central carbon metabolism could be linked to uncontrolled cell proliferation. For this, but also for several other reasons, some of which out of the scope of this chapter, the central carbon metabolism of cancer cells remained, for almost a century, a highly controversial field of research.

In 1955, the discovery of intratumoral hypoxia [55] provided a plausible and much more consensual explanation for the upregulation of lactic acid fermentation, although not for the upregulation of "aerobic glycolysis". To support their growth, tumors recruit blood vessels to their microenvironment. However, the development of the neovasculature is slower than that of the tumor. Moreover, this neovasculature is disorganized and does not deliver blood efficiently [56]. As the absence of an adequate oxygen supply compromises respiration, cancer cells in a hypoxic microenvironment become strongly dependent on lactic acid fermentation for ATP production. Thus, rather than being a driver of carcinogenesis, the increased fermentation rates of tumors appeared to most cancer researchers as an adaptive change to tumor hypoxia, *i.e.*, as a mere epiphenomenon of an already ongoing carcinogenic process. Another important consequence of the inefficacy of the newly formed network of blood vessels is the accumulation of large amounts of lactate produced by fermentation [57], leading to tumor acidification.

Warburg addressed the question of hypoxia in a much cited paper, published in Science in 1956 [58]. In this paper, Warburg showed that cultures of ascite cancer cells, which live free in suspension, thus in a well-aerated environment, exhibited high rates of "aerobic glycolysis", deriving up to 50% of their energy from lactic acid fermentation [58]. Thus, at least for these cancer cells, the Warburg effect could not be due to hypoxia.

In the 1980s, a novel imaging technique, ^{18}F-deoxyglucose positron emission tomography ([18]FDG–PET), was implemented in the clinic. This metabolic technique, which soon found a wide success in the diagnosis and staging of a wide variety of tumors, confirmed the avidity of cancer cells for glucose. Moreover, it confirmed Warburg's allegation that glucose uptake correlates with tumor aggressiveness and a poor prognosis [59].

Although [18]FDG–PET made a strong contribution to the rediscovery of the Warburg effect, the fundamental question of whether this effect is a driver of carcinogenesis or a mere epiphenomenon remained unresolved. In 1992, the identification of the transcription factor HIF-1 [60] tipped the scale in favor of the latter hypothesis. This transcription factor is stabilized by hypoxia (section 2) and, among other actions, promotes lactic acid fermentation by triggering a complex transcriptional program that results in the increased expression of all glycolytic enzymes (hexokinase (HK), phosphoglucose isomerase, PFK-1, aldolase, triose phosphate isomerase, glyceraldehyde-3-phosphate dehydrogenase (GAPDH), phosphoglycerate kinase, phosphoglucomutase, enolase, pyruvate kinase (PK)), LDH, two glucose transporters (glucose transporter 1 (GLUT1) and glucose transporter 3 (GLUT3)), and inhibitors of mitochondrial metabolism, such as PDK1 (section 2) [61].

As mentioned in the beginning of this section, prejudice against Warburg's ideas stemmed, to a significant extent, from unawareness of any links between central carbon metabolism and cell proliferation, cell death and tissue homeostasis. In fact, central carbon metabolism had mostly been viewed as a homeostatic, self-regulating network of reactions essentially disconnected from signaling pathways [62]. However, by the end of the 1990s, several findings began to seriously challenge this perception. One of them was the demonstration that cytochrome c, a mobile electron carrier of the mitochondrial respiratory chain, participates actively in apoptosis [63]. Another was the discovery that a metabolic gene, *LDHA*, which encodes LDHA, was transactivated by the transcription factor Myc [64]. Both findings represented major breakthroughs, as, up to then, cytochrome c and Myc had strictly been associated with, respectively, cellular respiration and cell cycle regulation and apoptosis [65]. Later, it was shown that Myc also activates glycolytic and glutaminolytic genes and stimulates mitochondrial biogenesis [66], playing a critical role in the regulation of central carbon metabolism.

The discovery of these unsuspected links between signal transduction and central carbon metabolism led to a reappraisal of Warburg's findings and ideas and to a resurgence of interest in this branch of biochemistry that had had its golden age in the first half of the 20th century, but had since been mostly neglected. Evidence further reinforcing the idea of an intimate link between central carbon metabolism and cell signaling pathways accumulated rapidly. Namely, it soon became known that the expression of genes related to central carbon metabolism is not only regulated by Myc, but also by other oncogenes and oncosuppressor proteins (*e.g.*, p53, HIF and NF-κB). Of note, it was also shown that these transcription factors play an important role in the metabolic rewiring that takes place during carcinogenesis [67]. For instance, the inactivation of the tumor suppressor p53, as observed in over 50% of all cancers [68], abrogates the repression that this transcription factor exerts on the transcription of GLUT1 and GLUT4 [69]. This might constitute a growth advantage in a situation of limited glucose availability, as frequently encountered in the tumor microenvironment [52 - 54]. An analogous effect can be achieved through oncogenic mutations in RAS and BRAF, as these are also associated with increased GLUT1 levels [70, 71].

In the last decade, the discovery that some forms of cancer exhibit recurrent loss-of-function mutations in two genes coding for TCA cycle enzymes, fumarate hydratase (FH; mutated in familial leimyomatosis and kidney cancer) and succinate dehydrogenase (SDH; mutated in pheochromocytomas and paragangliomas) (Fig. **1**) [72] suggested yet another biochemical mechanism for the shift of cancer cells to "aerobic glycolysis". Importantly, these two enzymes behave as classic tumor suppressors, thus contradicting the still common perception that all oncogenes and tumor suppressor genes are involved in signaling pathways specifically involved in cell proliferation, cell death and tissue homeostasis. It has been proposed that the increased levels of succinate and fumarate that result from the oncogenic disruption of the enzymatic activity of SDH and FH could drive oncogenesis [72], but the exact molecular basis of this process is still controversial.

More recently, two other metabolic genes, those encoding isoforms 1 and 2 of isocitrate dehydrogenase (IDH1 and IDH2), were found to be recurrently mutated in patients with glioma, glioblastoma and acute myeloid leukemia. Mutations were also found in a significant number of intrahepatic cholangiocarcinomas and cartilaginous tumors [73 - 76]. Contrary to what was observed for FH and FDH, IDH1 and IDH2 mutations do not result in loss of function, but rather in a neomorphic activity, specifically the conversion of α-ketoglutarate (α-KG) to 2-hydroxyglutarate (2-HG) [77, 78]. It is of note that, although all three isoforms of IDH catalyze the same reaction, *i.e.*, the conversion of isocitrate to 2-HG, IDH1 and IDH2 are not, strictly speaking, TCA cycle enzymes. In fact, IDH1 is located in the cytosol and both IDH1 and IDH2 are $NADP^+$-dependent, whereas the TCA cycle occurs in the mitochondrial matrix and is NAD^+-dependent (Fig. **1**). Nonetheless, these two isoforms consume a TCA cycle intermediate and it has been recently shown that the accumulation of 2-HG inhibits the TCA cycle and upregulates lipid metabolism [79]. 2-HG is now viewed as an oncometabolite, *i.e.*, a tumor-promoting metabolite, but the mechanisms of its actions are far from being unequivocally established [77].

Another mechanism that seems to play a critical role in the metabolic rewiring that accompanies neoplastic transformation is the preferential expression of specific isoforms of metabolic enzymes and transporters.

The existence of more than one molecular form of a given enzyme was first reported, in the late 1950s, for LDH [80]. Soon, this finding was extended to many other enzymes and it was further found that each molecular form of a given enzyme, *i.e.*, each isozyme, has unique kinetic properties that are specifically suited for the role played by that form. These findings prompted cancer researchers to investigate the isoform-specific expression of glycolytic enzymes in tumors. In 1963, an "anomaly" in the ratio of aldolase activities in primary liver cancer was observed, which suggested the expression of an aldolase form similar to the more dedifferentiated fetal or embryonic aldolases [81]. Six years later, it was found that, in Morris hepatomas, the expression of glucokinase (one of the isoforms of HK) tended to disappear with increased malignancy, whereas that of the other forms of HK increased markedly [82]. In 1972, a similar shift in isozyme-specific expression was reported for PK [83]. It is now known that HK2 is the isoform most often expressed in malignant cells [84]. Among the specific characteristics of this isoform is its insensitivity to feedback inhibition by glucose 6-phosphate and its association with the cytosolic face of the mitochondrial inner membrane. It is now appreciated that the isoform-specific expression of a very large number of metabolic enzymes is a general feature of tumors. In the case of PK, which catalyses the last step of glycolysis, the sole isoform expressed in tumor cells (as well as in embryonic cells and in other proliferating cells) is the splicing variant PKM2. Significantly, by replacing PKM2 with the adult isoform, *i.e.*, isoform PKM1, in the human cancer cell lines H1299, A549 and SN12C, it was possible to reverse the Warburg effect. Moreover, this replacement reduced the ability to form tumors in nude mouse xenografts, suggesting that M2 expression provides tumor cells with a selective growth advantage *in vivo* [85].

There is now a generalized consensus that the metabolic rewiring that accompanies the process of neoplastic transformation extends well beyond the Warburg effect. This rewiring also includes, but is not restricted to, a high glutamine utilization, an elevated flux through the pentose phosphate pathway (PPP) and increased rates of lipid biosynthesis [86, 87]. However, a detailed description of tumor metabolic phenotypes other than those directly involved in the Warburg effect is out of the scope of this review, as are efforts to target them for cancer therapy. Also, our description will be mostly restricted to direct targets, *i.e.*, metabolic enzymes and protein complexes. Indirect targets, *i.e.*, the signaling pathways that might contribute to the Warburg effect, will not be discussed and the reader is referred to recent reviews for information on this topic [86 - 89].

Nonetheless, this chapter does discuss other cancer therapeutic avenues potentially related to the Warburg effect, namely caloric restriction and ketogenic diets.

4. CURRENT AND PAST EFFORTS AT TARGETING THE WARBURG EFFECT FOR CANCER THERAPY

The idea of targeting the metabolic specificities of cancer cells for cancer therapy is not recent. In fact, this therapeutic approach was proposed by Warburg himself. Already in the 1950s, awareness of the glucose avidity of cancer cells led to several studies aimed at assessing the potential of glucose antimetabolites for cancer treatment [90, 91]. One of these antimetabolites, 2-deoxy-D-glucose (2-DG), demonstrated some efficacy in inhibiting the growth of certain, but not all, tumors in mice [91]. In 1958, Dean Burk, one of the earliest fervent supporters of Warburg's metabolic theory of cancer, conducted a small exploratory study at the National Cancer Institute in which five cancer patients were treated with 2-DG [90]. However, it was only by the early 2000s, when more detailed information on tumor metabolism became available, that the pharmaceutical industry made the first forays into the field of metabolic cancer interventions [92] (Fig. **2**). Table **1** contains the official titles and sponsors of completed and ongoing clinical trials aimed at assessing the anticancer potential of drugs and dietary interventions targeting the Warburg effect that were identified in the ClinicalTrials.gov website.

Table 1. Official title and sponsors of the clinical trials described in Tables 2, 3 and 4.

ClinicalTrials.gov identifier[1]	Official title	Sponsor
NCT00096707	Phase I Dose Escalation Trial of 2-Deoxy-D-Glucose (2DG) Alone and in Combination With Docetaxel in Subjects With Advanced Solid Malignancies	Threshold Pharmaceuticals
NCT00237536	A Randomized, Double-Blind, Placebo-Controlled, Dose Comparison Study of the Efficacy and Safety of Lonidamine for the Treatment of Symptomatic Benign Prostatic Hyperplasia	Threshold Pharmaceuticals
NCT00422786	Phase II Study of CAP-232 in Patients With Refractory Metastatic Renal Cell Carcinoma	Thallion Pharmaceuticals

(Table 1) contd.....

ClinicalTrials.gov identifier[1]	Official title	Sponsor
NCT00435448	A Randomized Phase 3, Double-Blind, Placebo-Controlled Study of the Efficacy and Safety of Lonidamine for the Treatment of Symptomatic Benign Prostatic Hyperplasia	Threshold Pharmaceuticals
NCT00444054	Pilot Feasibility Study Of A Low Carbohydrate Diet In Patients With Advanced Cancer	Albert Einstein College of Medicine of Yeshiva University
NCT00540176	A Phase II Open-labeled, Double-arm Clinical Study of Dichloroacetate (DCA) in Malignant Gliomas and Glioblastome Multiforme (GBM) Patients	University of Alberta
NCT00566410	A Phase I, Open-Labeled, Single-Arm, Dose Escalation, Clinical and Pharmacology Study of Dichloroacetate (DCA) in Patients with Recurrent and/or Metastatic Solid Tumours	AHS Cancer Control Alberta
NCT00575146	Ketogenic Diet for Patients With Recurrent Glioblastoma	University Hospital Tuebingen
NCT00633087	A Phase I/II Trial of 2-Deoxyglucose (2DG) for the Treatment of Advanced Cancer and Hormone Refractory Prostate Cancer	Rutgers, The State University of New Jersey
NCT00659568	A Phase I Study of Temsirolimus in Combination With Metformin in Advanced Solid Tumours	London Regional Cancer Program at London Health Sciences Centre
NCT00735332	A Phase IIa Study of TLN-232 as Second-line Therapy for Patients With Metastatic Melanoma	Thallion Pharmaceuticals
NCT00881725	A Phase II, Open Label Assessment of Neoadjuvant Intervention With Metformin Against Tumour Expression of Signaling	University Health Network, Toronto
NCT00897884	Clinical and Biologic Effects of Metformin in Early Stage Breast Cancer	Mount Sinai Hospital, Canada
NCT00930579	Phase II Pre-Surgical Intervention Study for Evaluating the Effect of Metformin on Breast Cancer Proliferation	Columbia University
NCT00933309	The Impact of Obesity and Obesity Treatments on Breast Cancer: A Phase I Trial of Exemestane With Metformin and Rosiglitazone for Postmenopausal Obese Women With ER+ Metastatic Breast Cancer	M.D. Anderson Cancer Center
NCT00984490	Pre-Surgical Trial of Metformin in Patients With Operable Breast Cancer	Vanderbilt-Ingram Cancer Center
NCT01029925	A Multicenter, Phase II Open-Labeled, Single-Arm Clinical and Pharmacology Study of Dichloroacetate (DCA) in Patients With Previously Treated Metastatic Breast or Non-Small Cell Lung Cancer	Jonsson Comprehensive Cancer Center

(Table 1) contd.....

ClinicalTrials.gov identifier[1]	Official title	Sponsor
NCT01042379	I-SPY 2 Trial (Investigation of Serial Studies to Predict Your Therapeutic Response With Imaging And molecular Analysis 2)	QuantumLeap Healthcare Collaborative
NCT01087983	A Phase 1 Trial of Lapatinib in Combination With 1) Sirolimus or 2) Metformin in Advanced Cancer	M.D. Anderson Cancer Center
NCT01101438	A Phase III Randomized Trial of Metformin *Versus* Placebo on Recurrence and Survival in Early Stage Breast Cancer	NCIC Clinical Trials Group
NCT01111097	Phase 1, Open-Label, Single-Arm, Clinical and Metabolomics Study of Dichloroacetate (DCA) in Adults With Recurrent Malignant Brain Tumors	University of Florida
NCT01163487	Phase I Trial of Metabolic Reprogramming Therapy for Treatment of Recurrent Head and Neck Cancers	Daniel T. Chang
NCT01167738	A Randomized Phase II Study of Chemotherapy ±Metformin in Metastatic Pancreatic Cancer	IRCCS San Raffaele
NCT01205672	Evaluation of the Molecular Effects of Metformin on the Endometrium in Patients With Endometrial Cancer	M.D. Anderson Cancer Center
NCT01210911	A Phase II, Randomized, Placebo Controlled Study to Evaluate the Efficacy of the Combination of Gemcitabine, Erlotinib and Metformin in Patients With Locally Advanced and Metastatic Pancreatic Cancer	Academisch Medisch Centrum - Universiteit van Amsterdam (AMC-UvA)
NCT01215032	Prospective Study of Metformin in Castration-Resistant Prostate Cancer	Massachusetts General Hospital
NCT01243385	Metformin in Castration Resistant Prostate Cancer. A Multicenter Phase II Trial	Swiss Group for Clinical Cancer Research
NCT01310231	A Randomized Phase II, Double Blind, Trial of Standard Chemotherapy With Metformin (*vs* Placebo) in Women With Metastatic Breast Cancer Receiving First or Second Line Chemotherapy With Anthracycline, Taxane, Platinum or Capecitabine Based Regimens	Ozmosis Research Inc.
NCT01324180	A Phase I Window, Dose Escalating and Safety Trial of Metformin in Combination With Induction Chemotherapy in Relapsed Refractory Acute Lymphoblastic Leukemia: Metformin With Induction Chemotherapy of Vincristine, Dexamethasone, Doxorubicin, and PEG-asparaginase (VPLD)	H. Lee Moffitt Cancer Center and Research Institute
NCT01333852	Randomized Phase II Study of Paclitaxel Plus Metformin or Placebo for the Treatment of Platinum-refractory, Recurrent or Metastatic Head and Neck Neoplasms	Lucas Vieira dos Santos

(Table 1) contd.....

ClinicalTrials.gov identifier[1]	Official title	Sponsor
NCT01341886	Effect of Metformin on Decrement in Levothyroxin Dose Required for Thyroid Stimulating Hormone (TSH) Suppression in Patients With Differentiated Thyroid Cancer	Mashhad University of Medical Sciences
NCT01386632	Phase II Study of DCA in Combination With Cisplatin and Definitive Radiation in Stage III-IV Squamous Cell Carcinoma of the Head and Neck	Sanford Health
NCT01419483	A Phase I Trial of a Ketogenic Diet With Concurrent Chemoradiation for Pancreatic Cancer	University of Iowa
NCT01419587	A Phase I Trial of a Ketogenic Diet With Concurrent Chemoradiation for Non-small Cell Lung Cancer	University of Iowa
NCT01430351	A Phase I lead-in to a 2x2x2 Factorial Trial of Dose Dense Temozolomide, Memantine, Mefloquine, and Metformin As Post-Radiation Adjuvant Therapy of Glioblastoma Multiforme	M.D. Anderson Cancer Center
NCT01433913	Phase II Study of Metformin in a Pre-prostatectomy Prostate Cancer Cohort	National Cancer Institute (NCI)
NCT01440127	Randomized Clinical Trial Evaluating the Impact of Pretreatment With Metformin on Colorectal Cancer Stem Cells (CCSC) and Related Pharmacodynamic Markers	Tufts Medical Center
NCT01442870	Prospective Evaluation of Clinical Safety of Combining Metformin With Anticancer Chemotherapy	Tufts Medical Center
NCT01477060	Modulation of Response to Hormonal Therapy With Lapatinib and/or Metformin in Patients With HER2-negative, ER and/or PgR Positive Metastatic Brest Cancer With Progressive Disease After First-line Therapy	Fondazione Michelangelo
NCT01488552	A Phase II Study of Induction Consolidation and Maintenance Approach for Patients With Advanced Pancreatic Cancer	Pancreatic Cancer Research Team
NCT01523639	A Randomized, Placebo-controlled, Double-blind Multicenter Phase II Study to Investigate the Protectivity and Efficacy of Metformin Against Steatosis in Combination With FOLFIRI and Cetuximab in Subjects With First-line Palliative Treated, KRAS-Wild-Type, Metastatic Colorectal Cancer	Austrian Breast & Colorectal Cancer Study Group
NCT01528046	A Phase I Trial of Dose Escalation of Metformin in Combination With Vincristine, Irinotecan, and Temozolomide in Children With Relapsed or Refractory Solid Tumors	H. Lee Moffitt Cancer Center and Research Institute
NCT01529593	Phase I Study of Temsirolimus in Combination With Metformin in Patients With Advanced Cancers	M.D. Anderson Cancer Center
NCT01535911	Pilot Study of a Metabolic Nutritional Therapy for the Management of Primary Brain Tumors	Michigan State University

(Table 1) contd.....

ClinicalTrials.gov identifier[1]	Official title	Sponsor
NCT01561482	Open-Label Study Of Metformin In Combination With Simvastatin For Men With Prostate Carcinoma And A Rising Serum Prostate-Specific Antigen Level After Radical Prostatectomy And/Or Radiation Therapy	Nicholas Mitsiades
NCT01578551	A Randomized Phase II Study of Metformin Plus Paclitaxel/Carboplatin/Bevacizumab in Patients With Previously Untreated Advanced/Metastatic Pulmonary Adenocarcinoma	Sidney Kimmel Comprehensive Cancer Center
NCT01579812	A Phase II Evaluation of Metformin, Targeting Cancer Stem Cells for the Prevention of Relapse in Patients With Stage IIC/III/IV Ovarian, Fallopian Tube, and Primary Peritoneal Cancer	Ronald Buckanovich
NCT01589367	Phase II Randomized Study of Neoadjuvant Metformin Plus Letrozole *vs* Placebo Plus Letrozole for ER-positive Postmenopausal Breast Cancer	Seoul National University Hospital
NCT01620593	Castration Compared to Castration Plus Metformin as First Line Treatment for Patients With Advanced Prostate Cancer	Devalingam Mahalingam
NCT01627067	Circulating FGF21 Levels and Efficacy of Exemestane, Everolimus and Metformin in Postmenopausal Women With Hormone Receptor Positive Metastatic Breast Cancer and BMI $>/= 25$	M.D. Anderson Cancer Center
NCT01632020	Pilot Study: Effect of Metformin on Biomarkers of Colorectal Tumor Cell Growth	University of Arkansas
NCT01638676	A Phase I/II Trial of Vemurafenib and Metformin to Unresectable Stage IIIC and Stage IV BRAF.V600E+ Melanoma Patients	James Graham Brown Cancer Center
NCT01650506	Phase I Study of Erlotinib and Metformin in Triple Negative Breast Cancer	Columbia University
NCT01666730	A Phase II Study of Metformin Plus Modified FOLFOX 6 in Patients With Metastatic Pancreatic Cancer	Case Comprehensive Cancer Center
NCT01677897	Impact of the Addition of Metformin to Abiraterone in Pre-docetaxel Metastatic Castration-resistant Prostate Cancer Patients Progressing on Abiraterone Treatment (MetAb-Pro): a Phase II Pilot Study	Kantonsspital GraubÜnden
NCT01686126	A Phase II Randomised Clinical Trial of Mirena® ±Metformin ±Weight Loss Intervention in Patients With Early Stage Cancer of the Endometrium	Queensland Centre for Gynaecological Cancer
NCT01750567	A Phase II Pilot Study of Metformin Therapy in Patients With Relapsed Chronic Lymphocytic Leukemia and Untreated CLL Patients With Genomic Deletion 11q	University of Michigan Cancer Center

(Table 1) contd.....

ClinicalTrials.gov identifier[1]	Official title	Sponsor
NCT01754350	Calorie-restricted, Ketogenic Diet and Transient Fasting *vs.* Standard Nutrition During Reirradiation for Patients With Recurrent Glioblastoma: the ERGO2 Study	Johann Wolfgang Goethe University Hospitals
NCT01791595	A Cancer Research United Kingdom Phase I Trial of AZD3965, a Monocarboxylate Transporter 1 Inhibitor (MCT1) in Patients With Advanced Cancer	Cancer Research UK
NCT01796028	A Multicentric, Randomized, Phase II Study Evaluating the Combination of METFORMIN With TAXOTERE®+Metformine Placebo *Versus* TAXOTERE®+Metformin for the Treatment of Metastatic Hormone-refractory Prostate Cancer.	Centre Antoine Lacassagne
NCT01797523	A Phase II, Single-Arm Study of RAD001 (Everolimus), Letrozole, and Metformin in Patients With Advanced or Recurrent Endometrial Carcinoma	M.D. Anderson Cancer Center
NCT01816659	An Open-Labeled Pilot Study of Biomarker Response in Patients With Colorectal Cancer or Endoscopically Non-Resectable Adenomas Following Short-Term Exposure to Metformin Extended Release (ER)	M.D. Anderson Cancer Center
NCT01819233	A Feasibility Pilot Trial Evaluating Caloric Restriction for Oncology Research in Early Stage Breast Cancer Patients	Thomas Jefferson University
NCT01849276	A Phase I Study of Metformin and Cytarabine for the Treatment of Relapsed/Refractory Acute Myeloid Leukemia	Northwestern University
NCT01864681	A Phase II, Randomized, Placebo Controlled Study to Evaluate the Efficacy of the Combination of Gefitinib and Metformin in Patients With Locally Advanced and Metastatic Non-Small-Cell-Lung-Cancer	Daping Hospital and the Research Institute of Surgery of the Third Military Medical University
NCT01865162	Ketogenic Diet as Adjunctive Treatment in Refractory/End-stage Glioblastoma Multiforme: a Pilot Study	Mid-Atlantic Epilepsy and Sleep Center, LLC
NCT01877564	A Randomized Pilot Study to Evaluate the Effects of a Short Course of Metformin *Versus* No Therapy in the Period Prior to Hysterectomy for Grade 1-2 Adenocarcinoma of the Endometrium in Obese Non-Diabetic Women	University of Arkansas
NCT01885013	MYME: Phase II Comparative Study Of Myocet Plus Cyclophosphamide Plus Metformin *Versus* Myocet Plus Cyclophosphamide In First Line Treatment Of HER2 Negative Metastatic Breast Cancer Patients	Istituto Scientifico Romagnolo per lo Studio e la cura dei Tumori
NCT01911247	Preoperative Window Study of Metformin for the Treatment of Endometrial Cancer	UNC Lineberger Comprehensive Cancer Center

(Table 1) contd.....

ClinicalTrials.gov identifier[1]	Official title	Sponsor
NCT01915498	A Phase 1, Multicenter, Open-Label, Dose-Escalation, Safety, Pharmacokinetic, Pharmacodynamic, and Clinical Activity Study of Orally Administered AG-221 in Subjects With Advanced Hematologic Malignancies With an IDH2 Mutation	Agios Pharmaceuticals, Inc.
NCT01926769	A Phase II Study to Determine the Safety and Efficacy of Second-line Treatment With Metformin and Chemotherapy (FOLFOX6 or FOFIRI) in the Second Line Treatment of Advanced Colorectal Cancer	Gachon University Gil Medical Center
NCT01929811	Neoadjuvant Treatment of TEC *Versus* TEC Plus Metformin in Breast Cancer: A Prospective, Randomized Trial	Shanghai Jiao Tong University School of Medicine
NCT01930864	Phase II Trial of Metformin Combined to Irinotecan for Refractory Metastatic or Recurrent Colorectal Cancer	Barretos Cancer Hospital
NCT01941953	Phase II Study of Metformin and 5-fluorouracil in Patients With Advanced Colorectal Cancer Previously Treated With Oxaliplatin and Irinotecan Based Chemotherapy.	Instituto do Cancer do Estado de São Paulo
NCT01954732	A Pharmacodynamic Study of Metformin in Patients With Resectable Pancreatic Cancer	Case Comprehensive Cancer Center
NCT01954836	Short-Term Fasting During Chemotherapy in Patients With Gynecological Cancer- a Randomized Controlled Cross-over Trial	Charite University, Berlin, Germany
NCT01968317	Megestrol Acetate Plus Metformin to Megestrol Acetate in Patients With Endometrial Atypical Hyperplasia or Early Stage Endometrial Adenocarcinoma	Xiaojun Chen
NCT01971034	A Prospective Study to Evaluate the Combination of Metformin With Paclitaxel in the Treatment of Patients With Advanced Pancreatic Cancer After Gemcitabine Failure	Instituto do Cancer do Estado de São Paulo
NCT01975766	A Phase I Trial of a Ketogenic Diet With Concurrent Chemoradiation for Head and Neck Cancer	University of Iowa
NCT01980823	Pre-Surgical "Window of Opportunity" Trial of the Combination of Metformin and Atorvastatin in Newly Diagnosed Operable Breast Cancer	Columbia University
NCT01997775	A Phase II Trial to Examine the Effect of Metformin on Plasma IL-6 Level in Patients With Advanced Non-Small Cell Lung Cancer	National Cheng-Kung University Hospital
NCT02005419	A Phase II, Randomized, Double-blind, Placebo Controlled Study to Evaluate the Efficacy and Safety of the Combination of Gemcitabine and Metformin in Treating Patients With Pancreatic Cancer After Curative Resection	Xian-Jun Yu

(Table 1) contd.....

ClinicalTrials.gov identifier[1]	Official title	Sponsor
NCT02019979	Metformin With a Carbohydrate Restricted Diet In Combination With Platinum Based Chemotherapy In Stage IIIB/IV Non-Squamous Non-Small Cell Lung Cancer (NS-NSCLC) - METRO Study	Beth Israel Medical Center
NCT02035787	Metformin With the Levonorgestrel-Releasing Intrauterine Device for the Treatment of Complex Atypical Hyperplasia (CAH) and Endometrial Cancer (EC) in Non-surgical Patients	UNC Lineberger Comprehensive Cancer Center
NCT02040376	Placebo Controlled Double Blind Crossover Trial of Metformin for Brain Repair in Children With Cranial-Spinal Radiation for Medulloblastoma	The Hospital for Sick Children
NCT02042495	A Clinical Trial to Evaluate Endometrial Cancer Biomarker Changes Following Exposure to the Insulin Sensitizer Metformin	Jewish General Hospital
NCT02046187	Phase I/II Prospective Trial for Newly Diagnosed GBM, With Upfront Gross or Subtotal Resection, Followed by Ketogenic Diet With Radiotherapy and Concurrent Temodar(R) Chemotherapy Followed by Adjuvant Temodar(R) Chemotherapy.	St. Joseph's Hospital and Medical Center, Phoenix
NCT02048384	An Exploratory Study of Metformin With or Without Rapamycin as Maintenance Therapy After Induction Chemotherapy in Subjects With Metastatic Pancreatic Adenocarcinoma	Sidney Kimmel Comprehensive Cancer Center
NCT02050009	The Use and Safety of Metformin, Carboplatin and Paclitaxel in Non-Diabetic Patients With Recurrent, Platinum Sensitive Ovarian Cancer and the Feasibility of Using a Core Biopsy for RNA-Seq	Fox Chase Cancer Center
NCT02065687	A Randomized Phase II/III Study of Paclitaxel/Carboplatin/Metformin (NSC#91485) *Versus* Paclitaxel/Carboplatin/Placebo as Initial Therapy for Measurable Stage III or IVA, Stage IVB, or Recurrent Endometrial Cancer	Gynecologic Oncology Group
NCT02073994	A Phase 1, Multicenter, Open-Label, Dose-Escalation, Safety, Pharmacokinetic, Pharmacodynamic, and Clinical Activity Study of Orally Administered AG-120 in Subjects With Advanced Solid Tumors, Including Glioma, With an IDH1 Mutation	Agios Pharmaceuticals, Inc.
NCT02074839	A Phase I, Multicenter, Open-Label, Dose-Escalation, Safety, Pharmacokinetic, Pharmacodynamic, and Clinical Activity Study of Orally Administered AG-120 in Subjects With Advanced Hematologic Malignancies With an IDH1 Mutation	Agios Pharmaceuticals, Inc.

(Table 1) contd.....

ClinicalTrials.gov identifier[1]	Official title	Sponsor
NCT02115464	A Phase II Study to Investigate a Combination of Metformin With Chemo-Radiotherapy in Patients With Locally Advanced Non-Small Cell Lung Cancer	Ontario Clinical Oncology Group (OCOG)
NCT02122185	A Randomized Placebo Controlled Phase II Trial of Metformin in Conjunction With Chemotherapy Followed by Metformin Maintenance Therapy in Advanced Stage Ovarian, Fallopian Tube and Primary Peritoneal Cancer	University of Chicago
NCT02126449	Dietary Restriction as an Adjunct to Neoadjuvant ChemoTherapy for HER2 Negative Breast Cancer	Leiden University Medical Center
NCT02143050	A Phase I/II Trial of Dabrafenib, Trametinib and Metformin Administered to Unresectable Stage IIIC and Stage IV BRAF V600E + Melanoma Patients	James Graham Brown Cancer Center
NCT02145559	A Pharmacodynamic Study of Sirolimus and Metformin in Patients With Advanced Solid Tumors	University of Chicago
NCT02149459	Improving the Response of Recurrent Glioma to Radiation Therapy Through Metabolic Intervention	Sheba Medical Center
NCT02153450	A Pilot Trial of Stereotactic Body Radiation Therapy and Metformin for Borderline-Resectable and Locally-Advanced Pancreatic Adenocarcinomas	Case Comprehensive Cancer Center
NCT02176161	Phase II Clinical Study of Effect of Metformin on Prostate Specific Antigen Doubling Time	Winthrop University Hospital
NCT02186847	Randomized Phase II Trial of Concurrent Chemoradiotherapy +/- Metformin HCL in Locally Advanced NSCLC	NRG Oncology
NCT02190838	Phase II Multicenter Randomized Study to Compare Dacarbazine With Melatonin or Metformin *Versus* Dacarbazine in the First Line Therapy of Disseminated Melanoma	Petrov Research Institute of Oncology
NCT02254512	Metformin With a Carbohydrate Restricted Diet in Combination With Platinum Based Chemotherapy in Stage IIIB/IV Non-squamous Non-small Cell Lung Cancer (NS-NSCLC) - METRO Study	Beth Israel Medical Center
NCT02273739	Study of Orally Administered AG-221 in Subjects With Advanced Solid Tumors, Including Glioma, and With Angioimmunoblastic T-cell Lymphoma, With an IDH2 Mutation	Agios Pharmaceuticals, Inc.
NCT02278965	Pilot Biomarker Modulation Study of Metformin and Omega-3 Fatty Acids in Woman With a History of Early Stage Breast Cancer	Katherine D. Crew
NCT02279758	A Phase II Pilot Study Of Metformin Treatment In Patients With Well-Differentiated Neuroendocrine Tumors	Instituto do Cancer do Estado de São Paulo

(Table 1) contd.....

ClinicalTrials.gov identifier[1]	Official title	Sponsor
NCT02285855	Tumor Mutation Status Will Predict Metabolic Response to Metformin in Non Small Cell Lung Cancer (NSCLC)	M.D. Anderson Cancer Center
NCT02286167	The Feasibility and Biologic Effect of a Modified Atkins-based Intermittent Fasting Diet in Patients With Glioblastoma (GBM)	Sidney Kimmel Comprehensive Cancer Center
NCT02294006	Activity and Safety of Everolimus in Combination With Octreotide LAR and Metformin in Patients With Advanced Pancreatic Well-differentiated Neuroendocrine Tumors (pWDNETs): a Phase II, Open, Monocentric, Prospective Study	Fondazione IRCCS Istituto Nazionale dei Tumori, Milano
NCT02302235	Ketogenic Diet Treatment Adjunctive to Radiation and Chemotherapy in Glioblastoma Multiforme: a Pilot Study	Mid-Atlantic Epilepsy and Sleep Center, LLC
NCT02312661	Phase Ib Study of Metformin in Combination With Carboplatin/Paclitaxel Chemotherapy in Patients With Advanced Ovarian Cancer	University Medical Centre Groningen
NCT02325401	A Phase I Dose-finding Study of Metformin in Combination With Concurrent Cisplatin and Radiation in Patients With Locally Advanced Head and Neck Squamous Cell Carcinoma	University of Cincinnati
NCT02336087	Pilot Trial of Gemcitabine, Abraxane, Metformin and a Standardized Dietary Supplement (DS) in Patients With Metastatic Pancreatic Cancer	City of Hope Medical Center
NCT02339168	Enzalutamide and Metformin Combination Therapy to Overcome Autophagy Resistance in Castration Resistant Prostate Cancer	University of California, Davis
NCT02360059	Metformin for Reduction of Paclitaxel Treatment-Related Neuropathy in Patients With Breast Cancer: A Randomized Pilot Study	M.D. Anderson Cancer Center
NCT02360618	A Window of Opportunity Study to Evaluate the Role of the Combination of Metformin and Simvastatin as a Neoadjuvant Therapy in Invasive Bladder Cancer	London Health Sciences Centre
NCT02379585	A Pilot Study of Short-term Fasting on Neoadjuvant Chemotherapy in Patients With Newly Diagnosed Breast Cancer (STEFNE Study)	Western Regional Medical Center

[1] Trials have been presented by increasing number of their identifiers.

As can be appreciated in Table **2**, in spite of significant pre-clinical data supporting an important role in carcinogenesis for a large number of central carbon metabolism enzymes, such as glycolytic enzymes [93, 94], TCA cycle enzymes [95], LDH [96] and monocarboxylate transporters [97], attempts to

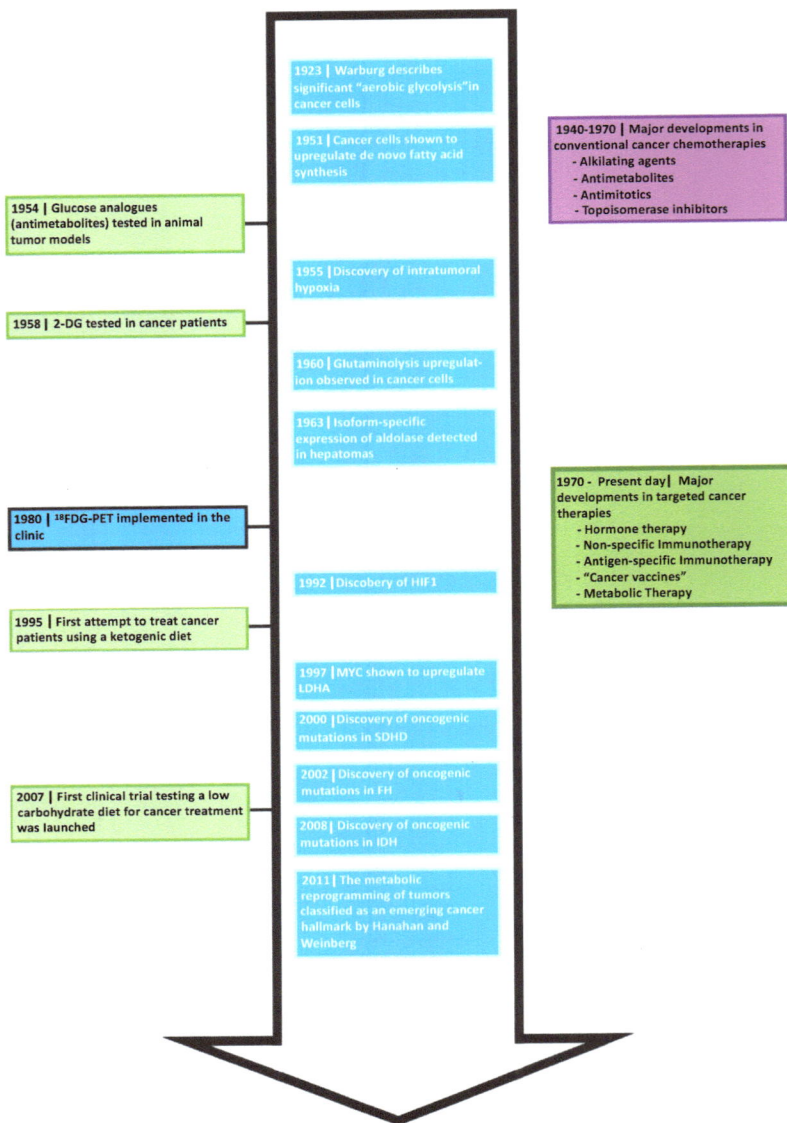

Fig. (2). Milestones in our knowledge of the Warburg effect and of its molecular basis. On the left-hand side of the arrow are summarized significant advances towards the clinical exploitation of this effect. Information on the right-hand size of the arrow contextualizes the clinical exploitation of the Warburg effect in the light of other major advances in cancer conventional chemotherapy and cancer targeted therapies. 2-DG, 2-deoxy-D-glucose; ^{18}FDG–PET, ^{18}F-deoxyglucose positron emission tomography; FH, fumarate hydratase; HIF1, hypoxia-inducible transcription factor 1; IDH, isocitrate dehydrogenase; LDHA, lactate dehydrogenase A; SDH, succinate dehydrogenase.

translate these findings into the clinic have been, so far, rather timid. In fact, only five drugs (2-DG, lonidamine (TH-070), TLN-232, AZD3965 and dichloroacetate (DCA)) have entered clinical trials, clearly showing that the pharmaceutical industry still regards metabolic cancer therapy as a high-risk field [92].

Table 2. Clinical trials aimed at assessing the anticancer potential of drugs targeting the Warburg effect.

| Target | | Compound | Indication[1] | Phase | Status | ClinicalTrials.gov identifier | Results (whenever published) |
Metabolic pathway / Process	Biomolecule						
Glycolysis	HK II	2-DG	Advanced solid malignancies	I	Completed	NCT00096707	[98]
		Lonidamine (TH-070)	Hormone refractory prostate cancer	I/II	Terminated[2]	NCT00633087	
			Symptomatic benign prostatic hyperplasia	II	Terminated	NCT00237536	
				III	Terminated[3]	NCT00435448	[100, 101]
	PKM2	TLN-232	Metastatic melanoma	II	Terminated[4]	NCT00735332	[103]
			Metastatic renal cell carcinoma	II	Completed	NCT00422786	[102]
Lactate transport	MCT1	AZD3965	Prostate cancer, gastric cancer or diffuse large B cell lymphoma	I	Recruiting	NCT01791595	
Lactic acid fermentation and aerobic respiration	PDK	DCA	Brain tumor; glioblastoma	I	Completed	NCT01111097	[106]
			Malignant gliomas, glioblastoma multiforme	II	Completed	NCT00540176	[105]
			Metastatic breast or non-small cell lung cancer (NSCLC)	II	Terminated[5]	NCT01029925	[107]
			Head and neck cancers	I	Recruiting	NCT01163487	
			Squamous cell carcinoma of the head and neck	II	Ongoing	NCT01386632	
			Metastatic solid tumours	I	Ongoing	NCT00566410	
	IDH1	AG-120	Advanced solid tumors with an IDH1 mutation	I	Recruiting	NCT02073994	
			Advanced hematologic malignancies with an IDH1 mutation	I	Recruiting	NCT02074839	[108]
	IDH2	AG-221	Advanced hematologic malignancies with an IDH2 mutation	I	Recruiting	NCT01915498	[109, 110]
			Advanced solid tumors with an IDH2 Mutation	I/II	Recruiting	NCT02273739	

[1] For more information, see Table **1**. [2] This study was terminated due to slow accrual. [3] This trial was discontinued based on safety concerns and negative efficacy results. [4] This trial was terminated due to license termination. [5] The Data Safety and Monitoring Board (DSMB) monitoring this study determined that due to higher than expected risk and safety concerns the study should be closed. 2-DG, 2-deoxy-D-glucose; DCA, dichloroacetate; HKII, isoform II of hexokinase; IDH1, isoform 1 of isocitrate dehydrogenase; IDH2, isoform 2 of isocitrate dehydrogenase; MCT1, isoform 1 of monocarboxylate transporter; NSCLC, non-small cell lung cancer; PDK, pyruvate dehydrogenase kinase; PKM2, isoform M2 of pyruvate kinase.

2-DG, one of the compounds that entered clinical trials, targets isoform II of HK (Fig. **3**). Two Phase I studies have now been completed. In one of them (NCT00096707), the aim was to evaluate the safety, tolerability, pharma-cokinetics and biologic effect of daily oral doses of 2-DG, with and without weekly docetaxel, in subjects with advanced solid tumors. The recommended Phase II 2-DG dose, in combination with weekly docetaxel, that emerged from this study was 63 mg/kg/day [98], with tolerable adverse effects. This dose is close to that found in the other completed study (45 mg/kg; study not identified in the ClinicalTrials.gov Web site), in which 2-DG as a single agent was evaluated in patients with castrate-resistant prostate cancer and advanced malignancies [99]. Not surprisingly, both 2-DG doses are much superior to those used in ^{18}FDG-PET, which employs radioactively labelled 2-DG. The fact that only one partial response (out of 34 patients) was observed in the trial using 2-DG in combination with docetaxel and no activity was observed when it was administered as a single agent [92] may have discouraged the sponsors from proceeding to Phase II trials. It has been suggested that these failures might be due, at least partially, to the high 2-DG doses that are likely necessary to inhibit HK *in vivo* [92].

A Phase I/II trial of 2-DG for the treatment of advanced cancer and hormone refractory prostate cancer was registered in 2008, but has meanwhile been terminated. This was due to slow accrual, a fate shared by several of the clinical trials compiled in Tables **2** and **3**.

In the mid-2000s, a Phase II (NCT00237536) and a Phase III (NCT00435448) clinical trial were launched by the same sponsor to test lonidamine (TH-070), another drug targeting HK, in subjects with symptomatic benign prostatic hyperplasia (BPH). Based on their safety and efficacy results, in particular the observation of severe hepatic adverse effects in six patients [100, 101], both trials were terminated in 2006.

TLN-232, a synthetic cyclic heptapeptide that inhibits PKM2, has been the subject of two clinical trials. One of these trials, a Phase II study in patients with refractory metastatic renal cell carcinoma (NCT00422786), has been completed and, according to the sponsors, TLN-232 was generally safe and well tolerated [102]. The same sponsor launched a Phase IIa study of this drug as second-line therapy for patients with metastatic melanoma (NCT00735332), but this trial was terminated due to an ongoing dispute with the licensor [103].

A Phase I clinical trial has been launched to test AZD3965, an inhibitor of the isoform 1 of the monocarboxylate transporter (MCT1). This trial is still recruiting participants and, as yet, no results have been made available.

Table 3. Clinical trials aimed at assessing the anticancer potential of metformin.

Target		Compound	Indication[1]	Phase	Status	ClinicalTrials.gov identifier	Results (whenever published)
Metabolic pathway / Process	Biomolecule						
Glycolysis and mitochondrial respiration	HKI, HKII and complex I of the ETC	Metformin	Acute myeloid leukemia	I	Recruiting	NCT01324180	
				I	Recruiting	NCT01849276	
			Advanced cancer	II	Ongoing	NCT01087983	
				I	Recruiting	NCT01529593	
			Bladder cancer	III	Not yet recruiting	NCT02360618	
			Breast cancer	Undisclosed	Completed	NCT00897884	
				II	Ongoing	NCT00930579	[130]
				Undisclosed	Terminated[2]	NCT00984490	
				II	Recruiting	NCT01042379	
				III	Ongoing	NCT01101438	[127]
				II	Recruiting	NCT01929811	
				0	Recruiting	NCT01980823	
				Undisclosed	Recruiting	NCT02278965	
				II	Not yet recruiting	NCT02360059	
			ER+ metastatic breast cancer	I	Completed	NCT00933309	[125]
			ER+ postmenopausal breast cancer	II	Recruiting	NCT01589367	[131]
			Metastatic breast cancer	II	Recruiting	NCT01310231	
				II	Terminated[2]	NCT01477060	
				II	Ongoing	NCT01627067	
				II	Recruiting	NCT01885013	
			Triple negative breast cancer	I	Recruiting	NCT01650506	
			Relapsed chronic lymphocytic leukemia	II	Recruiting	NCT01750567	
			Colon cancer	I	Terminated[2]	NCT01440127	
			Colorectal cancer	II	Ongoing	NCT01632020	
				I	Terminated[2]	NCT01816659	
				II	Not yet recruiting	NCT01930864	
				II	Recruiting	NCT01941953	[134]
			Advanced colorectal cancer	II	Recruiting	NCT01926769	
			Metastatic colorectal cancer	II	Terminated[2]	NCT01523639	
			Endometrial adenocarcinoma	II	Recruiting	NCT01877564	
				II	Recruiting	NCT01968317	
			Endometrial cancer	Undisclosed	Ongoing	NCT01205672	
				II	Recruiting	NCT01686126	

(Table 3) contd.....

Metabolic pathway / Process	Biomolecule	Compound	Indication[1]	Phase	Status	ClinicalTrials.gov identifier	Results (whenever published)
				II	Recruiting	NCT01797523	
				0	Completed	NCT01911247	
				II	Not yet recruiting	NCT02042495	
				II/III	Recruiting	NCT02065687	
			Complex atypical hyperplasia and endometrial cancer	Undisclosed	Recruiting	NCT02035787	
			Glioblastoma multiforme	I	Recruiting	NCT01430351	
			Glioma	I	Not yet recruiting	NCT02149459	
			Advanced head and neck squamous cell carcinoma	I	Not yet recruiting	NCT02325401	
			Metastatic head and neck cancer	II	Terminated[2]	NCT01333852	[124]
			Medulloblastoma	III	Recruiting	NCT02040376	
			Melanoma	I/II	Recruiting	NCT01638676	
				I/II	Recruiting	NCT02143050	
				II	Recruiting	NCT02190838	
			Neuroendocrine tumors	II	Recruiting	NCT02279758	
				II	Recruiting	NCT02294006	
			Non-small cell lung cancer (NSCLC)	II	Not yet recruiting	NCT02285855	
			Advanced NSCLC	II	Recruiting	NCT01997775	
				II	Recruiting	NCT02115464	
				II	Recruiting	NCT02186847	
			Metastatic NSCLC	II	Recruiting	NCT01864681	
			Nonsquamous NSCLC	II	Recruiting	NCT02019979	
				II	Recruiting	NCT02254512	
			Advanced ovarian cancer	I	Not yet recruiting	NCT02312661	
			Advanced stage ovarian, fallopian tube and primary peritoneal cancer	II	Recruiting	NCT01579812	
				I	Not yet recruiting	NCT02050009	
				II	Not yet recruiting	NCT02122185	
			Pancreatic cancer	II	Ongoing	NCT01243385	[114]
				I	Recruiting	NCT01954732	
				II	Completed	NCT01971034	[126]
				II	Recruiting	NCT02005419	
			Advanced pancreatic cancer	II	Recruiting	NCT01488552	[135]
				Undisclosed	Not yet recruiting	NCT02153450	
			Advanced and metastatic pancreatic cancer	II	Completed	NCT01210911	
			Metastatic pancreatic adenocarcinoma	I/II	Recruiting	NCT02048384	
			Metastatic pancreatic cancer	II	Ongoing	NCT01167738	
				II	Recruiting	NCT01666730	
				I	Not yet recruiting	NCT02336087	
			Prostate cancer	II	Terminated[2]	NCT00881725	[128, 129]
				Undisclosed	Terminated[3]	NCT01215032	
				II	Ongoing	NCT01433913	
				II	Recruiting	NCT01561482	
				II	Recruiting	NCT01677897	
				II	Recruiting	NCT01796028	
				II	Recruiting	NCT02176161	
				I	Not yet recruiting	NCT02339168	
			Advanced prostate cancer	II	Recruiting	NCT01620593	
			Metastatic pulmonary adenocarcinoma	II	Recruiting	NCT01578551	
			Solid tumors	I	Completed	NCT01442870	[132]
				I	Recruiting	NCT01528046	
			Advance solid tumors	I	Completed	NCT00659568	[133]
				I	Recruiting	NCT02145559	
			Thyroid cancer	Undisclosed	Completed	NCT01341886	

[1] For a more complete description, see Table **1**. [2] This trial was terminated due to slow accrual. [3] This trial was terminated due to slow accrual and competing clinical trials. ETC, mitochondrial electron transport chain; HKI, isoform I of hexokinase; HKII, isoform II of hexokinase; NSCLC, non-small cell lung cancer.

Great hopes have been placed in DCA, a drug that has long been used for the treatment of hereditary lactic acidosis [104]. Its low cost and oral availability make this drug quite attractive. On the other hand, as it is not a novel compound, it cannot be patented, discouraging the pharmaceutical companies from sponsoring clinical trials aimed at testing its therapeutic potential. By inhibiting PDK1, DCA ultimately inhibits the phosphorylation of PDH, preventing its inactivation (section 2 and Fig. **1**). Thus, DCA favors the conversion of pyruvate to acetyl CoA and, indirectly, prevents its conversion to lactate.

In its first clinical trial (NCT00540176), DCA was tested in patients with glioblastoma multiform. The results for five patients were encouraging, as four patients were still alive 18 months after starting DCA [105]. However, these results must be interpreted with care, as some patients also received another chemotherapy drug (temozolomide; brand names Temodar™, Temodal™) and there was no control group. This trial, which was sponsored by academia, has been suspended due, at least in part, to lack of financial support.

Meanwhile, five other clinical trials of DCA were launched, but only one of them has been completed (NCT01111097). This was a Phase I trial in patients with brain tumors. According to the published results, chronic, oral DCA, in the dose range established for metabolic diseases, was feasible and well-tolerated [106]. The authors of the study also confirmed the importance of genetic-based dosing, which should likely be the case for all metabolic cancer therapies. It must be emphasized that DCA has a low potency, requiring concentrations in the high micromolar range to inhibit PDK *in vivo* [92]. This requirement may compromise its use as an anticancer drug. There is hope, though, that combined with other anticancer drugs, DCA may have significant synergistic effects and could, therefore, be of use to complement other therapies.

Importantly, one of the five DCA studies (NCT01029925), an open label Phase II trial designed to determine the response rate, safety and tolerability of oral DCA in patients with metastatic breast cancer and advanced stage non-small cell lung cancer (NSCLC), was closed by the Data Safety and Monitoring Board (DSMB) that was monitoring it due to the lack of clinical benefit observed along with higher than expected risk and safety concerns (two of the seven patients enrolled died suddenly) [107].

The discovery that several common and lethal cancers harbor mutations in IDH1 and IDH2 (section 3) boosted the interest of pharmaceutical companies in cancer metabolic interventions. Presently, two inhibitors targeting the oncologically mutated forms of IDH1 and IDH2, AG-120 and AG-221, respectively, are being tested in advanced solid tumors (NCT02073994 and NCT02273739, respectively) and advanced hematologic malignancies (NCT02074839 and NCT01915498, respectively). Importantly, AG-120 is being tested specifically in patients with IDH1 mutations and AG-221 in patients with IDH2 mutations. Considering that these mutated forms are not present in normal cells, they fulfill one the requirements of an ideal drug target: its uniqueness to cancer cells. It remains to be proved whether, as is the case with the Abelson kinase, they fulfill the second, *i.e.*, whether they play an essential role in these cells.

Early results from the Phase I clinical trial of AG-120 in AML patients with IDH1 mutations are encouraging, showing that the drug is well tolerated and has clinical activity [108]. Results from the Phase I trial of AG-221 in patients with advanced hematologic malignancies harboring IDH2 mutations are also encouraging [109, 110].

As can be appreciated in Table **3**, the anticancer activity of metformin is currently being assessed for many different cancers in a large number of clinical trials. Metformin has been used for decades as a first-line treatment for type II (non-insulin-dependent) diabetes mellitus by over 120 million people worldwide. Interest in this drug in the context of cancer therapy spurred from retrospective studies clearly showing a significant reduction (by ca. 30%) in cancer incidence and cancer-specific mortality across many tumor types in diabetic patients treated with this antihyperglycemic agent [111 - 113]. In addition, metformin fulfills many criteria for an ideal drug, such as a low cost, a well-characterized pharmacodynamic profile and clinical safety. Indeed, the safety of this drug in nondiabetic patients has already been demonstrated in clinical trials, such as that evaluating its efficacy in patients with castration-resistant prostate cancer (CRPC) (NCT01243385) [114].

At the organismal level, this biguanide exerts its well-described antihyper-glycemic effects by downregulating liver gluconeogenesis and stimulating the uptake of glucose in skeletal muscle. Whether the observed anticancer and cancer preventive activities result from whole-body systemic changes (*e.g.*, reduced blood glucose and insulin levels), from alterations produced in individual cancer cells or from a combination of the two remains to be elucidated. The molecular mechanisms underlying the effects of metformin are not fully understood. It has been known since the early 2000s that metformin activates AMP-activated protein kinase (AMPK) [115]. This serine/threonine protein kinase is generally regarded as a critical energy sensor, ensuring proper cellular function under conditions of energy restriction, namely by upregulating catabolism and downregulating anabolic processes and, ultimately, growth [116]. As this kinase is activated by elevated AMP:ATP ratios, it is conceivable that AMPK activation by metformin might be an indirect effect of a disrupted energy metabolism produced by metformin. In fact, there is some evidence that it inhibits both HK [117, 118] and complex I of the ETC (Fig. **1**) [119]. Inhibition of HK might have the potential to reverse the Warburg effect. This potential might be further reinforced by metformin's capacity to reduce hypoxia-induced HIF stabilization [120] and, ultimately, downregulate the expression of all glycolytic genes, as well as those encoding LDH, GLUT1, GLUT3 and PDK1 (section 3). Thus, metformin might be particular effective against cancer cells experiencing hypoxia. On the other hand, metformin's capacity to inhibit complex I may account for its efficacy against tumors with a strong reliance on aerobic respiration for the generation of metabolic energy. It must be noted, though, that translations of *in vitro* findings to *in vivo* situations must be done with care, as the concentrations used in the *in vitro* studies are several orders of magnitude higher than those found in the plasma and peripheral tissues of diabetic patients under metformin treatment [121].

Preclinical studies suggest other mechanisms by which metformin might exert its anticancer effects, namely cell cycle arrest (through a reduction of cyclin D1 protein levels) [122, 123], but a discussion of these mechanisms is out of the scope of this chapter.

Although there are now 13 published results of clinical trials evaluating the anticancer potential of metformin [114, 124 - 135], it is too early to draw any conclusions, as all but one refer to Phase I and/or Phase II studies. In fact, only four Phase II/III or Phase III have been launched so far. One is ongoing (NCT01101438), two are recruiting (NCT02065687 and NCT02040376) and there is also one study that is not yet recruiting (NCT02360618). Early results from the ongoing study, a Phase III randomized trial of metformin *versus* placebo in early stage breast cancer, showed that metformin significantly improved weight and levels of insulin, glucose, leptin and C-reactive protein at 6 months [127].

Fig. (**3**) summarizes the targets (metabolic pathway/process and biomolecule) for the drugs whose clinical trials have just been discussed.

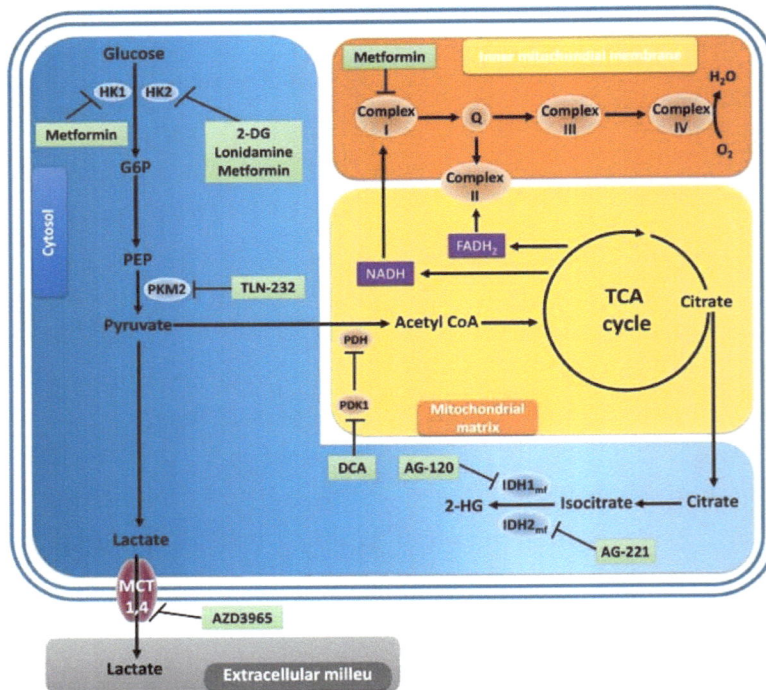

Fig. (3). Targets of drugs with the potential to revert the Warburg effect that have entered clinical trials as putative cancer drugs. The potential of these drugs to revert the Warburg effect emanates from their ability to impact on glycolysis (2-DG, lonidamine, metformin and TLN-232), lactate extrusion (AZD3965), the conversion of pyruvate to acetyl CoA (DCA), the TCA cycle (AG-120 and AG-221; indirect action, through substrate depletion) and OXPHOS (metformin). The number of arrows in the different pathways represented does not reflect the corresponding number of steps, neither do the sizes of these arrows (for a complete description of the pathways, see Fig. (**1**). Blocked lines indicate inhibition. Acetyl CoA, acetyl coenzyme A; 2-DG, 2-deoxy-D-glucose; DCA, dicholoroacetate; G6P, glucose-6-phosphate; HK, hexokinase; 2-HG, 2-hydroxyglutarate; IDH$_{mf}$, isocitrate dehydrogenase mutated form; MCT, monocarboxylate transporter; OXPHOS, oxidative phosphorylation; PDH, pyruvate dehydrogenase; PDK, pyruvate dehydrogenase kinase; PEP, phosphoenolpyruvate; PK, pyruvate kinase; Q, ubiquinone; TCA, tricarboxylic acid.

Another type of metabolic cancer therapy being tested in clinical trials is based on specific diets aimed at reducing blood glucose levels and/or by-passing glycolysis. This approach was suggested by two different, but possibly interconnected, observations. One of these was the frequently observed association between metabolic conditions characterized by elevated blood glucose levels (*e.g.*, hyperglycemia, diabetes and obesity) and an increased risk of cancer development and/or a poor prognosis for cancer patients [136, 137]. The other observation was an inhibition of the growth of tumors implanted in mice when these animals were subjected to caloric restriction.

The first evidence of a connection between food intake and cancer growth was reported in 1909, *i.e.*, prior to Warburg's seminal studies on cancer metabolism. This study showed that transplanted tumors did not grow in mice under caloric restriction [138], an effect that has since been repeatedly observed [139, 140]. Evidence from *in vitro* studies, animal model studies and a few clinical case reports suggests that, in humans, lowering the intake of carbohydrates might also have beneficial effects on cancer treatment and prevention [137], but this causal link remains to be firmly established [139]. In fact, it is not always easy to convince patients, most of them already in an extremely debilitated state, to adhere and follow restrictive diets which are often associated with weight loss and cachexia [139].

The molecular basis of these associations between cancer and metabolic conditions and/or diet is still elusive, but it might be related, at least to some extent, to the metabolic plasticity of some cell types, enabling them to adjust their metabolism to different glucose availabilities, namely through the use of ketone bodies as a preferential energy source, which circumvents glycolysis (section 2). This metabolic plasticity is the rationale behind several diets, namely the so-called ketogenic diets and caloric restriction.

In the ketogenic diet, the shift to the preferential use of ketone bodies is produced through a severely reduced percentage of dietary carbohydrates, while that of fatty acids is greatly increased. In caloric restriction and fasting, the use of alternative fuels is promoted by diminishing the overall energy intake, thus depleting the carbohydrate intracellular reservoirs [141]. Another principle underlying fasting diets is the so-called differential stress resistance. Very briefly, fasting is thought to protect normal cells against oxidative stress, whereas this protective effects is not observed for most of cancer cells [139].

Table **4** summarizes past and current clinical trials aimed at evaluating the potential of these types of diets in cancer therapy. As can be appreciated, most of them are still recruiting patients.

Table 4. Clinical trials assessing the anticancer potential of distinct dietary interventions targeting the Warburg effect.

Dietary intervention	Indication[1]	Phase	Status	ClinicalTrials.gov identifier	Results (whenever published)
Ketogenic diet	Glioblastoma multiforme	Undisclosed	Recruiting	NCT01535911	[145]
		I	Recruiting	NCT01865162	
		I/II	Recruiting	NCT02046187	
		Undisclosed	Recruiting	NCT02286167	
		II	Recruiting	NCT02302235	
	Recurrent glioblastoma	I	Completed	NCT00575146	[144]
		Undisclosed	Recruiting	NCT01754350	
	Head and neck cancer	I	Recruiting	NCT01975766	
	Pancreatic cancer	I	Suspended[2]	NCT01419483	
	Non-small cell lung cancer	I	Suspended[2]	NCT01419587	
Low carbohydrate diet	Breast, colon, cervical, uterine and ovarian Cancer	Undisclosed	Completed	NCT00444054	[148]
Fasting mimicking diet	Breast cancer	II/III	Recruiting	NCT02126449	
Fasting	Breast and ovarian cancer	Undisclosed	Recruiting	NCT01954836	
	Breast cancer	I/II	Recruiting	NCT02379585	

(Table 4) contd.....

Dietary intervention	Indication[1]	Phase	Status	ClinicalTrials.gov identifier	Results (whenever published)
Caloric restriction	Breast cancer	Undisclosed	Recruiting	NCT01819233	

[1] For more information, see Table **1**. [2] This trial has been suspended pending protocol amendment.

It is worth noting that, with one single exception, all clinical trials of ketogenic diets have been designed to be evaluated in glioblastomas. The rationale behind this bias is likely related to the differential capacity of normal and cancer brain cells to use ketone bodies, which is much reduced in the case of the latter [142, 143]. This inability, which has been linked to inactivating mutations in genes coding for the enzymes involved in the catabolism of ketone bodies, namely, β-ketoacyl-CoA transferase (Fig. **1**) [142], should make brain cancer cells unable to compensate for the reduction in glucose levels that this type of diet might induce, ultimately translating into cell death. The fact that this type of diet has already proven its value in the treatment of other neurological disorders, especially refractory childhood epilepsy [143], may also have contributed to the above-mentioned bias.

Of the two clinical trials already completed, one was a prospective trial aimed at assessing the feasibility and safety of a ketogenic diet in patients with glioblastoma (NCT00575146). According to its sponsors, the ketogenic diet under evaluation is feasible and safe, but did not show significant activity when used as a single agent [144]. The sponsors further hypothesized that this lack of significant activity might be related to the fact that, although most patients had stable ketosis, a significant reduction of blood glucose levels was not achieved. Similar results were obtained for two patients enrolled in an ongoing clinical trial (NCT01535911), as described in a recently published case report [145]. This publication reviewed the literature available on the use of ketogenic diets for the treatment of primary aggressive brain cancer [145].

In the case of the clinical trials testing the anticancer potential of the other diets described in Table **4**, the bias is mostly towards breast cancer. Two interrelated observations might account for this fact: caloric restriction was found to consistently reduce circulating sex hormones in laboratory animals [146] and the suggestion that alterations in the metabolism of these hormones might mediate the association between excess body weight or increases in abdominal fat and the increased risk of developing breast cancer (as well as endometrium and colon cancers) [147].

The second of the completed trials was a pilot study aimed at assessing the feasibility of a low carbohydrate diet in patients with advanced breast, colon, cervical, uterine and ovarian cancer (NCT00444054). Only preliminary data, presented in 2012 and relative to ten patients, is currently available. Stabilization or a partial remission of the disease was obtained in five patients, and a correlation was observed between the extent of ketosis and these beneficial effects [148].

CONCLUDING REMARKS

Neglected for many decades, the Warburg effect is now repeatedly presented as a promising target for cancer therapy. Nonetheless, as this review shows, only a small number of pharmaceutical companies have ventured into this area and only a few of the possible approaches have already entered clinical development. From the very small number of drugs that have reached Phase III clinical trials, it is still not possible to conclude whether the promise will materialize. Future successes will undoubtedly depend critically on a more detailed and accurate definition of the true metabolic makeup of tumors than that currently available and on the elucidation of which of the established metabolic perturbations actually drive malignancy.

It is rather ironic that, although there is now a general consensus as to the relevance of Warburg's findings, the actual findings and concepts developed by Warburg are rarely discussed, at least in exact terms. For instance, it is frequently stated or implied in the literature that, save for the production of the oncometabolite 2-HG, the energy metabolism of cancer cells is simply that of any normal (*i.e.*, non-transformed) highly proliferating cell [88, 149, 150]. However, Warburg's seminal experiments clearly showed that, while normal proliferating cells, such as those of the chick embryo, exhibited high rates of lactic acid fermentation in the absence of oxygen, their rates of "aerobic glycolysis" were very low, *i.e.*, they produced very little lactate in the presence of oxygen.

It must be added that the quest for metabolic targets sits on somewhat weak foundations. Indeed, since the "molecular revolution" of the 1950s, biochemical research has focused mostly on genetics and molecular biology, whereas metabolic pathways were "for many years relegated to the backbenches of biochemistry lecture halls", as put in a 2012 editorial of Nature Reviews Molecular Cell Biology. This is well exemplified in the general misconception found in the literature concerning the nature of "aerobic glycolysis". At the time of Warburg's seminal findings, the term glycolysis referred specifically to the production of lactate from glucose, *i.e.*, to what is now known as lactic acid fermentation, whereas the term fermentation was restricted to alcohol fermentation. In fact, as the reactions of these two energy-yielding processes were still mostly unknown, it was not appreciated that they share the first ten steps, *i.e.*, the conversion of glucose to pyruvate (Fig. **1**). Thus, Warburg's aerobic glycolysis referred to lactic acid fermentation in the presence of oxygen and should not be mistaken for glycolysis, a component of both lactic acid fermentation and aerobic respiration. This distinction may prove to have important implications in terms of cancer metabolic therapies, as the inhibition of glycolysis compromises not only lactic acid fermentation, but also aerobic respiration, whereas the inhibition of the last step of lactic acid fermentation, *i.e.*, the reduction of pyruvate to lactate, does not compromise the latter.

It is also important to bear in mind that, although cancer cells rely more strongly on fermentation than their normal counterparts, there are certain types of cells in our organism (*e.g.*, erythrocytes; section 2) that have also a strong reliance, or even a complete reliance, on fermentation. Therefore, the inhibition of fermentation may produce serious side effects. However, one cannot exclude the possibility of therapeutic regimens whose side effects are reversible and well-tolerated by the patient.

To repeat the remarkable success of imatinib, it will be important to identify targets that are both unique and fundamental to the cancer cell. Overexpressed enzymes might not be good targets, as they are also present in normal cells. To this day, perhaps the most promising discovery in the context of metabolic cancer therapy was the neomorphic activity of the mutated isoforms of IDH1 and IDH2. Therapies aimed at these targets are currently being tested clinically and the outcomes of these clinical trials will hopefully give us important information as to whether the mutated enzymes play a crucial role in carcinogenesis. Still, it is important to bear in mind that the IDH1 and IDH2 mutations have only been found in certain types of cancer. This will, in all likelihood, be the case for most, if not all, cancer-associated metabolic alterations, when examined at the molecular level. Thus, as is the case with other types of personalized, precision cancer therapies, the success of therapies targeting the Warburg effect will, in all likelihood, depend on the identification of the patient's specific pattern of DNA mutations and other alterations, such as epigenetic alterations, as well as on his/hers specific metabolic phenotype.

NOTES

[1]Certain cancer drugs, such as methotrexate, tamoxifen and flutamine, have more than 20 commercial names. For these and other cancer drugs commercialized under more than two different brand names, only one US brand name and one non-US brand name will be indicated.

CONFLICT OF INTEREST

The authors confirm that they have no conflict of interest to declare for this publication.

ACKNOWLEDGEMENTS

AMU research is supported by Fundação para a Ciência e a Tecnologia (FCT) (grant UID/MULTI/00070/2013) and by Centro de Investigação em Meio Ambiente, Genética e Oncobiologia (CIMAGO) (Grants 26/07 and 16/12).

ABBREVIATIONS

ALL   = Acute lymphoblastic leukemia
ATP   = Adenosine triphosphate
CML   = Chronic myelogenous leukemia
CoA   = Coenzyme A

DCA	=	Dichloroacetate
2-DG	=	2-Deoxy-ᴅ-glucose
DHFR	=	Dihydrofolate reductase
ETC	=	Mitochondrial electron transport chain
FDA	=	Food and drug administration
^{18}FDG–PET	=	^{18}F-Deoxyglucose positron emission tomography
FH	=	Fumarate hydratase
GLUT	=	Glucose transporter
2-HG	=	2-Hydroxyglutarate
HIF-1	=	Hypoxia-inducible transcription factor 1
HK	=	Hexokinase
IDH	=	Isocitrate dehydrogenase
INF	=	Interferon
α-KG	=	α-Ketoglutarate
LDH	=	Lactate dehydrogenase
NSCLC	=	Non-small cell lung cancer
OXPHOS	=	Oxidative phosphorylation
PDH	=	Pyruvate dehydrogenase
PDK	=	Pyruvate dehydrogenase kinase
PFK-1	=	6-Phosphofructo-1-kinase
PK	=	Pyruvate kinase
RNAi	=	RNA interference
SDH	=	Succinate dehydrogenase
TCA	=	Tricarboxylic acid
WHO	=	World health organization

REFERENCES

[1]   The American Cancer Society. The history of cancer 2010. Available from: www.cancer.org/acs/groups/cid/documents/webcontent/002048-pdf.pdf. [March 2011]

[2]   Hajdu SI. Greco-Roman thought about cancer. Cancer 2004; 100(10): 2048-51. [http://dx.doi.org/10.1002/cncr.20198] [PMID: 15139045]

[3]   Papac RJ. Origins of cancer therapy. Yale J Biol Med 2001; 74(6): 391-8. [PMID: 11922186]

[4]   Gilman A. The initial clinical trial of nitrogen mustard. Am J Surg 1963; 105: 574-8. [http://dx.doi.org/10.1016/0002-9610(63)90232-0] [PMID: 13947966]

[5]   Wills L, Clutterbuck PW, Evans BD. A new factor in the production and cure of macrocytic anaemias and its relation to other haemopoietic principles curative in pernicious anaemia. Biochem J 1937; 31(11): 2136-47.
[http://dx.doi.org/10.1042/bj0312136] [PMID: 16746555]

[6]   Farber S, Diamond LK. Temporary remissions in acute leukemia in children produced by folic acid antagonist, 4-aminopteroyl-glutamic acid. N Engl J Med 1948; 238(23): 787-93.
[http://dx.doi.org/10.1056/NEJM194806032382301] [PMID: 18860765]

[7]   Chabner BA, Roberts TG Jr. Timeline: Chemotherapy and the war on cancer. Nat Rev Cancer 2005; 5(1): 65-72.
[http://dx.doi.org/10.1038/nrc1529] [PMID: 15630416]

[8]   Hitchings GH, Elion GB. The chemistry and biochemistry of purine analogs. Ann N Y Acad Sci 1954; 60(2): 195-9.
[http://dx.doi.org/10.1111/j.1749-6632.1954.tb40008.x] [PMID: 14350523]

[9]   Skipper HE, Thomson JR, Elion GB, Hitchings GH. Observations on the anticancer activity of 6-mercaptopurine. Cancer Res 1954; 14(4): 294-8.
[PMID: 13160953]

[10]   Johnson IS, Armstrong JG, Gorman M, Burnett JP Jr. The Vinca Alkaloids: A New Class of Oncolytic Agents. Cancer Res 1963; 23: 1390-427.
[PMID: 14070392]

[11]   Oberlies NH, Kroll DJ. Camptothecin and taxol: historic achievements in natural products research. J Nat Prod 2004; 67(2): 129-35.
[http://dx.doi.org/10.1021/np030498t] [PMID: 14987046]

[12]   Pratt WB, Pratt WB. The anticancer drugs. 2nd ed.. New York: Oxford University Press 1994; p. viii, 352s.

[13]   Povirk LF, Shuker DE. DNA damage and mutagenesis induced by nitrogen mustards. Mutat Res 1994; 318(3): 205-26.
[http://dx.doi.org/10.1016/0165-1110(94)90015-9] [PMID: 7527485]

[14]   Huennekens FM. The methotrexate story: a paradigm for development of cancer chemotherapeutic agents. Adv Enzyme Regul 1994; 34: 397-419.
[http://dx.doi.org/10.1016/0065-2571(94)90025-6] [PMID: 7942284]

[15]   Jordan MA. Mechanism of action of antitumor drugs that interact with microtubules and tubulin. Curr Med Chem Anticancer Agents 2002; 2(1): 1-17.
[http://dx.doi.org/10.2174/1568011023354290] [PMID: 12678749]

[16]   Liu LF, Desai SD, Li TK, Mao Y, Sun M, Sim SP. Mechanism of action of camptothecin. Ann N Y Acad Sci 2000; 922: 1-10.
[http://dx.doi.org/10.1111/j.1749-6632.2000.tb07020.x] [PMID: 11193884]

[17]   Wang JC. Cellular roles of DNA topoisomerases: a molecular perspective. Nat Rev Mol Cell Biol 2002; 3(6): 430-40.
[http://dx.doi.org/10.1038/nrm831] [PMID: 12042765]

[18]   Urruticoechea A, Alemany R, Balart J, Villanueva A, Viñals F, Capellá G. Recent advances in cancer
        therapy: an overview. Curr Pharm Des 2010; 16(1): 3-10.
        [http://dx.doi.org/10.2174/138161210789941847] [PMID: 20214614]

[19]   Hanahan D, Weinberg RA. Hallmarks of cancer: the next generation. Cell 2011; 144(5): 646-74.
        [http://dx.doi.org/10.1016/j.cell.2011.02.013] [PMID: 21376230]

[20]   Hanahan D, Weinberg RA. The hallmarks of cancer. Cell 2000; 100(1): 57-70.
        [http://dx.doi.org/10.1016/S0092-8674(00)81683-9] [PMID: 10647931]

[21]   Kamb A, Wee S, Lengauer C. Why is cancer drug discovery so difficult? Nat Rev Drug Discov 2007;
        6(2): 115-20.
        [http://dx.doi.org/10.1038/nrd2155] [PMID: 17159925]

[22]   Devi GR. siRNA-based approaches in cancer therapy. Cancer Gene Ther 2006; 13(9): 819-29.
        [http://dx.doi.org/10.1038/sj.cgt.7700931] [PMID: 16424918]

[23]   Rothschild SI. microRNA therapies in cancer. Mol Cell Ther 2014; 2(1): 7.
        [http://dx.doi.org/10.1186/2052-8426-2-7] [PMID: 26056576]

[24]   Dao TL, Huggins C. Bilateral adrenalectomy in the treatment of cancer of the breast. AMA Arch Surg
        1955; 71(5): 645-57.
        [http://dx.doi.org/10.1001/archsurg.1955.01270170003002] [PMID: 13268210]

[25]   Pearson OH, Ray BS. Results of hypophysectomy in the treatment of metastatic mammary carcinoma.
        Cancer 1959; 12(1): 85-92.
        [http://dx.doi.org/10.1002/1097-0142(195901/02)12:1<85::AID-CNCR2820120114>3.0.CO;2-G]
        [PMID: 13618860]

[26]   Jordan VC. Tamoxifen: A most unlikely pioneering medicine. Nat Rev Drug Discov 2003; 2(3): 205-
        13.
        [http://dx.doi.org/10.1038/nrd1031] [PMID: 12612646]

[27]   Belardelli F, Ferrantini M, Proietti E, Kirkwood JM. Interferon-alpha in tumor immunity and
        immunotherapy. Cytokine Growth Factor Rev 2002; 13(2): 119-34.
        [http://dx.doi.org/10.1016/S1359-6101(01)00022-3] [PMID: 11900988]

[28]   Adams GP, Weiner LM. Monoclonal antibody therapy of cancer. Nat Biotechnol 2005; 23(9): 1147-
        57.
        [http://dx.doi.org/10.1038/nbt1137] [PMID: 16151408]

[29]   Maloney DG. Mechanism of action of rituximab. Anticancer Drugs 2001; 12 (Suppl. 2): S1-4.
        [PMID: 11508930]

[30]   Nahta R, Esteva FJ. Trastuzumab: Triumphs and tribulations. Oncogene 2007; 26(25): 3637-43.
        [http://dx.doi.org/10.1038/sj.onc.1210379] [PMID: 17530017]

[31]   Hsieh AC, Moasser MM. Targeting HER proteins in cancer therapy and the role of the non-target
        HER3. Br J Cancer 2007; 97(4): 453-7.
        [http://dx.doi.org/10.1038/sj.bjc.6603910] [PMID: 17667926]

[32]   Reichert JM. Marketed therapeutic antibodies compendium. MAbs 2012; 4(3): 413-5.
        [http://dx.doi.org/10.4161/mabs.19931] [PMID: 22531442]

[33]   Scott AM, Wolchok JD, Old LJ. Antibody therapy of cancer. Nat Rev Cancer 2012; 12(4): 278-87.
       [http://dx.doi.org/10.1038/nrc3236] [PMID: 22437872]

[34]   Mellman I, Coukos G, Dranoff G. Cancer immunotherapy comes of age. Nature 2011; 480(7378): 480-9.
       [http://dx.doi.org/10.1038/nature10673] [PMID: 22193102]

[35]   Groffen J, Stephenson JR, Heisterkamp N, de Klein A, Bartram CR, Grosveld G. Philadelphia chromosomal breakpoints are clustered within a limited region, bcr, on chromosome 22. Cell 1984; 36(1): 93-9.
       [http://dx.doi.org/10.1016/0092-8674(84)90077-1] [PMID: 6319012]

[36]   Lugo TG, Pendergast AM, Muller AJ, Witte ON. Tyrosine kinase activity and transformation potency of bcr-abl oncogene products. Science 1990; 247(4946): 1079-82.
       [http://dx.doi.org/10.1126/science.2408149] [PMID: 2408149]

[37]   Rowley JD. Letter: A new consistent chromosomal abnormality in chronic myelogenous leukaemia identified by quinacrine fluorescence and Giemsa staining. Nature 1973; 243(5405): 290-3.
       [http://dx.doi.org/10.1038/243290a0] [PMID: 4126434]

[38]   Druker BJ, Talpaz M, Resta DJ, *et al.* Efficacy and safety of a specific inhibitor of the BCR-ABL tyrosine kinase in chronic myeloid leukemia. N Engl J Med 2001; 344(14): 1031-7.
       [http://dx.doi.org/10.1056/NEJM200104053441401] [PMID: 11287972]

[39]   Urbano AM, Ferreira LM, Cerveira JF, Rodrigues CF, Alpoim MC. DNA Damage, Repair and Misrepair in Cancer and in Cancer Therapy. DNA Repair and Human Health . 2011. [Internet]. InTech.

[40]   Krebs HA. The Pasteur effect and the relations between respiration and fermentation. Essays Biochem 1972; 8: 1-34.
       [PMID: 4265190]

[41]   Park HJ, Lyons JC, Ohtsubo T, Song CW. Acidic environment causes apoptosis by increasing caspase activity. Br J Cancer 1999; 80(12): 1892-7.
       [http://dx.doi.org/10.1038/sj.bjc.6690617] [PMID: 10471036]

[42]   Williams AC, Collard TJ, Paraskeva C. An acidic environment leads to p53 dependent induction of apoptosis in human adenoma and carcinoma cell lines: implications for clonal selection during colorectal carcinogenesis. Oncogene 1999; 18(21): 3199-204.
       [http://dx.doi.org/10.1038/sj.onc.1202660] [PMID: 10359525]

[43]   Ramaiah A. Pasteur effect and phosphofructokinase. Curr Top Cell Regul 1974; 8(0): 297-345.
       [http://dx.doi.org/10.1016/B978-0-12-152808-9.50014-6] [PMID: 4370999]

[44]   Sola-Penna M, Da Silva D, Coelho WS, Marinho-Carvalho MM, Zancan P. Regulation of mammalian muscle type 6-phosphofructo-1-kinase and its implication for the control of the metabolism. IUBMB Life 2010; 62(11): 791-6.
       [http://dx.doi.org/10.1002/iub.393] [PMID: 21117169]

[45]   Fell D. Understanding the control of metabolism. UK: Portland Press Ltd. 1997.

[46]   Kim JW, Tchernyshyov I, Semenza GL, Dang CV. HIF-1-mediated expression of pyruvate dehydrogenase kinase: a metabolic switch required for cellular adaptation to hypoxia. Cell Metab

2006; 3(3): 177-85.
[http://dx.doi.org/10.1016/j.cmet.2006.02.002] [PMID: 16517405]

[47]   Kolobova E, Tuganova A, Boulatnikov I, Popov KM. Regulation of pyruvate dehydrogenase activity through phosphorylation at multiple sites. Biochem J 2001; 358(Pt 1): 69-77.
[http://dx.doi.org/10.1042/bj3580069] [PMID: 11485553]

[48]   Warburg O. The metabolism of tumors. London: Constable & Co. Ltd 1930.

[49]   Racker E. Bioenergetics and the problem of tumor growth. Am Sci 1972; 60(1): 56-63.
[PMID: 4332766]

[50]   Krebs HA. Otto Warburg: Cell Physiologist, Biochemist and Eccentric. New York: Oxford University Press 1981; p. 141. Available at: http://trove.nla.gov.au/version/30605906

[51]   Warburg O, Minami S. Versuche an Überlebendem Carcinom-gewebe. Klin Wochenschr 1923; 2(17): 776-7.
[http://dx.doi.org/10.1007/BF01712130]

[52]   Cori CF, Cori GT. The carbohydrate metabolism of tumors: I. The free sugar, lactic acid, and glycogen content of malignant tumors. J Biol Chem 1925; 64(1): 11-22.

[53]   Cori CF, Cori GT. The Carbohydrate Metabolism Of Tumors: Ii. Changes In The Sugar, Lactic Acid, And Co2-Combining Power Of Blood Passing Through A Tumor. J Biol Chem 1925; 65(2): 397-405.

[54]   Warburg O, Wind F, Negelein E. The Metabolism of Tumors in the Body. J Gen Physiol 1927; 8(6): 519-30.
[http://dx.doi.org/10.1085/jgp.8.6.519] [PMID: 19872213]

[55]   Thomlinson RH, Gray LH. The histological structure of some human lung cancers and the possible implications for radiotherapy. Br J Cancer 1955; 9(4): 539-49.
[http://dx.doi.org/10.1038/bjc.1955.55] [PMID: 13304213]

[56]   Semenza GL. HIF-1 mediates metabolic responses to intratumoral hypoxia and oncogenic mutations. J Clin Invest 2013; 123(9): 3664-71.
[http://dx.doi.org/10.1172/JCI67230] [PMID: 23999440]

[57]   Brizel DM, Schroeder T, Scher RL, *et al.* Elevated tumor lactate concentrations predict for an increased risk of metastases in head-and-neck cancer. Int J Radiat Oncol Biol Phys 2001; 51(2): 349-53.
[http://dx.doi.org/10.1016/S0360-3016(01)01630-3] [PMID: 11567808]

[58]   Warburg O. On the origin of cancer cells. Science 1956; 123(3191): 309-14.
[http://dx.doi.org/10.1126/science.123.3191.309] [PMID: 13298683]

[59]   Kelloff GJ, Hoffman JM, Johnson B, *et al.* Progress and promise of FDG-PET imaging for cancer patient management and oncologic drug development. Clin Cancer Res 2005; 11(8): 2785-808.
[http://dx.doi.org/10.1158/1078-0432.CCR-04-2626] [PMID: 15837727]

[60]   Semenza GL, Wang GL. A nuclear factor induced by hypoxia *via* de novo protein synthesis binds to the human erythropoietin gene enhancer at a site required for transcriptional activation. Mol Cell Biol 1992; 12(12): 5447-54.
[http://dx.doi.org/10.1128/MCB.12.12.5447] [PMID: 1448077]

[61]   Semenza GL. HIF-1: upstream and downstream of cancer metabolism. Curr Opin Genet Dev 2010; 20(1): 51-6.
[http://dx.doi.org/10.1016/j.gde.2009.10.009] [PMID: 19942427]

[62]   Thompson CB. Rethinking the regulation of cellular metabolism. Cold Spring Harb Symp Quant Biol 2011; 76: 23-9.
[http://dx.doi.org/10.1101/sqb.2012.76.010496] [PMID: 22429931]

[63]   Liu X, Kim CN, Yang J, Jemmerson R, Wang X. Induction of apoptotic program in cell-free extracts: requirement for dATP and cytochrome c. Cell 1996; 86(1): 147-57.
[http://dx.doi.org/10.1016/S0092-8674(00)80085-9] [PMID: 8689682]

[64]   Shim H, Dolde C, Lewis BC, *et al.* c-Myc transactivation of LDH-A: implications for tumor metabolism and growth. Proc Natl Acad Sci USA 1997; 94(13): 6658-63.
[http://dx.doi.org/10.1073/pnas.94.13.6658] [PMID: 9192621]

[65]   Zörnig M, Evan GI. Cell cycle: on target with Myc. Curr Biol 1996; 6(12): 1553-6.
[http://dx.doi.org/10.1016/S0960-9822(02)70769-0] [PMID: 8994810]

[66]   Dang CV. MYC on the path to cancer. Cell 2012; 149(1): 22-35.
[http://dx.doi.org/10.1016/j.cell.2012.03.003] [PMID: 22464321]

[67]   Levine AJ, Puzio-Kuter AM. The control of the metabolic switch in cancers by oncogenes and tumor suppressor genes. Science 2010; 330(6009): 1340-4.
[http://dx.doi.org/10.1126/science.1193494] [PMID: 21127244]

[68]   Vogelstein B, Lane D, Levine AJ. Surfing the p53 network. Nature 2000; 408(6810): 307-10.
[http://dx.doi.org/10.1038/35042675] [PMID: 11099028]

[69]   Schwartzenberg-Bar-Yoseph F, Armoni M, Karnieli E. The tumor suppressor p53 down-regulates glucose transporters GLUT1 and GLUT4 gene expression. Cancer Res 2004; 64(7): 2627-33.
[http://dx.doi.org/10.1158/0008-5472.CAN-03-0846] [PMID: 15059920]

[70]   Ying H, Kimmelman AC, Lyssiotis CA, *et al.* Oncogenic Kras maintains pancreatic tumors through regulation of anabolic glucose metabolism. Cell 2012; 149(3): 656-70.
[http://dx.doi.org/10.1016/j.cell.2012.01.058] [PMID: 22541435]

[71]   Yun J, Rago C, Cheong I, *et al.* Glucose deprivation contributes to the development of KRAS pathway mutations in tumor cells. Science 2009; 325(5947): 1555-9.
[http://dx.doi.org/10.1126/science.1174229] [PMID: 19661383]

[72]   Gottlieb E, Tomlinson IP. Mitochondrial tumour suppressors: A genetic and biochemical update. Nat Rev Cancer 2005; 5(11): 857-66.
[http://dx.doi.org/10.1038/nrc1737] [PMID: 16327764]

[73]   Borger DR, Tanabe KK, Fan KC, *et al.* Frequent mutation of isocitrate dehydrogenase (IDH)1 and IDH2 in cholangiocarcinoma identified through broad-based tumor genotyping. Oncologist 2012; 17(1): 72-9.
[http://dx.doi.org/10.1634/theoncologist.2011-0386] [PMID: 22180306]

[74]   Parsons DW, Jones S, Zhang X, *et al.* An integrated genomic analysis of human glioblastoma multiforme. Science 2008; 321(5897): 1807-12.
[http://dx.doi.org/10.1126/science.1164382] [PMID: 18772396]

[75] Razumilava N, Gores GJ. Cholangiocarcinoma. Lancet 2014; 383(9935): 2168-79.
   [http://dx.doi.org/10.1016/S0140-6736(13)61903-0] [PMID: 24581682]

[76] Wang P, Dong Q, Zhang C, *et al.* Mutations in isocitrate dehydrogenase 1 and 2 occur frequently in intrahepatic cholangiocarcinomas and share hypermethylation targets with glioblastomas. Oncogene 2013; 32(25): 3091-100.
   [http://dx.doi.org/10.1038/onc.2012.315] [PMID: 22824796]

[77] Ward PS, Patel J, Wise DR, *et al.* The common feature of leukemia-associated IDH1 and IDH2 mutations is a neomorphic enzyme activity converting alpha-ketoglutarate to 2-hydroxyglutarate. Cancer Cell 2010; 17(3): 225-34.
   [http://dx.doi.org/10.1016/j.ccr.2010.01.020] [PMID: 20171147]

[78] Dang L, White DW, Gross S, *et al.* Cancer-associated IDH1 mutations produce 2-hydroxyglutarate. Nature 2009; 462(7274): 739-44.
   [http://dx.doi.org/10.1038/nature08617] [PMID: 19935646]

[79] Miyata S, Urabe M, Gomi A, *et al.* An R132H mutation in isocitrate dehydrogenase 1 enhances p21 expression and inhibits phosphorylation of retinoblastoma protein in glioma cells. Neurol Med Chir (Tokyo) 2013; 53(10): 645-54.
   [http://dx.doi.org/10.2176/nmc.oa2012-0409] [PMID: 24077277]

[80] Markert CL, Møller F. Multiple forms of enzymes: tissue, ontogenetic, and species specific patterns. Proc Natl Acad Sci USA 1959; 45(5): 753-63.
   [http://dx.doi.org/10.1073/pnas.45.5.753] [PMID: 16590440]

[81] Schapira F, Dreyfus JC, Schapira G. Anomaly of aldolase in primary liver cancer. Nature 1963; 200: 995-7.
   [http://dx.doi.org/10.1038/200995a0] [PMID: 14097745]

[82] Shatton JB, Morris HP, Weinhouse S. Kinetic, electrophoretic, and chromatographic studies on glucose-ATP phosphotransferases in rat hepatomas. Cancer Res 1969; 29(6): 1161-72.
   [PMID: 4307780]

[83] Weinhouse S. Glycolysis, respiration, and anomalous gene expression in experimental hepatomas: G.H.A. Clowes memorial lecture. Cancer Res 1972; 32(10): 2007-16.
   [PMID: 4343003]

[84] Wolf A, Agnihotri S, Micallef J, *et al.* Hexokinase 2 is a key mediator of aerobic glycolysis and promotes tumor growth in human glioblastoma multiforme. J Exp Med 2011; 208(2): 313-26.
   [http://dx.doi.org/10.1084/jem.20101470] [PMID: 21242296]

[85] Christofk HR, Vander Heiden MG, Harris MH, *et al.* The M2 splice isoform of pyruvate kinase is important for cancer metabolism and tumour growth. Nature 2008; 452(7184): 230-3.
   [http://dx.doi.org/10.1038/nature06734] [PMID: 18337823]

[86] Schulze A, Harris AL. How cancer metabolism is tuned for proliferation and vulnerable to disruption. Nature 2012; 491(7424): 364-73.
   [http://dx.doi.org/10.1038/nature11706] [PMID: 23151579]

[87] Cairns RA, Harris IS, Mak TW. Regulation of cancer cell metabolism. Nat Rev Cancer 2011; 11(2): 85-95.

[http://dx.doi.org/10.1038/nrc2981] [PMID: 21258394]

[88] Galluzzi L, Kepp O, Vander Heiden MG, Kroemer G. Metabolic targets for cancer therapy. Nat Rev Drug Discov 2013; 12(11): 829-46.
[http://dx.doi.org/10.1038/nrd4145] [PMID: 24113830]

[89] Ward PS, Thompson CB. Metabolic reprogramming: A cancer hallmark even warburg did not anticipate. Cancer Cell 2012; 21(3): 297-308.
[http://dx.doi.org/10.1016/j.ccr.2012.02.014] [PMID: 22439925]

[90] Landau BR, Laszlo J, Stengle J, Burk D. Certain metabolic and pharmacologic effects in cancer patients given infusions of 2-deoxy-D-glucose. J Natl Cancer Inst 1958; 21(3): 485-94.
[PMID: 13576102]

[91] Ely JO. 2-deoxy-d-glucose as an inhibitor of cancerous growth in animals. J Franklin Inst 1954; 258(2): 157-60.
[http://dx.doi.org/10.1016/0016-0032(54)90946-1]

[92] Garber K. Oncology's energetic pipeline. Nat Biotechnol 2010; 28(9): 888-91.
[http://dx.doi.org/10.1038/nbt0910-888] [PMID: 20829819]

[93] Shoshan MC. 3-Bromopyruvate: targets and outcomes. J Bioenerg Biomembr 2012; 44(1): 7-15.
[http://dx.doi.org/10.1007/s10863-012-9419-2] [PMID: 22298255]

[94] Kumagai S, Narasaki R, Hasumi K. Glucose-dependent active ATP depletion by koningic acid kills high-glycolytic cells. Biochem Biophys Res Commun 2008; 365(2): 362-8.
[http://dx.doi.org/10.1016/j.bbrc.2007.10.199] [PMID: 17997978]

[95] Gaude E, Frezza C. Defects in mitochondrial metabolism and cancer. Cancer Metab 2014; 2: 10.
[http://dx.doi.org/10.1186/2049-3002-2-10] [PMID: 25057353]

[96] Le A, Cooper CR, Gouw AM, et al. Inhibition of lactate dehydrogenase A induces oxidative stress and inhibits tumor progression. Proc Natl Acad Sci USA 2010; 107(5): 2037-42.
[http://dx.doi.org/10.1073/pnas.0914433107] [PMID: 20133848]

[97] Birsoy K, Wang T, Possemato R, et al. MCT1-mediated transport of a toxic molecule is an effective strategy for targeting glycolytic tumors. Nat Genet 2013; 45(1): 104-8.
[http://dx.doi.org/10.1038/ng.2471] [PMID: 23202129]

[98] Raez LE, Papadopoulos K, Ricart AD, et al. A phase I dose-escalation trial of 2-deoxy-D-glucose alone or combined with docetaxel in patients with advanced solid tumors. Cancer Chemother Pharmacol 2013; 71(2): 523-30.
[http://dx.doi.org/10.1007/s00280-012-2045-1] [PMID: 23228990]

[99] Stein M, Lin H, Jeyamohan C, et al. Targeting tumor metabolism with 2-deoxyglucose in patients with castrate-resistant prostate cancer and advanced malignancies. Prostate 2010; 70(13): 1388-94.
[http://dx.doi.org/10.1002/pros.21172] [PMID: 20687211]

[100] Porporato PE, Dhup S, Dadhich RK, Copetti T, Sonveaux P. Anticancer targets in the glycolytic metabolism of tumors: A comprehensive review. Front Pharmacol 2011; 2: 49.
[http://dx.doi.org/10.3389/fphar.2011.00049] [PMID: 21904528]

[101] Powell D. Phase 2 and Phase 3 Clinical Trials of TH-070 in Benign Prostatic Hyperplasia (BPH) Do Not Meet Primary Endpoint , 2006 [[cited 2015 January]]; Available from:

http://investor.thresholdpharm.com/releasedetail.cfm?ReleaseID=203917

[102] Thallion Presents Final Phase II TLN-232 Results in Advanced Kidney Cancer Patients at the ESMO Congress , 2008 [cited 2015 January]; Available from: http://www.drugs.com/clinical_trials/ thallion-presents-final-phase-ii-tln-232-results-advanced-kidney-cancer-patients-esmo-congress-5545.html

[103] Thallion Suspends Patient Enrollment of TLN-232 Metastatic Melanoma Trial Over Licensing Dispute , 2009 [cited 2015 January]; Available from: http://www.fiercebiotech.com/press-releases/ thallion-suspends-patient-enrollment-tln-232-metastatic-melanoma-trial-over-licensing

[104] Michelakis ED, Webster L, Mackey JR. Dichloroacetate (DCA) as a potential metabolic-targeting therapy for cancer. Br J Cancer 2008; 99(7): 989-94.
[http://dx.doi.org/10.1038/sj.bjc.6604554] [PMID: 18766181]

[105] Michelakis ED, Sutendra G, Dromparis P, *et al.* Metabolic modulation of glioblastoma with dichloroacetate. Sci Transl Med 2010; 2(31): 31ra34.
[http://dx.doi.org/10.1126/scitranslmed.3000677] [PMID: 20463368]

[106] Dunbar EM, Coats BS, Shroads AL, *et al.* Phase 1 trial of dichloroacetate (DCA) in adults with recurrent malignant brain tumors. Invest New Drugs 2014; 32(3): 452-64.
[http://dx.doi.org/10.1007/s10637-013-0047-4] [PMID: 24297161]

[107] Garon EB, Christofk HR, Hosmer W, *et al.* Dichloroacetate should be considered with platinum-based chemotherapy in hypoxic tumors rather than as a single agent in advanced non-small cell lung cancer. J Cancer Res Clin Oncol 2014; 140(3): 443-52.
[http://dx.doi.org/10.1007/s00432-014-1583-9] [PMID: 24442098]

[108] Pollyea D. Clinical safety and activity in a phase I trial of AG-221, a first in class, potent inhibitor of the IDH2-mutant protein, in patients with IDH2 mutant positive advanced hematologic malignancies [abstract CT103]. Proceedings of the 105th Annual Meeting of the American Association for Cancer Research. San Diego, CA. 2014.

[109] Stein E, Tallman M, Pollyea DA, Eds. Clinical safety and activity in a phase I trial of AG-120, a first in class, selective, potent inhibitor of the IDH1-mutant protein, in patients with IDH1 mutant positive advanced hematologic malignancies. 26th EORTC-NCI-AACR SYMPOSIUM - Molecular Targets and Cancer Therapeutics. Barcelona, Spain. 2014.
[http://dx.doi.org/10.1158/1538-7445.AM2014-CT103]

[110] Agresta S, Stein EM, Tallman MS, *et al.* A PHASE I STUDY OF AG-221, A First In Class, Potent Inhibitor Of The Idh2-Mutant Protein, In Patients With Idh2 Mutant Positive Advanced Hematologic Malignancies [abstract LB-6156]. EHA 19th Congress. Milan, Italy. 2014.

[111] Evans JM, Donnelly LA, Emslie-Smith AM, Alessi DR, Morris AD. Metformin and reduced risk of cancer in diabetic patients. BMJ 2005; 330(7503): 1304-5.
[http://dx.doi.org/10.1136/bmj.38415.708634.F7] [PMID: 15849206]

[112] Li D, Yeung SC, Hassan MM, Konopleva M, Abbruzzese JL. Antidiabetic therapies affect risk of pancreatic cancer. Gastroenterology 2009; 137(2): 482-8.
[http://dx.doi.org/10.1053/j.gastro.2009.04.013] [PMID: 19375425]

[113] Gandini S, Puntoni M, Heckman-Stoddard BM, *et al.* Metformin and cancer risk and mortality: A systematic review and meta-analysis taking into account biases and confounders. Cancer Prev Res

(Phila) 2014; 7(9): 867-85.
[http://dx.doi.org/10.1158/1940-6207.CAPR-13-0424] [PMID: 24985407]

[114] Rothermundt C, Hayoz S, Templeton AJ, *et al*. Metformin in chemotherapy-naive castration-resistant prostate cancer: A multicenter phase 2 trial (SAKK 08/09). Eur Urol 2014; 66(3): 468-74.
[http://dx.doi.org/10.1016/j.eururo.2013.12.057] [PMID: 24412228]

[115] Zhou G, Myers R, Li Y, *et al*. Role of AMP-activated protein kinase in mechanism of metformin action. J Clin Invest 2001; 108(8): 1167-74.
[http://dx.doi.org/10.1172/JCI13505] [PMID: 11602624]

[116] Hardie DG, Ross FA, Hawley SA. AMPK: A nutrient and energy sensor that maintains energy homeostasis. Nat Rev Mol Cell Biol 2012; 13(4): 251-62.
[http://dx.doi.org/10.1038/nrm3311] [PMID: 22436748]

[117] Marini C, Salani B, Massollo M, *et al*. Direct inhibition of hexokinase activity by metformin at least partially impairs glucose metabolism and tumor growth in experimental breast cancer. Cell Cycle 2013; 12(22): 3490-9.
[http://dx.doi.org/10.4161/cc.26461] [PMID: 24240433]

[118] Salani B, Marini C, Rio AD, *et al*. Metformin impairs glucose consumption and survival in Calu-1 cells by direct inhibition of hexokinase-II. Sci Rep 2013; 3: 2070.
[http://dx.doi.org/10.1038/srep02070] [PMID: 23797762]

[119] Owen MR, Doran E, Halestrap AP. Evidence that metformin exerts its anti-diabetic effects through inhibition of complex 1 of the mitochondrial respiratory chain. Biochem J 2000; 348(Pt 3): 607-14.
[http://dx.doi.org/10.1042/bj3480607] [PMID: 10839993]

[120] Wheaton WW, Weinberg SE, Hamanaka RB, *et al*. Metformin inhibits mitochondrial complex I of cancer cells to reduce tumorigenesis. eLife 2014; 3: e02242.
[http://dx.doi.org/10.7554/eLife.02242] [PMID: 24843020]

[121] Luengo A, Sullivan LB, Heiden MG. Understanding the complex-I-ty of metformin action: limiting mitochondrial respiration to improve cancer therapy. BMC Biol 2014; 12: 82.
[http://dx.doi.org/10.1186/s12915-014-0082-4] [PMID: 25347702]

[122] Ben Sahra I, Laurent K, Loubat A, *et al*. The antidiabetic drug metformin exerts an antitumoral effect *in vitro* and *in vivo* through a decrease of cyclin D1 level. Oncogene 2008; 27(25): 3576-86.
[http://dx.doi.org/10.1038/sj.onc.1211024] [PMID: 18212742]

[123] Zhuang Y, Miskimins WK. Cell cycle arrest in Metformin treated breast cancer cells involves activation of AMPK, downregulation of cyclin D1, and requires p27Kip1 or p21Cip1. J Mol Signal 2008; 3: 18.
[http://dx.doi.org/10.1186/1750-2187-3-18] [PMID: 19046439]

[124] Dos Santos LV, Viana LD, Lima JP, *et al*. Metformin plus paclitaxel for metastatic or recurrent head and neck cancer: final results of the randomised prospective mettax trial (NCT01333852). Ann Oncol 2014; 25 (Suppl. 4): iv345.

[125] Esteva FJ, Moulder SL, Gonzalez-Angulo AM, *et al*. Phase I trial of exemestane in combination with metformin and rosiglitazone in nondiabetic obese postmenopausal women with hormone receptor-positive metastatic breast cancer. Cancer Chemother Pharmacol 2013; 71(1): 63-72.

[http://dx.doi.org/10.1007/s00280-012-1977-9] [PMID: 23053261]

[126] Ferrari AC, Pfiffer TE, Alex AK, Eds. Phase II trial of metformin and paclitaxel for patients with gemcitabine-refractory advanced adenocarcinoma of the pancreas. J Clin Oncol 2014; 32 (suppl; abstr e15196) 2014 ASCO Annual Meeting

[127] Goodwin PJ, Parulekar W, Gelmon KA, *et al.* Effect of metformin *versus* placebo on weight and metabolic factors in initial patients enrolled onto NCIC CTG MA.32, a multicenter adjuvant randomized controlled trial in early-stage breast cancer (BC). J Clin Oncol 2013; 31 (suppl; abstr 1033) 2013 ASCO Annual Meeting

[128] Joshua AM, Zannella VE, Downes MR, *et al.* A pilot 'window of opportunity' neoadjuvant study of metformin in localised prostate cancer. Prostate Cancer Prostatic Dis 2014; 17(3): 252-8.
[http://dx.doi.org/10.1038/pcan.2014.20] [PMID: 24861559]

[129] Joshua AM, Zannella VE, Downes MR, Eds. Final results of a phase II study of neoadjuvant metformin in prostatic carcinoma. J Clin Oncol 2013; 31 (suppl; abstr 5070) 2013 ASCO Annual Meeting

[130] Kalinsky K, Crew KD, Refice S, *et al.* Presurgical trial of metformin in overweight and obese patients with newly diagnosed breast cancer. Cancer Invest 2014; 32(4): 150-7.
[http://dx.doi.org/10.3109/07357907.2014.889706] [PMID: 24605899]

[131] Kim J, Lim W, Kim EK, *et al.* Phase II randomized trial of neoadjuvant metformin plus letrozole *versus* placebo plus letrozole for estrogen receptor positive postmenopausal breast cancer (METEOR). BMC Cancer 2014; 14: 170.
[http://dx.doi.org/10.1186/1471-2407-14-170] [PMID: 24612502]

[132] Kritharis A, Caplain J, Rajagopal S, Eds. A phase I study of metformin and chemotherapy in solid tumors. J Clin Oncol 2013; 32:5s (suppl; abstr 2560) 2014 ASCO Annual Meeting

[133] MacKenzie MJ, Ernst S, Johnson C, Winquist E. A phase I study of temsirolimus and metformin in advanced solid tumours. Invest New Drugs 2012; 30(2): 647-52.
[http://dx.doi.org/10.1007/s10637-010-9570-8] [PMID: 20978924]

[134] Miranda VC, Faria LD. A phase II trial of metformin and fluorouracil (MetFU) for patients (pts) with metastatic colorectal cancer (mCRC) refractory to standard treatment. J Clin Oncol 2014; 32 (suppl 3; abstr 601) 2014 Gastrointestinal Cancers Symposium

[135] Ramanathan RK, Lee P, Leach JW, Eds. Phase II study of induction therapy with gemcitabine and nab-paclitaxel followed by consolidation with mFOLFIRINOX in patients with metastatic pancreatic cancer. J Clin Oncol 2013; 31 (suppl 4; abstr 233) 2013 Gastrointestinal Cancers Symposium

[136] Dang CV. Links between metabolism and cancer. Genes Dev 2012; 26(9): 877-90.
[http://dx.doi.org/10.1101/gad.189365.112] [PMID: 22549953]

[137] Klement RJ, Kämmerer U. Is there a role for carbohydrate restriction in the treatment and prevention of cancer? Nutr Metab (Lond) 2011; 8: 75.
[http://dx.doi.org/10.1186/1743-7075-8-75] [PMID: 22029671]

[138] Moreschi C. Beziehungen zwischen Erna"hrung und Tumorwachstum. Z fur Immunitatsforsch 1909; 2: 651-75.

[139] Lee C, Longo VD. Fasting *vs* dietary restriction in cellular protection and cancer treatment: from model organisms to patients. Oncogene 2011; 30(30): 3305-16.
[http://dx.doi.org/10.1038/onc.2011.91] [PMID: 21516129]

[140] Hursting S, Smith S, Harvey A, Lashinger L. Calories and Cancer: The Role of Insulin-Like Growth Factor-1. In: LeRoith D, Ed. Insulin-like Growth Factors and Cancer. Springer, US: Cancer Drug Discovery and Development 2012; pp. 231-43.
[http://dx.doi.org/10.1007/978-1-4614-0598-6_12]

[141] Berg JM, Tymoczko JL, Stryer L. Biochemistry. 7th ed., New York: W. H. Freeman 2012. Available at: http://bcs.whfreeman.com/berg7e/#t_644431

[142] Maurer GD, Brucker DP, Bähr O, *et al.* Differential utilization of ketone bodies by neurons and glioma cell lines: a rationale for ketogenic diet as experimental glioma therapy. BMC Cancer 2011; 11: 315.
[http://dx.doi.org/10.1186/1471-2407-11-315] [PMID: 21791085]

[143] Seyfried TN, Kiebish M, Mukherjee P, Marsh J. Targeting energy metabolism in brain cancer with calorically restricted ketogenic diets. Epilepsia 2008; 49 (Suppl. 8): 114-6.
[http://dx.doi.org/10.1111/j.1528-1167.2008.01853.x] [PMID: 19049606]

[144] Rieger J, Bähr O, Maurer GD, *et al.* ERGO: a pilot study of ketogenic diet in recurrent glioblastoma. Int J Oncol 2014; 44(6): 1843-52.
[PMID: 24728273]

[145] Schwartz K, Chang HT, Nikolai M, *et al.* Treatment of glioma patients with ketogenic diets: report of two cases treated with an IRB-approved energy-restricted ketogenic diet protocol and review of the literature. Cancer Metab 2015; 3: 3.
[http://dx.doi.org/10.1186/s40170-015-0129-1] [PMID: 25806103]

[146] Cangemi R, Friedmann AJ, Holloszy JO, Fontana L. Long-term effects of calorie restriction on serum sex-hormone concentrations in men. Aging Cell 2010; 9(2): 236-42.
[http://dx.doi.org/10.1111/j.1474-9726.2010.00553.x] [PMID: 20096034]

[147] Bianchini F, Kaaks R, Vainio H. Overweight, obesity, and cancer risk. Lancet Oncol 2002; 3(9): 565-74.
[http://dx.doi.org/10.1016/S1470-2045(02)00849-5] [PMID: 12217794]

[148] Fine EJ, Segal-Isaacson CJ, Feinman RD, *et al.* Targeting insulin inhibition as a metabolic therapy in advanced cancer: A pilot safety and feasibility dietary trial in 10 patients. Nutrition 2012; 28(10): 1028-35.
[http://dx.doi.org/10.1016/j.nut.2012.05.001] [PMID: 22840388]

[149] Altman BJ, Dang CV. Normal and cancer cell metabolism: lymphocytes and lymphoma. FEBS J 2012; 279(15): 2598-609.
[http://dx.doi.org/10.1111/j.1742-4658.2012.08651.x] [PMID: 22672505]

[150] Michalek RD, Rathmell JC. The metabolic life and times of a T-cell. Immunol Rev 2010; 236: 190-202.
[http://dx.doi.org/10.1111/j.1600-065X.2010.00911.x] [PMID: 20636818]

CHAPTER 5

Immunotherapy Strategies in Follicular Lymphoma: Antibodies, Vaccines and Cells

Nicolás Martínez-Calle[1], Ascensión López Díaz de Cerio[1], Susana Inogés[1], Esther Pena[3], Ricardo García-Muñoz[2], Carlos Panizo[1,*]

[1] *Hematology Department, Clínica Universidad de Navarra, Pamplona, Spain*

[2] *Hematology Department, Hospital San Pedro, Logroño, Spain*

[3] *Hematology Department, Complejo Hospitalario de Navarra, Pamplona, Spain*

Abstract: Follicular lymphoma (FL) is the most frequent indolent non-Hodgkin lymphoma. Therapeutic strategies vary from withholding treatment to aggressive chemoimmunotherapy regimes, and stem cell transplantation, depending on the stage and risk stratification at diagnosis. A prominent role of the microenvironment in FL-cell survival and lymphomagenesis has been brought to light and consequently the manipulation of the FL-cell niche is progressively becoming an important therapeutic tool in FL. Chemotherapy agents are no longer under the spotlight, leaving the main role to immunotherapeutic strategies and targeted therapy that aim towards disease control with minimal side-effects and sequelae. Immunotherapy with monoclonal antibodies, radioimmunotherapy and vaccines, has resulted in increased response rates and survival in FL patients.

Adoptive immunotherapy is an emerging strategy for FL treatment, aiming to exploit the immune system's natural tendency to attack tumoral cells. AntiCD20 monoclonal antibodies have become the backbone of first line and relapse treatments combined with chemotherapy regimens. Anti-idiotype vaccines are the best developed active immunotherapy strategy, with proven efficacy in patients with FL on first relapse. The other vaccine types (Dentritic cells, proteoliposomal or DNA) are still in preclinical development. Adoptive cell transfer (NK cells, LAK and effector T-lymphocytes), chimeric-antigen receptor (CAR) engineered T-cells and Bi-specific T-cell engaging

---

* **Corresponding author Carlos Panizo:** Hematology Department, Clínica Universidad de Navarra, Av. Pío, XII, 36 31008 Pamplona, Navarra, Spain; Tel: +34 948 396 397; Fax: +34 948 396 676; Email: cpanizo@unav.es

Atta-ur-Rahman (Ed.)

antibodies (BiTE) for passive immunotherapy remain also experimental approaches, although promising pre-clinical results have recently become available.

The following chapter will summarize FL biology and conventional treatment with immunochemotherapy, with a final section focusing specifically on novel immunotherapy strategies (active and passive) for the treatment of FL.

Keywords: Adoptive cell-therapy, Anti-idiotype vaccines, Dentritic-cell vaccines, Follicular lymphoma, Immunotherapy, LAK cells, Monoclonal antibodies, NK cells, Radioimmunotherapy, Vaccines.

1. INTRODUCTION

Follicular lymphoma (FL) is the most frequent indolent non-Hodgkin's lymphoma (NHL), it is known to arise from the follicular B lymphocytes and typically features an indolent clinical course consisting of relapses followed by prolonged remissions. FL was originally named Brill-Symmers disease, it was first described in 1925 as a benign adenopatic disorder, typical of the elder [1]. FL is the second most common NHL in United States and Eastern Europe, representing 20-40% of all NHL and 70% of indolent lymphomas, with a yearly incidence of 3/100.000 [2, 3]. Definitive cure of FL seems to occur rarely [4], although patient survival continues to improve with a current average above 10 years [5 - 8].

Improvements in the outcome of FL have been driven by the appearance of novel biologic agents [9] together with a better risk assessment at diagnosis, which combines the traditional FLIPI (Follicular Lymphoma International Prognostic Index) [10] with genetic and molecular biomarkers [11]. These tools have helped clinicians to individualize treatment intensity, reduce unnecessary treatment-related toxicity and ultimately achieve durable complete remissions [12, 13]. Immunotherapy (*e.g.* anti CD20 antibodies, radioimmunotherapy or idiotypic vaccination) have probably been the greatest advance in FL treatment over the past 50 years, contributing to the extension of disease free intervals and challenging some of the oldest paradigms about FL treatment, such as incurability or the use of front-line aggressive treatment to extend survival [14].

2. BIOLOGY OF FOLLICULAR LYMPHOMA

2.1. Histopathology of FL

FL is a neoplasm composed of germinal center B cells (also known as follicle center cells), typically both centrocytes and centroblasts, maintaining at least partially the follicular histologic pattern. FL is characterized by the t(14;18)(q32;q21) translocation resulting in overexpression of anti-apoptotic BCL2 protein [15 - 17]. The World Health Organization (WHO) classification of malignant lymphomas defines three histologic grades of FL (1, 2 and 3), based on the number of centroblasts per high power field, using the cell counting method developed by Mann and Bernard [18]. More than 15 centroblasts per high power field defines grade 3 which is subsequently classified into grades 3a and 3b (3a representing an admixture of centrocytes and centroblasts and 3b predominant sheets of centroblasts). Grade 3 FL is heterogeneous, with increasing aggressiveness and less survival correlating with increasing centroblast counts [19]. In fact, clinical course of grade 3b FL overlaps with that of aggressive NHL and therefore should be treated as such [15]. FL tumor cells express surface immunglobulin (SIg+: IgM, IgD, IgG or rarely IgA) and also express typical B cell associated antigens (CD19, CD20, CD22, CD79a). Other phenotypic features include BCL2+, BCL6+, CD10+, CD5-, CD43+/- [20, 21]. Some cases, especially grade 3b, may lack CD10 but retain BCL6 expression. CD43 is a common marker of grade 3 FL [22, 23].

2.2. Follicular Lymphoma-cell Origin

The t(14;18)(q32;q21) translocation involves BCL2 and IGH genes, the breakpoint is located at the 5′ end of J heavy-chain (JH) gene, suggesting that the event occurs at the DH to JH rearrangement stage; such event occurs in bone marrow lymphoid progenitors or B cell precursors (pro-B and pre-B cells) [24 - 28]. Furthermore, FL-cells occasionally display class-switch recombination (CSR), suggesting altogether an origin between lymphoid progenitors in bone marrow and late germinal center follicular cells [29, 30].

After the immortalization event, FL-cells are thought to continue their normal differentiation path through the germinal center in spite of the BCL2-IGH translocation. In fact, FL-cell maturation after the translocation may explain the presence of different FL clones, with heterogeneous IG sequences and multiple isotypes as a consequence of divergent somatic hypermutation (SHM) and somatic recombination of the original mother clone [31, 32]. Moreover, FL clones may experience further variations in the pattern of SHM during disease progression [33].

BCR signaling is thought to be a driver of FL lymphomagenesis. Approximately 20% of cases of follicular lymphoma (FL) have non-canonical BCR activation, triggered through binding to common self-antigens in the ECM (*e.g.* N-terminal region of vimentin) [34 - 37]. Activation of the FL BCR has also been proposed to occur by non-antigenic mechanisms, as mutations on the IgH scaffold regions may lead to abnormal sites of N-glycosylation that bind to stromal lecithin and trigger BCR signaling without antigenic binding [38 - 40]. The FL-cell dependency on BCR have led to the design of novel molecules with the ability to inhibit or diminish BCR signaling/recognition (Discussed in 6) [41 - 45], some of which have successfully been translated into the clinical use and should become available for FL treatment in the upcoming decade [37].

2.3. Follicular Lymphoma Microenvironment

Only 50% of cell mass in FL is composed of neoplastic B-cells [46] This finding has led to a profound study of the accompanying non-tumoral cell types present in the neoplastic lymph nodes, a population that altogether constitute the FL-cell niche. These non-tumoral cells have been shown to interact actively with the neoplastic clone [47, 48] and may have a direct impact on treatment response and clinical outcome [49 - 51].

Different cell types have been identified by immunohistochemistry, including stromal cells [52, 53], mesenchymal cells, [54, 55], follicular dendritic cells (FDCs) [56, 57], T cells [58 - 60] and macrophages [61 - 63]; most of them are found in the normal germinal center microenvironment [64]. Spatially, nodular aggregates of FDCs are found outlining the neoplastic follicles, identified by CD21 or CD23 expression [16], whereas neoplastic follicles contain the remaining cell types (T cells, macrophages and stromal mesenchymal cells) [65, 66].

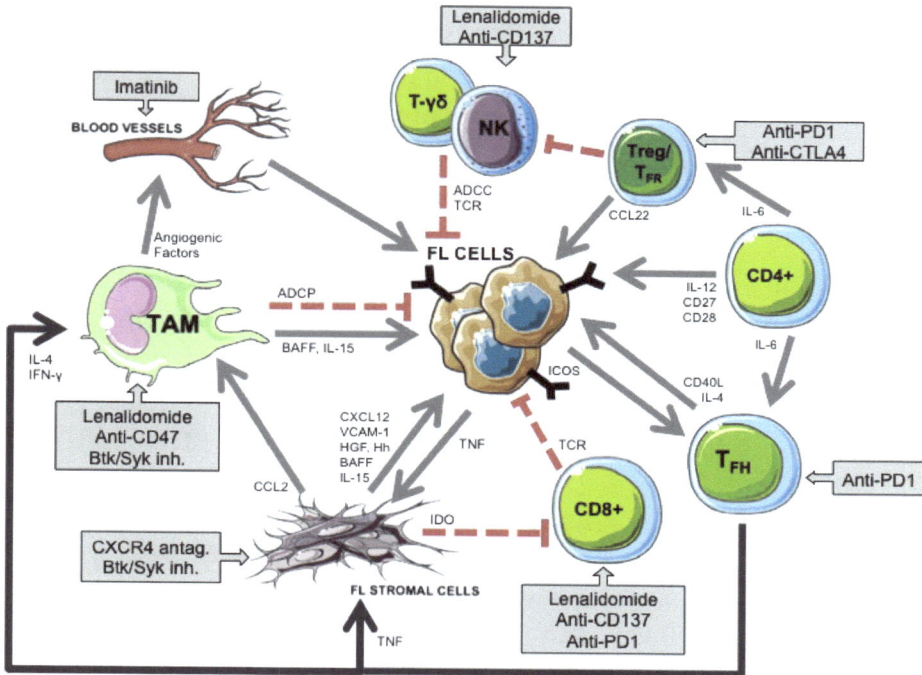

Fig. (1). Complexity of FL microenvironment. **1)** NK/Tγδ, CD8+ CTL (Cytotoxic-cell lymphocytes) and TAM (Tumor-associated macrophages) are the 3 main elements of native immune response against FL cells, all of which are inhibited by FL microenvironment. **2)** FL cells subvert microenvironment, shifting signals towards survival and proliferation, through ICOS-mediated follicular T-helper cells (T^{FH}) stimulation. **3)** The remaining microenvironment cell types (T-CD4+ lymphocytes, T-regs, TAM and stromal cells) provide cytokine and/or BCR mediated cell survival signals to FL-cells. TAM also stimulate angiogenesis. **4)** Almost all of the microenvironment networks can be pharmacologically manipulated. *Solid gray arrows denote supportive signals, whereas dashed red arrows denote inhibitory signals. The cytokines that are known to mediate each effect are shown. Gray boxes denote therapeutic strategies available to either potentiate immune response towards FL cells or block the supportive signaling. ADCC: Antibody-mediated cellular cytotoxicity; ADCP: Antibody-mediated cellular phagocytosis; TCR: T-cell receptor; IDO: Indoleamine-2,3 deoxygenase; Hh: Hedgehog; BAFF: B-cell activating factor.*

The major role of microenvironment in FL is highlighted by the fact that FL cells survive better *in vitro* when co-cultured with stromal cells and CD40L ligand/cytokine [67]. Moreover, FL-cells might be themselves the main drivers of their local microenvironment modifications [68] and seem to have different degrees of dependency on the stromal support when settled on lymph nodes or bone marrow [46, 69].

The best-characterized cell population within the microenvironment are the T-lymphocytes population; gene expression profiling studies have shown that the non-tumoral cells in FL mainly upregulate cytokine and chemokine genes known to be involved in B-T cell interactions [70]. It has been shown that high levels of intratumoral T-CD8+ lymphocytes are correlated with a better prognosis [49, 71]. Furthermore, T-CD8+ effector lymphocytes appear to be regulated in part by another subset of T regulatory lymphocytes (FOXP3+ T regulatory cells, Tregs), that damp the immune response against the FL clone by inducing anergy and reducing nodal T-CD8+ cell numbers [72]. For T-CD4+ cells, a FL-cell supporting role has been attributed, as CD40L expression of follicular CD4+ cells can mediate FL B-cell proliferation [73, 74], while the PD-1 axis signaling through follicular T-helper cells (F_{TH}) has been suggested as a mechanism for blockade of innate anti-tumor immune response [75 - 77].

Myeloid compartment within FL-niche is mainly represented by tumor-associated macrophages (TAM), whose main role within lymph nodes is phagocytosis and antigen presentation to effector immune cells (B and T cells). The antigen presentation dynamics gather particular importance after CD20 monoclonal antibody treatment, as the antibody-mediated cellular phagocytosis (ADCP) is known to be one of the cardinal mechanisms of FL-cell clearance after treatment [62, 63]. There is evidence of phagocytosis evasion mediated by CD47 molecule expression in FL-cells, which has been successfully overcome by anti-CD47 antibodies in murine models of FL. Macrophages have also been shown to have a direct action over FL-cell fate sustaining angiogenesis and supporting survival of FL-cells in a CD40-independent manner [51].

Follicular dendritic cells (FDCs) are also thought to contribute to FL-cell survival with the production of TNF-α and lymphotoxin-α1β2, a feature that may be directly induced by FL-cells, creating a self-sustaining signaling loop; similarly, other proteins produced by FDCs have been implicated on paracrine apoptotic evasion of FL-cell (Hedgehog, Hepatocyte growth factor, CD106). Finally, FL-stromal cells also seem to help in the orchestration of the niche, triggering recruitment of other cell types such as monocytes and their differentiation to pro-angiogenic macrophages [78].

It appears to be clear that FL-niche has a fundamental role in FL-cell survival and proliferation, however, the overall effect of the stroma on FL-cells has been proven to be variable and sometimes antagonistic, with some cell types providing either apoptotic or survival/immune evading signals to FL-cells depending on the situation and the spatial localization [69]. The understanding FL-niche role has led to the design of some therapeutic strategies aiming to reverse or dampen the immune evasion mechanisms of FL-cells, as well as others to block or weaken the supportive signals provided by surrounding cell types [79 - 81]. As an example, the use of immunomodulatory drugs (IMiDs) such as Lenalidomide has been purposed as an adjuvant treatment that could balance the immune response towards FL-cell reactivity by restoring the B-T immunological synapse [82 - 85]. Given the importance that FL-cell niche seems to have in tumor progression and immune evasion, it is not surprising that the greatest advancements in therapy for FL have been achieved in the field of immunotherapy; such improvements seek to potentiate the innate immune response towards FL-cells either by adoptive cell therapy, targeted drug therapy or monoclonal antibodies (Discussed in 6 and 7; Fig. (**1**)).

3. PREVIOUS CONSIDERATIONS BEFORE THERAPY

FL has a wide range of clinical presentations. It is often diagnosed during routine checkups or with a CT scan performed for a different purpose in asymptomatic patients, however, it may also come to light as advanced symptomatic disease with diffuse nodal compromise and even leukemization [4]. Bone Marrow (BM) infiltration is seen in 40-70% of cases. B-symptoms are found in less than 20% of patients, blood biochemistry abnormalities are also rare, with only 20% of cases with raised lactate dehydrogenase (LDH). Extranodal tissues are seldom affected and usually associated with advanced stage disease [12, 15].

3.1. Who should be Treated, and When?

As mentioned above, due to the indolent course of FL, patients are frequently asymptomatic at diagnosis. Decision to treat should be based on symptomatic disease or end-organ compromise at diagnosis. GELF criteria (Groupe d'Etude des

Lymphomes Folliculaires), published in 1997, [86 - 89] have been the mainstay of risk stratification for FL treatment (Table **1**). These criteria attempt to select patients that bear a truly indolent disease and benefit from deferred therapy, an approach known as "watch and wait", from those rapidly progressing that will require treatment either immediately or in the near future. Constant disease progression over a 6-month period might be added to these criteria, as a compelling indication for treatment [90, 91].

Table 1. Summary of GELF[a] criteria for FL[b] treatment[c].

Any of the following is a criterion to start active treatment:
• 3 or more nodal areas involved, each larger than 3cm.   • Any nodal or extranodal mass larger than 7cm.   • Presence of B symptoms (night fever or night sweating).   • Splenomegaly.   • Pleural effusion or ascites.   • Cytopenia (Leucocytes < 1.0 x10^9/L and/or platelets <100 x10^9/L).   • Leukemia (>5.0 x10^9/L malignant lymphocytes).

[a]GELF: Groupe d'Etude des Lymphomes Folliculaires; [b]FL: Follicular Lymphoma; [c]Solal-Céligny P, *et al.* (Reference [10]).

It is worth noting that the watch and wait strategy was established when modern biologic therapies were not available, the introduction of highly effective monoclonal antibodies could potentially modify the use of GELF criteria, as patients with low disease burden formerly chosen to a watch and wait approach might be safely treated with single-agent monoclonal antibodies. In this matter, Ardeshna *et al.* have recently reported an open label, randomized, phase III trial, enrolling 484 asymptomatic patients with low-tumor-burden follicular lymphoma. Patients were randomized to watchful waiting, Rituximab induction or Rituximab induction followed by maintenance with Rituximab. The early initiation of rituximab induction resulted in improved progression free survival (PFS) (80% *vs.* 48%, p<0.001), but the benefit on long-term survival is yet to be determined [92]; Rituximab maintenance in this setting has shown doubtful advantages [93]. Low toxicity and few contraindications for Rituximab monotherapy seem to validate it´s use in unfit patients; however, it remains a matter of debate whether this is acceptable from the risk/cost/benefit perspective in light of an unproven survival benefit [91, 94].

3.2. How to define Treatment Intensity

When the choice of active treatment is made, tumor eradication should be the objective, tailoring treatment intensity according to tolerance, fitness, disease burden and comorbidities. For unfit or older patients, quality of life should be given highest importance, adapting, or even withholding treatment in the setting of a voluminous disease with slow progression [94, 95]. Alternatives in such cases include low-intensity rituximab monotherapy [92, 96 - 99], reduced intensity chemoimmunotherapy (fewer cycles or lower doses) and other low toxic regimens such as Rituximab-chlorambucil or single-agent cyclophosphamide [100, 101].

On the contrary, for younger and fit patients a chemoimmunotherapy induction regimen should be considered aiming towards complete remission of measurable disease, with a consolidation strategy that varies according to the disease status at the end of the induction regimen and the tolerance to previous treatment.

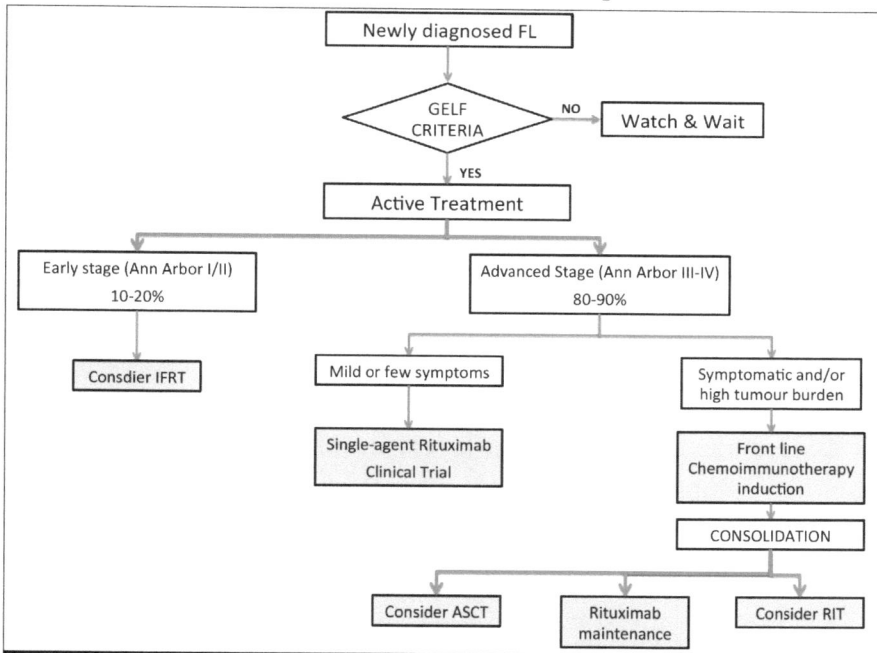

Fig. (2). Treatment algorithm for newly diagnosed Follicular Lymphoma (FL) patients based on current ESMO (European Society of Medical Oncology) and NCCN (National Comprehensive Cancer Network) guidelines. IFRT: Involved-field radiotherapy; ASCT: Autologous stem cell transplantation; RIT: Radioimmunotherapy.

4. FIRST LINE TREATMENT

As mentioned before, the goal of treatment is complete remission with the induction treatment, which is typically followed by a consolidation strategy aiming to extend the remission period as much as possible. It is thought that a small proportion of patients can achieve cure after the first line of treatment, however late relapses have been reported after complete remissions of more than 10 years [102]. Curability of FL is still a matter of debate, therefore, treatment strategies still aim to the longest possible remission period with the least possible toxicity. Treatment regimen should be selected according to the disease stage at diagnosis and the prognostic scoring; the following section reviews first line treatment strategies, which are further summarized in a treatment algorithm (Fig. **2**)

4.1. Early-stage Disease

Less than 10% of patients are diagnosed in stage I/II [15]. Involved-field radiotherapy (IFRT), chemoimmunotherapy and "watch and wait" approach can all be considered for these patients. Up to 40% of patients can achieve long-term remission with IFRT [103 - 106]. Localized FL is the only setting in which radiotherapy might be curative, with 10-year overall survival (OS) of 60-80% and a median survival of 19 years [107, 108]. The recommendation for radiation dosage is 25-30 Gy for subclinical disease and 36-40 Gy for clinically symptomatic areas.

The largest early-stage FL treatment follow-up trial involves 6000 patients of whom 34% were treated with upfront IFRT. Results prove that IFRT extends OS at 5 years when compared to standard chemotherapy (90 *vs.* 81%) and maintains the effect over 20 years (63 *vs.* 51%) [106, 109]. Despite robust scientific evidence, many patients do not receive IFRT at diagnosis, this phenomenon could be partially explained by physicians´ intention to avoid local morbidity related to IFRT in otherwise asymptomatic individuals [103]. A conservative watch and wait approach also seems to be reasonable for these patients, as 63% remain treatment free after 7 years [95].

Chemotherapy alone has proven to be ineffective to prevent disease relapse and thus, offers no benefit over the conservative approach or IFRT in early-stage disease. Immunochemotherapy with Rituximab is likely to improve chemotherapy efficacy and has proven superior disease-free and survival benefit when compared to IFRT [110]. Any patient with early-stage FL fulfilling GELF criteria should be offered treatment; the least toxic option will be the optimal choice in most cases. Well-designed comparative studies are lacking, thus, an individualized strategy should be adopted. In practice, a combination of strategies is most frequently adopted for early-stage FL [111].

4.2. Induction Treatment for Advanced Stages

Rituximab (R) should be included in the regimens of patients with advanced stage FL requiring treatment; however, the optimal drug choice for chemoimmuno-therapy regimens is yet to be clarified. Many regimens are available with comparable OS benefit; thus, choice should take into account both the physician and medical center experience with the different regimens. Available chemoimmunotherapy regimens are summarized in Table **2** [14, 112].

Rituximab has contributed to boost the efficacy of chemotherapy regimes, increasing complete response rates and extending the duration of response in advanced FL. The effect of rituximab treatment is thought to be long lasting, even after progression, making relapses less aggressive. Four prospective first-line trials [113 - 116], two salvage trials [117, 118] and a systematic meta-analysis [119] have confirmed an improved overall response, PFS and OS with the addition of rituximab to chemotherapy.

R-CHOP has been the most frequently used first line regimen for FL patients and has been the traditional standard of care for anthracycline based therapy [120 - 122]. R-CVP is an alternative to R-CHOP, usually proposed to non-fit patients or patients with cardiac disease in which anthracycline should be avoided [123]. One of the advantages of R-CHOP is the stem cell sparing capacity, which facilitates consolidation with autologous SCT, as it does not compromise mobilization compared to other regimens (*i.e.* Fludarabine based) [124, 125]. Anthracycline-based regimens should always be preferred in case of histological or clinical transformation to aggressive lymphoma [122].

FOLL05 trial, recently communicated by Federico *et al.*, is a randomized, multicenter and open-label trial which enrolled 524 previously untreated FL (stages II-IV) patients, to prospectively compare efficacy of R-CHOP *vs.* R-CVP *vs.* R-FM. The overall response rates were 88%, 93%, and 91% for R-CVP, R-CHOP, and R-FM, respectively (p= 0.2). After a median follow-up of 34 months, 3-year time to treatment failure (TTFs) rates were 46%, 62%, and 59% for the respective treatment groups (R-CHOP v R-CVP, p= 0.003; R-FM v R-CVP, p= 0.006; R-FM v R-CHOP, p=0.7). Three-year PFS rates were 52%, 68%, and 63% respectively (overall p= 0.01). Three-year OS was 95% for the whole series [126].

Fludarabine-based regimens are not the first choice in most centers, the higher risk of treatment-related infections and the long term B-cell depletion have reduced the use of fludarabine within the first line approach, despite comparable efficacy to anthracycline-based regimens [127 - 131].

Bendamustine is an old alkylating agent that is also a purine analogue, it has been successfully combined with Rituximab in FL, showing efficacy and limited toxicity. Early trials showed complete response in 60% of FL patients together with a median PFS of 24 months [132].

These encouraging results let to the design of a randomized phase III trial to compare efficacy and safety of Bendamustine-R (R-B) *versus* CHOP plus Rituximab (CHOP-R) as first-line therapy for patients with follicular (FL). The trial was conducted by the StIL grup (Study Indolent Lymphomas Group, Germany); 549 patients were enrolled, preliminary results showed higher rates of complete responses (40% *vs.* 30%) and less grade 4 adverse events on the Bendamustine arm [133]. Results have been updated in 2013 with a median follow-up of 45 months, median PFS was significantly longer in the R-B group than in the R-CHOP group (69.5 months *vs.* 31.2 months; p<0·0001). Bendamustine plus rituximab was better tolerated than R-CHOP, with lower rates of alopecia (0 *vs.* 100%; p<0·0001), hematological toxicity (30% *vs.* 68%; p<0·0001), infections (37% *vs.* 50%); p=0·002), peripheral neuropathy (7% *vs.* 29%; p<0·0001) and stomatitis (6% *vs.* 19%; p<0·0001) [134].

Another large trial, the BRIGHT study, is a randomized phase III study of non-inferiority evaluating the efficacy and safety of R-B (n= 224) *vs.* standard R-CHOP/R-CVP (n=223) for treatment-naive patients with indolent non-Hodgkin's lymphoma. R-B was non-inferior to R-CHOP/R-CVP, as assessed by the primary end point of complete response rate (31% *vs.* 25%, respectively; p= 0.02 for non-inferiority). The overall response rates for R-B and R-CHOP/R-CVP were 97% and 91%, respectively [135].

These results suggest an advantage of R-B over R-CHOP for first line therapy; however, long-term survival and side effects of R-B remain to be investigated. It seems obvious that R-B should be considered among first-line treatment options for patients with previously untreated FL [91]; in the near future, bendamustine-based regimens are expected to consolidate as the gold standard for first line immunochemotherapy in FL patients.

Table **2** also summarizes induction treatment alternatives for patients unable to tolerate standard chemoimmunotherapy regimens (*i.e.* "unfit patients").

Table 2. Chemoimmunotherapy options for first line treatment of FL[a, b].

Young and fit patients				Elderly and/or unfit			
Regimen	*ORR[c]*	*PFS[d]*	*OS[e]*	*Regimen*	*ORR[c]*	*PFS[d]*	*OS[e]*
R[f]- Bendamustine Rummel *et al.[i]*	90%	54m*	84% (4yr)	Rituximab[l,m] [231, 78]	74%	23m	90% (5yr)
R-CHOP[g] Hiddemman *et al.[j]*	96%	82m	97% (3yr)	Cyclophosphamide Peterson *et al.[o]*	66%	50m	104m
R-CVP[h] Marcus *et al.[k]*	81%	34m	83% (4yr)	Radioimmunotherapy (Y[90]-Ibritumumab tiuxetan) Morschhauser *et al.[p]*	87%	26m	95% (30m)
Rituximab Ardeshna *et al[l].,* Hainsworth *et al.[m]*	74%	23m	90% (5yr)	Chlorambucil + R Martinelli *et al.[q]*	97%	71% (5yr)	98% (5yr)
R + Lenalidomide Fowler *et al.[n]*	98%	NR (40m)	94% (3yr)				

[a]FL: Follicular Lymphoma; [b]Based on 2012 National Comprehensive Cancer Network (NCCN) guidelines, reference No. 137; [c]ORR: Overall response rate; [d]PFS: Progression-free survival; [e]OS: Overall survival; [f]R: Rituximab; [g]CHOP: Cyclophosphamide, Vincristine, Adriamycin, Prednisone; [h]CVP: Cyclophosphamide, Vincristine, Prednisone. [i]Reference [134]; [j]Reference [113]; [k]Reference [115]; [l]Reference [92]; [m]Reference [99]; [n]Reference [193]; [o]Reference [101]; [p]References [163] & [165]; [q]Reference [100].

4.3. Consolidation Treatment

The response rate is high among FL patients but relapses are frequent, patients tend to accumulate several lines of therapy throughout their lives. To overcome this clinical dilemma three main strategies have been designed to consolidate response and lengthen the disease free period: 1) maintenance treatment; 2) radioimmunotherapy and 3) autologous stem cell transplantation (ASCT). Consolidation treatment should have a good balance between efficacy and toxicity, to control undetectable residual disease and maintain an acceptable performance status.

4.3.1. Interferon Maintenance

Interferon (IFN) maintenance was historically the first attempt for immunotherapy in FL. Randomized trials have shown improvements in PFS and meta-analyses have shown significant improvements in both PFS (HR 0,6) and OS (HR 0,79) [136, 137]. However, it is worth noting that IFN maintenance trials have been conducted before the Rituximab era and thus, the survival benefit shown is compared to chemotherapy alone. No trials have been conducted comparing IFN to placebo after Rituximab containing induction regimens as well as no trials comparing directly Rituximab to IFN maintenance are available.

It seems that the good results of IFN maintenance have been eclipsed by the efficacy of Rituximab that offers a significantly better safety profile. Results of Rituximab maintenance have made the use of interferon anecdotal [138], however, but it should be always recognized as the pioneer attempt for immunotherapy against FL-cells.

4.3.2. Rituximab Maintenance

The first studies of Rituximab maintenance were done in FL and chronic lymphocytic leukemia with an induction schema of 4 weekly doses, extending treatment to 4 biannual treatment courses for those who responded to the first cycle (2 years) [98]. Median time to progression was 52 months in FL patients [99].

Subsequently, Rituximab maintenance was evaluated prospectively in randomized controlled trials. The SAAK trial was a placebo-controlled trial of newly diagnosed or relapsed FL, which found a significant improvement in PFS after a 35-month follow up [139, 140]. The second trial, ECOG1496, was a randomized, placebo-controlled study of Rituximab maintenance after response to upfront CVP. Significant improvement on PFS was seen after 36 months of follow-up, with a trend to higher survival rates on the Rituximab arm [141]. Neither of these studies included patients treated with Rituximab in the induction regimen.

The PRIMA study was the first trial to evaluate the benefit of Rituximab as maintenance therapy after first-line Rituximab-based regimens. Only patients with complete or partial response were included, and were randomized to receive 2-year Rituximab maintenance therapy every 8 weeks or placebo. PFS was 75% for the Rituximab arm compared to 58% in the placebo arm after 36-month follow up [142]. No survival benefit was seen in the initial analysis; a recent update on follow up after 6 years has shown sustained improvement on PFS and a 50% reduction (HR 0,63) of the risk of needing a new line of treatment; survival is still equivalent in both cohorts [143].

A slight increment in treatment-related infections was seen in the maintenance treatment arm due to B-cell depletion. Although life-threatening complications occurred rarely during Rituximab treatment, a small risk of morbid infections such as hepatitis B or JC virus should always be taken into account. Indeed, prophylaxis against hepatitis B has been recommended during maintenance treatment in patients at high risk of reactivation [144, 145].

The lack of survival benefit of Rituximab in maintenance trials only reflects the indolent nature of the disease and the relatively short follow-up time [146], furthermore, survival in FL is always biased by response to subsequent lines of therapy, which are typically able to induce another period of remission. Although a substantial benefit on survival has not been shown with maintenance treatment, risk/benefit ratio seems to be fare if 50% of patients are treatment free after 6 years. As a result of these data, Rituximab maintenance is starting to become standard of care for FL patients. It is worth noting that some authors still consider Rituximab maintenance inappropriate unless survival benefit is undeniably demonstrated [141, 142, 147].

4.3.3. Autologous Stem-cell Transplantation

Several randomized trials have investigated ASCT consolidation of FL in first complete response [148 - 151], however, the utility of this strategy after initial rituximab-chemotherapy induction remains to be established.

Hiddemann *et al.* have published in 2013 the results of a composite cohort of 940 patients treated in prospective randomized trials of The German Low Grade Lymphoma Study Group (GLSG) [152]. Patients with advanced stage FL were randomized for treatment with ASCT *versus* IFN-alpha maintenance in first remission after MCP, CHOP or R-CHOP in two consecutive trials. Promising results for ASCT were observed in the pre-rituximab era, with significant improvements in disease free survival, however, these results could not be confirmed when Rituximab was included in the induction regimen. After a median follow up of more than 6 years, in the 423 patient cohort assigned to R-CHOP, only a small improvement in time to treatment failure could be observed for ASCT compared to IFN-alpha maintenance.

Another meta-analysis, 941 pooled patients from the 4 major European studies showed a questionable benefit in PFS, with a non-significant increase in OS [153]. Noteworthy a slight increase in second malignancies was seen within the ASCT group, despite the short follow-up period.

Short and long-term toxicity added to the modest PFS benefit in the Rituximab era, seem to suggest that ASCT has a questionable benefit for patients with FL in first remission. Many clinicians choose Rituximab maintenance as the first line consolidation strategy, leaving ASCT for relapses where it seems to maintain a survival benefit [154, 155].

4.3.4. Radioimmunotherapy

In the setting of first-line treatment consolidation, both 131I-tositumomab and 90Yi-ibritumomab have been shown to induce high response rates and long-term remissions [156 - 159], some patients from these trials have achieved complete remission (CR) after being treatment-refractory [160]. The early proof of concept trials were performed with 131I-tositumomab, in 76 treatment-naïve FL patients.

Excellent responses were seen with a PFS of 59% and an OS of 89% after a 5-year follow-up period [161].

Phase III trials have also been conducted, SWOG S0016 is a Phase III Randomized Trial [162] comparing CHOP Plus Rituximab With CHOP Chemotherapy Plus 131I-Tositumomab. The trial enrolled 554 previously untreated FL patients, after a median follow-up period of 4.9 years, the 2-year estimate of PFS was 76% on the CHOP-R arm and 80% on the CHOP-RIT arm (P = .11). The 2-year estimated OS was 97% on the CHOP-R arm and 93% on the CHOP-RIT arm (P = .08); concluding that there was no evidence of a significant improvement in PFS comparing CHOP-RIT with CHOP-R.

Phase III trials with 90Yi-ibritumomab tiuxetan (Zevalin®) have also been conducted. The largest trial compared 90Yi-ibritumomab to placebo for patients achieving a CR or PR, demonstrating a 24-month increment in PFS [163]. The beneficial effect of 90Yi-ibritumomab tiuxetan as consolidation treatment is highest after the first complete remission, when compared to treatment after 2nd or 3rd line treatments [164].

In 2013, updated results of the phase III trial of 90Y-ibritumomab tiuxetan *vs.* placebo were presented with median follow-up of 7.3 years. 90Y-ibritumomab consolidation after achieving PR or CR/Cru to induction in patients with advanced-stage FL confers 3-year benefit in median PFS (p<0.01) and an improvement in time to new treatment (TTNT) of 5.1 years (p<0.01) [165].

The Spanish group PETHEMA/GELTAMO/GELCAB also conducted a randomized phase II trial comparing consolidation with a single dose of 90Yi-ibritumomab tiuxetan to Rituximab maintenance in patients with FL who responded to R-CHOP (ZAR2007 study). Enrollment was completed with 146 patients, results show that Rituximab maintenance is superior to consolidation with Ibritumomab in terms of PFS, with no differences in OS at the current follow-up (37 months). Nearly 50% of patients in partial response after R-CHOP achieved complete response during maintenance in both study arms [166]. Altogether, there is still lack of consolidated evidence about the benefit of radioimmunotherapy after an induction regimen with Rituximab.

5. RELAPSE TREATMENT

As previously stated, FL relapse after first line therapy is frequent. Recurrent disease is known for maintaining chemosensitivity and rarely transforming into high grade disease. Early relapse (< 12 months) is a sign of aggressive disease and bad prognosis, and should be treated aggressively and promptly. On the contrary, patients with late relapses, low disease burden and an indolent course may be considered for watch and wait strategy.

A new histopathologic study should be considered at relapse, as disease may evolve to a higher histologic grade or may transform into an aggressive NHL [91].

5.1. Choice of Rescue Treatment

Choice of rescue treatment depends on the patient's age, fitness, prognostic markers, disease burden, accumulated dose of chemotherapy drugs, medullary reserve capacity and suitability for autologous or allogeneic SCT.

Selection of rescue induction treatment should be non-cross resistant for early relapsed patients; additionally, stem cell sparing regimens must be prioritized if autologous transplantation is considered. R-CHOP or Rituximab-Bendamustine are suitable choices for induction treatment at relapse [14, 91, 160].

A previous response to Rituximab containing regimens lasting more than 6 months should encourage Rituximab use in the salvage regimen. Autologous stem cell transplantation should be strongly considered for relapsed disease, alternatively Radioimmunotherapy can be considered for consolidation in elderly or unfit patients [167]. Rituximab 2-year maintenance treatment after response to salvage therapy must be considered, as it has been shown to provide better clinical outcomes and prolong both PFS and OS [146, 168].

5.2. Bortezomib for FL Relapse

Bortezomib has recently gained attention in the field of NHL treatment. Bortezomib inhibits the ubiquitination of the proteasomal pathway, even though it has been extensively studied for multiple myeloma, it has shown efficacy in many types of NHL, including FL and mantle-cell lymphoma [169 - 172]. Several trials have demonstrated the efficacy of Bortezomib in relapsed/refractory FL, alone or combined with chemotherapy and/or Rituximab-based chemoimmunotherapy. Two regimens for Bortezomib administration are available, either as weekly injection or on days 1/4/8/11 of a 3-week cycle; weekly schedule is typically better tolerated with less adverse events (mainly peripheral neuropathy) [173].

Based on preliminary results, studies were designed to evaluate the Bortezomib and Rituximab combination in relapsed FL. LYM 3001 was a randomized phase III trial comparing standard Rituximab doses for 5 cycles of 35 days, with the same drug plus Bortezomib in days 1/8/15/22. A 1.8 month difference in PFS was seen, with a median follow up of 33.9 months [174].

Another two major trials have been published combining Bendamustine, Bortezomib and Rituximab, a highly effective regimen with low toxicity for unfit elderly patients with FL relapse [175, 176]. VERTICAL study was the first to evaluate this drug combination, a phase II trial with an overall response rate (ORR) of 84% and 47% of CR [175]. Friedberg *et al.* used a slightly lower dose of Bortezomib with similar ORR (84%) and CR (52%) and a reduction in adverse events, mainly thrombocytopenia [176]. No direct comparison of these regimens with Rituximab/Bendamustine has been conducted to date. The results of long term follow-up are awaited.

5.3. Autologous Stem-cell Transplantation for FL Relapse

EBMT registry data shows 10-year PFS and OS of 28% and 48% respectively, for patients receiving ASCT after CR2 [177]. The most frequently used conditioning regimens for FL patients undergoing ASCT include BEAM (carmustine, etoposide [VP-16], AraC, melphalan), BEAC (carmustine, VP-16, AraC, Cyclophosphamide [Cy]), and CBV (Cy, carmustine, VP-16) [178]. ASCT has been proven to extend PFS and OS in FL patients with early relapse, and thus it should be considered in this subset of patients if it has not previously been used [155, 179 - 181]. The ideal candidates for ASCT are patients in second relapse, at least in partial response after the induction regimen and a reasonably good performance status.

Randomized trials of ASCT consolidation in relapse disease have reported a PFS benefit of ASCT compared to best supportive care [179]. Rituximab maintenance has been shown to provide benefit after ASCT; no direct comparison of ASCT with Rituximab maintenance has been made to date.

It should be noted that ASCT confers a slight increase in the risk of late second tumors in the FL patient population, despite this fact, the survival benefit continues to be observed in long term follow-up studies [182]. Care should be taken in the post-remission follow up for the early detection of these complications [178].

5.4. Radioimmunotherapy for FL Relapse

The pivotal phase III trial for this indication included 143 patients with refractory/relapsed indolent NHL, comparing single-dose 90Yi-ibritumomab tiuxetan to a regime of 4 weekly doses of Rituximab [160, 183]. FL patient subgroup achieved the best ORR compared to Rituximab (86% *vs.* 55%), with a significant prolongation in time to new treatment. 90Yi-ibritumomab tiuxetan arm had also longer PFS when compared to Rituxmab (Median 14.2 months *vs.* 12.1 months) and a greater percentage of long-term remissions (>6 months). 131I-Tositumomab has been also recently reported to have high response rates (67%) with median PFS of 18 months and median OS of 32 months in a multicenter phase II trial including 142 patients [184]. No comparative trials of RIT and ASCT have been conducted in the relapse setting of FL, therefore RIT should be currently offered only to patients unfit for ASCT.

5.5. Rituximab Maintenance for FL Relapse

Current practice in relapsed FL includes the use of long-term Rituximab maintenance after response to salvage therapy and ASCT. The effect of Rituximab maintenance seems to be more evident in the relapse setting when compared to first line therapy, reducing long-term risk of relapse around 40% [185]. The largest trial published to date is the EORTC 20981, randomizing patients to rituximab maintenance after response to either CHOP or R-CHOP induction regimens, showing an improvement in PFS of more than 24 months in the maintenance arm, together with a 10% increment in 5-year OS [186]. Again, it should be noted that although generally safe, the combination of dose-intense rescue regimens with ASCT conditioning and Rituximab may induce a profound B-cell depletion that should be addressed during follow up, to manage infectious risks appropriately.

Results of a systematic meta-analysis [146] published in 2011, showed that rituximab maintenance for up to 2 years has a favorable side effect profile and prolongs PFS and OS in relapsed disease even after antibody containing induction regimens (pooled HR of death = 0.72, 95% CI = 0.57 to 0.91). However, it should be noted that the magnitude of PFS benefit was similar after maintenance in both first-line and relapse treatment.

A second maintenance treatment for patients previously progressing to a first-line maintenance treatment has not been investigated

5.6. Role of Allogeneic SCT

The number of FL patients requiring allogeneic SCT is generally low, thus, no prospective trials have been conducted in this setting. There is proven evidence of an effective graft *vs.* lymphoma effect (GVL) in FL patients, but there are no effective ways to predict response to allogeneic transplantation. Available trials have shown reduced recurrence rates and long term remission [181, 187 - 189]. The risk-benefit ratio should be carefully assessed, particularly because most of the patients are over 65 years of age and may have significant comorbidities.

Allogeneic SCT is usually for young patients in third remission or beyond, and only if an HLA-identical donor is found (familial or unrelated) [190, 191]. The role of novel, alternative-donor, allogeneic transplantation (*i.e.* haploidentical, cord blood), is yet to be established.

6. NOVEL AND EMERGING PHARMACOLOGICAL AGENTS

The immunomodulatory agent, lenalidomide, has been evaluated as single-agent therapy for NHL, obtaining a 27% ORR in FL, with a median duration of response of 16.5 months [192]. These results have been sufficient to promote the design of phase II trials of lenalidomide, combined with Rituximab (R^2 trials) for induction or maintenance therapy in FL. The trials for first-line induction treatment have shown outstanding preliminary results with 98% of responses and

94% of 3-year OS; long term follow-up is awaited [193].

Novel anti-CD20 antibodies are also under development, featuring greater avidity for the CD20 receptor and improved antibody-induced cytotoxicity. These novel antibodies have been shown to overcome Rituximab resistance and synergize with traditional chemotherapy. Ofatumumab is a novel second-generation of anti-CD20 antibody to be approved for use in relapsed/refractory FL; the pivotal trial has shown 42% of ORR, with 29.9 months of response duration [194]. Ofatumumab has been also combined with CHOP, with CR of 69% and ORR of 100% in phase II trials [195].

Obinutuzimab (GA-101) is another anti-CD20 antibody with an improved ADCC capacity [196]. GA-101 is currently approved only for CLL in combination with Chlorambucil, but Phase II and III trials are underway for other lymphoid malignancies. In FL, the GAUDI trial evaluated Obinutuzimab as part of the induction and the maintenance treatment in first line patients, with high response rates (70% after maintenance phase) and a 90% PFS at 32 month-follow up [197]. The GALLIUM study, comparing head to head Obinutuzimab *vs.* Rituximab as part of the induction and the maintenance regimen is underway, recruitment has already been completed.

The PI3K/Akt/mTOR pathway is widely known to play a significant role in FL pathogenesis. Temsirolimus and Everolimus are mTOR inhibitors that have been originally approved for renal carcinoma, but have also been tested for FL with acceptable results (50% ORR). The use of these agents in FL is currently limited to the clinical trial setting [198].

PI3K inhibitors are also in advanced clinical development, with recent published data of Idelalisib phase 2 trials in relapsed/refractory indolent B non-Hodgkin lymphoma. Results show a response rate of 54% for FL and a PFS of 11 months when Idelalisib was used in monotherapy [199]. These results will forward Idelalisib towards phase III trials in combination with other chemotherapy agents for FL. There are currently available results from phase I/II trials of Idelalisib combination with Rituximab/Bendamustine for refractory FL with 81% overall response, 39% complete response and 71% PFS at 24 months [173].

Ibrutinib (a first generation Bruton's tyrosine kinase inhibitor) is also in early clinical development for FL treatment. Small trials on monotherapy in FL have showed response rates of 30% in relapsed/refractory patients [200]. Phase I/II trials have also been published showing that Ibrutinib combination with R-CHOP or Bendamustine-R is safe and could increase efficacy of these regimens. Combination with Bendamustine-R yielded an ORR of 90% (50% complete responses) in FL patients [201, 202].

Vorinostat, a histone deacetylase inhibitor (HDACs), has been scarcely used specifically for FL and the first clinical trials are still to be concluded, preliminary results have shown an initial ORR of 47% [203].

7. INNOVATIVE IMMUNOTHERAPY STRATEGIES FOR TREATMENT OF FL

Treatment of follicular lymphoma has rapidly evolved in the last decades, however curability remains a challenge to overcome. Theoretically, the elimination of a microscopic population of residual FL cells after conventional treatment could be the key for the definitive cure. Immunotherapy with vaccines that induce a specific anti-tumor response is a promising strategy to remove these residual FL cells and thus avoid relapse.

Immunotherapy for lymphoid malignancies has evolved in of two parallel routes: on one hand the expansion of our knowledge about the function of the immune system and the interactions between tumor and immune cells, and on the other hand the development of technologies to manufacture biological products for immunotherapy.

Globally, two forms of immunotherapy can be distinguished: active immunotherapy, that attempts to activate "*in vivo*" the immune system and induce a competent immune response; and passive immunotherapy, that is based on the transfer of an previously generated immunity (usually *in vitro*). Both procedures may be antigen-specific or non-specific (a general activation of the immune system). The main advantage of active immunotherapy is the generation of immunologic memory, however, it requires a competent immune system to mount the desired effector and/or memory response.

The most common form of active immunotherapy is vaccination. There are different types of vaccines for cancer immunotherapy: dendritic cell (DCs) vaccines in all their forms (unloaded immature DCs, immature or mature DCs pulsed with tumor antigens), tumor cell vaccines, protein vaccines and DNA vaccines. Passive immunotherapy strategies include transfer of antibodies directed against tumor epitopes, *in vitro* activated T-cells against tumor antigens or a combination of both. The following sections review individually the most relevant immunotherapeutic strategies for FL.

7.1. Passive Immunotherapy: Adoptive Cell Therapy

As mentioned before, passive immunotherapy involves the transfer of a previously generated immunity, the two main elements that can be used for this purpose are antibodies and immune cells.

Adoptive cellular immunotherapy requires transfer of immunologically competent cells able to mediate antitumor activity, either directly or indirectly. Success of the technique relies on *in vitro* expansion of the effector cells, achieving a sufficient number to produce the desired therapeutic effect without toxicity.

The advantage of this form of immunotherapy is the activation of cells *in vitro*, avoiding the potential anergic influence of tumoral environment (*e.g.* IL-10 and TGF-beta production that inhibits the activation of immunocompetent cells) [204]. The most relevant cells types used for adoptive cell therapy will be discussed.

7.1.1. LAK Cells

LAK cells ("lymphokine activated cells") are generated from peripheral blood mononuclear cells stimulated with IL-2; cell types activated in this manner are a mixture of non-specific effector cells (mainly NK cells) and specific effector CTL (cytotoxic T lymphocytes), both proven to have significant *in vitro* cytolytic capacity against tumor cells, sparing normal cells [205]. LAK cells offer the advantage of not requiring prior exposure to the tumor to be effective [206]. Early proof of concept experiments showed that LAK were able to reduce metastatic tumor mass in humans [207].

LAK cells have been used for immunotherapy of several solid tumors as well as for the treatment of patients with lymphomas (Hodgkin´s and non-Hodgkin). Despite promising initial results, larger studies using only LAK cells in lymphoma have shown limited efficacy [208 - 210], thus, the role of LAK cells in FL will be likely limited to be the use in combinational strategies with other immunotherapy approaches.

7.1.2. NK Cells

NK cells have been demostrated to be an essential element of the innate immune response towards tumoral cells. NK cells are defined by the CD3-CD56+ phenotype, with the absence of CD19 and CD14; the effector functions can be either cytokine production or direct ADCC (antibody mediated cellular cytotoxicity).

Their mechanism of activation depends on extracellular signalling through transmembrane receptors, these receptors can be adhesion molecules or cytokine receptors and can have inhibitory or stimulatory effects depending on the context and the environment. The interaction of simultaneous signals through these receptors is complex and will ultimately determine activation or inhibition of NK cells.

NK cells have an important role in anti-cancer immunity, a decrease in peripheral blood NK activity has been linked to an increased risk of developing tumors [211] and the extent of intratumoral NK infiltration has also been linked to prognosis.

Large numbers of clinical trials have been designed attempting to exploit the innate tumor-lytic capacity of NK cells. Infusions of autologous or allogeneic NK cells for cancer therapy have been shown to be feasible and well-tolerated in cancer patients [212 - 214]. Although proven to be safe, clinical trials of autologous NK cells have shown scarse clinical benefits in solid tumors [215]. In the Hematology field, the first trials were done in AML with haploidentical NK cell transfer for relapsed patients, with a previous preparative regimen that contained Cyclophosphamide and Fludarabine; adequate expansion of transfered NK cells was observed and some complete responses were achieved without serious complications, however, the effect was always transitory and all patients eventually relapsed [216].

The combination of NK cells and monoclonal antibodies could be an interesting strategy to boost ADCC, indeed, several strategies are under investigation combining traditional monoclonal antibodies (Rituximab, Trastuzumab, Cetuximab) with addoptive NK cell transfer [217 - 219]. Another strategy for NK-related cell therapy are the recently described Bi-specific T-cell receptor enganging antibodies (BiTE), developed as a novel strategy for inducing NK reactivity towards tumor antigens. BiTE constitute a recombinant antibody construct that has a single-chain Fv directed against a tumor antigen, attached to a CD16 Fc for NK cell targeting. First in human trials have used CD16 x CD33 BiTE to target MDS clones in refactory patients, achieving succesful activation of host NK cells, safety and clinical outcomes are awaited to forward this strategy to other malignancies; for FL a CD16 x CD20 BiTE might be an interesting approach for immunotherapy [220].

7.1.3. Antigen-specific T Cells

Another strategy of passive immunotherapy is the transfer of T-cells genetically engineered to express receptors that specifically bind to antigens on tumoral B cells. There are two approaches for generating antigen-specific T cells by genetic modification: introducing genes encoding a natural T cell-receptor (TCRs) [221 - 223] or introducing genes encoding chimeric antigen receptors (CARs).

CARs are composed of an intracellular T-cell activation domain, one or more co-stimulatory domains, a hinge region, a transmembrane domain, and an antigen-recognition moiety that is typically derived from an antibody. CARs recognize intact-surface proteins and glycolipids and trigger a strong and stable activation of T-cells in an HLA-independent manner [224]. In the last 5 years, therapy with CARs has emerged, with many ongoing trials testing their efficacy. CAR therapy for hematological malignancies has pioneered this field of research, with at least 14 publications reporting clinical trials with CARs, probably due to the more extensive knowledge of surface antigens expressed in tumor cells.

CD19 has been the first CAR-T antigen that has been forwarded to clinical trials; CD19 is an attractive target as it is uniformly expressed in the vast majority of B-cell malignancies [225]. Importantly, expression of CD19 in normal tissues is restricted to mature B cells, B-cell precursors, plasma cells and some follicular dendritic cells [226, 227]. Treatment with CD19 CARs is being tested in hematologic malignancies such as ALL, CLL and follicular lymphomas. Preliminary results have been encouraging, many refractory patients in Phase I clinical trials have achieved and maintained complete remissions, hence, clinical development for B-cell neoplasms has moved ahead with over 25 clinical trials using CD19 CARs with different modifications.

Alongside the spectacular efficacy, the strength of the immune response that is generated by CD19 CARs can also have serious adverse effects. Some patients develop a cytokine release syndrome that can rapidly deteriorate clinical condition and lead to a life-threatening hemodynamic collapse. Other long-term side effects include hypogammaglobulinemia due to B-cell depletion, which could constrain patients to life-long immunoglobulin substitution therapy [228]. Strategies to overcome these issues are also under investigation; alternatives include the use of some monoclonal antibodies against cytokines to damp the inflammatory response and the use of a suicide gene that can be triggered to control CAR proliferation if complications arise [229, 230].

The design of CD20 CARs might be of particular interest for B-cell lymphomas, the trials are also underway with promising early clinical results. However, the use of CARs in indolent lymphomas demand a better security profile compared to that required for a CD19+ acute leukemia or a refractory aggressive lymphoma, therefore, clinical development for CD20 CARs is expected to arrive somewhat later.

Finally, beyond CD19 and CD20, attention has focused on other antigens for CAR development, such as Lewis-Y and CD33 for acute myeloid leukemia, or CD30 and Ig kappa light chain for FL [231]. CARs are likely to be the future in immunotherapy for hematologic malignancies, but nowadays remain an investigational strategy. As with any other treatment strategy, survival improvements must be demonstrated in phase II and III clinical trials and safety issues must be resolved before they can be incorporated into the routine clinical practice.

7.1.4. Treatment Combinations: Rituximab and Effector Cells

Combination studies have provided strong evidence that the administration of anti-CD20 monoclonal antibody with the induction and maintenance treatment prolongs the duration of remission and OS in patients with FL. However, some patients still relapse during the maintanenace treatment or soon after the end of treatment, suggesting the presence of residual FL cells that are resistant or non-responsive to Rituximab. Strategies to augment the efficacy of the anti-CD20 antbody are likely to improve clinical outcomes in these situations [232].

The main mechanism of action of Rituximab *in vivo* is ADCC. Noteworthy, succesful ADCC in not only dependant on the antibody, but also on a competent effector cell. CTLs and NK cells are the two main effector cells capable of mediating ADCC, both of which may show decreased activity in patients with cancer [233, 234]. In patients with B-cell ymphoma, ADCC activity is decreased compared to healthy controls and it can be further impaired after treatment with Rituximab, for reasons that are poorly understood [235].

An interesting strategy to improve the effectiveness of monoclonal antibodies might be enhancing the activity of the immune system effector arm. Rituximab has been combined with recombinant IL-2 that could promote expansion of NK cells and enhance ADCC. This has been demonstrated in murine models of lymphoma [236] and has led to development of various clinical trials in humans [237 - 239]. These trials demonstrated that IL-2 mediates an increase of circulating NK-cells and their cytotoxic effects, but failed to provide clinical benefit.

Another strategy could be the use of adoptive cell therapy with effector cells to potentiate ADCC (*e.g.* LAK cells with monoclonal antibodies), a combination that a priori would be easily translated to the clinic. LAK cells in combination with monoclonal antibodies have an enhanced antitumor activity in murine models [240]. In FL, LAK with anti-CD20 could induce a more potent lytic effect on CD20+ tumoral cells.

Berdeja *et al.,* [235] demonstrated that administration of systemic IL-2 and LAK cells improved ADCC in lymphoma patients treated with Rituximab. This is a small pilot study with 10 patients, that served as proof of concept. Currently, a clinical trial is being conducted to evaluate the efficacy of combined treatment with LAK cells and Rituximab during the maintenance phase in patients with FL, after achieveng complete response with conventional induction treatment.

7.2. Active Immunotherapy Strategies: Vaccines

The concept of vaccines in neoplastic diseases (hematologic and non-hematologic) is clearly different from the concept of infectious disease vaccination. Infectious diseases vaccines are directed against a well-known antigen, have a high immunogenic potential and a prophylactic purpose, whereas in the case of cancer, tumor antigens are not always known, many times the immunogenicity is weak and most importantly, the intent is therapeutic.

Advances in the identification of antigens expressed on tumor cells have permitted the development of vaccines specifically directed against them. In this regard it is important to distinguish between tumor-associated antigens (TAAs) that are localized in tumoral cells and some normal cells and tumor specific antigens (TEAs), which are expressed only in tumoral cells. TEAs are the obvious choice for immunotherapy strategies, if available.

FL represents an ideal tumor for the development of antigenic vaccines. All B cells express a surface clonal immunoglobulin, such clonality is determined by the idiotype (antigenic determinants located in the hypervariable region of immunoglobulin), thus, when a B lymphocyte transforms into a tumor cell, the idiotype becomes a TEA. Moreover, relatively large quantities of FL-cells are readily available from clinical samples, allowing *in vitro* manipulation to manufacture the specific idiotypic vaccines.

Production of soluble anti-idiotypic immunoglobulin is the key aspect of vaccine production in FL; it has been traditionally based on the hybridoma technique, which allows *in vitro* production of the tumor immunoglobulin but has some disadvantages such as a high cost and relatively slow rate of production. Recombinant technology is another method to obtaining soluble protein, two expression systems have been traditionally used: microorganisms and mammalian cells. Recently, another alternative method with the use of plants as bioreactors for the production of recombinant proteins has become available. The best and more reliable method for vaccine production remains to be established. The following sections will review individually the available vaccine subtypes for FL.

7.2.1. Idiotype Protein Vaccines

The Idiotype vaccines are constitued of a tumor specific immunoglobulin (*i.e.* the idiotype, [Id]), chemically conjugated with an immunogenic carrier protein (keyhole lipet hemocyanin [KLH] is the most frequently used) [241]. Adjuvant stimulation of the immune respose is required for vaccination, which is tipically done with GM-CSF protein co-administration [161, 242].

Kwak *et al.* [243] were the first to demonstrate that the idiotype vaccine (Id-KLH plus adjuvant SFA-1) was able to induce a specific immune response against the idiotype in seven of nine FL patients in situation of complete response (CR), or with evidence of persistent disease after chemotherapy. This study provided the first formal proof that humans could be immunized against an antigen derived from their own tumor (biological efficiency).

The same group reported some years later a long-term follow-up of 41 patients treated with the same idiotype vaccine formulation [244]. The results provided the first evidence that idiotype vaccine could have a relevant impact on the course of disease. Another similar study published by Bendandi *et al.* was conducted in 25 patients with FL in first remission, vaccinated with Id-KLH with adjuvant GM-CSF [245]. The most remarkable finding was the induction of long lasting vaccine-induced molecular remissions in 9 out of 12 evaluable patients (PCR monitoring of the t (14; 18) and bcl-2 rearrangements). This results suggest that vaccination can overcome chemotherapy resistance in residual FL cells. Outcomes of anti-idiotype vaccination have also been confirmed by other groups [246, 247].

Further studies have focused on PFS; Bendandi *et al.*, conducted a trial including 33 patients, showing that all patients who responded immunologically to the vaccine (20/25) had a second complete remission lasting longer than that expected with chemotherapy alone. Furthermore, in those patients with sufficient follow-up, the duration of the second complete remission exceeded that of the first remission [248]. The main limitation of these initial studies is that the number of patients is insufficient to obtain regulatory agencies approval. Three phase III clinical trials have been conducted seeking FDA approval of idiotypic vaccine in FL, however, the approval was denied because the results were not as positive as initially expected [249 - 252].

It might be concluded that idiotypic vaccines confer clinical benefit and generate anti-tumoral specific immune response, that might be translated into survival benefit only in the appropriate subgroup of patients. This is, patients with the least possible disease burden (*i.e.* CR after induction treatment) and a competent immune system able to develop immunologic memory after mounting an effective respose towards the idiotype.

7.2.2. DNA Vaccines

Naked DNA vaccines consist of bacterial DNA in which certain genes encoding the tumor protein are added [253, 254]. When a DNA vaccine is injected intramuscularly or subcutaneously, host cells (generally muscle cells, keratinocytes and fibroblasts) are transfected creating a zone of ectopic expression of the protein. The protein released by the target cell is captured by local presenting cells (which may also be transfected) and after being properly processed, it is presented to the immune system in secondary lymphoid organs [255]. The main advantage of DNA vaccines are the lower cost of production and the turnover time of the final vaccine product, that is substantially reduced compared to protein vaccines.

Bacterial DNA naturally contains immunostimulatory sequences that are not present in mammalian cells, which are able to activate the innate immune system through the release of cytokines (*e.g.* IFN-γ, IFN-α, IL-12 and IL-18) and also polarize the immune response towards a Th1 pattern [256, 257]. Despite these properties, DNA vaccines overall have a low immunogenic potential; to overcome this issue, immunomodulatory proteins or cytokines can be introduced into the plasmid construct to be co-expressed by transfected cells. Theoretically, the release of the stimulatory proteins together with the antigenic protein might increase the strength of the immune response.

For FL treatment, DNA vaccines consist of intramuscular or subcutaneous injections of a bacterial plasmid containing the sequence encoding the idiotype sFab. Initial studies in animal models have shown that vaccines are not immunogenic unless sFab sequences are fused with a carrier [258 - 261].

Another alternative to enhance the immunogenicity of idiotype sFab DNA vaccines is to fuse the antigen with ligands of receptors expressed in DCs, to boost the antigenic uptake and presentation. In this regard, MCP-3 or MIP-3a fused sFab vaccines have shown some efficacy in murine models of follicular lymphoma in both prophylactic and therapeutic strategies [262, 263]. No proof of concept trial has been published in humans so far.

7.2.3. Dendritic Cell Vaccines

The role of denritic cells (DCs) makes them very attractive for use in therapeutic vaccination strategies. The transport of antigens by dendritic cells is critical in the initiation of the immune response, even a small number of dendritic cells is sufficient to induce a potent immune response *in vivo*. Antigen presentation by DCs can induce the expansion of CTL and CD4+ helper T cells through antigen presentation *via* MHC-I or MHC-II respectively, DCs also modulate growth and differentiation of B cells and thus become involved in the humoral response.

The first milestone in dendritic cell vaccines was the possibility of growing large quantities of dendritic cells derived from monocytes, in the presence of GM-CSF and IL-4 [264]. The first assay published of a dendritic vaccine in FL employed autologous DCs pulsed *in vitro* with the Idiotype protein. Results demonstrated the induction of reactive T cells against the tumor in 4 patients, without detectable antibody response; more importantly, the procedure was proven to be clinically safe [265]. These preliminary results were updated in 2002, including a total of 35 patients; idiotype-pulsed DCs induced effective humoral and cellular immune responses that were translated into clinical response and durable tumor regressions [266].

Some authors have explored additional tumoral antigens for pulsed-DC vaccination, such as WT-1 protein, typically overexpressed in B-cell malignancies. Pilot studies have shown a fare safety profile and good clinical results, including some complete responses [267].

Vaccination with pulsed-DCs represents an interesting option for the design of active immunotherapy strategies, further development will likely be seen in the upcoming years. A clinical trial of pulsed-DC vaccination with tumoral lysates in FL is currently underway [268].

7.2.4. Membrane Proteoliposomal Vaccines

Liposomes are vesicles formed with a bilayer of phospholipids and cholesterol with an aqueous internal compartment. These structures are similar to phospholipid cell membranes and have many pharmaceutical applications. In the field of immunotherapy, liposomes have been shown to be effective as vaccine vehicles and as adjuvant agents [269].

Liposome-encapsulated-idiotype has been used as a model for FL vaccination, intraperitoneal injection of the compound in murine models has shown good results, extending animal survival. This approach has also been used in two Phase I clinical trials, with fare safety and near 50% of successful tumor-specific immune response, together with some complete responses in refractory patients [270, 271].

7.2.5. Strategies to Enhance Immunogenicity

Several mechanisms can counteract the vaccine-induced immune response and reduce clinical efficacy, thus, knlowledge and manipulation of these suppressor mechanisms could potentially improve the therapeutic effect of vaccines.

For example, CTL-4 and PD-1 are naturally occurring inhibitor receptors on the surface of activated T-cells. Under normal conditions, signalling through these receptors block T-cell activation, and dampen the immune reponse. This physiologic mechanism prevents autoimmunity and allows the organism to establish tolerance to self-antigens. However, CTL-4 and PD-1 ligand expresion by tumoral cells can become detrimental for anti-tumoral immune response, in fact, overexpression of such ligands in tumoral cells is a well known immune evasion mechanism of cancer [272]. PD-1 blockade with monoclonal antibodies is an emerging treatment for many hematologic malignancies with encougaring results; it remains to be shown if combination of these antibodies with vaccination is synergistic and translates into clinical benefit.

Pre-existing T-regulatory cells cells and myeloid suppressor cells in FL are other naturally occurring immunosupression mechanisms. Vaccination combined with strategies to block the effects of these immune-suppresant cell types cells could enhance the effects of vaccination. For example, IMiDs such as Lenalidomide or Pomalidomide which have antitumor properties by themselves, can also have an effect on T-regulatory and T-helper cells [273 - 276]. In fact, Lenalidomide increases the production of cytokines such as IL-2 and IFN-Ƴ by CD4+ T-helper 1 cells (Th1), enhancing antibody dependent cellular cytotoxicity, inhibiting the proliferation and altering functionality of regulatory T cells [277, 278]. Combination of IMiDs with vaccination could also be an interesting synergistic approach to improve efficacy.

7.3. New Targets for Immunotherapy

Important progress has been made on anti-idiotype vaccination strategies, the attractiveness of personalized medicine and the obvious advantage of a tumor specific antigen (*i.e.* the idiotype) has given these approaches much attention. However, some authors believe that the cost for large-scale application of anti-idiotype vaccination is still unacceptable.

Research continues towards the identification of universal FL antigens that would facilitate large-scale production of a "one-fits all" type of vaccine. The B-cell activating factor receptor (BAFF-R) has emerged as a potential candidate; BAFF-R is essential for B-cell maturation and survival, and is strongly expressed in most FL clones [279, 280].

Other candidates could be IGKV3 and IGKV3-20-50 proteins, which are detected in nearly 70% of HCV-related lymphomas. IGKV3 or IGKV3-20-15 light chains are also detected with a high degree of homology between different lymphomas including diffuse large B-cell lymphomas, marginal B-cell lymphoma, follicular lymphoma, multiple myeloma and chronic lymphocytic leukemia. IGKV3 proteins are immunogenic, inducing both humoral and cellular responses and thus, are another attractive target for vaccine development [281].

TCL-1 (T- cell leukemia/lymphoma 1) is an oncoprotein encoded by the TCL-1 gene which is selectively expressed on normal B lymphocytes and markedly overexpressed in many human B-cell lymphomas, including follicular lymphoma, mantle cell lymphoma, chronic lymphocytic leukemia, diffuse large B-cell lymphoma and splenic marginal zone B-cell lymphoma. Weng *et al.* have demonstrated that CD8+ T cells specific against TCL-1 are naturally generated and identified TCL-1$_{71-78}$ as the minimal epitope recognized by these T cells. TCL-1 specific lymphocytes are found in peripheral blood and tumor-infiltrating lymphocytes and can be isolated and expanded *in vitro*. These results suggest that TCL-1 is naturally processed and presented on the surface of lymphoma cells for recognition by cytotoxic T cells and may serve as another novel target for development of vaccines [282].

7.4. Future Directions in Vaccine Development

The results obtained in the field of active immunotherapy for FL are encouraging, many aspects remain to be solved and optimized before moving them to the clinical practice. The indolent nature of FL is probably the main obstacle for a more rapid development of this area, long-term benefit in survival must be demonstrated before approval, and as for any novel therapeutic strategy randomized trials with long-term follow up are needed.

Additionally, important aspects remain yet to be elucidated from the basic science perspective, such as the identification of a universal tumor-specific antigen, the definition of better tumor-associated antigens and epitopes, the optimal vaccine formulation and the best adjuvant therapy.

From the clinical point of view, the critical aspects that could help to achieve translation are: 1) Optimization of vaccine efficacy in terms of immune response, increasing immunogenicity and/or blocking the inhibitory mechanisms that prevent the generation of the immune response; 2) Development of biomarkers that may help identify which patients could have the greatest benefit with these treatment strategies; 3) Definition of the best antigen for vaccination in terms of clinical effectiveness; and 4) Definition of the best vaccination strategy in terms of turn-around time, logistics and cost.

CONCLUDING REMARKS

The current management of patients with FL involves the risk-stratification of patients at diagnosis to offer an appropriate and timely therapy; this is, dose-intense treatment for poor-risk disease and low toxicity treatments for low-risk patients. Therapy for FL will undoubtedly move in the years to come towards a "curative intent" with a multimodal approach. Immunotherapy is becoming an increasingly relevant therapeutic modality for the treatment of FL patients, thus, the careful and adequate use of modified immune cells, antibodies, vaccines and cytokines together with conventional treatments will almost certainly continue to improve the therapeutic outcome of patients with FL .

CONFLICT OF INTEREST

The authors confirm that they have no conflict of interest to declare for this publication.

ACKNOWLEDGEMENTS

Declared none.

REFERENCES

[1]   van Besien K, Schouten H. Follicular lymphoma: A historical overview. Leuk Lymphoma 2007; 48(2): 232-43.
        [http://dx.doi.org/10.1080/10428190601059746] [PMID: 17325883]

[2]   Groves FD, Linet MS, Travis LB, Devesa SS. Cancer surveillance series: non-Hodgkin's lymphoma incidence by histologic subtype in the United States from 1978 through 1995. J Natl Cancer Inst 2000; 92(15): 1240-51.
        [http://dx.doi.org/10.1093/jnci/92.15.1240] [PMID: 10922409]

[3]   Morton LM, Wang SS, Devesa SS, Hartge P, Weisenburger DD, Linet MS. Lymphoma incidence patterns by WHO subtype in the United States, 1992-2001. Blood 2006; 107(1): 265-76.
        [http://dx.doi.org/10.1182/blood-2005-06-2508] [PMID: 16150940]

[4]   Czuczman MS. Controversies in follicular lymphoma: "who, what, when, where, and why?" (not necessarily in that order!). Hematology (Am Soc Hematol Educ Program) 2006; 2006: 303-10.
        [http://dx.doi.org/10.1182/asheducation-2006.1.303] [PMID: 17124076]

[5]   Sacchi S, Pozzi S, Marcheselli L, *et al.* Italian Lymphoma Study Group. Introduction of rituximab in front-line and salvage therapies has improved outcome of advanced-stage follicular lymphoma patients. Cancer 2007; 109(10): 2077-82.
        [http://dx.doi.org/10.1002/cncr.22649] [PMID: 17394190]

[6]   Liu Q, Fayad L, Cabanillas F, *et al.* Improvement of overall and failure-free survival in stage IV
        follicular lymphoma: 25 years of treatment experience at The University of Texas M.D. Anderson
        Cancer Center. J Clin Oncol 2006; 24(10): 1582-9.
        [http://dx.doi.org/10.1200/JCO.2005.03.3696] [PMID: 16575009]

[7]   Swenson WT, Wooldridge JE, Lynch CF, Forman-Hoffman VL, Chrischilles E, Link BK. Improved
        survival of follicular lymphoma patients in the United States. J Clin Oncol 2005; 23(22): 5019-26.
        [http://dx.doi.org/10.1200/JCO.2005.04.503] [PMID: 15983392]

[8]   Fisher RI, LeBlanc M, Press OW, Maloney DG, Unger JM, Miller TP. New treatment options have
        changed the survival of patients with follicular lymphoma. J Clin Oncol 2005; 23(33): 8447-52.
        [http://dx.doi.org/10.1200/JCO.2005.03.1674] [PMID: 16230674]

[9]   Czuczman M, Straus D, Gribben J, Bredenfeld H, Friedberg J, Bollard C. Management options,
        survivorship, and emerging treatment strategies for follicular and Hodgkin lymphomas. Leuk
        Lymphoma 2010; 51 (Suppl. 1): 41-9.
        [http://dx.doi.org/10.3109/10428194.2010.500083] [PMID: 20658953]

[10]   Solal-Céligny P, Roy P, Colombat P, *et al.* Follicular lymphoma international prognostic index. Blood
        2004; 104(5): 1258-65.
        [http://dx.doi.org/10.1182/blood-2003-12-4434] [PMID: 15126323]

[11]   Relander T, Johnson NA, Farinha P, Connors JM, Sehn LH, Gascoyne RD. Prognostic factors in
        follicular lymphoma. J Clin Oncol 2010; 28(17): 2902-13.
        [http://dx.doi.org/10.1200/JCO.2009.26.1693] [PMID: 20385990]

[12]   Gribben JG. How I treat indolent lymphoma. Blood 2007; 109(11): 4617-26.
        [http://dx.doi.org/10.1182/blood-2006-10-041863] [PMID: 17311989]

[13]   Davies AJ. Clinical and molecular prognostic factors in follicular lymphoma. Curr Oncol Rep 2006;
        8(5): 359-67.
        [http://dx.doi.org/10.1007/s11912-006-0059-8] [PMID: 16901397]

[14]   Ghielmini M, Vitolo U, Kimby E, *et al.* Panel Members of the 1st ESMO Consensus Conference on
        Malignant Lymphoma. ESMO Guidelines consensus conference on malignant lymphoma 2011 part 1:
        diffuse large B-cell lymphoma (DLBCL), follicular lymphoma (FL) and chronic lymphocytic
        leukemia (CLL). Ann Oncol 2013; 24(3): 561-76.
        [http://dx.doi.org/10.1093/annonc/mds517] [PMID: 23175624]

[15]   Harris NH, Swerdlow SH, Jaffe ES, *et al.* Follicular Lymphoma. In: Swerdlow SH, Campo E, Lee
        Harris N, Eds. WHO Classification of tumours of haematopoietic and lymphoid tissues. 4th ed. Lyon,
        France: IARC press/World Health Organization 2008; pp. 229-32.

[16]   Harris NL, de Leval L, Ferry JA. Follicular Lymphoma. In: Jaffe E, Harris N, Vardiman J, Eds.
        Hematopathology. 1st ed. Philadelphia, PA: Saunders/Elsevier 2011; p. 267. [electronic resource]
        [http://dx.doi.org/10.1016/B978-0-7216-0040-6.00017-4]

[17]   Rohatiner AZ. Follicular Lymphoma. In: Magrath IT, Bathia K, Boffeta P, Eds. The lymphoid
        neoplasms. 3rd ed. London, UK: Hodder Arnold 2010; p. 1173.
        [http://dx.doi.org/10.1201/b13424-76]

[18]   Mann RB, Berard CW. Criteria for the cytologic subclassification of follicular lymphomas: a proposed

alternative method. Hematol Oncol 1983; 1(2): 187-92.
[http://dx.doi.org/10.1002/hon.2900010209] [PMID: 6376315]

[19]   Ott G, Katzenberger T, Lohr A, *et al.* Cytomorphologic, immunohistochemical, and cytogenetic profiles of follicular lymphoma: 2 types of follicular lymphoma grade 3. Blood 2002; 99(10): 3806-12.
[http://dx.doi.org/10.1182/blood.V99.10.3806] [PMID: 11986240]

[20]   de Leval L, Harris NL, Longtine J, Ferry JA, Duncan LM. Cutaneous b-cell lymphomas of follicular and marginal zone types: use of Bcl-6, CD10, Bcl-2, and CD21 in differential diagnosis and classification. Am J Surg Pathol 2001; 25(6): 732-41.
[http://dx.doi.org/10.1097/00000478-200106000-00004] [PMID: 11395550]

[21]   Harris NL, Nadler LM, Bhan AK. Immunohistologic characterization of two malignant lymphomas of germinal center type (centroblastic/centrocytic and centrocytic) with monoclonal antibodies. Follicular and diffuse lymphomas of small-cleaved-cell type are related but distinct entities. Am J Pathol 1984; 117(2): 262-72.
[PMID: 6437232]

[22]   Cattoretti G, Chang CC, Cechova K, *et al.* BCL-6 protein is expressed in germinal-center B cells. Blood 1995; 86(1): 45-53.
[PMID: 7795255]

[23]   Lai R, Weiss LM, Chang KL, Arber DA. Frequency of CD43 expression in non-Hodgkin lymphoma. A survey of 742 cases and further characterization of rare CD43+ follicular lymphomas. Am J Clin Pathol 1999; 111(4): 488-94.
[PMID: 10191768]

[24]   Raghavan SC, Swanson PC, Wu X, Hsieh CL, Lieber MR. A non-B-DNA structure at the Bcl-2 major breakpoint region is cleaved by the RAG complex. Nature 2004; 428(6978): 88-93.
[http://dx.doi.org/10.1038/nature02355] [PMID: 14999286]

[25]   Busslinger M. Transcriptional control of early B cell development. Annu Rev Immunol 2004; 22: 55-79.
[http://dx.doi.org/10.1146/annurev.immunol.22.012703.104807] [PMID: 15032574]

[26]   Willis TG, Dyer MJ. The role of immunoglobulin translocations in the pathogenesis of B-cell malignancies. Blood 2000; 96(3): 808-22.
[PMID: 10910891]

[27]   Stamatopoulos K, Kosmas C, Belessi C, *et al.* t(14;18) chromosomal translocation in follicular lymphoma: an event occurring with almost equal frequency both at the D to J(H) and at later stages in the rearrangement process of the immunoglobulin heavy chain gene locus. Br J Haematol 1997; 99(4): 866-72.
[http://dx.doi.org/10.1046/j.1365-2141.1997.4853290.x] [PMID: 9432035]

[28]   Jäger U, Böcskör S, Le T, *et al.* Follicular lymphomas' BCL-2/IgH junctions contain templated nucleotide insertions: novel insights into the mechanism of t(14;18) translocation. Blood 2000; 95(11): 3520-9.
[PMID: 10828038]

[29]   Martinez-Climent JA, Fontan L, Gascoyne RD, Siebert R, Prosper F. Lymphoma stem cells: enough evidence to support their existence? Haematologica 2010; 95(2): 293-302.

[http://dx.doi.org/10.3324/haematol.2009.013318] [PMID: 20139392]

[30]   Fenton JA, Vaandrager JW, Aarts WM, *et al.* Follicular lymphoma with a novel t(14;18) breakpoint involving the immunoglobulin heavy chain switch mu region indicates an origin from germinal center B cells. Blood 2002; 99(2): 716-8.
[http://dx.doi.org/10.1182/blood.V99.2.716] [PMID: 11781262]

[31]   Ottensmeier CH, Thompsett AR, Zhu D, Wilkins BS, Sweetenham JW, Stevenson FK. Analysis of VH genes in follicular and diffuse lymphoma shows ongoing somatic mutation and multiple isotype transcripts in early disease with changes during disease progression. Blood 1998; 91(11): 4292-9.
[PMID: 9596678]

[32]   Lossos IS, Alizadeh AA, Eisen MB, *et al.* Ongoing immunoglobulin somatic mutation in germinal center B cell-like but not in activated B cell-like diffuse large cell lymphomas. Proc Natl Acad Sci USA 2000; 97(18): 10209-13.
[http://dx.doi.org/10.1073/pnas.180316097] [PMID: 10954754]

[33]   Oeschger S, Bräuninger A, Küppers R, Hansmann ML. Tumor cell dissemination in follicular lymphoma. Blood 2002; 99(6): 2192-8.
[http://dx.doi.org/10.1182/blood.V99.6.2192] [PMID: 11877297]

[34]   Dighiero G, Hart S, Lim A, Borche L, Levy R, Miller RA. Autoantibody activity of immunoglobulins isolated from B-cell follicular lymphomas. Blood 1991; 78(3): 581-5.
[PMID: 1859876]

[35]   Sachen KL, Strohman MJ, Singletary J, *et al.* Self-antigen recognition by follicular lymphoma B-cell receptors. Blood 2012; 120(20): 4182-90.
[http://dx.doi.org/10.1182/blood-2012-05-427534] [PMID: 23024238]

[36]   Cha SC, Qin H, Kannan S, *et al.* Nonstereotyped lymphoma B cell receptors recognize vimentin as a shared autoantigen. J Immunol 2013; 190(9): 4887-98.
[http://dx.doi.org/10.4049/jimmunol.1300179] [PMID: 23536634]

[37]   Fowler N, Davis E. Targeting B-cell receptor signaling: changing the paradigm. Hematology Am Soc Hematol Educ Program 2013; 2013: 553-60.

[38]   McCann KJ, Ottensmeier CH, Callard A, *et al.* Remarkable selective glycosylation of the immunoglobulin variable region in follicular lymphoma. Mol Immunol 2008; 45(6): 1567-72.
[http://dx.doi.org/10.1016/j.molimm.2007.10.009] [PMID: 18022232]

[39]   Radcliffe CM, Arnold JN, Suter DM, *et al.* Human follicular lymphoma cells contain oligomannose glycans in the antigen-binding site of the B-cell receptor. J Biol Chem 2007; 282(10): 7405-15.
[http://dx.doi.org/10.1074/jbc.M602690200] [PMID: 17197448]

[40]   Coelho V, Krysov S, Ghaemmaghami AM, *et al.* Glycosylation of surface Ig creates a functional bridge between human follicular lymphoma and microenvironmental lectins. Proc Natl Acad Sci USA 2010; 107(43): 18587-92.
[http://dx.doi.org/10.1073/pnas.1009388107] [PMID: 20937880]

[41]   Irish JM, Czerwinski DK, Nolan GP, Levy R. Altered B-cell receptor signaling kinetics distinguish human follicular lymphoma B cells from tumor-infiltrating nonmalignant B cells. Blood 2006; 108(9): 3135-42.

[http://dx.doi.org/10.1182/blood-2006-02-003921] [PMID: 16835385]

[42] Blum KA, Christian B, Flynn JM, *et al.* A Phase I Trial of the Bruton's Tyrosine Kinase (BTK) Inhibitor, Ibrutinib (PCI-32765), in Combination with Rituximab (R) and Bendamustine in Patients with Relapsed/Refractory Non-Hodgkin's Lymphoma (NHL). ASH Annual Meeting Abstracts. 120(21): 1643.

[43] Fowler NH, de Vos S, Schreeder MT, *et al.* Combinations of the Phosphatidylinositol 3-Kinase-Delta (PI3K{delta}) Inhibitor Gs-1101 (CAL-101) with Rituximab and/or Bendamustine Are Tolerable and Highly Active in Previously Treated, Indolent Non-Hodgkin Lymphoma: Results From a Phase I Study. ASH Annual Meeting Abstracts. 120(21): 3645.

[44] Fowler NH, Advani RH, Sharman J, *et al.* The bruton's tyrosine kinase inhibitor ibrutinib (PCI-32765) is active and tolerated in relapsed follicular lymphoma. ASH Annual Meeting Abstracts. 120(21): 156.

[45] Kheirallah S, Caron P, Gross E, *et al.* Rituximab inhibits B-cell receptor signaling. Blood 2010; 115(5): 985-94.
[http://dx.doi.org/10.1182/blood-2009-08-237537] [PMID: 19965664]

[46] de Jong D, Fest T. The microenvironment in follicular lymphoma. Best Pract Res Clin Haematol 2011; 24(2): 135-46.
[http://dx.doi.org/10.1016/j.beha.2011.02.007] [PMID: 21658614]

[47] Carbone A, Gloghini A, Cabras A, Elia G. The Germinal centre-derived lymphomas seen through their cellular microenvironment. Br J Haematol 2009; 145(4): 468-80.
[http://dx.doi.org/10.1111/j.1365-2141.2009.07651.x] [PMID: 19344401]

[48] Wahlin BE, Sander B, Christensson B, *et al.* Entourage: the immune microenvironment following follicular lymphoma. Blood Cancer J 2012; 2(1): e52.
[http://dx.doi.org/10.1038/bcj.2011.53] [PMID: 22829236]

[49] Wahlin BE, Sundström C, Holte H, *et al.* T cells in tumors and blood predict outcome in follicular lymphoma treated with rituximab. Clin Cancer Res 2011; 17(12): 4136-44.
[http://dx.doi.org/10.1158/1078-0432.CCR-11-0264] [PMID: 21518780]

[50] Sweetenham JW, Goldman B, LeBlanc ML, *et al.* Prognostic value of regulatory T cells, lymphoma-associated macrophages, and MUM-1 expression in follicular lymphoma treated before and after the introduction of monoclonal antibody therapy: a Southwest Oncology Group Study. Ann Oncol 2010; 21(6): 1196-202.
[http://dx.doi.org/10.1093/annonc/mdp460] [PMID: 19875761]

[51] Dave SS, Wright G, Tan B, *et al.* Prediction of survival in follicular lymphoma based on molecular features of tumor-infiltrating immune cells. N Engl J Med 2004; 351(21): 2159-69.
[http://dx.doi.org/10.1056/NEJMoa041869] [PMID: 15548776]

[52] Binder M, Léchenne B, Ummanni R, *et al.* Stereotypical chronic lymphocytic leukemia B-cell receptors recognize survival promoting antigens on stromal cells. PLoS One 2010; 5(12): e15992.
[http://dx.doi.org/10.1371/journal.pone.0015992] [PMID: 21209908]

[53] Lanemo Myhrinder A, Hellqvist E, Sidorova E, *et al.* A new perspective: molecular motifs on oxidized LDL, apoptotic cells, and bacteria are targets for chronic lymphocytic leukemia antibodies. Blood 2008; 111(7): 3838-48.

[http://dx.doi.org/10.1182/blood-2007-11-125450] [PMID: 18223168]

[54]   Guilloton F, Caron G, Ménard C, *et al.* Mesenchymal stromal cells orchestrate follicular lymphoma cell niche through the CCL2-dependent recruitment and polarization of monocytes. Blood 2012; 119(11): 2556-67.
[http://dx.doi.org/10.1182/blood-2011-08-370908] [PMID: 22289889]

[55]   Amé-Thomas P, Maby-El Hajjami H, Monvoisin C, *et al.* Human mesenchymal stem cells isolated from bone marrow and lymphoid organs support tumor B-cell growth: role of stromal cells in follicular lymphoma pathogenesis. Blood 2007; 109(2): 693-702.
[http://dx.doi.org/10.1182/blood-2006-05-020800] [PMID: 16985173]

[56]   Alvaro T, Lejeune M, Salvadó MT, *et al.* Immunohistochemical patterns of reactive microenvironment are associated with clinicobiologic behavior in follicular lymphoma patients. J Clin Oncol 2006; 24(34): 5350-7.
[http://dx.doi.org/10.1200/JCO.2006.06.4766] [PMID: 17135637]

[57]   Glas AM, Knoops L, Delahaye L, *et al.* Gene-expression and immunohistochemical study of specific T-cell subsets and accessory cell types in the transformation and prognosis of follicular lymphoma. J Clin Oncol 2007; 25(4): 390-8.
[http://dx.doi.org/10.1200/JCO.2006.06.1648] [PMID: 17200149]

[58]   Carreras J, Lopez-Guillermo A, Roncador G, *et al.* High numbers of tumor-infiltrating programmed cell death 1-positive regulatory lymphocytes are associated with improved overall survival in follicular lymphoma. J Clin Oncol 2009; 27(9): 1470-6.
[http://dx.doi.org/10.1200/JCO.2008.18.0513] [PMID: 19224853]

[59]   Lee AM, Clear AJ, Calaminici M, *et al.* Number of CD4+ cells and location of forkhead box protein P3-positive cells in diagnostic follicular lymphoma tissue microarrays correlates with outcome. J Clin Oncol 2006; 24(31): 5052-9.
[http://dx.doi.org/10.1200/JCO.2006.06.4642] [PMID: 17033038]

[60]   Carreras J, Lopez-Guillermo A, Fox BC, *et al.* High numbers of tumor-infiltrating FOXP3-positive regulatory T cells are associated with improved overall survival in follicular lymphoma. Blood 2006; 108(9): 2957-64.
[http://dx.doi.org/10.1182/blood-2006-04-018218] [PMID: 16825494]

[61]   Canioni D, Salles G, Mounier N, *et al.* High numbers of tumor-associated macrophages have an adverse prognostic value that can be circumvented by rituximab in patients with follicular lymphoma enrolled onto the GELA-GOELAMS FL-2000 trial. J Clin Oncol 2008; 26(3): 440-6.
[http://dx.doi.org/10.1200/JCO.2007.12.8298] [PMID: 18086798]

[62]   Farinha P, Masoudi H, Skinnider BF, *et al.* Analysis of multiple biomarkers shows that lymphoma-associated macrophage (LAM) content is an independent predictor of survival in follicular lymphoma (FL). Blood 2005; 106(6): 2169-74.
[http://dx.doi.org/10.1182/blood-2005-04-1565] [PMID: 15933054]

[63]   Alvaro T, Lejeune M, Camacho FI, *et al.* The presence of STAT1-positive tumor-associated macrophages and their relation to outcome in patients with follicular lymphoma. Haematologica 2006; 91(12): 1605-12.
[PMID: 17145596]

[64]   Gloghini A, Carbone A. The nonlymphoid microenvironment of reactive follicles and lymphomas of follicular origin as defined by immunohistology on paraffin-embedded tissues. Hum Pathol 1993; 24(1): 67-76.
[http://dx.doi.org/10.1016/0046-8177(93)90065-O] [PMID: 8418015]

[65]   Poppema S, Bhan AK, Reinherz EL, McCluskey RT, Schlossman SF. Distribution of T cell subsets in human lymph nodes. J Exp Med 1981; 153(1): 30-41.
[http://dx.doi.org/10.1084/jem.153.1.30] [PMID: 6450262]

[66]   Harris NL, Bhan AK. Distribution of T-cell subsets in follicular and diffuse lymphomas of B-cell type. Am J Pathol 1983; 113(2): 172-80.
[PMID: 6605689]

[67]   Johnson PW, Watt SM, Betts DR, *et al.* Isolated follicular lymphoma cells are resistant to apoptosis and can be grown *in vitro* in the CD40/stromal cell system. Blood 1993; 82(6): 1848-57.
[PMID: 7691240]

[68]   Amé-Thomas P, Tarte K. The yin and the yang of follicular lymphoma cell niches: role of microenvironment heterogeneity and plasticity. Semin Cancer Biol 2014; 24: 23-32.
[http://dx.doi.org/10.1016/j.semcancer.2013.08.001] [PMID: 23978491]

[69]   Bognár A, Csernus B, Bödör C, *et al.* Clonal selection in the bone marrow involvement of follicular lymphoma. Leukemia 2005; 19(9): 1656-62.
[http://dx.doi.org/10.1038/sj.leu.2403844] [PMID: 15973453]

[70]   Husson H, Carideo EG, Neuberg D, *et al.* Gene expression profiling of follicular lymphoma and normal germinal center B cells using cDNA arrays. Blood 2002; 99(1): 282-9.
[http://dx.doi.org/10.1182/blood.V99.1.282] [PMID: 11756183]

[71]   Wahlin BE, Sander B, Christensson B, Kimby E. CD8+ T-cell content in diagnostic lymph nodes measured by flow cytometry is a predictor of survival in follicular lymphoma. Clin Cancer Res 2007; 13(2 Pt 1): 388-97.
[http://dx.doi.org/10.1158/1078-0432.CCR-06-1734] [PMID: 17255259]

[72]   Yang ZZ, Novak AJ, Ziesmer SC, Witzig TE, Ansell SM. Attenuation of CD8(+) T-cell function by CD4(+)CD25(+) regulatory T cells in B-cell non-Hodgkin's lymphoma. Cancer Res 2006; 66(20): 10145-52.
[http://dx.doi.org/10.1158/0008-5472.CAN-06-1822] [PMID: 17047079]

[73]   Schmitter D, Koss M, Niederer E, Stahel RA, Pichert G. T-cell derived cytokines co-stimulate proliferation of CD40-activated germinal centre as well as follicular lymphoma cells. Hematol Oncol 1997; 15(4): 197-207.
[http://dx.doi.org/10.1002/(SICI)1099-1069(199711)15:4<197::AID-HON614>3.0.CO;2-V] [PMID: 9722891]

[74]   Travert M, Ame-Thomas P, Pangault C, *et al.* CD40 ligand protects from TRAIL-induced apoptosis in follicular lymphomas through NF-kappaB activation and up-regulation of c-FLIP and Bcl-xL. J Immunol 2008; 181(2): 1001-11.
[http://dx.doi.org/10.4049/jimmunol.181.2.1001] [PMID: 18606651]

[75]   Amé-Thomas P, Le Priol J, Yssel H, *et al.* Characterization of intratumoral follicular helper T cells in

follicular lymphoma: role in the survival of malignant B cells. Leukemia 2012; 26(5): 1053-63.
[http://dx.doi.org/10.1038/leu.2011.301] [PMID: 22015774]

[76]   Pangault C, Amé-Thomas P, Ruminy P, *et al.* Follicular lymphoma cell niche: identification of a preeminent IL-4-dependent T(FH)-B cell axis. Leukemia 2010; 24(12): 2080-9.
[http://dx.doi.org/10.1038/leu.2010.223] [PMID: 20944673]

[77]   Sage PT, Francisco LM, Carman CV, Sharpe AH. The receptor PD-1 controls follicular regulatory T cells in the lymph nodes and blood. Nat Immunol 2013; 14(2): 152-61.
[http://dx.doi.org/10.1038/ni.2496] [PMID: 23242415]

[78]   Park CS, Choi YS. How do follicular dendritic cells interact intimately with B cells in the germinal centre? Immunology 2005; 114(1): 2-10.
[http://dx.doi.org/10.1111/j.1365-2567.2004.02075.x] [PMID: 15606789]

[79]   Kiaii S, Clear AJ, Ramsay AG, *et al.* Follicular lymphoma cells induce changes in T-cell gene expression and function: potential impact on survival and risk of transformation. J Clin Oncol 2013; 31(21): 2654-61.
[http://dx.doi.org/10.1200/JCO.2012.44.2137] [PMID: 23775959]

[80]   Rawal S, Chu F, Zhang M, *et al.* Cross talk between follicular Th cells and tumor cells in human follicular lymphoma promotes immune evasion in the tumor microenvironment. J Immunol 2013; 190(12): 6681-93.
[http://dx.doi.org/10.4049/jimmunol.1201363] [PMID: 23686488]

[81]   Dorfman DM, Schultze JL, Shahsafaei A, *et al. In vivo* expression of B7-1 and B7-2 by follicular lymphoma cells can prevent induction of T-cell anergy but is insufficient to induce significant T-cell proliferation. Blood 1997; 90(11): 4297-306.
[PMID: 9373240]

[82]   Ramsay AG, Clear AJ, Kelly G, *et al.* Follicular lymphoma cells induce T-cell immunologic synapse dysfunction that can be repaired with lenalidomide: implications for the tumor microenvironment and immunotherapy. Blood 2009; 114(21): 4713-20.
[http://dx.doi.org/10.1182/blood-2009-04-217687] [PMID: 19786615]

[83]   Rawal S, Fowler N, Zhang M, *et al.* Activation of T and NK Cells Following Lenalidomide Therapy in Patients with Follicular Lymphoma. ASH Annual Meeting Abstracts. 120(21): 2766.

[84]   Fowler NH, Neelapu SS, Hagemeister FB, *et al.* Lenalidomide and Rituximab for Untreated Indolent Lymphoma: Final Results of a Phase II Study. ASH Annual Meeting Abstracts. 120(21): 901.

[85]   Qi L, Yu C, Li X-D, *et al.* Correlative analysis and clinical update of a phase II study using lenalidomide and rituximab in patients with indolent non-hodgkin lymphoma. Blood 2013; 122(21): 249.

[86]   Ardeshna KM, Smith P, Norton A, *et al.* British National Lymphoma Investigation. Long-term effect of a watch and wait policy *versus* immediate systemic treatment for asymptomatic advanced-stage non-Hodgkin lymphoma: a randomised controlled trial. Lancet 2003; 362(9383): 516-22.
[http://dx.doi.org/10.1016/S0140-6736(03)14110-4] [PMID: 12932382]

[87]   Horning SJ, Rosenberg SA. The natural history of initially untreated low-grade non-Hodgkin's lymphomas. N Engl J Med 1984; 311(23): 1471-5.

[http://dx.doi.org/10.1056/NEJM198412063112303] [PMID: 6548796]

[88]   Solal-Céligny P, Lepage E, Brousse N, *et al.* Doxorubicin-containing regimen with or without interferon alfa-2b for advanced follicular lymphomas: final analysis of survival and toxicity in the Groupe d'Etude des Lymphomes Folliculaires 86 Trial. J Clin Oncol 1998; 16(7): 2332-8.
[PMID: 9667247]

[89]   Brice P, Bastion Y, Lepage E, *et al.* Comparison in low-tumor-burden follicular lymphomas between an initial no-treatment policy, prednimustine, or interferon alfa: a randomized study from the Groupe d'Etude des Lymphomes Folliculaires. Groupe d'Etude des Lymphomes de l'Adulte. J Clin Oncol 1997; 15(3): 1110-7.
[PMID: 9060552]

[90]   Zelenetz AD, Abramson JS, Advani RH, *et al.* NCCN Clinical Practice Guidelines in Oncology: non-Hodgkin's lymphomas. J Natl Compr Canc Netw 2010; 8(3): 288-334.
[PMID: 20202462]

[91]   Zelenetz AD, Wierda WG, Abramson JS, *et al.* Non-Hodgkin's Lymphomas, version 3.2012. J Natl Compr Canc Netw 2012; 10(12): 1487-98.
[PMID: 23221787]

[92]   Ardeshna KM, Qian W, Smith P, *et al.* Rituximab *versus* a watch-and-wait approach in patients with advanced-stage, asymptomatic, non-bulky follicular lymphoma: an open-label randomised phase 3 trial. Lancet Oncol 2014; 15(4): 424-35.
[http://dx.doi.org/10.1016/S1470-2045(14)70027-0] [PMID: 24602760]

[93]   Kahl BS, Hong F, Williams ME, *et al.* Results of Eastern Cooperative Oncology Group Protocol E4402 (RESORT): A Randomized Phase III Study Comparing Two Different Rituximab Dosing Strategies for Low Tumor Burden Follicular Lymphoma. ASH Annual Meeting Abstracts. 118(21): LBA-6.

[94]   Young RC, Longo DL, Glatstein E, Ihde DC, Jaffe ES, DeVita VT Jr. The treatment of indolent lymphomas: watchful waiting v aggressive combined modality treatment. Semin Hematol 1988; 25(2) (Suppl. 2): 11-6.
[PMID: 2456618]

[95]   Advani R, Rosenberg SA, Horning SJ. Stage I and II follicular non-Hodgkin's lymphoma: long-term follow-up of no initial therapy. J Clin Oncol 2004; 22(8): 1454-9.
[http://dx.doi.org/10.1200/JCO.2004.10.086] [PMID: 15024027]

[96]   Witzig TE, Vukov AM, Habermann TM, *et al.* Rituximab therapy for patients with newly diagnosed, advanced-stage, follicular grade I non-Hodgkin's lymphoma: a phase II trial in the North Central Cancer Treatment Group. J Clin Oncol 2005; 23(6): 1103-8.
[http://dx.doi.org/10.1200/JCO.2005.12.052] [PMID: 15657404]

[97]   Hainsworth JD, Litchy S, Barton JH, *et al.* Minnie Pearl Cancer Research Network. Single-agent rituximab as first-line and maintenance treatment for patients with chronic lymphocytic leukemia or small lymphocytic lymphoma: a phase II trial of the Minnie Pearl Cancer Research Network. J Clin Oncol 2003; 21(9): 1746-51.
[http://dx.doi.org/10.1200/JCO.2003.09.027] [PMID: 12721250]

[98]   Hainsworth JD, Litchy S, Burris HA III, *et al.* Rituximab as first-line and maintenance therapy for

patients with indolent non-hodgkin's lymphoma. J Clin Oncol 2002; 20(20): 4261-7.
[http://dx.doi.org/10.1200/JCO.2002.08.674] [PMID: 12377971]

[99] Hainsworth JD, Litchy S, Morrissey LH, *et al.* Rituximab plus short-duration chemotherapy as first-line treatment for follicular non-Hodgkin's lymphoma: a phase II trial of the minnie pearl cancer research network. J Clin Oncol 2005; 23(7): 1500-6.
[http://dx.doi.org/10.1200/JCO.2005.05.004] [PMID: 15632411]

[100] Martinelli G, Laszlo D, Bertolini F, *et al.* Chlorambucil in combination with induction and maintenance rituximab is feasible and active in indolent non-Hodgkin's lymphoma. Br J Haematol 2003; 123(2): 271-7.
[http://dx.doi.org/10.1046/j.1365-2141.2003.04586.x] [PMID: 14531908]

[101] Peterson BA, Petroni GR, Frizzera G, *et al.* Prolonged single-agent *versus* combination chemotherapy in indolent follicular lymphomas: a study of the cancer and leukemia group B. J Clin Oncol 2003; 21(1): 5-15.
[http://dx.doi.org/10.1200/jco.2003.05.128] [PMID: 12506163]

[102] Lunning M, Armitage JO. The curability of follicular lymphoma. Transfus Apheresis Sci 2007; 37(1): 31-5.
[http://dx.doi.org/10.1016/j.transci.2007.04.012] [PMID: 17936072]

[103] Haas RL, Poortmans P, de Jong D, *et al.* High response rates and lasting remissions after low-dose involved field radiotherapy in indolent lymphomas. J Clin Oncol 2003; 21(13): 2474-80.
[http://dx.doi.org/10.1200/JCO.2003.09.542] [PMID: 12829665]

[104] Tezcan H, Vose JM, Bast M, Bierman PJ, Kessinger A, Armitage JO. Limited stage I and II follicular non-Hodgkin's lymphoma: the Nebraska Lymphoma Study Group experience. Leuk Lymphoma 1999; 34(3-4): 273-85.
[http://dx.doi.org/10.3109/10428199909050952] [PMID: 10439364]

[105] Wilder RB, Jones D, Tucker SL, *et al.* Long-term results with radiotherapy for Stage I-II follicular lymphomas. Int J Radiat Oncol Biol Phys 2001; 51(5): 1219-27.
[http://dx.doi.org/10.1016/S0360-3016(01)01747-3] [PMID: 11728680]

[106] Friedberg JW, Taylor MD, Cerhan JR, *et al.* Follicular lymphoma in the United States: first report of the national LymphoCare study. J Clin Oncol 2009; 27(8): 1202-8.
[http://dx.doi.org/10.1200/JCO.2008.18.1495] [PMID: 19204203]

[107] Guadagnolo BA, Li S, Neuberg D, *et al.* Long-term outcome and mortality trends in early-stage, Grade 1-2 follicular lymphoma treated with radiation therapy. Int J Radiat Oncol Biol Phys 2006; 64(3): 928-34.
[http://dx.doi.org/10.1016/j.ijrobp.2005.08.010] [PMID: 16243446]

[108] Heinzelmann F, Ottinger H, Engelhard M, Soekler M, Bamberg M, Weinmann M. Advanced-stage III/IV follicular lymphoma: treatment strategies for individual patients. Strahlenther Onkol 2010; 186(5): 247-54.
[http://dx.doi.org/10.1007/s00066-010-2091-8] [PMID: 20437015]

[109] Pugh TJ, Ballonoff A, Newman F, Rabinovitch R. Improved survival in patients with early stage low-grade follicular lymphoma treated with radiation: a Surveillance, Epidemiology, and End Results database analysis. Cancer 2010; 116(16): 3843-51.

[http://dx.doi.org/10.1002/cncr.25149] [PMID: 20564102]

[110] Ha CS, Cabanillas F, Lee MS, *et al.* A prospective randomized study to compare the molecular response rates between central lymphatic irradiation and intensive alternating triple chemotherapy in the treatment of stage I-III follicular lymphoma. Int J Radiat Oncol Biol Phys 2005; 63(1): 188-93.
[http://dx.doi.org/10.1016/j.ijrobp.2005.01.027] [PMID: 16111588]

[111] Seymour JF, Pro B, Fuller LM, *et al.* Long-term follow-up of a prospective study of combined modality therapy for stage I-II indolent non-Hodgkin's lymphoma. J Clin Oncol 2003; 21(11): 2115-22.
[http://dx.doi.org/10.1200/JCO.2003.07.111] [PMID: 12775737]

[112] López-Guillermo A, Caballero D, Canales M, Provencio M, Rueda A, Salar A. Spanish Hematology and Hemotherapy Association; Oncological Group for the Treatment of Lymphatic Diseases; Spanish Lymphomas/Autologous Bone Marrow Transplant Group. Clinical practice guidelines for first-line/after-relapse treatment of patients with follicular lymphoma. Leuk Lymphoma 2011; 52 (Suppl. 3): 1-14.
[http://dx.doi.org/10.3109/10428194.2011.629897] [PMID: 22149349]

[113] Hiddemann W, Kneba M, Dreyling M, *et al.* Frontline therapy with rituximab added to the combination of cyclophosphamide, doxorubicin, vincristine, and prednisone (CHOP) significantly improves the outcome for patients with advanced-stage follicular lymphoma compared with therapy with CHOP alone: results of a prospective randomized study of the German Low-Grade Lymphoma Study Group. Blood 2005; 106(12): 3725-32.
[http://dx.doi.org/10.1182/blood-2005-01-0016] [PMID: 16123223]

[114] Herold M, Haas A, Srock S, *et al.* East German Study Group Hematology and Oncology Study. Rituximab added to first-line mitoxantrone, chlorambucil, and prednisolone chemotherapy followed by interferon maintenance prolongs survival in patients with advanced follicular lymphoma: an East German Study Group Hematology and Oncology Study. J Clin Oncol 2007; 25(15): 1986-92.
[http://dx.doi.org/10.1200/JCO.2006.06.4618] [PMID: 17420513]

[115] Marcus R, Imrie K, Solal-Celigny P, *et al.* Phase III study of R-CVP compared with cyclophosphamide, vincristine, and prednisone alone in patients with previously untreated advanced follicular lymphoma. J Clin Oncol 2008; 26(28): 4579-86.
[http://dx.doi.org/10.1200/JCO.2007.13.5376] [PMID: 18662969]

[116] Salles G, Mounier N, de Guibert S, *et al.* Rituximab combined with chemotherapy and interferon in follicular lymphoma patients: results of the GELA-GOELAMS FL2000 study. Blood 2008; 112(13): 4824-31.
[http://dx.doi.org/10.1182/blood-2008-04-153189] [PMID: 18799723]

[117] Rehwald U, Schulz H, Reiser M, *et al.* German Hodgkin Lymphoma Study Group (GHSG). Treatment of relapsed CD20+ Hodgkin lymphoma with the monoclonal antibody rituximab is effective and well tolerated: results of a phase 2 trial of the German Hodgkin Lymphoma Study Group. Blood 2003; 101(2): 420-4.
[http://dx.doi.org/10.1182/blood.V101.2.420] [PMID: 12509381]

[118] Davis TA, White CA, Grillo-López AJ, *et al.* Single-agent monoclonal antibody efficacy in bulky non-Hodgkin's lymphoma: results of a phase II trial of rituximab. J Clin Oncol 1999; 17(6): 1851-7.
[PMID: 10561225]

[119] Schulz H, Bohlius JF, Trelle S, *et al.* Immunochemotherapy with rituximab and overall survival in patients with indolent or mantle cell lymphoma: a systematic review and meta-analysis. J Natl Cancer Inst 2007; 99(9): 706-14.
[http://dx.doi.org/10.1093/jnci/djk152] [PMID: 17470738]

[120] Czuczman MS, Weaver R, Alkuzweny B, Berlfein J, Grillo-López AJ. Prolonged clinical and molecular remission in patients with low-grade or follicular non-Hodgkin's lymphoma treated with rituximab plus CHOP chemotherapy: 9-year follow-up. J Clin Oncol 2004; 22(23): 4711-6.
[http://dx.doi.org/10.1200/JCO.2004.04.020] [PMID: 15483015]

[121] Rigacci L, Federico M, Martelli M, *et al.* Intergruppo Italiano Linfomi. The role of anthracyclines in combination chemotherapy for the treatment of follicular lymphoma: retrospective study of the Intergruppo Italiano Linfomi on 761 cases. Leuk Lymphoma 2003; 44(11): 1911-7.
[http://dx.doi.org/10.1080/1042819031000123564] [PMID: 14738142]

[122] Ganti AK, Weisenburger DD, Smith LM, *et al.* Patients with grade 3 follicular lymphoma have prolonged relapse-free survival following anthracycline-based chemotherapy: the Nebraska Lymphoma Study Group Experience. Ann Oncol 2006; 17(6): 920-7.
[http://dx.doi.org/10.1093/annonc/mdl039] [PMID: 16524969]

[123] Nabhan C. It is follicular... . so, why CHOP? J Clin Oncol 2007; 25(7): 915-6.
[http://dx.doi.org/10.1200/JCO.2006.09.5950] [PMID: 17327620]

[124] Nickenig C, Dreyling M, Hoster E, *et al.* German Low-Grade Lymphoma Study Group. Initial chemotherapy with mitoxantrone, chlorambucil, prednisone impairs the collection of stem cells in patients with indolent lymphomas--results of a randomized comparison by the German Low-Grade Lymphoma Study Group. Ann Oncol 2007; 18(1): 136-42.
[http://dx.doi.org/10.1093/annonc/mdl348] [PMID: 17071931]

[125] Nickenig C, Dreyling M, Hoster E, *et al.* German Low-Grade Lymphoma Study Group. Combined cyclophosphamide, vincristine, doxorubicin, and prednisone (CHOP) improves response rates but not survival and has lower hematologic toxicity compared with combined mitoxantrone, chlorambucil, and prednisone (MCP) in follicular and mantle cell lymphomas: results of a prospective randomized trial of the German Low-Grade Lymphoma Study Group. Cancer 2006; 107(5): 1014-22.
[http://dx.doi.org/10.1002/cncr.22093] [PMID: 16878325]

[126] Federico M, Luminari S, Dondi A, *et al.* R-CVP *versus* R-CHOP *versus* R-FM for the initial treatment of patients with advanced-stage follicular lymphoma: results of the FOLL05 trial conducted by the Fondazione Italiana Linfomi. J Clin Oncol 2013; 31(12): 1506-13.
[http://dx.doi.org/10.1200/JCO.2012.45.0866] [PMID: 23530110]

[127] Zinzani PL, Pulsoni A, Perrotti A, *et al.* Fludarabine plus mitoxantrone with and without rituximab *versus* CHOP with and without rituximab as front-line treatment for patients with follicular lymphoma. J Clin Oncol 2004; 22(13): 2654-61.
[http://dx.doi.org/10.1200/JCO.2004.07.170] [PMID: 15159414]

[128] Vitolo U, Ladetto M, Boccomini C, *et al.* Rituximab maintenance compared with observation after brief first-line R-FND chemoimmunotherapy with rituximab consolidation in patients age older than 60 years with advanced follicular lymphoma: a phase III randomized study by the Fondazione Italiana Linfomi. J Clin Oncol 2013; 31(27): 3351-9.

[http://dx.doi.org/10.1200/JCO.2012.44.8290] [PMID: 23960180]

[129]   McLaughlin P. Management options for follicular lymphoma: observe; R-CHOP; B-R; others? Clin Lymphoma Myeloma Leuk 2011; 11 (Suppl. 1): S91-5.
[http://dx.doi.org/10.1016/j.clml.2011.04.006] [PMID: 22035757]

[130]   Gill S, Carney D, Ritchie D, *et al.* The frequency, manifestations, and duration of prolonged cytopenias after first-line fludarabine combination chemotherapy. Ann Oncol 2010; 21(2): 331-4.
[http://dx.doi.org/10.1093/annonc/mdp297] [PMID: 19625344]

[131]   Anderson VR, Perry CM. Fludarabine: a review of its use in non-Hodgkin's lymphoma. Drugs 2007; 67(11): 1633-55.
[http://dx.doi.org/10.2165/00003495-200767110-00008] [PMID: 17661532]

[132]   Rummel MJ, Al-Batran SE, Kim SZ, *et al.* Bendamustine plus rituximab is effective and has a favorable toxicity profile in the treatment of mantle cell and low-grade non-Hodgkin's lymphoma. J Clin Oncol 2005; 23(15): 3383-9.
[http://dx.doi.org/10.1200/JCO.2005.08.100] [PMID: 15908650]

[133]   Rummel MJ, Niederle N, Maschmeyer G, *et al.* Bendamustine Plus Rituximab Is Superior in Respect of Progression Free Survival and CR Rate When Compared to CHOP Plus Rituximab as First-Line Treatment of Patients with Advanced Follicular, Indolent, and Mantle Cell Lymphomas: Final Results of a Randomized Phase III Study of the StiL (Study Group Indolent Lymphomas, Germany). ASH Annual Meeting Abstracts. 114(22): 405.

[134]   Rummel MJ, Niederle N, Maschmeyer G, *et al.* Study group indolent Lymphomas (StiL). Bendamustine plus rituximab *versus* CHOP plus rituximab as first-line treatment for patients with indolent and mantle-cell lymphomas: an open-label, multicentre, randomised, phase 3 non-inferiority trial. Lancet 2013; 381(9873): 1203-10.
[http://dx.doi.org/10.1016/S0140-6736(12)61763-2] [PMID: 23433739]

[135]   Flinn IW, van der Jagt R, Kahl BS, *et al.* Randomized trial of bendamustine-rituximab or R-CHOP/-CVP in first-line treatment of indolent NHL or MCL: the BRIGHT study. Blood 2014; 123(19): 2944-52.
[http://dx.doi.org/10.1182/blood-2013-11-531327] [PMID: 24591201]

[136]   Hiddemann W, Griesinger F, Unterhalt M. Interferon alfa for the treatment of follicular lymphomas. Cancer J Sci Am 1998; 4 (Suppl. 2): S13-8.
[PMID: 9672770]

[137]   Rohatiner AZ, Gregory WM, Peterson B, *et al.* Meta-analysis to evaluate the role of interferon in follicular lymphoma. J Clin Oncol 2005; 23(10): 2215-23.
[http://dx.doi.org/10.1200/JCO.2005.06.146] [PMID: 15684317]

[138]   Baldo P, Rupolo M, Compagnoni A, *et al.* Interferon-alpha for maintenance of follicular lymphoma. Cochrane Database Syst Rev 2010; (1): CD004629.
[PMID: 20091564]

[139]   Ghielmini M, Schmitz SF, Cogliatti SB, *et al.* Prolonged treatment with rituximab in patients with follicular lymphoma significantly increases event-free survival and response duration compared with the standard weekly x 4 schedule. Blood 2004; 103(12): 4416-23.
[http://dx.doi.org/10.1182/blood-2003-10-3411] [PMID: 14976046]

[140] Martinelli G, Schmitz SF, Utiger U, *et al.* Long-term follow-up of patients with follicular lymphoma receiving single-agent rituximab at two different schedules in trial SAKK 35/98. J Clin Oncol 2010; 28(29): 4480-4.
[http://dx.doi.org/10.1200/JCO.2010.28.4786] [PMID: 20697092]

[141] Salles G, Seymour JF, Offner F, *et al.* Rituximab maintenance for 2 years in patients with high tumour burden follicular lymphoma responding to rituximab plus chemotherapy (PRIMA): a phase 3, randomised controlled trial. Lancet 2011; 377(9759): 42-51.
[http://dx.doi.org/10.1016/S0140-6736(10)62175-7] [PMID: 21176949]

[142] Michallet AS, Coiffier B, Salles G. Maintenance therapy in follicular lymphoma. Curr Opin Oncol 2011; 23(5): 449-54.
[http://dx.doi.org/10.1097/CCO.0b013e3283490515] [PMID: 21734580]

[143] Seymour JF, Feugier P, Offner F, *et al.* Updated 6 Year Follow-Up Of The PRIMA Study Confirms The Benefit Of 2-Year Rituximab Maintenance In Follicular Lymphoma Patients Responding To Frontline Immunochemotherapy. Blood 2013; 122(21): 509.

[144] Gea-Banacloche JC. Rituximab-associated infections. Semin Hematol 2010; 47(2): 187-98.
[http://dx.doi.org/10.1053/j.seminhematol.2010.01.002] [PMID: 20350666]

[145] Artz AS, Somerfield MR, Feld JJ, *et al.* American Society of Clinical Oncology provisional clinical opinion: chronic hepatitis B virus infection screening in patients receiving cytotoxic chemotherapy for treatment of malignant diseases. J Clin Oncol 2010; 28(19): 3199-202.
[http://dx.doi.org/10.1200/JCO.2010.30.0673] [PMID: 20516452]

[146] Vidal L, Gafter-Gvili A, Salles G, *et al.* Rituximab maintenance for the treatment of patients with follicular lymphoma: an updated systematic review and meta-analysis of randomized trials. J Natl Cancer Inst 2011; 103(23): 1799-806.
[http://dx.doi.org/10.1093/jnci/djr418] [PMID: 22021664]

[147] Cheson BD. Hematology: The case against rituximab maintenance. Nat Rev Clin Oncol 2009; 6(11): 622-4.
[http://dx.doi.org/10.1038/nrclinonc.2009.161] [PMID: 19861992]

[148] Lenz G, Dreyling M, Schiegnitz E, *et al.* German Low-Grade Lymphoma Study Group. Myeloablative radiochemotherapy followed by autologous stem cell transplantation in first remission prolongs progression-free survival in follicular lymphoma: results of a prospective, randomized trial of the German Low-Grade Lymphoma Study Group. Blood 2004; 104(9): 2667-74.
[http://dx.doi.org/10.1182/blood-2004-03-0982] [PMID: 15238420]

[149] Gyan E, Foussard C, Bertrand P, *et al.* Groupe Ouest-Est des Leucémies et des Autres Maladies du Sang (GOELAMS). High-dose therapy followed by autologous purged stem cell transplantation and doxorubicin-based chemotherapy in patients with advanced follicular lymphoma: a randomized multicenter study by the GOELAMS with final results after a median follow-up of 9 years. Blood 2009; 113(5): 995-1001.
[http://dx.doi.org/10.1182/blood-2008-05-160200] [PMID: 18955565]

[150] Sebban C, Mounier N, Brousse N, *et al.* Standard chemotherapy with interferon compared with CHOP followed by high-dose therapy with autologous stem cell transplantation in untreated patients with advanced follicular lymphoma: the GELF-94 randomized study from the Groupe d'Etude des

Lymphomes de l'Adulte (GELA). Blood 2006; 108(8): 2540-4.
[http://dx.doi.org/10.1182/blood-2006-03-013193] [PMID: 16835383]

[151] Ladetto M, De Marco F, Benedetti F, *et al.* Gruppo Italiano Trapianto di Midollo Osseo (GITMO); Intergruppo Italiano Linfomi (IIL). Prospective, multicenter randomized GITMO/IIL trial comparing intensive (R-HDS) *versus* conventional (CHOP-R) chemoimmunotherapy in high-risk follicular lymphoma at diagnosis: the superior disease control of R-HDS does not translate into an overall survival advantage. Blood 2008; 111(8): 4004-13.
[http://dx.doi.org/10.1182/blood-2007-10-116749] [PMID: 18239086]

[152] Dreyling MH, Metzner B, Pfreundschuh M, *et al.* Evaluation of myeloablative therapy followed by autologous stem cell transplantation in first remission in patients with advanced stage follicular lymphoma after initial immuno-chemotherapy (R-CHOP) or chemotherapy alone: analysis of 940 patients treated. Blood 2013; 122(21): 419.

[153] Al Khabori M, de Almeida JR, Guyatt GH, Kuruvilla J, Crump M. Autologous stem cell transplantation in follicular lymphoma: a systematic review and meta-analysis. J Natl Cancer Inst 2012; 104(1): 18-28.
[http://dx.doi.org/10.1093/jnci/djr450] [PMID: 22190633]

[154] Rohatiner AZ, Nadler L, Davies AJ, *et al.* Myeloablative therapy with autologous bone marrow transplantation for follicular lymphoma at the time of second or subsequent remission: long-term follow-up. J Clin Oncol 2007; 25(18): 2554-9.
[http://dx.doi.org/10.1200/JCO.2006.09.8327] [PMID: 17515573]

[155] Schouten HC, Qian W, Kvaloy S, *et al.* High-dose therapy improves progression-free survival and survival in relapsed follicular non-Hodgkin's lymphoma: results from the randomized European CUP trial. J Clin Oncol 2003; 21(21): 3918-27.
[http://dx.doi.org/10.1200/JCO.2003.10.023] [PMID: 14517188]

[156] Zinzani PL, Tani M, Pulsoni A, *et al.* Fludarabine and mitoxantrone followed by yttrium-90 ibritumomab tiuxetan in previously untreated patients with follicular non-Hodgkin lymphoma trial: a phase II non-randomised trial (FLUMIZ). Lancet Oncol 2008; 9(4): 352-8.
[http://dx.doi.org/10.1016/S1470-2045(08)70039-1] [PMID: 18342572]

[157] Jacobs SA, Swerdlow SH, Kant J, *et al.* Phase II trial of short-course CHOP-R followed by 90Y-ibritumomab tiuxetan and extended rituximab in previously untreated follicular lymphoma. Clin Cancer Res 2008; 14(21): 7088-94.
[http://dx.doi.org/10.1158/1078-0432.CCR-08-0529] [PMID: 18981007]

[158] Leonard JP, Coleman M, Kostakoglu L, *et al.* Abbreviated chemotherapy with fludarabine followed by tositumomab and iodine I 131 tositumomab for untreated follicular lymphoma. J Clin Oncol 2005; 23(24): 5696-704.
[http://dx.doi.org/10.1200/JCO.2005.14.803] [PMID: 16110029]

[159] Link BK, Martin P, Kaminski MS, Goldsmith SJ, Coleman M, Leonard JP. Cyclophosphamide, vincristine, and prednisone followed by tositumomab and iodine-131-tositumomab in patients with untreated low-grade follicular lymphoma: eight-year follow-up of a multicenter phase II study. J Clin Oncol 2010; 28(18): 3035-41.
[http://dx.doi.org/10.1200/JCO.2009.27.8325] [PMID: 20458031]

[160] Dreyling M, Trümper L, von Schilling C, *et al.* Results of a national consensus workshop: therapeutic algorithm in patients with follicular lymphoma--role of radioimmunotherapy. Ann Hematol 2007; 86(2): 81-7.
[http://dx.doi.org/10.1007/s00277-006-0207-0] [PMID: 17068667]

[161] Kaminski MS, Kitamura K, Maloney DG, Levy R. Idiotype vaccination against murine B cell lymphoma. Inhibition of tumor immunity by free idiotype protein. J Immunol 1987; 138(4): 1289-96. [PMID: 3492546]

[162] Press OW, Unger JM, Rimsza LM, *et al.* Phase III randomized intergroup trial of CHOP plus rituximab compared with CHOP chemotherapy plus (131)iodine-tositumomab for previously untreated follicular non-Hodgkin lymphoma: SWOG S0016. J Clin Oncol 2013; 31(3): 314-20.
[http://dx.doi.org/10.1200/JCO.2012.42.4101] [PMID: 23233710]

[163] Morschhauser F, Radford J, Van Hoof A, *et al.* Phase III trial of consolidation therapy with yttrium-90-ibritumomab tiuxetan compared with no additional therapy after first remission in advanced follicular lymphoma. J Clin Oncol 2008; 26(32): 5156-64.
[http://dx.doi.org/10.1200/JCO.2008.17.2015] [PMID: 18854568]

[164] Press OW. Evidence mounts for the efficacy of radioimmunotherapy for B-cell lymphomas. J Clin Oncol 2008; 26(32): 5147-50.
[http://dx.doi.org/10.1200/JCO.2008.18.5447] [PMID: 18854559]

[165] Morschhauser F, Radford J, Van Hoof A, *et al.* 90Yttrium-ibritumomab tiuxetan consolidation of first remission in advanced-stage follicular non-Hodgkin lymphoma: updated results after a median follow-up of 7.3 years from the International, Randomized, Phase III First-LineIndolent trial. J Clin Oncol 2013; 31(16): 1977-83.
[http://dx.doi.org/10.1200/JCO.2012.45.6400] [PMID: 23547079]

[166] Canales MA, Dlouhy I, Briones J, *et al.* A Randomized Phase II Study Comparing Consolidation With a Single Dose Of 90y Ibritumomab Tiuxetan (Zevalin®) (Z) *vs.* Maintenance With Rituximab (R) For Two Years In Patients With Newly Diagnosed Follicular Lymphoma (FL) Responding To R-CHOP. Preliminary…. Blood 2013; 122(21): 369.

[167] Dreyling M, Ghielmini M, Marcus R, Salles G, Vitolo U. ESMO Guidelines Working Group. Newly diagnosed and relapsed follicular lymphoma: ESMO Clinical Practice Guidelines for diagnosis, treatment and follow-up. Ann Oncol 2011; 22 (Suppl. 6): vi59-63.
[http://dx.doi.org/10.1093/annonc/mdr388] [PMID: 21908506]

[168] van Oers MH, Klasa R, Marcus RE, *et al.* Rituximab maintenance improves clinical outcome of relapsed/resistant follicular non-Hodgkin lymphoma in patients both with and without rituximab during induction: results of a prospective randomized phase 3 intergroup trial. Blood 2006; 108(10): 3295-301.
[http://dx.doi.org/10.1182/blood-2006-05-021113] [PMID: 16873669]

[169] O'Connor OA, Wright J, Moskowitz C, *et al.* Phase II clinical experience with the novel proteasome inhibitor bortezomib in patients with indolent non-Hodgkin's lymphoma and mantle cell lymphoma. J Clin Oncol 2005; 23(4): 676-84.
[http://dx.doi.org/10.1200/JCO.2005.02.050] [PMID: 15613699]

[170] Goy A, Younes A, McLaughlin P, *et al.* Phase II study of proteasome inhibitor bortezomib in relapsed

or refractory B-cell non-Hodgkin's lymphoma. J Clin Oncol 2005; 23(4): 667-75.
[http://dx.doi.org/10.1200/JCO.2005.03.108] [PMID: 15613697]

[171] Di Bella N, Taetle R, Kolibaba K, *et al.* Results of a phase 2 study of bortezomib in patients with relapsed or refractory indolent lymphoma. Blood 2010; 115(3): 475-80.
[http://dx.doi.org/10.1182/blood-2009-08-233155] [PMID: 19965689]

[172] Fisher RI, Bernstein SH, Kahl BS, *et al.* Multicenter phase II study of bortezomib in patients with relapsed or refractory mantle cell lymphoma. J Clin Oncol 2006; 24(30): 4867-74.
[http://dx.doi.org/10.1200/JCO.2006.07.9665] [PMID: 17001068]

[173] de Vos S, Wagner-Johnston ND, Coutre SE, *et al.* Durable responses following treatment with the PI3K-delta inhibitor idelalisib in combination with rituximab, bendamustine, or both, in recurrent indolent non-hodgkin lymphoma: phase I/II results. Blood 2014; 124(21): 3063.

[174] Coiffier B, Osmanov EA, Hong X, *et al.* LYM-3001 study investigators. Bortezomib plus rituximab *versus* rituximab alone in patients with relapsed, rituximab-naive or rituximab-sensitive, follicular lymphoma: a randomised phase 3 trial. Lancet Oncol 2011; 12(8): 773-84.
[http://dx.doi.org/10.1016/S1470-2045(11)70150-4] [PMID: 21724462]

[175] Fowler N, Kahl BS, Lee P, *et al.* Bortezomib, bendamustine, and rituximab in patients with relapsed or refractory follicular lymphoma: the phase II VERTICAL study. J Clin Oncol 2011; 29(25): 3389-95.
[http://dx.doi.org/10.1200/JCO.2010.32.1844] [PMID: 21810687]

[176] Friedberg JW, Vose JM, Kelly JL, *et al.* The combination of bendamustine, bortezomib, and rituximab for patients with relapsed/refractory indolent and mantle cell non-Hodgkin lymphoma. Blood 2011; 117(10): 2807-12.
[http://dx.doi.org/10.1182/blood-2010-11-314708] [PMID: 21239695]

[177] Montoto S, Canals C, Rohatiner AZ, *et al.* EBMT Lymphoma Working Party. Long-term follow-up of high-dose treatment with autologous haematopoietic progenitor cell support in 693 patients with follicular lymphoma: an EBMT registry study. Leukemia 2007; 21(11): 2324-31.
[http://dx.doi.org/10.1038/sj.leu.2404850] [PMID: 17637813]

[178] Kim SW. Hematopoietic stem cell transplantation for follicular lymphoma: optimal timing and indication. J Clin Exp Hematop 2014; 54(1): 39-47.
[http://dx.doi.org/10.3960/jslrt.54.39] [PMID: 24942945]

[179] Sebban C, Brice P, Delarue R, *et al.* Impact of rituximab and/or high-dose therapy with autotransplant at time of relapse in patients with follicular lymphoma: a GELA study. J Clin Oncol 2008; 26(21): 3614-20.
[http://dx.doi.org/10.1200/JCO.2007.15.5358] [PMID: 18559872]

[180] Bierman PJ, Vose JM, Anderson JR, Bishop MR, Kessinger A, Armitage JO. High-dose therapy with autologous hematopoietic rescue for follicular low-grade non-Hodgkin's lymphoma. J Clin Oncol 1997; 15(2): 445-50.
[PMID: 9053464]

[181] van Besien K, Loberiza FR Jr, Bajorunaite R, *et al.* Comparison of autologous and allogeneic hematopoietic stem cell transplantation for follicular lymphoma. Blood 2003; 102(10): 3521-9.
[http://dx.doi.org/10.1182/blood-2003-04-1205] [PMID: 12893748]

[182] Friedberg JW, Neuberg D, Stone RM, *et al.* Outcome in patients with myelodysplastic syndrome after autologous bone marrow transplantation for non-Hodgkin's lymphoma. J Clin Oncol 1999; 17(10): 3128-35.
[PMID: 10506609]

[183] Witzig TE, Gordon LI, Cabanillas F, *et al.* Randomized controlled trial of yttrium-90-labeled ibritumomab tiuxetan radioimmunotherapy *versus* rituximab immunotherapy for patients with relapsed or refractory low-grade, follicular, or transformed B-cell non-Hodgkin's lymphoma. J Clin Oncol 2002; 20(10): 2453-63.
[http://dx.doi.org/10.1200/JCO.2002.11.076] [PMID: 12011122]

[184] Leahy MF, Turner JH. Radioimmunotherapy of relapsed indolent non-Hodgkin lymphoma with 131I-rituximab in routine clinical practice: 10-year single-institution experience of 142 consecutive patients. Blood 2011; 117(1): 45-52.
[http://dx.doi.org/10.1182/blood-2010-02-269753] [PMID: 20864582]

[185] Pettengell R, Schmitz N, Gisselbrecht C, *et al.* Rituximab purging and/or maintenance in patients undergoing autologous transplantation for relapsed follicular lymphoma: a prospective randomized trial from the lymphoma working party of the European group for blood and marrow transplantation. J Clin Oncol 2013; 31(13): 1624-30.
[http://dx.doi.org/10.1200/JCO.2012.47.1862] [PMID: 23547078]

[186] van Oers MH, Van Glabbeke M, Giurgea L, *et al.* Rituximab maintenance treatment of relapsed/resistant follicular non-Hodgkin's lymphoma: long-term outcome of the EORTC 20981 phase III randomized intergroup study. J Clin Oncol 2010; 28(17): 2853-8.
[http://dx.doi.org/10.1200/JCO.2009.26.5827] [PMID: 20439641]

[187] van Besien K, Sobocinski KA, Rowlings PA, *et al.* Allogeneic bone marrow transplantation for low-grade lymphoma. Blood 1998; 92(5): 1832-6.
[PMID: 9716615]

[188] Forrest DL, Thompson K, Nevill TJ, Couban S, Fernandez LA. Allogeneic hematopoietic stem cell transplantation for progressive follicular lymphoma. Bone Marrow Transplant 2002; 29(12): 973-8.
[http://dx.doi.org/10.1038/sj.bmt.1703573] [PMID: 12098065]

[189] Toze CL, Barnett MJ, Connors JM, *et al.* Long-term disease-free survival of patients with advanced follicular lymphoma after allogeneic bone marrow transplantation. Br J Haematol 2004; 127(3): 311-21.
[http://dx.doi.org/10.1111/j.1365-2141.2004.05194.x] [PMID: 15491292]

[190] Khouri IF, McLaughlin P, Saliba RM, *et al.* Eight-year experience with allogeneic stem cell transplantation for relapsed follicular lymphoma after nonmyeloablative conditioning with fludarabine, cyclophosphamide, and rituximab. Blood 2008; 111(12): 5530-6.
[http://dx.doi.org/10.1182/blood-2008-01-136242] [PMID: 18411419]

[191] Khouri IF, Saliba RM, Giralt SA, *et al.* Nonablative allogeneic hematopoietic transplantation as adoptive immunotherapy for indolent lymphoma: low incidence of toxicity, acute graft-*versus*-host disease, and treatment-related mortality. Blood 2001; 98(13): 3595-9.
[http://dx.doi.org/10.1182/blood.V98.13.3595] [PMID: 11739162]

[192] Witzig TE, Wiernik PH, Moore T, *et al.* Lenalidomide oral monotherapy produces durable responses

in relapsed or refractory indolent non-Hodgkin's Lymphoma. J Clin Oncol 2009; 27(32): 5404-9.
[http://dx.doi.org/10.1200/JCO.2008.21.1169] [PMID: 19805688]

[193]   Fowler NH, Davis RE, Rawal S, *et al*. Safety and activity of lenalidomide and rituximab in untreated
        indolent lymphoma: an open-label, phase 2 trial. Lancet Oncol 2014; 15(12): 1311-8.
        [http://dx.doi.org/10.1016/S1470-2045(14)70455-3] [PMID: 25439689]

[194]   Czuczman MS, Fayad L, Delwail V, *et al*. 405 Study Investigators. Ofatumumab monotherapy in
        rituximab-refractory follicular lymphoma: results from a multicenter study. Blood 2012; 119(16):
        3698-704.
        [http://dx.doi.org/10.1182/blood-2011-09-378323] [PMID: 22389254]

[195]   Czuczman MS, Hess G, Gadeberg OV, *et al*. 409 Study Investigators. Chemoimmunotherapy with
        ofatumumab in combination with CHOP in previously untreated follicular lymphoma. Br J Haematol
        2012; 157(4): 438-45.
        [http://dx.doi.org/10.1111/j.1365-2141.2012.09086.x] [PMID: 22409295]

[196]   Cameron F, McCormack PL. Obinutuzumab: first global approval. Drugs 2014; 74(1): 147-54.0
        [http://dx.doi.org/10.1007/s40265-013-0167-3] [PMID: 24338113]

[197]   Dyer MJ, Grigg AP, González Díaz M, *et al*. Obinutuzumab (GA101) in combination with CHOP
        (cyclophosphamide, doxorubicin, vincristine and prednisone) or bendamustine for the first-line
        treatment of follicular non-hodgkin lymphoma: final results from the maintenance phase of the phase
        ib GAUDI study. Blood 2014; 124(21): 1743.

[198]   Smith SM, van Besien K, Karrison T, *et al*. Temsirolimus has activity in non-mantle cell non-
        Hodgkin's lymphoma subtypes: The University of Chicago phase II consortium. J Clin Oncol 2010;
        28(31): 4740-6.
        [http://dx.doi.org/10.1200/JCO.2010.29.2813] [PMID: 20837940]

[199]   Gopal AK, Kahl BS, de Vos S, *et al*. PI3Kδ inhibition by idelalisib in patients with relapsed indolent
        lymphoma. N Engl J Med 2014; 370(11): 1008-18.
        [http://dx.doi.org/10.1056/NEJMoa1314583] [PMID: 24450858]

[200]   Bartlett NL, LaPlant BR, Qi J, *et al*. Ibrutinib Monotherapy in Relapsed/Refractory Follicular
        Lymphoma (FL): Preliminary Results of a Phase 2 Consortium (P2C) Trial. Blood 2014; 124(21): 800.

[201]   Maddocks K, Christian B, Jaglowski S, *et al*. A phase 1/1b study of rituximab, bendamustine, and
        ibrutinib in patients with untreated and relapsed/refractory non-Hodgkin lymphoma. Blood 2015;
        125(2): 242-8.
        [http://dx.doi.org/10.1182/blood-2014-08-597914] [PMID: 25355819]

[202]   Younes A, Thieblemont C, Morschhauser F, *et al*. Combination of ibrutinib with rituximab,
        cyclophosphamide, doxorubicin, vincristine, and prednisone (R-CHOP) for treatment-naive patients
        with CD20-positive B-cell non-Hodgkin lymphoma: a non-randomised, phase 1b study. Lancet Oncol
        2014; 15(9): 1019-26.
        [http://dx.doi.org/10.1016/S1470-2045(14)70311-0] [PMID: 25042202]

[203]   Cheson BD. New agents in follicular lymphoma. Best Pract Res Clin Haematol 2011; 24(2): 305-12.
        [http://dx.doi.org/10.1016/j.beha.2011.03.006] [PMID: 21658626]

[204]   Seo N, Hayakawa S, Takigawa M, Tokura Y. Interleukin-10 expressed at early tumour sites induces

subsequent generation of CD4(+) T-regulatory cells and systemic collapse of antitumour immunity. Immunology 2001; 103(4): 449-57.
[http://dx.doi.org/10.1046/j.1365-2567.2001.01279.x] [PMID: 11529935]

[205] Rayner AA, Grimm EA, Lotze MT, Chu EW, Rosenberg SA. Lymphokine-activated killer (LAK) cells. Analysis of factors relevant to the immunotherapy of human cancer. Cancer 1985; 55(6): 1327-33.
[http://dx.doi.org/10.1002/1097-0142(19850315)55:6<1327::AID-CNCR2820550628>3.0.CO;2-O] [PMID: 3871657]

[206] Ettinghausen SE, Lipford EH III, Mulé JJ, Rosenberg SA. Recombinant interleukin 2 stimulates *in vivo* proliferation of adoptively transferred lymphokine-activated killer (LAK) cells. J Immunol 1985; 135(5): 3623-35.
[PMID: 3900213]

[207] Lafreniere R, Rosenberg SA. Adoptive immunotherapy of murine hepatic metastases with lymphokine activated killer (LAK) cells and recombinant interleukin 2 (RIL 2) can mediate the regression of both immunogenic and nonimmunogenic sarcomas and an adenocarcinoma. J Immunol 1985; 135(6): 4273-80.
[PMID: 3877766]

[208] Weber JS, Yang JC, Topalian SL, Schwartzentruber DJ, White DE, Rosenberg SA. The use of interleukin-2 and lymphokine-activated killer cells for the treatment of patients with non-Hodgkin's lymphoma. J Clin Oncol 1992; 10(1): 33-40.
[PMID: 1727923]

[209] Margolin KA, Aronson FR, Sznol M, *et al.* Phase II trial of high-dose interleukin-2 and lymphokine-activated killer cells in Hodgkin's disease and non-Hodgkin's lymphoma. J Immunother (1991) 1991; 10(3): 214-20.

[210] Bernstein ZP, Vaickus L, Friedman N, *et al.* Interleukin-2 lymphokine-activated killer cell therapy of non-Hodgkin's lymphoma and Hodgkin's disease. J Immunother (1991) 1991; 10(2): 141-6.

[211] Seidel UJ, Schlegel P, Lang P. Natural killer cell mediated antibody-dependent cellular cytotoxicity in tumor immunotherapy with therapeutic antibodies. Front Immunol 2013; 4: 76.
[http://dx.doi.org/10.3389/fimmu.2013.00076] [PMID: 23543707]

[212] Lister J, Rybka WB, Donnenberg AD, *et al.* Autologous peripheral blood stem cell transplantation and adoptive immunotherapy with activated natural killer cells in the immediate posttransplant period. Clin Cancer Res 1995; 1(6): 607-14.
[PMID: 9816022]

[213] deMagalhaes-Silverman M, Donnenberg A, Lembersky B, *et al.* Posttransplant adoptive immunotherapy with activated natural killer cells in patients with metastatic breast cancer. J Immunother 2000; 23(1): 154-60.
[http://dx.doi.org/10.1097/00002371-200001000-00018] [PMID: 10687148]

[214] Bachanova V, Burns LJ, McKenna DH, *et al.* Allogeneic natural killer cells for refractory lymphoma. Cancer Immunol Immunother 2010; 59(11): 1739-44.
[http://dx.doi.org/10.1007/s00262-010-0896-z] [PMID: 20680271]

[215] Ishikawa E, Tsuboi K, Saijo K, *et al.* Autologous natural killer cell therapy for human recurrent

malignant glioma. Anticancer Res 2004; 24(3b): 1861-71.
[PMID: 15274367]

[216] Miller JS, Soignier Y, Panoskaltsis-Mortari A, *et al.* Successful adoptive transfer and *in vivo* expansion of human haploidentical NK cells in patients with cancer. Blood 2005; 105(8): 3051-7.
[http://dx.doi.org/10.1182/blood-2004-07-2974] [PMID: 15632206]

[217] Roberti MP, Rocca YS, Amat M, *et al.* IL-2- or IL-15-activated NK cells enhance Cetuximab-mediated activity against triple-negative breast cancer in xenografts and in breast cancer patients. Breast Cancer Res Treat 2012; 136(3): 659-71.
[http://dx.doi.org/10.1007/s10549-012-2287-y] [PMID: 23065032]

[218] Moga E, Alvarez E, Cantó E, *et al.* NK cells stimulated with IL-15 or CpG ODN enhance rituximab-dependent cellular cytotoxicity against B-cell lymphoma. Exp Hematol 2008; 36(1): 69-77.
[http://dx.doi.org/10.1016/j.exphem.2007.08.012] [PMID: 17959301]

[219] Miller JS. Therapeutic applications: natural killer cells in the clinic. Hematology Am Soc Hematol Educ Program 2013; 2013: 247-53.
[http://dx.doi.org/10.1182/asheducation-2013.1.247] [PMID: 24319187]

[220] Gleason MK, Ross JA, Warlick ED, *et al.* CD16xCD33 bispecific killer cell engager (BiKE) activates NK cells against primary MDS and MDSC CD33+ targets. Blood 2014; 123(19): 3016-26.
[http://dx.doi.org/10.1182/blood-2013-10-533398] [PMID: 24652987]

[221] Kerkar SP, Sanchez-Perez L, Yang S, *et al.* Genetic engineering of murine CD8+ and CD4+ T cells for preclinical adoptive immunotherapy studies. J Immunother 2011; 34(4): 343-52.
[http://dx.doi.org/10.1097/CJI.0b013e3182187600] [PMID: 21499127]

[222] Abad JD, Wrzensinski C, Overwijk W, *et al.* T-cell receptor gene therapy of established tumors in a murine melanoma model. J Immunother 2008; 31(1): 1-6.
[http://dx.doi.org/10.1097/CJI.0b013e31815c193f] [PMID: 18157006]

[223] Morgan RA, Dudley ME, Wunderlich JR, *et al.* Cancer regression in patients after transfer of genetically engineered lymphocytes. Science 2006; 314(5796): 126-9.
[http://dx.doi.org/10.1126/science.1129003] [PMID: 16946036]

[224] Sadelain M, Brentjens R, Rivière I. The promise and potential pitfalls of chimeric antigen receptors. Curr Opin Immunol 2009; 21(2): 215-23.
[http://dx.doi.org/10.1016/j.coi.2009.02.009] [PMID: 19327974]

[225] Nadler LM, Anderson KC, Marti G, *et al.* B4, a human B lymphocyte-associated antigen expressed on normal, mitogen-activated, and malignant B lymphocytes. J Immunol 1983; 131(1): 244-50.
[PMID: 6408173]

[226] Uckun FM, Jaszcz W, Ambrus JL, *et al.* Detailed studies on expression and function of CD19 surface determinant by using B43 monoclonal antibody and the clinical potential of anti-CD19 immunotoxins. Blood 1988; 71(1): 13-29.
[PMID: 3257143]

[227] Scheuermann RH, Racila E. CD19 antigen in leukemia and lymphoma diagnosis and immunotherapy. Leuk Lymphoma 1995; 18(5-6): 385-97.
[http://dx.doi.org/10.3109/10428199509059636] [PMID: 8528044]

[228] Kochenderfer JN, Rosenberg SA. Treating B-cell cancer with T cells expressing anti-CD19 chimeric antigen receptors. Nat Rev Clin Oncol 2013; 10(5): 267-76.
[http://dx.doi.org/10.1038/nrclinonc.2013.46] [PMID: 23546520]

[229] Aktipis CA, Ellis BJ, Nishimura KK, Hiatt RA. Modern reproductive patterns associated with estrogen receptor positive but not negative breast cancer susceptibility. Evol Med Public Health 2014; 2015(1): 52-74.
[http://dx.doi.org/10.1093/emph/eou028] [PMID: 25389105]

[230] Maude SL, Barrett D, Teachey DT, Grupp SA. Managing cytokine release syndrome associated with novel T cell-engaging therapies. Cancer J 2014; 20(2): 119-22.
[http://dx.doi.org/10.1097/PPO.0000000000000035] [PMID: 24667956]

[231] Maus MV, Grupp SA, Porter DL, June CH. Antibody-modified T cells: CARs take the front seat for hematologic malignancies. Blood 2014; 123(17): 2625-35.
[http://dx.doi.org/10.1182/blood-2013-11-492231] [PMID: 24578504]

[232] Bendandi M. Aiming at a curative strategy for follicular lymphoma. CA Cancer J Clin 2008; 58(5): 305-17.
[http://dx.doi.org/10.3322/CA.2008.0011] [PMID: 18755938]

[233] Jakóbisiak M, Janowska-Wieczorek A, Dobaczewska H, *et al.* Decreased antibody-dependent cellular cytotoxicity in various types of leukaemia in man. Scand J Haematol 1981; 27(3): 181-5.
[http://dx.doi.org/10.1111/j.1600-0609.1981.tb00470.x] [PMID: 6947403]

[234] Saijo N, Shimizu E, Irimajiri N, *et al.* Analysis of natural killer activity and antibody-dependent cellular cytotoxicity in healthy volunteers and in patients with primary lung cancer and metastatic pulmonary tumors. J Cancer Res Clin Oncol 1982; 102(3): 195-214.
[http://dx.doi.org/10.1007/BF00411340] [PMID: 7061569]

[235] Berdeja JG, Hess A, Lucas DM, *et al.* Systemic interleukin-2 and adoptive transfer of lymphokine-activated killer cells improves antibody-dependent cellular cytotoxicity in patients with relapsed B-cell lymphoma treated with rituximab. Clin Cancer Res 2007; 13(8): 2392-9.
[http://dx.doi.org/10.1158/1078-0432.CCR-06-1860] [PMID: 17438098]

[236] Eisenbeis CF, Grainger A, Fischer B, *et al.* Combination immunotherapy of B-cell non-Hodgkin's lymphoma with rituximab and interleukin-2: a preclinical and phase I study. Clin Cancer Res 2004; 10(18 Pt 1): 6101-10.
[http://dx.doi.org/10.1158/1078-0432.CCR-04-0525] [PMID: 15447996]

[237] McLaughlin P, Grillo-López AJ, Link BK, *et al.* Rituximab chimeric anti-CD20 monoclonal antibody therapy for relapsed indolent lymphoma: half of patients respond to a four-dose treatment program. J Clin Oncol 1998; 16(8): 2825-33.
[PMID: 9704735]

[238] Gluck WL, Hurst D, Yuen A, *et al.* Phase I studies of interleukin (IL)-2 and rituximab in B-cell non-hodgkin's lymphoma: IL-2 mediated natural killer cell expansion correlations with clinical response. Clin Cancer Res 2004; 10(7): 2253-64.
[http://dx.doi.org/10.1158/1078-0432.CCR-1087-3] [PMID: 15073100]

[239] Khan KD, Emmanouilides C, Benson DM Jr, *et al.* A phase 2 study of rituximab in combination with

recombinant interleukin-2 for rituximab-refractory indolent non-Hodgkin's lymphoma. Clin Cancer Res 2006; 12(23): 7046-53.
[http://dx.doi.org/10.1158/1078-0432.CCR-06-1571] [PMID: 17145827]

[240] Schultz KR, Klarnet JP, Peace DJ, *et al.* Monoclonal antibody therapy of murine lymphoma: enhanced efficacy by concurrent administration of interleukin 2 or lymphokine-activated killer cells. Cancer Res 1990; 50(17): 5421-5.
[PMID: 2386946]

[241] Hurvitz SA, Timmerman JM. Recombinant, tumour-derived idiotype vaccination for indolent B cell non-Hodgkin's lymphomas: a focus on FavId. Expert Opin Biol Ther 2005; 5(6): 841-52.
[http://dx.doi.org/10.1517/14712598.5.6.841] [PMID: 15952914]

[242] Inoges S, de Cerio AL, Villanueva H, Pastor F, Bendandi M. Idiotype vaccine production using hybridoma technology. Methods Mol Biol 2014; 1139: 367-87.
[http://dx.doi.org/10.1007/978-1-4939-0345-0_30] [PMID: 24619694]

[243] Kwak LW, Campbell MJ, Czerwinski DK, Hart S, Miller RA, Levy R. Induction of immune responses in patients with B-cell lymphoma against the surface-immunoglobulin idiotype expressed by their tumors. N Engl J Med 1992; 327(17): 1209-15.
[http://dx.doi.org/10.1056/NEJM199210223271705] [PMID: 1406793]

[244] Hsu FJ, Caspar CB, Czerwinski D, *et al.* Tumor-specific idiotype vaccines in the treatment of patients with B-cell lymphoma--long-term results of a clinical trial. Blood 1997; 89(9): 3129-35.
[PMID: 9129015]

[245] Bendandi M, Gocke CD, Kobrin CB, *et al.* Complete molecular remissions induced by patient-specific vaccination plus granulocyte-monocyte colony-stimulating factor against lymphoma. Nat Med 1999; 5(10): 1171-7.
[http://dx.doi.org/10.1038/13928] [PMID: 10502821]

[246] Barrios Y, Cabrera R, Yáñez R, *et al.* Anti-idiotypic vaccination in the treatment of low-grade B-cell lymphoma. Haematologica 2002; 87(4): 400-7.
[PMID: 11940484]

[247] Yáñez R, Barrios Y, Ruiz E, Cabrera R, Díaz-Espada F. Anti-idiotypic Immunotherapy in follicular lymphoma patients: results of a long follow-up study. J Immunother 2008; 31(3): 310-2.
[http://dx.doi.org/10.1097/CJI.0b013e31816a8116] [PMID: 18317357]

[248] Inogès S, Rodrìguez-Calvillo M, Zabalegui N, *et al.* Grupo Español de Linfomas/Trasplante Autologo de Medula Oseo study group; Programa para el Estudio y Tratamiento de Hemopatias Malignas study group. Clinical benefit associated with idiotypic vaccination in patients with follicular lymphoma. J Natl Cancer Inst 2006; 98(18): 1292-301.
[http://dx.doi.org/10.1093/jnci/djj358] [PMID: 16985248]

[249] Neelapu SS, Gause BL, Nikcevich DA, *et al.* Phase III randomized trial of patient-specific vaccination for previously untreated patients with follicular lymphoma in first complete remission: protocol summary and interim report. Clin Lymphoma 2005; 6(1): 61-4.
[http://dx.doi.org/10.3816/CLM.2005.n.031] [PMID: 15989711]

[250] Bendandi M. Idiotype vaccines for lymphoma: proof-of-principles and clinical trial failures. Nat Rev Cancer 2009; 9(9): 675-81.

[http://dx.doi.org/10.1038/nrc2717] [PMID: 19701243]

[251] Bendandi M. Clinical benefit of idiotype vaccines: too many trials for a clever demonstration? Rev Recent Clin Trials 2006; 1(1): 67-74.
[http://dx.doi.org/10.2174/157488706775246120] [PMID: 18393782]

[252] de Cerio AL, Inogés S. Future of idiotypic vaccination for B-cell lymphoma. Expert Rev Vaccines 2009; 8(1): 43-50.
[http://dx.doi.org/10.1586/14760584.8.1.43] [PMID: 19093772]

[253] Hawkins RE, Zhu D, Ovecka M, *et al.* Idiotypic vaccination against human B-cell lymphoma. Rescue of variable region gene sequences from biopsy material for assembly as single-chain Fv personal vaccines. Blood 1994; 83(11): 3279-88.
[PMID: 8193363]

[254] Wolff JA, Malone RW, Williams P, *et al.* Direct gene transfer into mouse muscle *in vivo.* Science 1990; 247(4949 Pt 1): 1465-8.
[http://dx.doi.org/10.1126/science.1690918] [PMID: 1690918]

[255] Davis HL, Millan CL, Watkins SC. Immune-mediated destruction of transfected muscle fibers after direct gene transfer with antigen-expressing plasmid DNA. Gene Ther 1997; 4(3): 181-8.
[http://dx.doi.org/10.1038/sj.gt.3300380] [PMID: 9135731]

[256] Klinman DM, Yi AK, Beaucage SL, Conover J, Krieg AM. CpG motifs present in bacteria DNA rapidly induce lymphocytes to secrete interleukin 6, interleukin 12, and interferon gamma. Proc Natl Acad Sci USA 1996; 93(7): 2879-83.
[http://dx.doi.org/10.1073/pnas.93.7.2879] [PMID: 8610135]

[257] Sato Y, Roman M, Tighe H, *et al.* Immunostimulatory DNA sequences necessary for effective intradermal gene immunization. Science 1996; 273(5273): 352-4.
[http://dx.doi.org/10.1126/science.273.5273.352] [PMID: 8662521]

[258] Syrengelas AD, Chen TT, Levy R. DNA immunization induces protective immunity against B-cell lymphoma. Nat Med 1996; 2(9): 1038-41.
[http://dx.doi.org/10.1038/nm0996-1038] [PMID: 8782465]

[259] Hakim I, Levy S, Levy R. A nine-amino acid peptide from IL-1beta augments antitumor immune responses induced by protein and DNA vaccines. J Immunol 1996; 157(12): 5503-11.
[PMID: 8955200]

[260] Spellerberg MB, Zhu D, Thompsett A, King CA, Hamblin TJ, Stevenson FK. DNA vaccines against lymphoma: promotion of anti-idiotypic antibody responses induced by single chain Fv genes by fusion to tetanus toxin fragment C. J Immunol 1997; 159(4): 1885-92.
[PMID: 9257853]

[261] King CA, Spellerberg MB, Zhu D, *et al.* DNA vaccines with single-chain Fv fused to fragment C of tetanus toxin induce protective immunity against lymphoma and myeloma. Nat Med 1998; 4(11): 1281-6.
[http://dx.doi.org/10.1038/3266] [PMID: 9809552]

[262] Biragyn A, Surenhu M, Yang D, *et al.* Mediators of innate immunity that target immature, but not mature, dendritic cells induce antitumor immunity when genetically fused with nonimmunogenic

tumor antigens. J Immunol 2001; 167(11): 6644-53.
[http://dx.doi.org/10.4049/jimmunol.167.11.6644] [PMID: 11714836]

[263] Biragyn A, Tani K, Grimm MC, Weeks S, Kwak LW. Genetic fusion of chemokines to a self tumor antigen induces protective, T-cell dependent antitumor immunity. Nat Biotechnol 1999; 17(3): 253-8.
[http://dx.doi.org/10.1038/6995] [PMID: 10096292]

[264] Sallusto F, Lanzavecchia A. Efficient presentation of soluble antigen by cultured human dendritic cells is maintained by granulocyte/macrophage colony-stimulating factor plus interleukin 4 and downregulated by tumor necrosis factor alpha. J Exp Med 1994; 179(4): 1109-18.
[http://dx.doi.org/10.1084/jem.179.4.1109] [PMID: 8145033]

[265] Timmerman JM, Singh G, Hermanson G, et al. Immunogenicity of a plasmid DNA vaccine encoding chimeric idiotype in patients with B-cell lymphoma. Cancer Res 2002; 62(20): 5845-52.
[PMID: 12384547]

[266] Timmerman JM, Czerwinski DK, Davis TA, et al. Idiotype-pulsed dendritic cell vaccination for B-cell lymphoma: clinical and immune responses in 35 patients. Blood 2002; 99(5): 1517-26.
[http://dx.doi.org/10.1182/blood.V99.5.1517] [PMID: 11861263]

[267] Ogasawara M. Vaccination of malignant lymphoma patients with WT1 peptide-pulsed dendritic cells induces immunological and clinical responses: a pilot study. Blood 2013; 122(21): 4403.

[268] Lin Y, Atwell T, Weisbrod A, et al. Dendritic cell vaccine treatment for B-cell non-hodgkin lymphoma: clinical trial in progress. Blood 2014; 124(21): 4474.

[269] Richards RL, Alving CR, Wassef NM. Liposomal subunit vaccines: effects of lipid A and aluminum hydroxide on immunogenicity. J Pharm Sci 1996; 85(12): 1286-9.
[http://dx.doi.org/10.1021/js9601593] [PMID: 8961140]

[270] Neelapu SS, Gause BL, Harvey L, et al. A novel proteoliposomal vaccine induces antitumor immunity against follicular lymphoma. Blood 2007; 109(12): 5160-3.
[http://dx.doi.org/10.1182/blood-2006-12-063594] [PMID: 17339422]

[271] Neelapu SS, Baskar S, Gause BL, et al. Human autologous tumor-specific T-cell responses induced by liposomal delivery of a lymphoma antigen. Clin Cancer Res 2004; 10(24): 8309-17.
[http://dx.doi.org/10.1158/1078-0432.CCR-04-1071] [PMID: 15623607]

[272] Yamamoto R, Nishikori M, Kitawaki T, et al. PD-1-PD-1 ligand interaction contributes to immunosuppressive microenvironment of Hodgkin lymphoma. Blood 2008; 111(6): 3220-4.
[http://dx.doi.org/10.1182/blood-2007-05-085159] [PMID: 18203952]

[273] Hideshima T, Chauhan D, Shima Y, et al. Thalidomide and its analogs overcome drug resistance of human multiple myeloma cells to conventional therapy. Blood 2000; 96(9): 2943-50.
[PMID: 11049970]

[274] Mitsiades N, Mitsiades CS, Poulaki V, et al. Apoptotic signaling induced by immunomodulatory thalidomide analogs in human multiple myeloma cells: therapeutic implications. Blood 2002; 99(12): 4525-30.
[http://dx.doi.org/10.1182/blood.V99.12.4525] [PMID: 12036884]

[275] Verhelle D, Corral LG, Wong K, et al. Lenalidomide and CC-4047 inhibit the proliferation of malignant B cells while expanding normal CD34+ progenitor cells. Cancer Res 2007; 67(2): 746-55.

[http://dx.doi.org/10.1158/0008-5472.CAN-06-2317] [PMID: 17234786]

[276] Corral LG, Muller GW, Moreira AL, *et al.* Selection of novel analogs of thalidomide with enhanced tumor necrosis factor alpha inhibitory activity. Mol Med 1996; 2(4): 506-15.
[PMID: 8827720]

[277] Davies FE, Raje N, Hideshima T, *et al.* Thalidomide and immunomodulatory derivatives augment natural killer cell cytotoxicity in multiple myeloma. Blood 2001; 98(1): 210-6.
[http://dx.doi.org/10.1182/blood.V98.1.210] [PMID: 11418482]

[278] Galustian C, Meyer B, Labarthe MC, *et al.* The anti-cancer agents lenalidomide and pomalidomide inhibit the proliferation and function of T regulatory cells. Cancer Immunol Immunother 2009; 58(7): 1033-45.
[http://dx.doi.org/10.1007/s00262-008-0620-4] [PMID: 19009291]

[279] Novak AJ, Grote DM, Stenson M, *et al.* Expression of BLyS and its receptors in B-cell non-Hodgkin lymphoma: correlation with disease activity and patient outcome. Blood 2004; 104(8): 2247-53.
[http://dx.doi.org/10.1182/blood-2004-02-0762] [PMID: 15251985]

[280] Rodig SJ, Shahsafaei A, Li B, Mackay CR, Dorfman DM. BAFF-R, the major B cell-activating factor receptor, is expressed on most mature B cells and B-cell lymphoproliferative disorders. Hum Pathol 2005; 36(10): 1113-9.
[http://dx.doi.org/10.1016/j.humpath.2005.08.005] [PMID: 16226112]

[281] Martorelli D, Guidoboni M, De Re V, *et al.* IGKV3 proteins as candidate "off-the-shelf" vaccines for kappa-light chain-restricted B-cell non-Hodgkin lymphomas. Clin Cancer Res 2012; 18(15): 4080-91.
[http://dx.doi.org/10.1158/1078-0432.CCR-12-0763] [PMID: 22705988]

[282] Weng J, Rawal S, Chu F, *et al.* TCL1: a shared tumor-associated antigen for immunotherapy against B-cell lymphomas. Blood 2012; 120(8): 1613-23.
[http://dx.doi.org/10.1182/blood-2011-09-382838] [PMID: 22645177]

CHAPTER 6

Epigenetics and Cancer Cell Metabolism: Cross-talk and Therapeutic Opportunities

Chi Chun Wong[*], Jun Yu[*]

Department of Medicine and Therapeutics, State Key Laboratory of Digestive Disease, Li Ka Shing Institute of Health Sciences, Shenzhen Research Institute, The Chinese University of Hong Kong, Hong Kong

Abstract: Epigenetics is increasingly recognized to play an important role in tumorigenesis. The epigenome encompasses a multitude of elements that regulate gene expression, including DNA methylation, histone modification, microRNA, and more recently, non-coding RNA. Aberrant regulation of the epigenome has been implicated in altered gene expression and function, which contribute to cancer development and progression *via* the promotion of cellular transformation, metastatic spread, and drug resistance. Emerging evidence indicates that the activities of key epigenetic regulators including DNA methyltransferases and histone modification enzymes are sensitive to cellular metabolism. The efficiency of these metabolic enzymes depends on the availability of substrates and/or co-factors that can be profoundly altered in cancer. Mutations in metabolic enzymes in cancer also generate oncometabolites that can lead to the dysfunction of DNA and histone demethylases. Conversely, through mediating aberrant expression of genes that are involved in cellular metabolism, epigenetic mechanisms could contribute to metabolic rewiring in cancer to confer a growth advantage to cancer cells. Understanding this cross-talk between epigenetics and cancer cell metabolism may unravel novel therapeutic opportunities. In this chapter, we will review recent discoveries linking epigenetics and cancer cell metabolism, their implications in oncogenesis, and highlight potential approaches to target these cancer-specific abnormities therapeutically.

[*] **Corresponding authors Chi Chun Wong and Jun Yu:** Institute of Digestive Disease and Department of Medicine and Therapeutics, Prince of Wales Hospital, The Chinese University of Hong Kong. Shatin, NT, Hong Kong; Tel: (852) 3763 6099; E-mails: chichun.wong@cuhk.edu.hk; junyu@cuhk.edu.hk

Atta-ur-Rahman (Ed.)

Keywords: Acetyl-coenzyme A, Cancer, Cancer metabolism, DNA methylation, Epigenetics, Fumarate hydratase, Gene expression, Glutaminolysis, Glycolysis, Histone acetylation, Histone demethylase, Histone methylation, Isocitrate dehydrogenase, MicroRNA, Mitochondrial succinate dehydrogenase, Non-coding RNA, S-adenosylmethionine, TET methyl-cytosine dioxygenase, Tricarboxylic acid cycle, Warburg hypothesis.

INTRODUCTION

Epigenetics is defined as heritable changes in gene expression that are not resulted from change(s) in the underlying DNA sequence. Epigenetic regulation of gene expression can be highly dynamic and of a transient nature, or can be relatively stable and be passed to offspring through the germline. Given its role in the regulation of gene expression, it is increasingly recognized that epigenetics play an important role in cell growth, differentiation and development. The human 'epigenome' encompasses three major elements that interact with each other to co-operatively to either activate or silence gene expression, which involves direct chemical modification of DNA by methylation, alteration of DNA accessibility by histone modifications, and the selective silencing of mRNA levels by noncoding RNA.

The tight regulation of the epigenome is essential in normal cellular processes. Consequently, disruption of the epigenetic machinery can cause the inappropriate activation or silencing of genes, leading to the development of numerous diseases. The notion that epigenetic disruptions may be associated with cancer development was first proposed in the 1980's [1, 2]. Extensive research over the past two decades has clearly demonstrated that epigenetic dysregulation contributes to tumorigenesis by silencing of tumor suppressor genes [3 - 5]. With the advent of next-generation sequencing in conjunction with chromatin immunoprecipitation (ChIP-Seq) [6] and microarray technologies (*e.g.* Illumina 27K and 450K) [7], we are just beginning to appreciate the impact of epigenetic dysregulation in the development of cancers on a genome-wide scale [8].

Comprehensive molecular characterization of the cancer genome, transcriptome, epigenome and proteome by the Cancer Genome Atlas (TCGA) has further highlighted the role of aberrant epigenetics across different types of cancer, such as promoter DNA hypermethylation in a subset of colorectal cancers [9] and extreme hypermethylation in Epstein-Barr virus (EBV)-associated gastric cancer [10]. Moreover, whole genome sequencing has unraveled a number of epigenetic regulators, such as chromatin modification enzymes, that are recurrently mutated in various cancers, indicating that they may be driver mutations in carcinogenesis [11].

Recent studies have revealed an intricate relationship between epigenetics and cancer metabolism [12 - 14]. Cancer cells exhibit metabolic alterations to support an increased biosynthesis [15] and adaptations to allow their proliferation under an adverse microenvironment [16]. For example, cancer cells consume more glucose than normal cells through aerobic glycolysis, an inefficient pathway that generates much less ATP than oxidative phosphorylation, a phenomenon also known as the 'Warburg's effect' [17]. Such a metabolic re-programming is crucial for cancer cell survival, and is activated by oncogenic signaling cascades such as PI3K-AKT-mTOR [18] and transcription factors such as the hypoxia-inducible factor (HIF) and MYC [19], and the inactivation of tumor suppressor signaling, *e.g.* LKB-AMPK [20].

Metabolic sensing by the epigenetic machinery represents a built-in mechanism to regulate cellular activities in response to environmental clues, and it is frequently deregulated in cancers [12, 16]. There exists a four-way cross-talk between epigenetics and metabolism in cancer: epigenetic dysfunction that 1) directly affects expression of metabolic enzymes; and 2) indirectly alters signaling transduction cascades involved in the control of cell metabolism; and metabolic alternations that 3) influence the availability of substrates and cofactors necessary for the proper functioning of epigenetic modification enzymes; and 4) result in the production of oncometabolites that act as agonists or antagonists for epigenetic modification enzymes. In this chapter, we will provide a brief background on the epigenetic and metabolic dysregulation in human cancers, followed by a detailed account of the cross-talk between epigenetics and cancer metabolism, its underlying cause, clinical significance and potential therapeutic implications.

CANCER EPIGENETICS AND ROLE IN CARCINOGENESIS

DNA Methylation

DNA methylation is the most extensively characterized and the best understood epigenetic alteration in human cancers. DNA methylation involves the covalent addition of a methyl group to the 5C of cytosine to form 5-methylcytosine (5mC). In mammalian genomes, DNA methylation is highly specific and it occurs at CpG sites, where a cytosine nucleotide is located next to a guanine nucleotide and linked by a phosphate group. DNA methylation is mediated by members of the DNA methyltransferase (DNMT) family that catalyzes the transfer of a methyl group from S-adenosylmethionine to the 5C of cytosine. Three major DNMT isoforms, DNMT1, DNMT3A and DNMT3B, are active in DNA methylation in the human [21]. DNMT1 is a maintenance DNMT that recognizes and methylates hemi-methylated DNA during the process of DNA replication [22]. On the other hand, DNMT3A and DNMT3B are '*denovo*' DNMTs that initiate DNA methylation at unmethylated CpG sites and therefore are critical for establishment of genomic methylation patterns, especially during development [23]. Numerous promoter-associated CpG islands are excessively methylated in human cancers and this represents a mechanism for silencing of gene expression [24 - 26]. Promoter DNA methylation at CpG islands contributes to gene silencing impeding transcription factor binding [27], the recruitment of transcriptional repressors [28] and the inhibition of RNA polymerase II [29].

DNMT1, DNMT3A and DNMT3B have all been shown to be overexpressed in cancers [30]. A large number of genes are silenced by promoter methylation, and they encode proteins involved in diverse functions, including transcription factors and repressors [31 - 34], DNA repair [35] and signal transduction [36, 37]. Analogous to driver mutations in cancer, identification of driver methylation events from passenger methylation has attracted considerable interest [38]. In cancer, driver methylation events typically involve silencing of tumor suppressor proteins that participate in the maintenance of genomic stability and DNA repair, thus contributing to gene mutations and carcinogenesis, including the O^6-methylguanine-DNA methyltransferase (MGMT; repair of mutagenic O^6-methylguanine lesion) [39], MutL homolog 1 (MLH1, DNA mismatch repair)

[40], and Breast cancer 1, early onset (BRCA1, chromosomal damage repair) [41] genes. Apart from the silencing of tumor suppressor genes, DNA methylation at miRNA promoters has been demonstrated to specifically silence the expression of tumor suppressor miRNAs. Therefore, DNA methylation-mediated gene silencing may promote the development of cancers. Small molecules targeting DNA methylation (DNMT inhibitors) azacitidine and decitabine are currently used in the treatment of myelodysplastic syndromes and acute myeloid leukemia. Aberrant DNA methylation is also a very useful non-invasive biomarker for cancer diagnosis and prognosis [42 - 44].

In the past, it was widely conceived that DNA methylation is a relatively stable phenomenon [45]. It was not until 2009 that mechanisms of DNA demethylation was resolved. Methylated cytosines can be demethylated in two sequential steps, first involving oxidation of 5mC to 5-hydroxymethylcytosine (5hmC), catalyzed by the ten-eleven translocation (TET 1-3) family of proteins [46 - 48], followed by reversion to cytosine through oxidation and base excision repair by thymine DNA glycosylase (TDG) [49]. DNA replication can also passively remove 5hmC. Given that promoter DNA methylation is a common feature in human cancers, it is not surprising that TET enzymes are tumor suppressors. Frequent inactivating TET2 mutations have been detected in myeloid lineage malignancies [50] and down-regulation of TET expression has been observed in various cancers [51 - 53]. Hence, a hyperactive methylation and a deactivated demethylation machinery may coordinately promote methylation of promoter DNA in human cancers.

Histone Modifications

Histone proteins are the main building blocks of nucleosome core particle that consists of ~147 base pairs of DNA wrapped around a histone octamer comprising two copies of histone 2A, 2B, 3 and 4 [54]. Nucleosomes in turn are folded into higher order structures that enable compaction of DNA into the nucleus. Histone proteins are regulated by a myriad of post-translational modifications including acetylation, methylation, phosphorylation, sumoylation and ubiquitylation [55]. Histone modifications allow a fine tuning of chromatin structure and contribute to the control of gene expression through influencing the compaction of DNA that affects its accessibility and the recruitment of transcription activators or repressors

[56]. Dysregulation of histone acetylation and methylation has been frequently documented in cancers, and they will be discussed further in the following section.

Histone acetylation involves the addition of an acetyl group to lysine residues. Acetylation of histone is dynamically regulated by opposing actions of histone acetyltransferases (HATs) and histone deacetylases (HDACs) which catalyze the addition and removal of the acetyl group, respectively. HATs are divided into GCN5/PCAF, p300/CBP and MYST (MOZ, Ybf2/Sas3, Sas2, Tip60) families, whereas HDACs are classified into four groups: the zinc-dependent class I, II and IV and NAD$^+$-dependent class III HDACs (also known as sirtuins). Addition of a negatively charged acetyl group diminishes the electrostatic interactions between the histones and the negatively charged DNA. Histone acetylation is thus associated with a more open chromatin structure that is permissive for gene transcription [57]. In contrast, deactylation leads to a compact structure that represses gene transcription. HDACs have well-recognized roles in cancers *via* transcriptional repression of tumor suppressor genes and their overexpression has been reported in different types of cancer [58, 59]. Among genes that are epigenetically silenced by HDACs include p21^{WAF1} [60] and E-cadherin [61], which leads to enhanced cell growth, invasion and metastasis. Some HATs are putative tumor suppressors and inactivating mutations of p300/CBP have been identified in breast, colorectal and gastric cancers [62, 63]. Other members of HATs have been implicated in neoplastic transformation, exemplified by chromosomal translocations of MLL-CBP [64] and MOZ-TIF2 [65] that drive hematological malignancies. HDACs have been actively pursued as drug targets. HDAC inhibitors (HDACi) such as Vorinostat and Romidepsin have been approved for treatment of cutaneous T cell lymphoma (CTCL), and HDACi are undergoing Phase II/III clinical trials for solid malignancies [66].

Histones are methylated on basic amino acid residues including arginine, lysine, and histidine. Lysines may be mono-, di-, or tri-methylated on their ε-amine group; arginine may be mono- or di-methylated and histidine can be mono-methylated. Lysine methylation is the most extensively studied among these amino acids, in particular at the following sites: histone H3 lysine 4 (H3K4), H3K9, H3K27, H3K36, H3K79 and H4K20. Given that there are 19 lysine residues on histone H3 alone that can be methylated and that each histone lysine can be mono-, di-, and tri-methylated, this gives rise to a highly complex histone methylation code [67]. Histone methylation is regulated by competing actions of histone methyltransferases (HMTs) and demethylases. HMTs comprise 3 enzyme families that catalyze the transfer of a methyl group donated from S-adenosylmethionine (SAM) to histones. Lysines are methylated by SET-domai--containing (SETD) and DOT1-like (DOT1L) proteins; arginines are methylated by protein arginine N-methyltransferases (PRMT) [68, 69]. Demethylation of lysine is mediated by flavin-dependent KDM1 family and jumonji C (JmjC)-domain-containing, iron-dependent dioxygenases [70]. Histone methylation at different sites may have opposing effects on gene expression. As an example, tri-methylation of H3K4 near promoter region is associated with active transcription [71], whereas tri-methylation of H3K9/H3K27 is a repressive mark implicated in transcriptional silencing [72]. A number of gene alterations in HMTs have been identified in human cancers. MLL (11q23) and WHSC1 t(4:14) translocations are main drivers of aberrant cell proliferation in MLL-rearranged leukemia and a subset of multiple myeloma, respectively [73, 74]. Gain-of-function mutations (Y641, A677 and A687) of EZH2 that greatly enhance its ability to be di- or tri-methylated at H3K27 are driver mutations in non-Hodgkin lymphoma (NHL) [75]. Drugs targeting DOT1L (EPZ-5676) [76] and EZH2 (EPZ-6438) [77] have been described and they have shown dramatic effects in preclinical models of MLL-rearranged leukemia and EZH2-mutant NHL, respectively. Various malignancies showed the amplification of certain demethylases, such as JMJD2C [78] and LSD1 [79], that are linked to tumorigenesis and resistance to therapeutic agents. Histone modifiers hold promise as potential therapeutic targets in cancers because of the reversible nature of epigenetic regulation. A better understanding of the functions of histone modifications will reveal novel targets as biomarkers or therapeutic targets for intervention.

Non-coding RNA

Non-coding RNAs (ncRNAs) are functional, non-translated RNA molecules that regulate gene expression at the transcriptional and posttranscriptional levels. NcRNAs that are involved in the epigenetic regulation of gene expression could be broadly classified into two categories: short ncRNAs (<30nts) and long ncRNAs (lncRNAs) (>200nts). Short ncRNAs include microRNAs (miRNAs), siRNAs and Piwi-interacting RNAs (piRNAs), of which miRNAs are functionally the most important in humans. LncRNAs consist of a diverse class of non-translated RNAs such as those that are involved in housekeeping functions (tRNAs and rRNAs) and others that regulate gene expression and protein synthesis. Over the past decade, numerous studies have documented the epigenetic influence of miRNAs and their contribution to tumorigenesis.

MiRNAs are post-transcriptional regulators that are ~22 nucleotides in length [80, 81]. Mature miRNAs mediate post-transcriptional gene silencing by binding to the 3'-untranslated regions (3'-UTR) of target mRNA sequences [82]. In humans, miRNAs can recognize partially complementary sequences 2 to 7 nucleotides in length and such interaction is sufficient to trigger silencing *via* the recruitment of the miRNA-induced silencing complex that inhibits translation and triggers mRNA degradation [83 - 85]. Due to their promiscuity, a single miRNA may repress the expression of multiple genes and it has been estimated that >30% of human genes may be regulated by a small number miRNAs [86]. Thus far, 2588 miRNAs have been described (Wellcome Trust Sanger Institute, as of December 2014). MiRNA dysregulation is a common feature in human cancers [87]. Depending on their gene targets, miRNAs can either be oncogenic or tumor suppressive. For example, miR-139-5p functions as a tumor suppressive miRNA by repression of oncogenic NOTCH1 [88]. In contrast, miR-19 and miR-21 are oncogenic miRNAs (oncomiR) that repress the expression of PTEN tumor suppressor and promote cancer cell growth and invasion [89, 90]. Given their frequent dysregulation in cancers, modulation of miRNAs may be potentially therapeutic [91]. MiRNA can be silenced by antisense mechanisms or expressed using synthetic miRNA mimics. Moreover, miRNA fingerprints are being developed as novel cancer biomarkers that may help predict cancer diagnosis, prognosis and resistance to therapy.

CANCER METABOLISM

The Warburg's Hypothesis: Deregulated Metabolism in Cancer

It has been appreciated since the early days of cancer research that the metabolism of tumor cells differs significantly from most normal cells. Tumor cells have high metabolic demands and they utilize nutrients with an altered metabolic program to support their high proliferative rates, as well as to adapt to the hostile tumor microenvironment. Adenosine triphosphate (ATP), a fundamental molecule required for all energy-dependent cellular processes, can be generated through two metabolic pathways utilizing glucose as a starting substrate. Glycolysis refers to non-oxidative metabolism of glucose to pyruvate, generating two units of ATP in the process. Pyruvate is then catabolized by oxidative phosphorylation *via* the tricarboxylic acid (TCA) cycle in the mitochondria, a highly efficient process that generates an additional 34 molecules of ATP. Under hypoxic conditions, pyruvate is converted to lactate, an inefficient process known as anaerobic glycolysis.

An abnormal tumor metabolism was first documented by Otto Warburg in 1920's, who observed that tumor cells, unlike normal cells, metabolize glucose through fermentation to form lactic acid, even in the presence of normal oxygen (O_2) levels [17, 92]. The "Warburg hypothesis" postulates that cancer cells derive their energy in the form of ATP from glucose utilizing the glycolytic pathway instead of oxidative phosphorylation in the mitochondria, while O_2 consumption remains unchanged. Warburg at that time reasoned that aerobic glycolysis in tumor cells is necessary due to a disturbance in oxidative respiration caused by defects in the mitochondria. Indeed, mitochondria respiratory stress signaling induced by partial mitochondrial DNA (mtDNA) depletion [93, 94] and mutant mtDNA (3243A>G heteroplasmy) are associated with metabolic re-programming in cancers [95] (Picard M *et al.* PNAS 2015). Whilst the "Warburg's effect" may develop as a consequence of mitochondrial DNA mutations, many cancer cells also retain functional oxidative phosphorylation in parallel with an abnormally high rate of glycolysis. Since the initial discovery, it has been recognized that tumor cells are highly dependent on glucose for growth [17, 96]. However, tumor cells also require building blocks that cannot be satisfied with glucose. Indeed, proliferation of cancer cells demands a robust supply of reduced nitrogen for the production of non-essential amino acids and nucleotides. Recent metabolic studies revealed that tumor cells depend heavily on the supply of glutamine for nitrogen anabolism [97].

Tumor cells, *via* a process known as glutaminolysis, divert a major fraction of the cellular glutamine to replenish the TCA cycle [98]. Glutamine is metabolized by glutaminase (GLS) to glutamate and then to α-ketoglutarate either by glutamine dehydrogenase or aminotransferases. α-Ketoglutarate enters the TCA cycle and generates reducing equivalents for oxidative phosphorylation and intermediates for anabolism. Another function of glutaminolysis in cancer is for maintenance of redox homeostasis [99, 100]. Glutamate is the precursor of glutathione (GSH), a major cellular antioxidant. Glutamine-derived aspartate is converted in the cytoplasm to pyruvate in a cascade of reactions which generate NADPH and increase NADPH/NAD$^+$ ratio necessary for regeneration of reduced glutathione and maintenance of redox balance. Apart from glucose and glutamine, recent studies have revealed diverse metabolism alteration in tumor cells that helps sustain their high proliferative demands, and in some cases, even to generate oncogenic metabolites that promote tumorigenesis.

Pathways Leading to Altered Metabolism in Tumors

The signaling mechanisms underlying the altered metabolism in cancer cells have been a subject of extensive research over the past three decades. Dysregulation of the phosphoinositide 3-kinase (PI3K)/mammalian target of rapamycin (mTOR), AMP-activated protein kinase (AMPK), c-Myc, hypoxia-inducible factor (HIF) and p53 pathways have been identified to have a profound effect on cellular metabolism in cancer cells. The PI3K/mTOR pathway is frequently deregulated in cancers [101]. Under normal conditions, PI3K is activated by phosphorylation upon binding of various growth factors, such as fibroblast growth factor (FGF), vascular endothelial cell growth factor (VEGF), human growth factor (HGF), angiopoietin I (Ang1), and insulin G-protein-coupled receptors or tyrosine kinase receptors (RTK) in its proximity. Active PI3K mediates phosphatidylinositol-3,4,5-triphosphates (PtdIns(3,4,5)P3) production to activate its downstream effector AKT1. Opposing the effect of PI3K is phosphatase and tensin homolog (PTEN) that dephosphorylates PtdIns(3,4,5)P3 to the inactive biphosphates [101, 102]. In many cancers, this pathway is aberrantly activated either by mutations in PI3K components (activating mutations in PIK3CA) [103], PTEN (inactivating) [102] and/or the hyperactivation of RTK. AKT1, the central effector of PI3K, stimulates glycolysis flux by promoting uptake of glucose and phosphorylation glycolytic enzymes including hexokinase and 6-phosphofructo-2-kinase/fructose

2,6-bisphosphatases (PFK-2/FBPase-2) [104]. Last but not least, AKT1 activates the mTOR kinase, a master regulator of metabolic regulation. An activated mTOR promotes biogenesis by stimulating ribosome synthesis, mRNA translation, lipogenesis and mitochondrial metabolism [105]. Thus, an aberrant PI3K-AK--mTOR axis is a major driver of metabolic alteration in cancers, and inhibitors against PI3K/AKT1 (Perifosine and Idelalisib), and mTOR (Rapamycin/Sirolimus and Everolimus) are in the advanced stages of clinical trials to evaluate their efficacy in the treatment of cancer.

AMPK is an AMP activated kinase that acts as a senor of energy status, consisting of a complex of a catalytic α-subunit and two regulatory β- and γ-subunits. During a low energy status, a low AMP/ADP to ATP ratio initiates the replacement of ATP molecules by an ADP at site 3 and/or by AMP at site 1 of the γ-subunit. This facilitates phosphorylation of the AMPK complex by the liver kinase B1 (STK11/LKB1), inducing a 100-fold increase in its activity [106]. In response to low energetic stress, activation of AMPK opposes the action of AKT1 and inhibits mTOR. AMPK promotes downstream signaling mechanisms that replenish the supply of cellular ATP, including oxidative phosphorylation and fatty acid oxidation and inhibit energy-consuming anabolic processes such as lipogenesis, gluconeogenesis and protein synthesis [107]. Moreover, activation of AMPK causes cell cycle arrest at the G1 phase *via* the activation of p53 [108] and up-regulation of cyclin-dependent kinase inhibitor 1A (CDKN1A; p21[WAF1]) [109], thereby serving as a molecular link between metabolic stress and reduced cell proliferation. Cancer cells actively suppress AMPK signaling in order to engage growth signaling pathways in the face of metabolic stress and promote a glycolytic phenotype *via* the unchecked activation of PI3K-AKT1-mTOR signaling. For example, LKB1, the upstream kinase of AMPK, is frequently inactivated in cancers [110]. Recurrent somatic mutations in LKB1 have been identified in various cancers such as lung, cervical, breast, intestinal, testicular and pancreatic cancers, leading to a reduced activation of AMPK signaling [111]. Anti-diabetic drugs metformin and phenformin are AMPK agonists that have been shown to re-activate AMPK activity in cancer cells, resulting in the reversion of the glycolytic phenotype and inhibition of tumorigenesis [112].

HIF are transcription factors that respond to low oxygen concentrations, also known as hypoxia. HIFs are heterodimers consisting of constitutive HIFβ and the hypoxia-sensitive HIF1α or HIF2α. Under normoxic conditions, HIFα subunits are hydrolxylated by oxygen-dependent HIF prolyl-hydroxylases, which marks them for ubiquitination by the VHL E3 ubiquitin ligase [113], followed by degradation in the proteasome. Hypoxic conditions inhibit the activity of prolyl-hydroxylases and HIFα subunits are stabilized. HIF1α plays a key role in the re-programming of cancer metabolism, as it activates the transcription of multiple genes involved in glucose uptake (glucose transporter (GLUT) 1 and GLUT3), glycolysis (hexokinase 1, hexokinase 2, aldolase A, phosphoglycerate kinase 1, pyruvate kinase M2) and lactate synthesis (lactate dehydrogenase) [114]. HIF1 also inactivates pyruvate dehydrogenase (PDH) *via* pyruvate dehydrogenase kinase [115], which shuttles pyruvate produced by glycolysis away from TCA cycle/oxidative phosphorylation to lactate fermentation, thereby contributing to the 'Warburg effect'. Besides hypoxia, HIF1α can be constitutively activated in cancer cells through oncogenic signaling pathways. The PI3K-AKT-mTOR pathway induces the phosphorylation of ribosomal protein S6 kinase and eIF-4E binding protein 1, which promotes HIF1α translation [116]. Thus, either the activating mutations in PI3K-AKT-mTOR, or inactivation of LKB1 will increase HIFα activity. Aberrant stabilization of HIFα in cancer can also be mediated by: 1) inactivating mutations in VHL E3 ubiquitin ligase [117], which attenuate HIFα ubiquitination; and 2) loss-of–function mutations in mitochondrial TCA cycle enzymes succinate dehydrogenase and fumarate hydratase, which promote the accumulation of succinate and fumarate, respectively, that in turn inhibits the activity of HIF prolyl-hydroxylases,leading to HIF1α stabilization [118]. Hence, diverse genetic abnormalities contribute to HIF1α activity and its associated metabolic alternations.

MYC is a transcription factor and proto-oncogene that mediates various metabolic alterations in cancer cells. MYC expression is frequently induced by upstream signaling cascades such as Wnt/β-catenin, MAPK/ERK and PI3K. Mutations in MYC, which lead to its constitutive activation, have been observed in specific types of cancers such as Burkitt's lymphoma and other hematologic malignancies [119, 120]. MYC forms a heterodimer with MAX and regulates gene expression. It was recognized early on that MYC stimulates cell growth and accumulation of cell mass. Cells overexpressing MYC produce significantly higher amounts of RNAs and proteins. In this regard, MYC broadly induced gene expression by inducing gene transcription and translation *via* stimulating RNA polymerase I and II and ribosome biogenesis [121]. Hand in hand with increased protein synthesis, MYC enhances literally all genes involved in glycolysis [122] and glutaminolysis [97] that contribute to energy production and maintenance of redox homeostasis. Of note, MYC expression favors the alternative splicing of pyruvate kinase (PK) gene to form PKM2 [123]. PKM2 is largely inactive in the conversion of PEP to pyruvate, which promotes the shuttling of intermediates of glycolysis to the pentose phosphate pathway to generate large quantities of reduced NADPH and macromolecules. These factors are required to support the rapid cell division in tumors. Accordingly, MYC-driven cancers exhibit strong dependence on glucose or glutamine, which may be targeted with metabolic inhibitors.

The classical tumor suppressor TP53, the guardian of the genome, is crucial for control of cell cycle and DNA repair. However, it has also an emerging role in the regulation of cell metabolism. In this regard, p53 imposes a metabolic phenotype that favors ATP generation from oxidative phosphorylation over glycolysis. P53 activates the transcription of multiple proteins involved in the electron transport chain [124]. In contrast, p53 suppresses glycolysis by transcriptional repression of glucose transporters (GLUT1, GLUT3 and GLUT4) [125] and up-regulates TP53-induced glycolysis regulator (TIGAR), an inhibitor of fructose-2,6-bisphosphate [126]. Fructose-2,6-bisphosphate is an allosteric activator of glycolysis by the concomitant activation phospho-fructokinase 1 (PFK-1), which catalyzes the "committed" step in glycolysis; and inhibition of fructose-1,6-bisphosphatase which catalyzes the reverse reaction of PFK-1. By blocking the effect of fructose-2,6-bisphosphate through TIGAR, p53 can reduce the glycolytic flux. Hence, the loss-of-function mutations in TP53 serve to promote a glycolytic phenotype in human cancer cells.

Epigenetics and Metabolism: Crosstalk

It is increasingly clear that mutations in oncogenes and tumor suppressors, as well as dysregulation of signaling pathways not only contribute to inappropriate growth signals and evasion of replicative senescence, but also to re-engineering of the cellular metabolic machinery to one that promotes biomass accumulation and nutrient uptake, which is permissive for an increased energy generation, macro-molecule synthesis and antioxidative defense. Emerging studies have provided ample evidence that epigenetics and cell metabolism are involved in a four-way crosstalk that drives carcinogenesis, as described in the introduction section. The diverse crosstalk between epigenetics and metabolism is believed to be an inherent mechanism for the regulation of gene expression in response to nutritional status. Meanwhile, there has also been increasing evidence that the crosstalk between epigenetics and metabolism is rewired in cancers to sustain cell growth and proliferation. In the following, we will describe examples of such a crosstalk and how its dysregulation may contribute to disease development.

MODULATION OF METABOLISM BY EPIGENETIC DYS-REGULATION

Modulation of Metabolism by DNA Methylation

DNA methylation at gene promoters is a frequently observed phenomenon in human cancers and it mediates stable silencing of tumor suppressors. Various metabolic pathways (glucose uptake and glycolysis) and inhibitors of oncogenic cascades (AKT, AMPK, HIF and p53) have been shown to be aberrantly silenced by promoter methylation, as described below.

DNA methylation indirectly contributes to increased glucose uptake in cancer cells *via* epigenetic silencing of Derlin-3 (DERL3), a gene involved in the endoplasmic reticulum-associated protein degradation pathway [127]. Silencing of DERL3 leads to overexpression of its downstream target glucose transporter 1 (GLUT1), which in turn, contributes to an increased glucose uptake. DNA methylation also has an impact on glycolysis. Fructose-1,6-bisphosphatase-1 (FBP1) antagonizes glycolysis and promotes gluconeogenesis by converting fructose-1,6-bisphosphate to fructose 6-phosphate. FBP1 is down-regulated in gastric cancer by promoter hypermethylation [128]. Expression of FBP1 in gastric cancer cell lines inhibited cell growth and cell cycle progression. FBP1 is thus a functional tumor suppressor and the promoter methylation of FBP1 was found to be an independent prognostic marker for gastric cancer patients. FBP1 is also silenced by promoter methylation in hepatocellular carcinoma and colon cancer [129]. In basal-like breast cancer, FBP1 promoter methylation is mediated by the Snail-G9a-DNMT1 complex, and FBP1 silencing induces glycolysis, resulting in increased glucose consumption, macromolecules biosynthesis, and maintenance of ATP production under hypoxia [130]. FBP1-loss induced metabolic reprogramming that promotes epithelial-to-mesenchymal transition (EMT) which confers a cancer stem cell-like property and tumorigenicity. An alternative isoform FBP2 is also silenced in gastric cancer by dense promoter methylation [131]. Lactate dehydrogenase B (LDH-B) has been shown to be silenced by promoter methylation in breast, colon, gastric and prostate cancers [132, 133]. The abrogation of LDH-B potentially suppresses the conversion of pyruvate to lactate and slows glycolysis; which seems to oppose metabolic alterations in cancer. However, LDH-B silencing can be accompanied by overexpression of the LDH-A subunit that promotes lactate production under hypoxia. Finally, promoter hypomethylation can aberrantly up-regulate glycolytic enzymes that contribute to a glycolytic phenotype. For example, overexpression of pyruvate kinase (PK), especially that of PK isozyme M2 (PKM2) is associated with hypomethylation of its promoter and first intron [134]. PK catalyzes the final step of glycolysis and serves as a regulatory point. PKM2 is an inactive PK isomer and it exerts an oncogenic effect by virtue of its ability to translocate to the nucleus to activate GLUT1 and lactate dehydrogenase. Hence, the differential DNA hypo- and hyper-methylation contribute to a glycolytic phenotypic in cancer.

Signaling cascades linked to tumor metabolism are also aberrantly deregulated by DNA methylation induced gene silencing. PTEN, repressor of PI3K/AKT/mTOR signaling pathway, is transcriptionally silenced by promoter DNA methylation in endometrial, gastric, lung, thyroid, breast and ovarian cancers [135 - 139]. In breast cancer, for example, PTEN promoter methylation can be detected in ~50% of the breast tumors, which correlates with a loss of PTEN immuno-reactivity (40%) [138]. Across different cancer types, there is a highly consistent correlation between promoter DNA methylation and PTEN expression, suggesting that DNA methylation contributes to PTEN loss during malignant transformation. PTEN loss is a driver that activates PI3K-AKT-mTOR signaling cascade in cancers. In melanoma, promoter methylation of PTEN is also associated with poor overall survival [140].

LKB1, a tumor suppressor involved in the activation of AMPK, is also silenced *via* methylation of its promoter. In patients with Peutz-Jeghers syndrome, 80-90% of the patients have a mutation that inactivates one copy of STK11/LKB1 gene and they are at greater risk of developing gastrointestinal cancers. Loss of the wild type allele can be resulted from its deletion, or promoter methylation [141]. In a survey of primary sporadic tumors from various cancers (*n*=195), LKB1 promoter methylation were rare events, only detected in colorectal (1/43), testicular (3/28) and papillary breast (5/11) carcinomas [142]. The loss of LKB1 may lead to repressed AMPK activity, resulting in the unchecked activation of PI3K-AK--mTOR signaling cascade.

HIFα subunits are rapidly hydroxylated by HIF prolyl-hydroxylases, followed by ubiquitination by the VHL E3 ubiquitin ligase that marks them for degradation under normoxic conditions. However, aberrant silencing of either HIF prolyl-hydroxylases or VHL by DNA methylation can result in inappropriate HIFα activation in tumors [143]. Mutations in VHL are associated with the Von Hippel–Lindau disease, a dominant hereditary cancer syndrome that predisposes to a high risk of clear cell renal cell carcinoma (RCC). In these patients, the second wild type allele is frequently inactivated *via* promoter methylation [144]. In sporadic RCCs, VHL promoter hypermethylation was also found in 19% (5/26) of the tumors examined, suggesting that DNA methylation-mediated gene silencing is a common mechanism of VHL inactivation in RCCs. Infrequent VHL methylation has also been detected in other cancers [145]. The prolyl-hydroxylase domain family of enzymes (PHD1-3) are involved in HIF hydroxylation. In plasma cell neoplasia and colon cancer, it was demonstrated that PHD3, but not PHD1/PHD2, was frequently methylated at its promoter [146]. In colon cancer, the reduced PHD3 expression was correlated with significantly increased DNA methylation in the CpG Island of the PHD3 promoter region [147]. In cancer cell lines of diverse anatomical origins, methylation of the PHD3 CpG islands was identified in prostate, breast, melanoma and RCC cell lines, resulting in a decreased PHD3 expression [148]. Thus, the epigenetic silencing of either VHL or PHDs can result in aberrant activation of HIF and its associated metabolic alterations.

Epigenetic silencing *via* promoter DNA methylation of the p53 gene is a potential mechanism for the inactivation of this tumor suppressor gene. While genetic mutations and/or deletions of p53 are the dominant mechanism for its inactivation in cancers, emerging evidence suggests that promoter methylation plays a role in cancers harboring wild type p53. In acute lymphoblastic leukemia (ALL) where p53 mutations are relatively rare (<3%), p53 promoter methylation is observed in a substantial portion of the patients (32%) [149]. In breast cancer (~20% of the patients harboring p53 mutations), p53 promoter was methylated in ~19% of the cases and promoter methylation appeared to be exclusive of mutations of p53, indicating that promoter methylation is an alternative pathway to p53 inactivation where there is no p53 mutations [150]. P53 promoter methylation has also been detected in human glioma [151], although conflicting results have been reported. Methylation of p53 promoter represents a rare event in many other cancers, and alternative mechanisms may predominate in the inactivation of p53

Modulation of Metabolism by Histone Modifications

Due to the complexity of the histone modification code, we are just beginning to understand its functional role in regulating gene expression. As described above, histone proteins can be modified by methylation, acetylation, phosphorylation, sumoylation and ubiquitylation. Among these diverse modifications, the role of histone acetylation/de-acetylation in cellular metabolism has been the most extensively described and will be reviewed below.

Sirtuins are class III HDACs that play functional roles in the aging process and development of cancer [152]. SIRT1 negatively regulates glycolysis and promotes gluconeogenesis by the deacetylation of non-histone targets such as peroxisome proliferator-activated receptor-γ co-activator 1α (PGC1α) [153], forkhead box O1 (FOXO1) [154] and HIF1α [155]. Emerging data indicate that SIRT6 regulates glucose homeostasis by directly modulating histone acetylation. *Sirt6*$^{-/-}$ mice are characterized by severe hypoglycemia and an increased glucose uptake in muscle and brown adipose tissue [156]. Moreover, *Sirt6*-deficient cells grown in nutrient replete media exhibit a shift towards a 'glycolytic phenotype' with an increased glucose uptake and lactate production and a decreased ATP production [156 - 158]. Notably, *Sirt6*-deficiency induces expression of glycolytic enzymes including GLUT1, PFK-1, aldolase and triose phosphate isomerase. In addition, *Sirt6*-deficiency inactivates PDH through activation of PDH kinase. Curiously, the metabolic effect of *Sirt6* deficiency mimics that of Hif1 activation. Indeed, *Sirt6* was found to interact with Hif1α and deacetylates histone H3K9 at Hif1α-targeted promoter regions, thereby inhibiting transcription. Remarkably, *in vitro* and *in vivo* treatment with a Hif1α inhibitor reversed the glycolytic phenotype, indicating that *Sirt6* regulates metabolism in a Hif1α-dependent manner.

Apart from Hif1α, SIRT6 was also identified to be a co-repressor of MYC transcriptional activity and tumor suppressor [159]. SIRT6 deficient cells were found to be tumorigenic and exhibit oncogene independent transformation. Chromatin immunoprecipitation-sequencing (ChIP-seq) showed that SIRT6 is associated with ribosomal and ribonucleoprotein genes. MYC, as a global regulator of ribosome biogenesis, shares a similar chromatin occupancy pattern on the ribosomal genes such as Rpl3, Rpl6, Rpl23 and Rps15a with SIRT6, suggesting that they may co-regulate the expression of these genes. In the context of MYC-mediated transcription, SIRT6 also acts as a transcriptional co-repressor through the deacetylation of histone H3K56. Hence, MYC-regulated metabolic genes, such as Rpl3, Rpl6, Rpl23 and Rps15a, were induced in SIRT6 deficient tumors. Moreover, MYC-targeted genes such as those involved in glutamine uptake and metabolism (*e.g.* GLS) were induced in the absence of SIRT6. *In vitro* and *in vivo* experiments further showed that *Sirt6* deletion was sufficient to induce tumor formation and promote cancer aggressiveness. *Sirt6* hence acts as a tumor suppressor by repressing Hif1α-dependent glycolytic switch and MYC-dependent ribosome biogenesis and glutaminolysis. Consistent with its role as a tumor suppressor, decreased SIRT6 expression and deletions have been detected in cancer cell lines and in colon, pancreatic and hepatocellular carcinomas [160].

SIRT7 is another sirtuin that can directly repress the function of MYC [161]. SIRT7 possesses a highly selective catalytic activity on peptides containing H3K18 acetylation, but with no activity on other histone acetylation sites [162]. A physical interaction was demonstrated between MYC and SIRT7, which targets the latter to the core promoters of ribosomal proteins. Given that H3K18 deacetylation is known to be associated with repression of gene expression, it is not surprising that SIRT7 opposes MYC-dependent gene regulation and therefore suppresses MYC-mediated metabolic alternations. In contrast to SIRT6/7, SIRT2 promotes oncogenesis through indirectly stabilizing MYC [163]. SIRT2 catalyzes deacetylation of histone H4K16 to directly repress gene transcription. A genome-wide profiling revealed the ubiquitin–protein ligase NEDD4 as the gene most significantly repressed by SIRT2. SIRT2 was subsequently found to directly bind to NEDD4 promoter, deacetylate at H4K16 and repress transcription. Importantly, NEDD4 was discovered to be a negative regulator of MYC proteins by targeting them for ubiquitination and degradation. SIRT2, by repressing NEDD4 expression, enhances the stability of MYC. Since SIRT2 is itself up-regulated by MYC in cancer cell lines, it forms a positive feedback loop that promotes MYC-dependent transcription and oncogenesis.

Despite these recent discoveries, much remains to be understood regarding the impact of histone modification, such as histone methylation and phosphorylation, on the metabolic reprogramming in cancer. Given that histone methylation plays a fundamental role in the regulation of gene transcription, and its potential modulation by cancer metabolism (as described below), it will be of importance to further uncover potential links between the dynamics of histone methylation and metabolic alterations in cancer.

Modulation of Metabolism by miRNAs

MiRNAs regulate the expression of genes involved in diverse cellular functions. Recent studies have demonstrated that miRNAs regulate enzymes involved in various metabolic pathways, and their dysregulation underlies altered metabolism in cancer. Several aspects of cell metabolism are regulated by miRNAs, including glycolysis and mitochondrial TCA cycle, thereby contributing to the Warburg's effect. Moreover, miRNAs have a major impact on the aberrant signal transduction *via* PI3K/AKT, AMPK, HIF, Myc and p53 that contribute to the metabolic phenotype in human cancers.

MiRNAs play a role in glucose metabolism. GLUTs govern the uptake of glucose and their gene expression has been shown to be regulated by miRNAs. Tumor suppressive miR-1291 is often down-regulated in renal cell carcinoma (RCC) [164]. MiR-1291 restoration in RCC cells inhibited their growth, migration and invasion. GLUT1 is identified as a direct target of miR-1291 *in vitro*. In clinical RCC samples a significant inverse correlation was observed between GLUT1 mRNA and miR-1291. Another facultative glucose transporter GLUT3 is directly targeted by miR-195-5p and miR-106a. MiR-195-5p is down-regulated in bladder cancer and its consequent GLUT3 up-regulation may contribute to tumorigenesis [165]. MiR-106a is down-regulated in Glioma and its decreased expression confers a poor prognosis in glioma patients [166]. Re-expression of either miRNAs decreased glucose uptake and attenuated cell proliferation. MiR-133 is a negative regulator of GLUT4 by suppressing the expression of its transcriptional activator, Krüppel-like factor KLF15 [167, 168]. GLUT4 mRNA is directly targeted by miR-93, whose expression is reduced in colon cancer [169]. Down-regulation of miRNAs might mediate the increased glucose uptake in cancer.

Studies also demonstrate that miRNAs regulate glycolysis. Hexokinases catalyze the first step of glycolysis, converting glucose to glucose-6-phosphate. Among the four hexokinase (HK) isoforms (I-IV), HKII is the principal inducible isoform that is upregulated in many cancers. Expression of HKII is under tight regulation by multiple miRNAs. MiR-143 directly represses HKII expression through a conserved miR-143 recognition motif located in 3'-UTR of HKII mRNA [170 - 175]. MiR-143 suppresses HKII expression in breast, colon, glioblastoma, head and neck, and lung cancers, where miR-143 levels are significantly reduced as compared to normal tissues. Re-expression of miR-143 in cancer cells reduced aerobic glycolysis (suppressed glucose consumption and lactate production), cell proliferation and colony formation. These effects are reversed upon ectopic expression of HKII, indicating that the down-regulation of HKII is an effector downstream of miR-143 [172]. MiR-145 forms a cluster with miR-143 and it also represses expression of HKII [175]. The p53-inducible miR-34a is an inhibitor of numerous glycolytic enzymes including HK1 and HK2 [176]. On the contrary, miR-155 acts to up-regulate HKII expression by the following two mechanisms [172]; first miR-155 activates STAT3, a transcription activator of HKII, and second, miR-155 represses the HKII-targeting miR-143 by suppressing C/EBPβ. The miR-155/miR-143 axis thus contribute to deregulation of glycolysis in cancers. Numerous other tumor suppressor miRNAs target other glycolytic enzymes and their expression is frequently silenced in cancers. Phosphoglucose isomerase, which catalyzes the second step in glycolysis, is a target of miR-200 [177]. The liver specific miR-122 negatively regulates expression of aldolase A [178]. Aldolase A is also thought to be regulated by miR-15a/16-1 in leukemia [179]. Oncogenic PKM2 is targeted by tumor suppressor miRNAs such as miR-326, miR133a and miR-133b [180, 181]. MiRNA dysregulation also contributes to increased lactate fermentation *via* aerobic glycolysis. The aberrant down-regulation of miR-375, which targets lactate dehydrogenase B, may enhance lactate production in cancers [182, 183].

Glutaminolysis and the flux in TCA cycle is significantly altered in cancers. MiR-23a and miR-23b target 3'UTR of gluaminase (GLS), which catalyzes conversion of glutamine to glutamate for further metabolism in the TCA cycle [184]. Myc, an oncogenic transcription factor, suppresses the expression of miR-23a and miR-23b, resulting in the greater expression of GLS [185]. This contributes to the increased glutamine catabolism *via* the TCA cycle to provide carbon skeletons for biosynthesis pathways and for the production of ATP. Increased production of glutamate also boosts the redox homeostasis in cancers by serving as a substrate for glutathione synthesis. MiR-210 is a hypoxia-inducible miRNA that suppresses expression of the iron-sulfur cluster assembly proteins (ISCU1 and ISCU2) [186]. ISCU1/2 are required for the assembly of iron-sulfur clusters and attenuation of their activity compromises the iron-sulfur clusters-dependent metabolic proteins in the electron transport chain (ETC) and the TCA cycle, including Complex I and aconitase. MiR-210, by repressing ISCU1/2 expression, reduces mitochondrial function and favors a shift towards a glycolytic phenotype and lactate production, critical for the adaptation of cancer cells to the hypoxic tumor microenvironment.

MiRNA dysregulation also affects the signaling transduction cascades involved in the metabolic reprogramming in cancers. Components of the PI3K/AKT/mTOR pathway have been shown to be regulated by miRNAs. Subunits of PI3K complex are targeted by miRNAs. PIK3CA encodes the p100α catalytic subunit and activation mutation(s) of this gene have been identified in a range of human cancers. MiRs that target the PIK3CA gene include miR-1 [187], miR-10a [188], miR-124 [189], miR-203 [190] and miR-375 [191]. MiR-1 is a tumor suppressor miRNA that is down-regulated in non-small cell lung cancer (NSCLC) that directly targets PIK3CA 3'UTR. In a NSCLC cohort, the low expression of miR-1 and PIK3CA over-expression were found to be useful biomarkers for increased risk of recurrence. MiR-124 and miR-375 were down-regulated in hepatocellular carcinoma and colon cancer, respectively, and overexpression of either of the two miRNAs resulted in the down-regulation of PIK3CA expression, suppression of PI3K/AKT signaling and inhibition of cell growth. PIK3CD (p100δ), another PI3K catalytic unit, is a target of miR-7 [192]. In hepatocellular carcinoma (HCC), miR-7 is suppressed and its overexpression inhibited HCC tumorigenesis. MiRNAs also regulate the expression of PI3K regulatory subunits. PIK3R1 (p85α) negatively regulates the PI3K/AKT pathway, and its 3'UTR is targeted by miR-155 for degradation [193]. Overexpression of miR-155 in B-cell lymphoma down-regulates PIK3R1, therefore leading to aberrant activation of PI3K/AKT signaling pathway. PIK3R2 (p85β) facilitates the propagation of PI3K signaling and it is negatively regulated by miR-126 [194]. MiR-126 is frequently lost in colon cancer and re-expression of this miRNA in colon cancer cells is accompanied by a significant reduction of phospho-AKT. PTEN expression is extensively regulated by miRNAs. MiR-21, a commonly overexpressed miRNA present in diverse malignancies, directly targets PTEN 3'UTR [195 - 200]. MiR-21 expression is associated with the silencing of PTEN in breast, colon, gastric, lung, and ovarian, pancreatic and renal cancers. Other miRNAs that negatively regulate PTEN expression include miR-19b [89], miR-23b [201], miR-26a [202], miR-32 [203], miR-92a [89], miRNA518c(*), miR-638 [204] and the miR-106b~25 cluster [205]. Many of these miRNAs function in a cell type- and contextual-specific manner. Among these miRNAs, miR-638 was found to be a multi-targeting miRNA that concomitantly regulates PTEN, p53 and BRCA1. Intriguingly, miR-638 precursor is located in the first intron of DNM2 oncogene, which acts co-operatively with miR-638 to promote tumorigenesis [204]. Other phosphatases that inactivate AKT, including PH domain leucine-rich repeat protein phosphatase, protein phosphatase 2A subunit B and protein phosphatase 2 regulatory subunit Aβ, are repressed by miR-190 [206], miR-221/222 [207] and miR-200C [208], respectively, and the expression of these miRNAs contributes to AKT activation in cancers.

AMPK pathway, a major sensor of cellular energetic status that suppresses tumor growth during metabolic stress, is regulated by the oncogenic miR-451 and miR-

19. In glioma patients, elevated miR-451 is associated with poor outcome [209]. MiR-451 plays an intricate role in modulating AMPK activity in response to the microenvironment. MiR-451 directly targets the 3'UTR of CAB39, a scaffolding protein that forms a protein complex with LKB1 and STAD, which induces LKB1-mediated phosphorylation and activation of AMPK. MiR-451 levels were found to fluctuate with glucose availability. MiR-451 expression is enhanced when glucose is plentiful, which leads to repression of CAB39 and reduced LKB1/AMPK activity. Suppressed AMPK activity, in turn, facilitates mTOR activation and cell proliferation. Under glucose limiting conditions, miR-451 is decreased resulting in the activation of LKB1/AMPK cascade, which contributes to adaptation, cell survival and increased migration and invasiveness. MiR-451 thus differentially regulates LKB1/AMPK pathway in response to altered energy availability. MiR-19 is an oncogenic miR that induces leukaemogenesis. MiR-19 promotes aberrant cell proliferation through co-ordinate targeting of AMPK, PTEN and PP2A, negative regulators of PI3K/AKT/mTOR cascades [210].

Recent studies have identified numerous miRNAs that modulate the expression of transcription factors HIF, MYC and p53. MYC 3'UTR has been shown to be targeted by let-7a [211], miR-24 [212], miR-34a [213], miR-145 [214], miR-184 [215], miR-196b [216] and miR-449c [217]. All these miRNAs mediate the repression of oncogenic MYC and their down-regulation in malignancies is associated with enhanced MYC transcriptional activity. Of note, p53 has been shown to inhibit MYC expression *via* a miRNA-dependent mechanism. P53 transcriptionally activates the expression of tumor suppressive miR-145 [214] and miR-34a [213] by interacting with p53 responsive elements. Both miR-145 and miR-34a then directly target MYC 3'UTR, thus serving as a link that mediates p53-induced repression of MYC.

HIF1 is directly targeted by miR-20b [218], miR-199-a-3p [219] and miR-17-92 [220] that repress expression of HIF1. These miRNAs are down-regulated in a low oxygen (O_2) microenvironment, thereby promoting the stabilization of HIF1 in hypoxia. Several miRNAs also contribute to HIF stabilization by indirect mechanisms. MiR-424 is up-regulated in hypoxia and it represses cullin 2 (CUL2), a scaffolding protein for the assembly of the ubiquitin ligase system [221]. Reduced CUL2 stabilizes HIF1 by suppressing its ubiquitination. Similarly, hypoxia-induced miR-210 contributes to stability of HIF1 by suppressing glycerol-3-phosphate dehydrogenase 1-like (GPD1L), which in turn, prevents the hyper-hydroxylation and degradation of HIF1 in the proteasome [222]. MiR-210 is a transcriptional target of HIF1, thus forming a positive feedback loop that propagates hypoxia-induced signaling, where HIF1 drives miR-210 expression and miR-210 then further stabilizes HIF1 activity.

TP53, a classical tumor suppressor, is under negative regulation by oncogenic miRNAs, including miR-25 [223], miR-30d [224], miR-33 [225], miR-125b [226], miR-380-5p [227], miR-504 [228], miR-1285 [229] by directly binding to its 3'UTR. Accordingly, ectopic expression of these miRNA induced phenotypes that are associated with p53 loss-of-function such as reduced cell cycle arrest and apoptosis. MiRNAs also positively regulate p53 *via* Mouse double minute 2 homolog (MDM2). MDM2 functions as an E3 ubiquitin ligase that promotes the degradation of p53. In a positive feedback loop, p53 induced tumor suppressive miRNAs such as miR-192, miR-194, miR-215 [230] and miR-605 [231] that target 3'UTR of MDM2. Repressed MDM2 expression by miRNAs further increased the stability and activation of p53. Co-ectopic expression of miR-192, miR-194 and miR-215 synergized with MDM2 inhibitors to attenuate tumor growth [230]. Acetylation of p53, a post-translational modification, is a regulatory mechanism that disrupts MDM2-p53 interaction. MiR-34 and miR-449 promote acetylation and stabilization of p53 through the repression of p53-targeting deacetylases SIRT1 [232] and HDAC1 [233], respectively. As miR-34a is itself up-regulated by p53, the p53-miR34a interaction constitutes a positive regulatory loop that facilitates tumor suppression. Hence, p53 is modulated by a miRNA network that fine-tunes its activity and its dysregulation contributes to tumorigenesis.

MiRNAs have a diverse impact on both the expression of metabolic enzymes and the pathways that contribute to metabolic alterations in human cancers. Altered miRNA profiles in cancers may therefore contribute to the aberrant production of certain metabolites or activation of metabolic pathways, such as glycolysis and glutaminolysis, which contribute to the Warburg phenotype in tumors. The dysregulation of pivotal metabolic signaling pathways such as PI3K/AKT/mTOR and LKB1-AMPK by miRNAs additionally contributes to altered metabolism in cancers. Development of miRNA mimetics or miRNA anti-sense oligonucleotides to reverse aberrant miRNA regulation, and suppress cancer cell metabolism is a promising therapeutic strategy.

EPIGENETIC REGULATION BY THE AVAILABILITY OF CO-SUBSTRATES

Epigenetic regulation is imparted on the human genome through the action of various enzymes, including DNMTs, TETs, HATs, HDACs, HMTs and HDMs. Activities of these epigenetic enzymes governed the availability of the metabolic substrates and cofactors. Many of these substrates and cofactors are the products of cellular metabolism, thereby serving as a sensing mechanism between epigenetic regulation of gene expression and nutrient status. However, as a result of the deregulated cellular metabolism in many cancers, the altered metabolic profiles may result in aberrant regulation of the epigenome and gene transcription. Below we will discuss the substrates or cofactors for epigenetics, such as acetyl-CoA and S-adenosylmethionine, the two cofactors for acetylation and methylation, respectively, their deregulated metabolism in cancers and potential impact on the epigenome.

Acetyl-CoA and Histone Acetylation

Acetyl-CoA is an important molecule in intermediary metabolism. It fuels the TCA cycle and it is at the crossroads of numerous metabolic pathways. Glycolytic metabolism generates pyruvate, which is catalyzed by pyruvate dehydrogenase complex to form acetyl-CoA, generating 1 NADH from NAD^+ and carbon dioxide. Acetyl-CoA is also produced from β-oxidation of fatty acids. Acetyl CoA then enters the TCA cycle and generates ATP *via* oxidative phosphorylation. In addition, acetyl CoA serves as the building blocks for the synthesis of fatty acids and cholesterol. Apart from the two major metabolic pathways that generate acetyl-CoA to provide energy, acetyl-CoA levels in the nucleus and cytoplasm are maintained by two other metabolic pathways, the direct synthesis of acetyl-CoA from acetate and CoA by acetyl-CoA synthetase short-chain family 1 (AceCS1); and the conversion from citrate to acetyl-CoA in the cytosol by ATP citrate lyase (ACL) [234]. The latter pathway relies on a steady supply of citrate from the mitochondria *via* the malate-citrate anti-porter. Cytoplasmic and nuclear acetyl-CoA is utilized extensively as a cofactor for enzymes that catalyze the transfer of an acetyl group, *i.e.* acetyltransferases. Presence of a high energy thioester bond (-31.5 kJ/mol) facilitates the transfer of the 'activated' acetyl group. HATs mediate histone acetylation and they utilize the acetyl group of acetyl-CoA to histone lysines to form ε-N-acetyl-lysine. The intracellular concentrations of acetyl-CoA can vary roughly ~10-fold under normal physiological conditions and it falls within the K_m range of histone acetyltransferases. Therefore, histone acetylation activity is, at least in part, influenced by availability of acetyl CoA.

Studies in yeast have shown that histone acetylation is highly sensitive to levels of acetyl-CoA produced by acetyl-CoA synthetase. Instead of the acetyl-CoA synthetase pathway, mammalian cells utilize ACL as the major pathway to generate acetyl-CoA using mitochondrial-derived citrate as the substrate [235]. ACL-mediated conversion of citrate to acetyl-CoA is critical for the maintenance of fatty acids, cholesterol, and isoprenoids pools to support the high rates of proliferation. Wellen *et al.* first described the regulation of HATs by cellular energetics in mammalian cells in an ACL-dependent manner [236]. ACL protein expression was detected in the nucleus, suggesting that its activity may contribute to the nuclear acetyl-CoA pool. Consistent with this hypothesis, RNAi-mediated silencing of ACL in HCT116 cells significantly suppressed histone acetylation levels for all the core histones but AceCS1 knockdown had no effect. Non-histone protein acetylation was apparently unaffected, suggesting that ACL-derived acetyl-CoA has a specific role in regulating histone acetylation. ACL-silencing blocked histone acetylation during cell cycle progression and differentiation, and selectively suppressed the expression of genes involved in glycolysis. Cancer cells often overexpress ACL [237] and this probably contributes to the nuclear acetyl-CoA pool that is necessary for histone acetylation and expression of glycolytic enzymes.

Cancer cells frequently display a high level of aerobic glycolytic flux that leads to an increased mitochondrial citrate that translocates to the cytosol. Cytosolic citrate is then converted to acetyl-CoA by ACL. Lee *et al.* identified the ratio of acetyl-CoA to coenzyme A as a determinant of histone acetylation in cancer cells by showing that even at high acetyl-CoA levels, addition of coenzyme A dose-dependently reduced histone acetylation in cancers [238]. Importantly, the authors have demonstrated that oncogene-driven metabolic reprogramming in cancers aberrantly increased global histone acetylation. Expression of a constitutively activated KRAS^{G12D} in mouse pancreas resulted in high levels of histone H3 and H4 acetylation in precancerous pancreatic intraepithelial neoplasia (PanIN) and pancreatic adenocarcinoma (PDA). Downstream of KRAS activation is AKT, a master regulator of metabolism. AKT promotes acetyl-CoA production and histone acetylation *via* two mechanisms: 1) it promotes glycolysis by up-regulating glucose uptake and its metabolism to acetyl-CoA *via* glycolysis; 2) it increases ACL phosphorylation (Ser455) and activation, thereby maintaining a high level of acetyl-CoA under glucose limiting conditions. Consequently, the ectopic expression of constitutively active AKT (myristoylated AKT) induced a rapid and pronounced increase in global histone acetylation. Conversely, the inhibition of AKT dramatically decreased acetyl-CoA:coenzyme A ratio and suppressed histone acetylation. In glioblastoma multiforme (GBM), activated p-AKT was positively correlated with acetylation at histone H4; in prostate cancer it was correlated with H3K18, H3K9 and H4K12 acetylation [238]. These observations indicate that oncogenic AKT activation drives global histone acetylation in tumors.

Acetyl-CoA synthesis in cells is also regulated by MYC. Myc has been shown to regulate the chromatin structure by up-regulation of HAT GCN5, which induced mono-, di-, tri-, and tetra-acetylation of histone H4 N-terminal [239]. Besides, MYC enhanced the gene expression of metabolic enzymes linked to acetyl-CoA synthesis, including glycolysis and glutaminolysis. In isogenic rat fibroblasts with *myc*$^{-/-}$ or *myc*$^{+/+}$, it was demonstrated that *myc* increased the mitochondrial export of acetyl-groups during cell division and ~50% of these acetyl equivalents were incorporated into histone H4-K16 [240]. This emphasizes the role of Myc in modulating both the expression of HATs and the availability of acetyl-CoA to support histone acetylation in response to proliferative signals.

S-adenosylmethionine and DNA and Histone Methylation

Methylation of DNA and histone by DNMTs and HMTs, respectively, utilizes the same methyl donor, S-adenosylmethionine (SAM). SAM serves as a methyl donor for the methylation of a myriad of cellular constituents, and is utilized by most methyl-transferase enzymes. Biosynthesis of SAM takes place *via* the methylation cycle [241]. In the first and the rate limiting step of the cycle, methionine adenosyltransferase (MAT) catalyzes SAM synthesis from dietary L-methionine and ATP. The methyl group of SAM is chemically activated by the positively charged sulfonium ion in SAM, and the donation of the methyl group invariably releases S-adenosyl-homocysteine (SAH) as the product. SAH is a potent inhibitor of methylation reactions that requires SAM as a cofactor, and hence the SAM/SAH ratio controls the activity of methyltransferase *in vivo*. SAH is physiologically maintained at low levels through its hydrolysis to homocysteine and adenosine by the SAH hydrolase. Methionine synthases complete the cycle by recycling of homocysteine back to methionine through the transfer of a methyl group from 5-methyltetrahydrofolate (N^5-MTHF). Moreover, homocysteine may be catabolized *via* alternative metabolic pathways to give amino acids, GSH and inorganic sulfate. N^5-MTHF, the biologically active form of folic acid, may act as a methyl donor; however, its methyl group is considerably less active than SAM and is insufficient for most biological methylation reactions. However, N^5-MTHF is critical for the maintenance of the methylation cycle and the levels of SAM available for biosynthetic reactions. Since DNMTs and HMTs require SAM as the methyl donor, fluctuations in its concentrations will have an impact on both their DNA and histone methylation.

The impact of SAM on aberrant DNA and histone methylation in cancers is a case of too much, but also too little, depending on the biological context and divergent effects at different stages of cancer development. For example, global DNA hypomethylation has been with a high frequency in various cancers, yet CpG islands around gene promoters are extensively methylated. Likewise, the impact of histone methylation or demethylation on gene expression depends upon the histone subunits and the specific lysine-residues in question. Studies in rodent animal models and epidemiological data have indicated a positive correlation between methyl-deficient diets that are lacking in methionine, one carbon compounds and choline, and genomic DNA hypomethylation [242, 243]. Polymorphisms in methylenetetrahydrofolate reductase required for the synthesis of N^5-MTHF (and methylation cycle) also contributes to a DNA hypomethylation phenotype [244]. Either of the above conditions decreases SAM to SAH ratio, thereby inhibiting DNMT activity and leading to DNA hypomethylation. Global DNA hypomethylation is associated with genomic instability including elevated mutation rates [245] and chromosomal instability [246], which is thought to promote carcinogenesis in colon and liver.

On the contrary, an excess of SAM may contribute to DNA hypermethylation at CpG islands and inappropriate silencing of tumor suppressor genes. Excessive SAM has been linked to an altered DNA methylation profile. Deficiency of glycine N-methyltransferase (GNMT) is a rare condition leading to over-production of SAM [247]. *Gnmt* KO mice showed a ~40-fold increase in hepatic SAM concentration and aberrant DNA methylation [248], supporting the hypothesis that SAM levels modulate DNA methylation. In cancer cells, hypermethylation of DNA at CpGs may be supported by an increased availability of SAM by 1) overexpression of amino acid transporters LAT1 (SLC7A5) [249] and LAT4 (SLC43A2) [250] that mediate cellular uptake of methionine; 2) overexpression of 3-phosphoglycerate dehydrogenase (PGDH) that diverts the glycolysis intermediates to the serine-glycine biosynthesis pathway [251, 252]. PGDH oxidizes 3-phospho-glycerate to produce 3-phosphohydroxy-pyruvate, followed by transamination by phospho-serine aminotransferase to form phosphoserine, which in turn, is hydrolyzed to serine by phosphoserine hydrolase. Serine participates in 1-carbon metabolism and in the methylation cycle by donating its side chain to tetrahydrofolate to form N^5,N^{10}-MTHF, a reaction catalyzed by serine hydroxymethyltransferase. N^5,N^{10}-MTHF is reduced by methylenetetrahydrofolate reductase to N^5-MTHF, a cofactor in the regeneration of methionine from homocysteine. PGDH, the rate limiting enzyme in serine synthesis, is often overexpressed in cancers. Silencing of PGDH in PGDH-overexpressing cells suppressed cell proliferation. By boosting N^5-MTHF pool, PGDH contributes to the overproduction of SAM.

Similar to DNMTs, HMTs utilize SAM as the methyl donor to methylate histones. Alterations in SAM and aberrant histone methylation have been observed in many cancers. Nicotinamide N-methyl-transferase (NNMT) is an enzyme that catalyzes the conversion of nicotinamide to 1-methylnicotinamide (1-MNA) using SAM as the methyl donor. NNMT is overexpressed in a variety of cancers, including lung, liver, kidney bladder and colon and it exerts an oncogenic effect by promoting migration, invasion and metastasis [253, 254]. Metabolomic analysis of NNMT overexpressing cells revealed two deregulated metabolites, 1-MNA and SAH, were up-regulated in response to NNMT overexpression [255]. The significant increase in SAH, coupled with a modest decrease of SAM, resulted in >50% reduction in the ratio of SAM to SAH. Such reduction can be attributed to the formation of 1-MNA, which is metabolically very stable and cannot enter the methylation cycle. 1-MNA thus essentially acts as a sink that depletes SAM in cells. As a consequence, cell lines overexpressing NNMT showed a substantial decrease in the methylation of histones H3K4, H3K9, H3K27 and H4K20. On the contrary, histone methylation increased with knockdown of NNMT. Alteration of histone methylation by NNMT is associated with the acquisition of a more aggressive phenotype. The impact of NNMT appears to be limited to the methylation of histone as global DNA methylation is unaffected. The apparent discrepancy between DNA and histone methylation may arise from the varying K_m values of these enzymes for SAM, as a high K_m value indicates a higher sensitivity to SAM levels.

Metabolism-influenced histone methylation also has a role in pluripotency in mouse embryonic stem cells (mESCs) [256]. In mESCs, threonine is the only amino acid that is essential for maintaining pluripotency. In murine cells, threonine is catabolized to acetyl CoA and glycine *via* a two-step reaction involving threonine dehydrogenase (TDH) and 2-amino-3-ketobutyrate (KBL). Glycine is then used by the mitochondrial glycine cleavage enzyme complex for synthesis of N^5-MTHF from THF. Given that a steady supply of N^5-MTHF is necessary for the re-generation of SAM in the methylation cycle, it is unsurprising that threonine restriction caused a reduction in the SAM/SAH ratio. The altered SAM/SAH ratio dramatically suppressed the di- and tri-methylation of H3K4; but it had little impact on the deposition of other histone marks. Tri-methylated H3K4 is critical for the self-renewal of pluripotent stem cells. By supplying SAM and also acetyl-CoA, threonine metabolism *via* TDH serves as a link between metabolic state and the epigenome in mESCs. Humans harbor a mutation in TDH that renders it inactive; however, human ES cells express a high level of enzymes involved in methionine metabolism. Methionine deprivation in human ES cells induced a rapid decrease in intracellular SAM and triggered differentiation [257]. Similar to mESCs, a low SAM/SAH ratio caused a rapid and specific decrease in histone H3K4me3 levels, which poise the ES cells for differentiation. A modest decrease in global DNA methylation was also observed. SAM is thus a critical regulator of stem cell pluripotency through its epigenomic influence. Much remains to be explored regarding the regulatory impact of SAM concentrations on the epigenome, especially in the context of carcinogenesis.

EPIGENETIC DYSREGULATION INDUCED BY ONCOMETABOLITES

In the past, intense research efforts primarily focused on oncogenic alterations at the genetic and/or epigenetic level. Advances in metabolite profiling technologies including liquid chromatography coupled to mass spectrometry (HPLC-MS) and nuclear magnetic resonance (NMR) have greatly facilitated high-resolution elucidation of alterations in cancer cells at the metabolome level. Recent studies have identified that cancer cells with specific genetic defects may gain the ability to accumulate metabolites that promote tumorigenesis or participate in oncogenic transformation. These metabolites, termed "oncometabolites", are currently in the spotlight as the key players in the development of cancer, and to date biochemical evidence indicates that some of the onco-metabolites act through modulating gene expression at the epigenetic level, such as 2-hydroxyl-glutarate, succinate and fumarate.

2-Hydroxylglutarate Production in IDH1 and IDH2 Mutant Cancers

Mutations in the metabolic enzyme isocitrate dehydrogenase (IDH) isoforms IDH1 and IDH2 are common in diverse cancer types including gliomas [258], and acute myeloid leukemia (AML) [259]. Wild type IDHs (1/2/3) are $NADP^+$-dependent metabolic enzymes that participate in the TCA cycle, catalyzing a two-step reaction for the oxidative decarboxylation of isocitrate to α-ketoglutarate [260]. The first reaction step involves the oxidation of isocitrate at the α-hydroxyl to give oxalosuccinate, with $NADP^+$ acting as the hydrogen acceptor. The second reaction step involves the decarboxylation of oxalosuccinate to produce α-ketoglutarate. Both IDH1 and IDH2 catalyze the reverse reactions, whilst IDH3 only catalyzes the forward reaction. IDH1 functions to generate α-ketoglutarate in the cytoplasm and peroxisomes and thereby promotes activity of dioxygenases utilizing α-ketoglutarate as a co-substrate. IDH2 participates in the TCA cycle and glutaminolysis by catalyzing conversion of α-ketoglutarate to isocitrate. IDH1 and IDH2 also generate reducing equivalents in the form of NADPH.

Mutations in IDH1 or IDH2 occur at the substrate binding arginine residues (IDH1: R132; IDH2: R140/172) and they abrogate the ability of IDH1/2 to convert isocitrate to α-ketoglutarate. Interestingly, the loss-of-function is accompanied by gain-of-function of IDH1/2 to catalyze the conversion of α-ketoglutarate to 2-R-hydroxyglutarate [261]. Mutant IDH1 is present in 80% of grade II–III gliomas and secondary glioblastomas [262]; IDH2 mutations are found in hematological malignancies, such as AML and angioimmunoblastic T-cell lymphoma [259, 263]. Notably, mutations in IDH1 and IDH2 are mutually exclusive [264]. Mutant IDH1 or IDH2 both possess oncogenic properties, and their ectopic expression enhanced cell proliferation, colony formation and inhibits cellular differentiation *in vitro* [261, 265]. However, IDH1 mutations alone are insufficient in the malignant transformation *in vivo*. Introduction of tissue specific mutant IDH1 (R132H) knockin failed to induce tumorigenesis in brain or hematopoietic lineage, but its expression increased the numbers of early haematopoietic progenitors in the latter model [266]. This suggests that mutant IDHs may co-operate with other specific mutations to generate a full malignant phenotype. Pivotal to the functional effects of mutant IDHs is 2-R-hydroxyglutarate. This oncometabolite accumulates to astonishingly high levels (5 to 35mM) in tumors expressing mutant IDHs. Indeed, treatment of TF-1 leukemia and murine 3T3-L1 fibroblasts (wild type IDH) with cell-permeable 2-R-hydroxyglutarate recapitulates the effect of mutant IDH1 [267, 268]. Moreover, small molecule inhibitors are able to reverse the phenotypical alterations in cells expressing mutant IDH1 and IDH2, further reaffirming the role of 2-R-hydroxyglutarate as an oncometabolite [269]. Recent studies have also highlighted the involvement of alternative pathways, such as MYC activation, that may drive 2-R-hydroxyglutarate accumulation in other cancers (*e.g.* breast) [270].

2-R-hydroxyglutarate is structurally similar to α-ketoglutarate and it acts as a competitive antagonist. Hence, enzymes that utilize α-ketoglutarate as a substrate are among the targets of 2-R-hydroxyglutarate. This includes dioxygenases, a large class of enzymes that hydroxylate diverse substrates and require both Fe(II) and α-ketoglutarate as cofactors. Since their discovery, >60 dioxygenases have been identified, and they hydroxylate proteins, RNA, DNA and lipids. Therefore, the accumulation of 2-R-hydroxyglutarate in tumors may have broad functional implications. Indeed, subsequent investigations showed that 2-R-hydroxyglutarate production has a profound impact on the epigenome, as described below.

2-Hydroxylglutarate Modulates DNA Methylation

TET enzymes (TET1, TET2 and TET3), which catalyze the first step in DNA demethylation (5mC to 5hmC), are α-ketoglutarate-dependent dioxygenases that are susceptible to inhibition by 2-R-hydroxyglutarate. Inhibition of the activity of TET may mediate aberrant DNA methylation and inappropriate gene silencing. TET-mediated conversion of 5mC to 5hmC, in particular the activity of TET2, appears to be a relevant target of 2-R-hydroxyglutarate [271]. Overexpression of TET1 or TET2 in human cells significantly increased the levels of 5hmC. However, co-transfection TET1 or TET2 with mutant IDH1 (R132H) reduced the levels of 5hmC drastically to barely detectable levels. A similar result was obtained by co-expressing TET1 or TET2 with either IDH2 (R140Q or R172K) mutants, indicating that mutations in either IDH1 or IDH2 can abrogate the hydroxylase activity of TET1 and TET2. *In vitro* enzymatic assay with TET1 and TET2 confirmed that 2-R-hydroxyglutarate acts as a competitive inhibitor of α-ketoglutarate-dependent hydroxylase activity [272]. The inhibitory effect of 2-R-hydroxyglutarate was especially pronounced for TET2, where it inhibited the activity of TET2 by 33% and 83% at 10mM and 50mM, respectively (0.1mM α-ketoglutarate as co-substrate).

Among glioma patients, those that harbor IDH1 mutations (*n*=10) had lower levels of 5hmC (~50% decrease) compared to patients with wild type IDH1. On the contrary, 5mC, the methylated cytosine nucleotide, was significantly increased in IDH1 mutant glioma [272]. These results are consistent with the finding that IDH1 mutations in glioma defines a distinct subgroup of patients with a CpG island methylator phenotype [273, 274] and that the ectopic expression of mutant IDH1 (R132H) into primary human astrocytes is sufficient to reproduce a CpG island methylator phenotype by inducing hypermethylation in a large number of genes. Similarly, mutations in IDH1 or IDH2 in an AML patient cohort were also associated with a hypermethylation phenotype [271]. Moreover, mutations in IDH1/2 and those in TET2 were mutually exclusive in a large AML cohort, and these mutations may be biologically redundant. AMLs with either IDH1/2 or TET2 displayed a hypermethylation signature affecting a large proportion of overlapping genes (>60%), suggesting that promotion of DNA methylation is a shared mechanism of action of the IDH1 or IDH2 and TET2 mutations. As a consequence, IDH1, IDH2 or TET2 can mediate leukemogenesis by increasing hematopoietic stem/progenitor cell population and have a similar impact on impairing myeloid differentiation. Notably, recent studies have demonstrated that DNA hypermethylation induced by 2-R-hydroxyglutarate is reversible, and therefore represents a viable therapeutic target in IDH-mutant cancers [271].

2-Hydroxylglutarate Modulates Histone Methylation

Apart from TET1/2, 2-R-hydroxyglutarate targets the epigenetic landscape by inhibiting histone demethylases [275]. JmjC-domain-containing, iron-dependent dioxygenases comprise the largest class of histone demethylases that catalyze the removal of a methyl group from mono-, di- or tri-methylated histone lysine modifications. JmjC demethylases have diverse site and substrate specificity and modulation of their activity will have a broad impact on epigenetic regulation of gene expression. For example, JHDM3 and JMJD2 demethylases are capable of removing H3K9 and H3K36 trimethylated lysine and their activities are required for the proliferation of cancer cells [276]. On the other hand, other JmjC histone demethylases exert tumor suppressive effects. PHF2, which demethylates H3K9-dimethylation, is frequently silenced in cancers either by chromosomal deletion or promoter hypermethylation [277]. PHF2 co-operates with p53 and enhances its transcription by demethylating the repressive H3K9 Me2 mark [277]. Many other tumor suppressive JmjC demethylases including JARID1C [278], JMJD3 [279], JMJD1B [280] and FBXL10 [281] are lost in cancers as a result of mutation, deletion or translocation. Chowdhury *et al.* [275] systematically evaluated the effect of R- and S-2-hydroxy glutarate on functionally diverse dioxygenases including HIF hydroxylases (PHD2/EGLN1 and FIH), fatty acid hydroxylase (BBOX1) and histone demethylases (JMJD2A/KDM4A, JMJD2C/KDM4C and JHDM1A/KDM2A). It was found that 2-R-hydroxyglutarate, the major product of mutant IDH1 or IDH2, most strongly inhibited KDM4A activity (IC_{50}: 24μM) and histone demethylases (KDM4C: 79μM, KDM2A: 106μM) were more susceptible to inhibition compared to other dioxygenases. Crystallographic analysis showed that S- or R-2-hydroxyglutarate both bind to the active site Fe(II) and compete with α-ketoglutarate for binding. JMJD2A/KDM4A showed structural resemblance to other JmjC histone demethylases, and thus it is likely that R-2-hydroxyglutarate can act as an inhibitor of histone demethylases at physiological levels induced by oncogenic mutations in IDH1 or IDH2 (5 to 35mM). Further studies identified R-2-hydroxyglutarate as a KDM7A inhibitor [267, 272] by binding to the catalytic core with close proximity to Fe(II) and competing with α-ketoglutarate. Hence, JmjC histone demethylase is a target of the oncometabolite R-2-hydroxyglutarate.

The functional significance of the R-2-hydroxyglutarate-mediated inhibition of histone demethylase remains largely unknown. The *In vitro* incubation with cell permeable R-2-hydroxyglutarate in U-87MG cells increased dimethylation of H3K9 and H3K79. Ectopic expression of mutant IDH1 (R132H) in the same cell line increased mono-methylation of H3K4, di-methylation of H3K9, H3K27 and H3K79, and tri-methylation of H3K4 [272]. These effects were mediated by the competitive inhibition of histone demethylases by R-2-hydroxyglutarate, since it could be reversed upon incubation with α-ketoglutarate. *In vitro* studies in adipocytes and astrocytes either with mutant IDH1 expression or R-2-hydroxyglutarate treatment resulted in the progressive accumulation of histone methylation, in particular H3K9 tri-methylation, which in turn, prevented terminal differentiation of lineage-specific progenitor cells [267]. H3K9 tri-methylation is a repressive histone mark and it contributes to a block in differentiation. The effect of IDH1/2 mutations on histone methylation has also been examined *in vivo*. Knockin of mutant IDH1 (R132H) in the haematopoietic cells or the myeloid lineage in mice was associated with increased di-methylation of H3K79 and tri-methylation of H3K4, H3K9, H3K27 and H3K36 [266]. In humans, primary glioma with mutant IDH1 (R132H, *n*=10) had elevated H3K79 dimethylation levels compared to those with wild type IDH1 (*n*=10) [272]. In another study, oligodendroglioma patients with IDH1 mutations also had higher H3K9me3 compared to those with wild type IDH1 and IDH2 [282]. Whilst it appears that R-2-hydroxyglutarate can mediate histone methylation in IDH1/2 mutant tumors and trigger a gene signature of progenitor cells that prevents differentiation, additional studies are required to determine the full spectrum of histone modifications caused by R-2-hydroxyglutarate. It is noteworthy that JmjC histone demethylases represent a large class of enzymes, some of which are tumor suppressive and others promote growth in a context dependent manner. Tumor promoting effect of R-2-hydroxyglutarate-induced histone methylation may depend on the relative expression of different demethylases in tumor tissues, the differential inhibitory potencies against different demethylase isoforms and the dependency of the specific tumor tissues on demethylase for growth/tumor suppression.

Succinate and Fumarate Modulate DNA and Histone Methylation

Inactivating mutations in Krebs cycle enzymes fumarate hydratase (FH) and succinate dehydrogenase (SDH) [283] were found in a subset of human cancers. SDH mutations have been identified in gastrointestinal stromal tumors (GISTs) [284], renal cell carcinoma [285], paraganglioma and pheochromocytoma [286 - 288]. SDH is an enzyme complex consisting of four subunits encoded by SDHA, SDHB, SDHC and SDHD and is located in the inner mitochondrial membrane. SDH participates in the TCA cycle by catalyzing the oxidation of succinate to fumarate, which is coupled to electron transfer to ubiquinone in the electron transport chain. Mutations in any of the four subunits can inactivate the SDH complex, leading the marked accumulation of succinate. Mutations in FH have been detected in hereditary leiomyomatosis and renal cell cancer (HLRCC) [289]. Mitochondrial FH mediates the reversible conversion between fumarate and malate, and loss-of-function of FH resulted in high levels of fumarate.

Early on it was thought that mutations in FH or SDH contributed to tumorigenesis by abrogating mitochondrial function and generating reactive oxygen species that induced DNA damage and genomic instability. Recent data have shed new light on the mechanisms of the tumor suppressor effect of FH and SDH. Both succinate and fumarate are structurally similar to α-ketoglutarate, and they may behave as antagonists of α-ketoglutarate. Succinate and fumarate (at 1-10mM) inhibited the activity of purified KDM2A and KDM4A, with succinate being the more potent inhibitor [290]. In HEK293T cells, succinate and fumarate increased mono-methylation of H3K4, di-methylation of H3K27 and H3K79 and tri-methylation of H3K4. Both of these metabolites also inhibited TET-catalyzed hydroxylation of 5mC. Ectopic expression of tumor specific FH and SDH mutants recapitulated the effect of succinate or fumarate administration. Furthermore, mouse chromaffin cells with genetic knockout of *Sdhb* exhibited a methylator phenotype, with an increased 5-mC/5-hmC ratio, and enhanced histone methylation at H3K9me3, H3K27me2, and H3K27me3 [291]. The methylome abnormalities in *Sdhb* knockout cells triggered a transcriptional program that down-regulated a set of genes implicated in differentiation and suppression of metastasis, leading to a more invasive phenotype with increased migration ability. These epigenetic and phenotypic alterations were reversed by the addition to α-ketoglutarate to the media, consistent with the notion that succinate competitively inhibits α-ketoglutarate-dependent TETs as the basis for methylator phenotype. These observations suggest that, in a similar manner to R-2-hydroxyglutarate, fumarate and succinate can be accumulated in tumors as a consequence of genetic mutations (FH and SDH, respectively), which inhibit the demethylation of DNA and histone lysines, thus altering the epigenetic landscape.

Genetic mutations in FH and SDH have been associated with a dysregulated epigenome. In GIST, tumorigenesis is either driven by activating mutations in the proto-oncogene c-KIT, or mutations that inactivate the SDH complex [292]. By stratifying GIST patients into c-KIT-mutated (n=39) and SDH-deficient (n=24) subtypes and analyzing their methylation profiles on a genome wide scale, the authors demonstrated that SDH deficient GISTs had genomic hypermethylation an order of magnitude greater than that of the c-KIT-mutated GISTs. Consistent with the inhibitory effect of succinate on TETs, SDH-deficient GIST tumors displayed a marked loss of 5-hmC nucleotides, indicating a loss of TET activity. Genomic hypermethylation was also observed in patients with SDH-mutant hereditary paraganglioma and pheochromocytoma (n=20) as compared to SDH wild type counterparts (n=9). Interestingly, genome wide methylation profiling of IDH1-mutant glioma revealed a comparable hypermethylation profile, implying that mutations in the 3 mitochondrial TCA cycle enzymes had a similar impact on cancer methylome. In an independent study, clinical impact of SDH-deficiency was examined in a large chohort of paraganglioma and pheochromocytoma [291], which showed that 16 out of 17 patients with CpG island methylator phenotype harbor SDH-inactivating mutations. Interestingly, germline and somatic mutations in FH were detected in the remaining case, suggesting that succinate or fumarate plays a role in epigenetic dysregulation in paraganglioma and pheochromocytoma. Finally, paraganglioma patients with SDH or FH-deficiency associated DNA methylator phenotype had a much worse prognosis compared with other molecular subtypes, indicating that epigenetic dysregulation contributes to tumor development and progression.

THERAPEUTIC OPPORTUNITIES

DNMT Inhibitors

DNA methylation can be therapeutically targeted using DNMT inhibitors that can inhibit DNA methylation and restore the expression of aberrantly silenced genes. Two DNMT inhibitors, 5-azacytidine and 5-aza-2'-deoxycytidine, have been clinically approved by the FDA for treatment of myelodysplastic syndrome. These two drugs are cytosine analogues that are incorporated into DNA and covalently inactivate DNMT1, DNMT3A and DNMT3B. Thus far, their use is limited to hematological malignancy but pre-clinical studies have demonstrated promising efficacy in solid tumors [293]. It is largely unknown whether DNMT inhibitors can have a metabolic effect on cancer. Given the non-specific nature of these DNA methylation inhibitors and their widespread effect on gene expression, it will be important to elucidate their role in cancer metabolism. On the other hand, DNMT inhibitors may be useful in reversing aberrant DNA methylation induced by metabolic alterations. As an example, IDH1/2-mutant cancers are driven by oncometabolite-induced epigenetic dysregulation, including DNA methylation. Hence, IDH-mutant cancers may be targeted using DNMT inhibitors. Both 5-azacytidine and 5-aza-2'-deoxycytidine demonstrated a promising efficacy in targeting IDH-mutant glioma in preclinical models. Borodovsky *et al.* [294] showed that 5-azacytidine induced tumor regression in a patient-derived IDH1 mutant glioma xenograft model. Meanwhile, Turcan and colleagues [295] showed that 5-aza-2'-deoxycytidine effectively inhibited growth in IDH-mutant glioma cells *in vitro* and in xenografts. In both of the studies, administration of DNMT inhibitors reversed the hypermethylator phenotype and resulted in induction of differentiation and reduced cell growth. In the latter study, 5-aza-2'-deoxycytidine was shown to be more effective than IDH inhibitors (discussed below) in inducing differentiation of IDH-mutant glioma cells. Hence, targeting the methylome may be a complementary approach to counteract the effect of oncometabolites in cancers.

HDAC Inhibitors (HDACi)

HDACi represent a diverse class of compounds that inhibit HDAC activity and they are being actively pursued for the treatment of cancers or as adjuvant therapy. Currently, two HDACi Vorinostat and Romidepsin are approved for treating cutaneous T cell lymphoma. Moreover, butyrate, a product of microbial fermentation in the gut, also regulates epigenetics by inhibiting HDACs. HDACi induce histone acetylation and reverse gene silencing by HDACs in human cancers. Emerging evidence suggests that inhibition of HDACs may impact cancer metabolism. In HT29 cells, treatment with an HDACi butyrate or trichostatin A was associated with a significant reduction of glucose uptake, glycolysis and lactate production [296]. In multiple myeloma cells, treatment with Vorinostat or valproic acid suppressed the expression of GLUT1 and the inhibition of HKI enzymatic activity [297]. In H460 lung cancer cells, butyrate or trichostatin A treatment suppressed glycolysis and triggered a shift in metabolism away from a glycolytic phenotype by activating mitochondrial metabolism [298]. Butyrate also attenuated glycolysis in breast cancer cells [299]. These results suggest that inhibition of HDAC may promote the reversion of Warburg's phenotype in cancer cells, and their effect on cancer cell metabolism warrants further investigation. Despite their importance in metabolic regulation in cancers, very limited attention has been paid to the potential use of sirtuin inhibitors to modulate cancer metabolism. Further investigations are required to define the effect of HDAC and sirtuin inhibitors on cancer metabolism and their role in cancer management.

miRNA Targeting Agents

Modulation of miRNAs holds great promise as therapeutic targets, and as discussed above, plays regulatory roles in metabolism dysregulation during the tumorigenic process. Currently, there are two approaches to target miRNAs. The first therapeutic approach is to restore the activity of aberrantly silenced miRNAs using synthetic miRNA mimics [300]. MiRNA mimics are chemically modified to increase their stability and to promote cellular uptake. The second approach involves the silencing of overexpressed mature miRNAs using either miRNA sponges [301] or antisense oligonucleotides (Anti-miRs) [302]. A sponge miRNA contains multiple target sites and can inhibit the activity of target miRNAs sharing a common seed. However, this approach requires transgene expression, which is useful in experimental models but has very limited therapeutic usage. Anti-miRs are single-stranded oligonucleotides that can target mature miRNAs with a fully complementary sequence. Anti-miRs can be administered *in vivo* and have shown effectiveness in suppression of miRNAs. As highlighted in the above sections, miRNAs extensively modulate both the gene expression of metabolic enzymes and signaling pathways that mediate altered metabolism in cancers. For instance, the re-expression of miR-143, which targets HKII, reversed the glycolytic phenotype and inhibited cancer growth [173]. On the other hand, oncogenic miRs that target AMPK/LKB or p53 tumor suppressive pathways may represent attractive targets for the design of therapeutic anti-miRs. A major challenge facing miRNA-targeting is the safe and efficient delivery of miRNA mimics and anti-miRs [303]. Advances in delivery technology will accelerate the realization of miRNA-based therapeutics in the clinic.

IDH1 and IDH2 Inhibitors

Inhibition of IDH1 and IDH2 has been pursued as a therapeutic strategy to suppress the production of oncometabolite 2-R-hydroxyglutarate. Rohle *et al.* [304] described the first selective inhibitor (AGI-5198) of mutant IDH1 (R132H), the most common IDH1 mutation (50 to 80%) observed in glioma. AGI-5198 selectively inhibited IDH1-R132H (IC_{50}=70nM), but not wildtype IDH1 or any of the IDH2 isoforms (IC_{50}>100μM). In the TS603 glioma cell line harboring IDH1-R132H, AGI-5198 dose-dependently inhibited 2-R-hydroxyglutarate production and the growth of IDH-R132H glioma cells *in vitro* and IDH-R132H xenografts *in vivo*. AGI-5198 impaired cell proliferation and induced the demethylation of H3K9me3 and H3K27me3. AGI-5198 had no effect on DNA methylation status. Hence, epigenetic effect of IDH1 inhibition only accounts partially for the effect of AGI-5198 on tumor growth. Another IDH1-R132H inhibitor, ML309, has also been described [305]. ML309 inhibited IDH1-R132H with an IC_{50} of 96nM and was inactive towards wild type IDH1. ML309 also inhibited 2-R-hydroxyglutarate production in U87 cells; however, its therapeutic efficacy awaits further investigation.

Wang and colleagues developed AGI-6780 that targets the mutant IDH2 (R140Q) (expressed in ~9% of AML patients) [306]. It exhibits a selective and nanomolar potency for 2-R-hydroxyglutarate inhibition against mutant IDH2-R140Q, but not its wild type counterpart. In cell lines expressing IDH2-R140Q, AGI-6780 inhibited 2-R-hydroxyglutarate production (IC_{50}<20nM). Treatment of TF-1 cells expressing IDH2-R140Q and primary human IDH2-R140Q AML leukemic cells with AGI-6780 induced differentiation in these cells. In a subsequent study, medium term AGI-6780 treatment was found to have a significant impact on the TF-1 (IDH2-R140Q) cell epigenome [307]. As compared to control TF-1 cells, TF-1 IDH-R140Q cells exhibited aberrant DNA hypermethylation. Treatment of TF-1 IDH-R140Q cells with AGI-6780 resulted in progressive demethylation over a period of several weeks; while the same treatment had no effect in control TF-1 cells. On the other hand, hypermethylation of several histone marks induced by IDH-R140Q was reversed rapidly in days. Correspondingly, gene signatures associated with DNA (leukemic tumorigenesis) and histone (differentiation block) hypermethylation were reversed upon AGI-6780 treatment. Overall, these proof-of-concept studies indicate that the targeting of mutant IDH1/IDH2 has potential clinical applications as a differentiation therapy in cancers bearing mutant forms of these proteins.

CONCLUDING REMARKS

Cross-talk between epigenetics and metabolism is a fundamental aspect of cellular adaptation to nutritional status [308]. As reviewed here, the human epigenome is dynamically regulated by products of metabolism, such as acetyl-CoA, SAM, SAH, succinate fumarate, and 2-R-hydroxyglutarate. Abnormal levels of these metabolites lead to epigenetic deregulation, which in turn, induces aberrant gene expression (Fig. **1**). On the other hand, epigenetic deregulation initiates altered metabolism by affecting the expression of metabolic genes. This cross-talk is frequently deregulated in human cancer. Human cancer genome sequencing project has unveiled a host of recurrent mutations in epigenetic modification and metabolic enzymes, indicating that both epigenetics and metabolism are drivers in carcinogenesis. Much remains to be understood regarding the biological mechanisms by which these metabolites can fine-tune the epigenome in normal tissues and how their altered levels contribute to human carcinogenesis. Moreover, whether epigenetics influence the metabolic rewiring in the stroma cells and immune cells of the host, and its potential role in promoting a tumorigenic micro-environment remains largely unknown. Epigenetic therapies have shown a promising efficacy in the treatment of various cancers. Given the close connections between aberrant epigenetics and cancer metabolism, epigenetic therapies may be more effective in cancer treatment in conjunction with therapeutics targeting aberrant tumor metabolism.

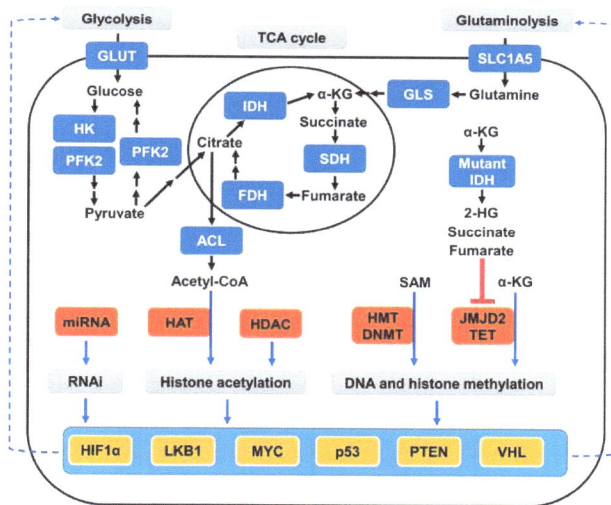

Fig. (1). Cross-talk between epigenetics and metabolism. The human epigenetic machinery is regulated by products of cellular metabolism. Aberrant metabolism in tumors leads to abnormal levels of acetyl-CoA, SAM, SAH, succinate fumarate, and 2-R-hydroxyglutarate. These metabolites act as co-factors and/or inhibitors of various DNA and histone modification enzymes to influence gene expression. On the other hand, epigenetic deregulation initiates altered metabolism, as metabolic genes and signal transduction genes (HIF1α, LKB1, MYC, p53, PTEN and VHL) have been shown to be targeted by epigenetic dysregulation. Cross-talk between epigenetics and metabolism thus forms a positive regulatory cycle that contributes to the altered metabolic phenotype in cancers.

Further elucidation of the network between oncogenic signaling, epigenetic deregulation and metabolism will unravel novel mechanisms in cancer development, and ultimately, uncover new therapeutic targets for intervention.

CONFLICT OF INTEREST

The authors confirm that they have no conflict of interest to declare for this publication.

ACKNOWLEDGEMENTS

Declared none.

REFERENCES

[1]   Feinberg AP, Vogelstein B. Hypomethylation distinguishes genes of some human cancers from their normal counterparts. Nature 1983; 301(5895): 89-92.
       [http://dx.doi.org/10.1038/301089a0] [PMID: 6185846]

[2]   Gama-Sosa MA, Slagel VA, Trewyn RW, *et al.* The 5-methylcytosine content of DNA from human tumors. Nucleic Acids Res 1983; 11(19): 6883-94.
       [http://dx.doi.org/10.1093/nar/11.19.6883] [PMID: 6314264]

[3]   Jones PA, Baylin SB. The epigenomics of cancer. Cell 2007; 128(4): 683-92.
       [http://dx.doi.org/10.1016/j.cell.2007.01.029] [PMID: 17320506]

[4]   Feinberg AP, Tycko B. The history of cancer epigenetics. Nat Rev Cancer 2004; 4(2): 143-53.
       [http://dx.doi.org/10.1038/nrc1279] [PMID: 14732866]

[5]   Jones PA, Baylin SB. The fundamental role of epigenetic events in cancer. Nat Rev Genet 2002; 3(6): 415-28.
       [PMID: 12042769]

[6]   Park PJ. ChIP-seq: Advantages and challenges of a maturing technology. Nat Rev Genet 2009; 10(10): 669-80.
       [http://dx.doi.org/10.1038/nrg2641] [PMID: 19736561]

[7]   Dedeurwaerder S, Defrance M, Calonne E, Denis H, Sotiriou C, Fuks F. Evaluation of the Infinium Methylation 450K technology. Epigenomics 2011; 3(6): 771-84.
       [http://dx.doi.org/10.2217/epi.11.105] [PMID: 22126295]

[8]   Weisenberger DJ. Characterizing DNA methylation alterations from The Cancer Genome Atlas. J Clin Invest 2014; 124(1): 17-23.
       [http://dx.doi.org/10.1172/JCI69740] [PMID: 24382385]

[9]   Muzny DM, Bainbridge MN, Chang K, *et al.* Cancer Genome Atlas Network. Comprehensive molecular characterization of human colon and rectal cancer. Nature 2012; 487(7407): 330-7.
       [http://dx.doi.org/10.1038/nature11252] [PMID: 22810696]

[10]   Bass AJ, Thorsson V, Shmulevich I, *et al.* Cancer Genome Atlas Research Network. Comprehensive molecular characterization of gastric adenocarcinoma. Nature 2014; 513(7517): 202-9.
[http://dx.doi.org/10.1038/nature13480] [PMID: 25079317]

[11]   Kandoth C, McLellan MD, Vandin F, *et al.* Mutational landscape and significance across 12 major cancer types. Nature 2013; 502(7471): 333-9.
[http://dx.doi.org/10.1038/nature12634] [PMID: 24132290]

[12]   Gupta V, Gopinath P, Iqbal MA, Mazurek S, Wellen KE, Bamezai RN. Interplay between epigenetics & cancer metabolism. Curr Pharm Des 2014; 20(11): 1706-14.
[http://dx.doi.org/10.2174/13816128113199990536] [PMID: 23888952]

[13]   Muñoz-Pinedo C, González-Suárez E, Portela A, Gentilella A, Esteller M. Exploiting tumor vulnerabilities: epigenetics, cancer metabolism and the mTOR pathway in the era of personalized medicine. Cancer Res 2013; 73(14): 4185-9.
[http://dx.doi.org/10.1158/0008-5472.CAN-13-0512] [PMID: 23687347]

[14]   Lu C, Thompson CB. Metabolic regulation of epigenetics. Cell Metab 2012; 16(1): 9-17.
[http://dx.doi.org/10.1016/j.cmet.2012.06.001] [PMID: 22768835]

[15]   Vander Heiden MG, Cantley LC, Thompson CB. Understanding the Warburg effect: the metabolic requirements of cell proliferation. Science 2009; 324(5930): 1029-33.
[http://dx.doi.org/10.1126/science.1160809] [PMID: 19460998]

[16]   Bristow RG, Hill RP. Hypoxia and metabolism. Hypoxia, DNA repair and genetic instability. Nat Rev Cancer 2008; 8(3): 180-92.
[http://dx.doi.org/10.1038/nrc2344] [PMID: 18273037]

[17]   Warburg O. On the origin of cancer cells. Science 1956; 123(3191): 309-14.
[http://dx.doi.org/10.1126/science.123.3191.309] [PMID: 13298683]

[18]   Elstrom RL, Bauer DE, Buzzai M, *et al.* Akt stimulates aerobic glycolysis in cancer cells. Cancer Res 2004; 64(11): 3892-9.
[http://dx.doi.org/10.1158/0008-5472.CAN-03-2904] [PMID: 15172999]

[19]   Gordan JD, Thompson CB, Simon MC. HIF and c-Myc: sibling rivals for control of cancer cell metabolism and proliferation. Cancer Cell 2007; 12(2): 108-13.
[http://dx.doi.org/10.1016/j.ccr.2007.07.006] [PMID: 17692803]

[20]   Faubert B, Vincent EE, Griss T, *et al.* Loss of the tumor suppressor LKB1 promotes metabolic reprogramming of cancer cells *via* HIF-1α. Proc Natl Acad Sci USA 2014; 111(7): 2554-9.
[http://dx.doi.org/10.1073/pnas.1312570111] [PMID: 24550282]

[21]   Rhee I, Bachman KE, Park BH, *et al.* DNMT1 and DNMT3b cooperate to silence genes in human cancer cells. Nature 2002; 416(6880): 552-6.
[http://dx.doi.org/10.1038/416552a] [PMID: 11932749]

[22]   Hermann A, Goyal R, Jeltsch A. The Dnmt1 DNA-(cytosine-C5)-methyltransferase methylates DNA processively with high preference for hemimethylated target sites. J Biol Chem 2004; 279(46): 48350-9.
[http://dx.doi.org/10.1074/jbc.M403427200] [PMID: 15339928]

[23]   Okano M, Bell DW, Haber DA, Li E. DNA methyltransferases Dnmt3a and Dnmt3b are essential for de novo methylation and mammalian development. Cell 1999; 99(3): 247-57.
[http://dx.doi.org/10.1016/S0092-8674(00)81656-6] [PMID: 10555141]

[24]   Ehrlich M. DNA methylation in cancer: too much, but also too little. Oncogene 2002; 21(35): 5400-13.
[http://dx.doi.org/10.1038/sj.onc.1205651] [PMID: 12154403]

[25]   Esteller M. Aberrant DNA methylation as a cancer-inducing mechanism. Annu Rev Pharmacol Toxicol 2005; 45: 629-56.
[http://dx.doi.org/10.1146/annurev.pharmtox.45.120403.095832] [PMID: 15822191]

[26]   Robertson KD. DNA methylation and human disease. Nat Rev Genet 2005; 6(8): 597-610.
[http://dx.doi.org/10.1038/nrg1655] [PMID: 16136652]

[27]   Watt F, Molloy PL. Cytosine methylation prevents binding to DNA of a HeLa cell transcription factor required for optimal expression of the adenovirus major late promoter. Genes Dev 1988; 2(9): 1136-43.
[http://dx.doi.org/10.1101/gad.2.9.1136] [PMID: 3192075]

[28]   Ng HH, Zhang Y, Hendrich B, et al. MBD2 is a transcriptional repressor belonging to the MeCP1 histone deacetylase complex. Nat Genet 1999; 23(1): 58-61.
[http://dx.doi.org/10.1038/12659] [PMID: 10471499]

[29]   Selvakumar T, Gjidoda A, Hovde SL, Henry RW. Regulation of human RNA polymerase III transcription by DNMT1 and DNMT3a DNA methyltransferases. J Biol Chem 2012; 287(10): 7039-50.
[http://dx.doi.org/10.1074/jbc.M111.285601] [PMID: 22219193]

[30]   Robertson KD, Uzvolgyi E, Liang G, et al. The human DNA methyltransferases (DNMTs) 1, 3a and 3b: coordinate mRNA expression in normal tissues and overexpression in tumors. Nucleic Acids Res 1999; 27(11): 2291-8.
[http://dx.doi.org/10.1093/nar/27.11.2291] [PMID: 10325416]

[31]   Liu W, Li X, Chu ES, et al. Paired box gene 5 is a novel tumor suppressor in hepatocellular carcinoma through interaction with p53 signaling pathway. Hepatology 2011; 53(3): 843-53.
[http://dx.doi.org/10.1002/hep.24124] [PMID: 21319196]

[32]   Wang S, Cheng Y, Du W, et al. Zinc-finger protein 545 is a novel tumour suppressor that acts by inhibiting ribosomal RNA transcription in gastric cancer. Gut 2013; 62(6): 833-41.
[http://dx.doi.org/10.1136/gutjnl-2011-301776] [PMID: 22580414]

[33]   Yu J, Liang QY, Wang J, et al. Zinc-finger protein 331, a novel putative tumor suppressor, suppresses growth and invasiveness of gastric cancer. Oncogene 2013; 32(3): 307-17.
[http://dx.doi.org/10.1038/onc.2012.54] [PMID: 22370639]

[34]   Yu J, Ma X, Cheung KF, et al. Epigenetic inactivation of T-box transcription factor 5, a novel tumor suppressor gene, is associated with colon cancer. Oncogene 2010; 29(49): 6464-74.
[http://dx.doi.org/10.1038/onc.2010.370] [PMID: 20802524]

[35]   Shen L, Kondo Y, Rosner GL, et al. MGMT promoter methylation and field defect in sporadic colorectal cancer. J Natl Cancer Inst 2005; 97(18): 1330-8.
[http://dx.doi.org/10.1093/jnci/dji275] [PMID: 16174854]

[36]	Du W, Wang S, Zhou Q, *et al.* ADAMTS9 is a functional tumor suppressor through inhibiting AKT/mTOR pathway and associated with poor survival in gastric cancer. Oncogene 2013; 32(28): 3319-28.
	[http://dx.doi.org/10.1038/onc.2012.359] [PMID: 22907434]

[37]	Choi GC, Li J, Wang Y, *et al.* The metalloprotease ADAMTS8 displays antitumor properties through antagonizing EGFR-MEK-ERK signaling and is silenced in carcinomas by CpG methylation. Mol Cancer Res 2014; 12(2): 228-38.
	[http://dx.doi.org/10.1158/1541-7786.MCR-13-0195] [PMID: 24184540]

[38]	Burgess DJ. Epigenetics. Dissecting driving DNA methylations. Nat Rev Cancer 2012; 12(7): 448-9.
	[http://dx.doi.org/10.1038/nrc3300] [PMID: 22673152]

[39]	Patel SA, Graunke DM, Pieper RO. Aberrant silencing of the CpG island-containing human O6-methylguanine DNA methyltransferase gene is associated with the loss of nucleosome-like positioning. Mol Cell Biol 1997; 17(10): 5813-22.
	[http://dx.doi.org/10.1128/MCB.17.10.5813] [PMID: 9315639]

[40]	Cunningham JM, Christensen ER, Tester DJ, *et al.* Hypermethylation of the hMLH1 promoter in colon cancer with microsatellite instability. Cancer Res 1998; 58(15): 3455-60.
	[PMID: 9699680]

[41]	Dobrovic A, Simpfendorfer D. Methylation of the BRCA1 gene in sporadic breast cancer. Cancer Res 1997; 57(16): 3347-50.
	[PMID: 9269993]

[42]	Carmona FJ, Azuara D, Berenguer-Llergo A, *et al.* DNA methylation biomarkers for noninvasive diagnosis of colorectal cancer. Cancer Prev Res (Phila) 2013; 6(7): 656-65.
	[http://dx.doi.org/10.1158/1940-6207.CAPR-12-0501] [PMID: 23694962]

[43]	Dadmehr M, Hosseini M, Hosseinkhani S, *et al.* DNA methylation detection by a novel fluorimetric nanobiosensor for early cancer diagnosis. Biosens Bioelectron 2014; 60: 35-44.
	[http://dx.doi.org/10.1016/j.bios.2014.03.033] [PMID: 24768860]

[44]	Qureshi SA, Bashir MU, Yaqinuddin A. Utility of DNA methylation markers for diagnosing cancer. Int J Surg 2010; 8(3): 194-8.
	[http://dx.doi.org/10.1016/j.ijsu.2010.02.001] [PMID: 20139036]

[45]	Baylin SB, Jones PA. A decade of exploring the cancer epigenome - biological and translational implications. Nat Rev Cancer 2011; 11(10): 726-34.
	[http://dx.doi.org/10.1038/nrc3130] [PMID: 21941284]

[46]	Guo JU, Su Y, Zhong C, Ming GL, Song H. Hydroxylation of 5-methylcytosine by TET1 promotes active DNA demethylation in the adult brain. Cell 2011; 145(3): 423-34.
	[http://dx.doi.org/10.1016/j.cell.2011.03.022] [PMID: 21496894]

[47]	Tahiliani M, Koh KP, Shen Y, *et al.* Conversion of 5-methylcytosine to 5-hydroxymethylcytosine in mammalian DNA by MLL partner TET1. Science 2009; 324(5929): 930-5.
	[http://dx.doi.org/10.1126/science.1170116] [PMID: 19372391]

[48]	Ito S, D'Alessio AC, Taranova OV, Hong K, Sowers LC, Zhang Y. Role of Tet proteins in 5mC to 5hmC conversion, ES-cell self-renewal and inner cell mass specification. Nature 2010; 466(7310):

1129-33.
[http://dx.doi.org/10.1038/nature09303] [PMID: 20639862]

[49]   Kohli RM, Zhang Y. TET enzymes, TDG and the dynamics of DNA demethylation. Nature 2013;
         502(7472): 472-9.
         [http://dx.doi.org/10.1038/nature12750] [PMID: 24153300]

[50]   Abdel-Wahab O, Mullally A, Hedvat C, *et al.* Genetic characterization of TET1, TET2, and TET3
         alterations in myeloid malignancies. Blood 2009; 114(1): 144-7.
         [http://dx.doi.org/10.1182/blood-2009-03-210039] [PMID: 19420352]

[51]   Gambichler T, Sand M, Skrygan M. Loss of 5-hydroxymethylcytosine and ten-eleven translocation 2
         protein expression in malignant melanoma. Melanoma Res 2013; 23(3): 218-20.
         [http://dx.doi.org/10.1097/CMR.0b013e32835f9bd4] [PMID: 23458759]

[52]   Yang H, Liu Y, Bai F, *et al.* Tumor development is associated with decrease of TET gene expression
         and 5-methylcytosine hydroxylation. Oncogene 2013; 32(5): 663-9.
         [http://dx.doi.org/10.1038/onc.2012.67] [PMID: 22391558]

[53]   Kudo Y, Tateishi K, Yamamoto K, *et al.* Loss of 5-hydroxymethylcytosine is accompanied with
         malignant cellular transformation. Cancer Sci 2012; 103(4): 670-6.
         [http://dx.doi.org/10.1111/j.1349-7006.2012.02213.x] [PMID: 22320381]

[54]   Mariño-Ramírez L, Kann MG, Shoemaker BA, Landsman D. Histone structure and nucleosome
         stability. Expert Rev Proteomics 2005; 2(5): 719-29.
         [http://dx.doi.org/10.1586/14789450.2.5.719] [PMID: 16209651]

[55]   Bannister AJ, Kouzarides T. Regulation of chromatin by histone modifications. Cell Res 2011; 21(3):
         381-95.
         [http://dx.doi.org/10.1038/cr.2011.22] [PMID: 21321607]

[56]   Karlić R, Chung HR, Lasserre J, Vlahovicek K, Vingron M. Histone modification levels are predictive
         for gene expression. Proc Natl Acad Sci USA 2010; 107(7): 2926-31.
         [http://dx.doi.org/10.1073/pnas.0909344107] [PMID: 20133639]

[57]   Eberharter A, Becker PB. Histone acetylation: A switch between repressive and permissive chromatin.
         Second in review series on chromatin dynamics. EMBO Rep 2002; 3(3): 224-9.
         [http://dx.doi.org/10.1093/embo-reports/kvf053] [PMID: 11882541]

[58]   Nakagawa M, Oda Y, Eguchi T, *et al.* Expression profile of class I histone deacetylases in human
         cancer tissues. Oncol Rep 2007; 18(4): 769-74.
         [PMID: 17786334]

[59]   Weichert W, Röske A, Gekeler V, *et al.* Histone deacetylases 1, 2 and 3 are highly expressed in
         prostate cancer and HDAC2 expression is associated with shorter PSA relapse time after radical
         prostatectomy. Br J Cancer 2008; 98(3): 604-10.
         [http://dx.doi.org/10.1038/sj.bjc.6604199] [PMID: 18212746]

[60]   Gui CY, Ngo L, Xu WS, Richon VM, Marks PA. Histone deacetylase (HDAC) inhibitor activation of
         p21WAF1 involves changes in promoter-associated proteins, including HDAC1. Proc Natl Acad Sci
         USA 2004; 101(5): 1241-6.
         [http://dx.doi.org/10.1073/pnas.0307708100] [PMID: 14734806]

[61]   Christofori G, Semb H. The role of the cell-adhesion molecule E-cadherin as a tumour-suppressor gene. Trends Biochem Sci 1999; 24(2): 73-6.
[http://dx.doi.org/10.1016/S0968-0004(98)01343-7] [PMID: 10098402]

[62]   Iyer NG, Ozdag H, Caldas C. p300/CBP and cancer. Oncogene 2004; 23(24): 4225-31.
[http://dx.doi.org/10.1038/sj.onc.1207118] [PMID: 15156177]

[63]   Gayther SA, Batley SJ, Linger L, *et al.* Mutations truncating the EP300 acetylase in human cancers. Nat Genet 2000; 24(3): 300-3.
[http://dx.doi.org/10.1038/73536] [PMID: 10700188]

[64]   Wang J, Iwasaki H, Krivtsov A, *et al.* Conditional MLL-CBP targets GMP and models therapy-related myeloproliferative disease. EMBO J 2005; 24(2): 368-81.
[http://dx.doi.org/10.1038/sj.emboj.7600521] [PMID: 15635450]

[65]   Huntly BJ, Shigematsu H, Deguchi K, *et al.* MOZ-TIF2, but not BCR-ABL, confers properties of leukemic stem cells to committed murine hematopoietic progenitors. Cancer Cell 2004; 6(6): 587-96.
[http://dx.doi.org/10.1016/j.ccr.2004.10.015] [PMID: 15607963]

[66]   Dokmanovic M, Clarke C, Marks PA. Histone deacetylase inhibitors: overview and perspectives. Mol Cancer Res 2007; 5(10): 981-9.
[http://dx.doi.org/10.1158/1541-7786.MCR-07-0324] [PMID: 17951399]

[67]   Zhang Y, Reinberg D. Transcription regulation by histone methylation: interplay between different covalent modifications of the core histone tails. Genes Dev 2001; 15(18): 2343-60.
[http://dx.doi.org/10.1101/gad.927301] [PMID: 11562345]

[68]   Feng Q, Wang H, Ng HH, *et al.* Methylation of H3-lysine 79 is mediated by a new family of HMTases without a SET domain. Curr Biol 2002; 12(12): 1052-8.
[http://dx.doi.org/10.1016/S0960-9822(02)00901-6] [PMID: 12123582]

[69]   Bedford MT. Arginine methylation at a glance. J Cell Sci 2007; 120(Pt 24): 4243-6.
[http://dx.doi.org/10.1242/jcs.019885] [PMID: 18057026]

[70]   Lan F, Nottke AC, Shi Y. Mechanisms involved in the regulation of histone lysine demethylases. Curr Opin Cell Biol 2008; 20(3): 316-25.
[http://dx.doi.org/10.1016/j.ceb.2008.03.004] [PMID: 18440794]

[71]   Sims RJ III, Millhouse S, Chen CF, *et al.* Recognition of trimethylated histone H3 lysine 4 facilitates the recruitment of transcription postinitiation factors and pre-mRNA splicing. Mol Cell 2007; 28(4): 665-76.
[http://dx.doi.org/10.1016/j.molcel.2007.11.010] [PMID: 18042460]

[72]   Derks S, Bosch LJ, Niessen HE, *et al.* Promoter CpG island hypermethylation- and H3K9me3 and H3K27me3-mediated epigenetic silencing targets the deleted in colon cancer (DCC) gene in colorectal carcinogenesis without affecting neighboring genes on chromosomal region 18q21. Carcinogenesis 2009; 30(6): 1041-8.
[http://dx.doi.org/10.1093/carcin/bgp073] [PMID: 19329758]

[73]   Poirel H, Rack K, Delabesse E, *et al.* Incidence and characterization of MLL gene (11q23) rearrangements in acute myeloid leukemia M1 and M5. Blood 1996; 87(6): 2496-505.
[PMID: 8630416]

[74]   Chesi M, Nardini E, Lim RS, Smith KD, Kuehl WM, Bergsagel PL. The t(4;14) translocation in myeloma dysregulates both FGFR3 and a novel gene, MMSET, resulting in IgH/MMSET hybrid transcripts. Blood 1998; 92(9): 3025-34.
[PMID: 9787135]

[75]   Morin RD, Mendez-Lago M, Mungall AJ, *et al.* Frequent mutation of histone-modifying genes in non-Hodgkin lymphoma. Nature 2011; 476(7360): 298-303.
[http://dx.doi.org/10.1038/nature10351] [PMID: 21796119]

[76]   Daigle SR, Olhava EJ, Therkelsen CA, *et al.* Potent inhibition of DOT1L as treatment of MLL-fusion leukemia. Blood 2013; 122(6): 1017-25.
[http://dx.doi.org/10.1182/blood-2013-04-497644] [PMID: 23801631]

[77]   Knutson SK, Kawano S, Minoshima Y, *et al.* Selective inhibition of EZH2 by EPZ-6438 leads to potent antitumor activity in EZH2-mutant non-Hodgkin lymphoma. Mol Cancer Ther 2014; 13(4): 842-54.
[http://dx.doi.org/10.1158/1535-7163.MCT-13-0773] [PMID: 24563539]

[78]   Wu J, Liu S, Liu G, *et al.* Identification and functional analysis of 9p24 amplified genes in human breast cancer. Oncogene 2012; 31(3): 333-41.
[http://dx.doi.org/10.1038/onc.2011.227] [PMID: 21666724]

[79]   Schulte JH, Lim S, Schramm A, *et al.* Lysine-specific demethylase 1 is strongly expressed in poorly differentiated neuroblastoma: implications for therapy. Cancer Res 2009; 69(5): 2065-71.
[http://dx.doi.org/10.1158/0008-5472.CAN-08-1735] [PMID: 19223552]

[80]   Lee RC, Feinbaum RL, Ambros V. The C. elegans heterochronic gene lin-4 encodes small RNAs with antisense complementarity to lin-14. Cell 1993; 75(5): 843-54.
[http://dx.doi.org/10.1016/0092-8674(93)90529-Y] [PMID: 8252621]

[81]   Pasquinelli AE, Reinhart BJ, Slack F, *et al.* Conservation of the sequence and temporal expression of let-7 heterochronic regulatory RNA. Nature 2000; 408(6808): 86-9.
[http://dx.doi.org/10.1038/35040556] [PMID: 11081512]

[82]   Nilsen TW. Mechanisms of microRNA-mediated gene regulation in animal cells. Trends Genet 2007; 23(5): 243-9.
[http://dx.doi.org/10.1016/j.tig.2007.02.011] [PMID: 17368621]

[83]   Mathonnet G, Fabian MR, Svitkin YV, *et al.* MicroRNA inhibition of translation initiation in vitro by targeting the cap-binding complex eIF4F. Science 2007; 317(5845): 1764-7.
[http://dx.doi.org/10.1126/science.1146067] [PMID: 17656684]

[84]   Gu S, Jin L, Zhang F, Sarnow P, Kay MA. Biological basis for restriction of microRNA targets to the 3′ untranslated region in mammalian mRNAs. Nat Struct Mol Biol 2009; 16(2): 144-50.
[http://dx.doi.org/10.1038/nsmb.1552] [PMID: 19182800]

[85]   Wu L, Fan J, Belasco JG. MicroRNAs direct rapid deadenylation of mRNA. Proc Natl Acad Sci USA 2006; 103(11): 4034-9.
[http://dx.doi.org/10.1073/pnas.0510928103] [PMID: 16495412]

[86]   Lewis BP, Burge CB, Bartel DP. Conserved seed pairing, often flanked by adenosines, indicates that thousands of human genes are microRNA targets. Cell 2005; 120(1): 15-20.

[http://dx.doi.org/10.1016/j.cell.2004.12.035] [PMID: 15652477]

[87]   Lu J, Getz G, Miska EA, *et al.* MicroRNA expression profiles classify human cancers. Nature 2005; 435(7043): 834-8.
       [http://dx.doi.org/10.1038/nature03702] [PMID: 15944708]

[88]   Zhang L, Dong Y, Zhu N, *et al.* microRNA-139-5p exerts tumor suppressor function by targeting NOTCH1 in colorectal cancer. Mol Cancer 2014; 13: 124.
       [http://dx.doi.org/10.1186/1476-4598-13-124] [PMID: 24885920]

[89]   Olive V, Bennett MJ, Walker JC, *et al.* miR-19 is a key oncogenic component of mir-17-92. Genes Dev 2009; 23(24): 2839-49.
       [http://dx.doi.org/10.1101/gad.1861409] [PMID: 20008935]

[90]   Iliopoulos D, Jaeger SA, Hirsch HA, Bulyk ML, Struhl K. STAT3 activation of miR-21 and miR-181b-1 *via* PTEN and CYLD are part of the epigenetic switch linking inflammation to cancer. Mol Cell 2010; 39(4): 493-506.
       [http://dx.doi.org/10.1016/j.molcel.2010.07.023] [PMID: 20797623]

[91]   Broderick JA, Zamore PD. MicroRNA therapeutics. Gene Ther 2011; 18(12): 1104-10.
       [http://dx.doi.org/10.1038/gt.2011.50] [PMID: 21525952]

[92]   Vander Heiden MG, Cantley LC, Thompson CB. Understanding the Warburg effect: the metabolic requirements of cell proliferation. Science 2009; 324(5930): 1029-33.
       [http://dx.doi.org/10.1126/science.1160809] [PMID: 19460998]

[93]   Guha M, Srinivasan S, Biswas G, Avadhani NG. Activation of a novel calcineurin-mediated insulin-like growth factor-1 receptor pathway, altered metabolism, and tumor cell invasion in cells subjected to mitochondrial respiratory stress. J Biol Chem 2007; 282(19): 14536-46.
       [http://dx.doi.org/10.1074/jbc.M611693200] [PMID: 17355970]

[94]   Guha M, Fang JK, Monks R, Birnbaum MJ, Avadhani NG. Activation of Akt is essential for the propagation of mitochondrial respiratory stress signaling and activation of the transcriptional coactivator heterogeneous ribonucleoprotein A2. Mol Biol Cell 2010; 21(20): 3578-89.
       [http://dx.doi.org/10.1091/mbc.E10-03-0192] [PMID: 20719961]

[95]   Picard M, Zhang J, Hancock S, *et al.* Progressive increase in mtDNA 3243A>G heteroplasmy causes abrupt transcriptional reprogramming. Proc Natl Acad Sci USA 2014; 111(38): E4033-42.
       [http://dx.doi.org/10.1073/pnas.1414028111] [PMID: 25192935]

[96]   Shaw RJ. Glucose metabolism and cancer. Curr Opin Cell Biol 2006; 18(6): 598-608.
       [http://dx.doi.org/10.1016/j.ceb.2006.10.005] [PMID: 17046224]

[97]   Hensley CT, Wasti AT, DeBerardinis RJ. Glutamine and cancer: cell biology, physiology, and clinical opportunities. J Clin Invest 2013; 123(9): 3678-84.
       [http://dx.doi.org/10.1172/JCI69600] [PMID: 23999442]

[98]   Wise DR, DeBerardinis RJ, Mancuso A, *et al.* Myc regulates a transcriptional program that stimulates mitochondrial glutaminolysis and leads to glutamine addiction. Proc Natl Acad Sci USA 2008; 105(48): 18782-7.
       [http://dx.doi.org/10.1073/pnas.0810199105] [PMID: 19033189]

[99]   Son J, Lyssiotis CA, Ying H, *et al.* Glutamine supports pancreatic cancer growth through a KRAS-

regulated metabolic pathway. Nature 2013; 496(7443): 101-5.
[http://dx.doi.org/10.1038/nature12040] [PMID: 23535601]

[100] Bryant KL, Mancias JD, Kimmelman AC, Der CJ. KRAS: feeding pancreatic cancer proliferation. Trends Biochem Sci 2014; 39(2): 91-100.
[http://dx.doi.org/10.1016/j.tibs.2013.12.004] [PMID: 24388967]

[101] Fruman DA, Rommel C. PI3K and cancer: lessons, challenges and opportunities. Nat Rev Drug Discov 2014; 13(2): 140-56.
[http://dx.doi.org/10.1038/nrd4204] [PMID: 24481312]

[102] Li J, Yen C, Liaw D, *et al.* PTEN, a putative protein tyrosine phosphatase gene mutated in human brain, breast, and prostate cancer. Science 1997; 275(5308): 1943-7.
[http://dx.doi.org/10.1126/science.275.5308.1943] [PMID: 9072974]

[103] Campbell IG, Russell SE, Choong DY, *et al.* Mutation of the PIK3CA gene in ovarian and breast cancer. Cancer Res 2004; 64(21): 7678-81.
[http://dx.doi.org/10.1158/0008-5472.CAN-04-2933] [PMID: 15520168]

[104] Robey RB, Hay N. Is Akt the "Warburg kinase"?-Akt-energy metabolism interactions and oncogenesis. Semin Cancer Biol 2009; 19(1): 25-31.
[http://dx.doi.org/10.1016/j.semcancer.2008.11.010] [PMID: 19130886]

[105] Mayer C, Grummt I. Ribosome biogenesis and cell growth: mTOR coordinates transcription by all three classes of nuclear RNA polymerases. Oncogene 2006; 25(48): 6384-91.
[http://dx.doi.org/10.1038/sj.onc.1209883] [PMID: 17041624]

[106] Lizcano JM, Göransson O, Toth R, *et al.* LKB1 is a master kinase that activates 13 kinases of the AMPK subfamily, including MARK/PAR-1. EMBO J 2004; 23(4): 833-43.
[http://dx.doi.org/10.1038/sj.emboj.7600110] [PMID: 14976552]

[107] Shackelford DB, Shaw RJ. The LKB1-AMPK pathway: metabolism and growth control in tumour suppression. Nat Rev Cancer 2009; 9(8): 563-75.
[http://dx.doi.org/10.1038/nrc2676] [PMID: 19629071]

[108] Jones RG, Plas DR, Kubek S, *et al.* AMP-activated protein kinase induces a p53-dependent metabolic checkpoint. Mol Cell 2005; 18(3): 283-93.
[http://dx.doi.org/10.1016/j.molcel.2005.03.027] [PMID: 15866171]

[109] Tiainen M, Vaahtomeri K, Ylikorkala A, Mäkelä TP. Growth arrest by the LKB1 tumor suppressor: induction of p21(WAF1/CIP1). Hum Mol Genet 2002; 11(13): 1497-504.
[http://dx.doi.org/10.1093/hmg/11.13.1497] [PMID: 12045203]

[110] Koivunen JP, Kim J, Lee J, *et al.* Mutations in the LKB1 tumour suppressor are frequently detected in tumours from Caucasian but not Asian lung cancer patients. Br J Cancer 2008; 99(2): 245-52.
[http://dx.doi.org/10.1038/sj.bjc.6604469] [PMID: 18594528]

[111] Launonen V. Mutations in the human LKB1/STK11 gene. Hum Mutat 2005; 26(4): 291-7.
[http://dx.doi.org/10.1002/humu.20222] [PMID: 16110486]

[112] Ben Sahra I, Le Marchand-Brustel Y, Tanti JF, Bost F. Metformin in cancer therapy: A new perspective for an old antidiabetic drug? Mol Cancer Ther 2010; 9(5): 1092-9.
[http://dx.doi.org/10.1158/1535-7163.MCT-09-1186] [PMID: 20442309]

[113] Ivan M, Kondo K, Yang H, *et al.* HIFalpha targeted for VHL-mediated destruction by proline hydroxylation: implications for O2 sensing. Science 2001; 292(5516): 464-8.
[http://dx.doi.org/10.1126/science.1059817] [PMID: 11292862]

[114] Semenza GL, Roth PH, Fang HM, Wang GL. Transcriptional regulation of genes encoding glycolytic enzymes by hypoxia-inducible factor 1. J Biol Chem 1994; 269(38): 23757-63.
[PMID: 8089148]

[115] Kim JW, Tchernyshyov I, Semenza GL, Dang CV. HIF-1-mediated expression of pyruvate dehydrogenase kinase: A metabolic switch required for cellular adaptation to hypoxia. Cell Metab 2006; 3(3): 177-85.
[http://dx.doi.org/10.1016/j.cmet.2006.02.002] [PMID: 16517405]

[116] Zhong H, Chiles K, Feldser D, *et al.* Modulation of hypoxia-inducible factor 1alpha expression by the epidermal growth factor/phosphatidylinositol 3-kinase/PTEN/AKT/FRAP pathway in human prostate cancer cells: implications for tumor angiogenesis and therapeutics. Cancer Res 2000; 60(6): 1541-5.
[PMID: 10749120]

[117] Kim WY, Kaelin WG. Role of VHL gene mutation in human cancer. J Clin Oncol 2004; 22(24): 4991-5004.
[http://dx.doi.org/10.1200/JCO.2004.05.061] [PMID: 15611513]

[118] Pollard PJ, Brière JJ, Alam NA, *et al.* Accumulation of Krebs cycle intermediates and over-expression of HIF1alpha in tumours which result from germline FH and SDH mutations. Hum Mol Genet 2005; 14(15): 2231-9.
[http://dx.doi.org/10.1093/hmg/ddi227] [PMID: 15987702]

[119] Bahram F, von der Lehr N, Cetinkaya C, Larsson LG. c-Myc hot spot mutations in lymphomas result in inefficient ubiquitination and decreased proteasome-mediated turnover. Blood 2000; 95(6): 2104-10.
[PMID: 10706881]

[120] Bhatia K, Spangler G, Gaidano G, Hamdy N, Dalla-Favera R, Magrath I. Mutations in the coding region of c-myc occur frequently in acquired immunodeficiency syndrome-associated lymphomas. Blood 1994; 84(3): 883-8.
[PMID: 8043869]

[121] van Riggelen J, Yetil A, Felsher DW. MYC as a regulator of ribosome biogenesis and protein synthesis. Nat Rev Cancer 2010; 10(4): 301-9.
[http://dx.doi.org/10.1038/nrc2819] [PMID: 20332779]

[122] Osthus RC, Shim H, Kim S, *et al.* Deregulation of glucose transporter 1 and glycolytic gene expression by c-Myc. J Biol Chem 2000; 275(29): 21797-800.
[http://dx.doi.org/10.1074/jbc.C000023200] [PMID: 10823814]

[123] David CJ, Chen M, Assanah M, Canoll P, Manley JL. HnRNP proteins controlled by c-Myc deregulate pyruvate kinase mRNA splicing in cancer. Nature 2010; 463(7279): 364-8.
[http://dx.doi.org/10.1038/nature08697] [PMID: 20010808]

[124] Matoba S, Kang JG, Patino WD, *et al.* p53 regulates mitochondrial respiration. Science 2006; 312(5780): 1650-3.

[http://dx.doi.org/10.1126/science.1126863] [PMID: 16728594]

[125] Schwartzenberg-Bar-Yoseph F, Armoni M, Karnieli E. The tumor suppressor p53 down-regulates glucose transporters GLUT1 and GLUT4 gene expression. Cancer Res 2004; 64(7): 2627-33.
[http://dx.doi.org/10.1158/0008-5472.CAN-03-0846] [PMID: 15059920]

[126] Bensaad K, Tsuruta A, Selak MA, *et al.* TIGAR, a p53-inducible regulator of glycolysis and apoptosis. Cell 2006; 126(1): 107-20.
[http://dx.doi.org/10.1016/j.cell.2006.05.036] [PMID: 16839880]

[127] Lopez-Serra P, Marcilla M, Villanueva A, *et al.* A DERL3-associated defect in the degradation of SLC2A1 mediates the Warburg effect. Nat Commun 2014; 5: 3608.
[http://dx.doi.org/10.1038/ncomms4608] [PMID: 24699711]

[128] Liu X, Wang X, Zhang J, *et al.* Warburg effect revisited: An epigenetic link between glycolysis and gastric carcinogenesis. Oncogene 2010; 29(3): 442-50.
[http://dx.doi.org/10.1038/onc.2009.332] [PMID: 19881551]

[129] Chen M, Zhang J, Li N, *et al.* Promoter hypermethylation mediated downregulation of FBP1 in human hepatocellular carcinoma and colon cancer. PLoS One 2011; 6(10): e25564.
[http://dx.doi.org/10.1371/journal.pone.0025564] [PMID: 22039417]

[130] Dong C, Yuan T, Wu Y, *et al.* Loss of FBP1 by Snail-mediated repression provides metabolic advantages in basal-like breast cancer. Cancer Cell 2013; 23(3): 316-31.
[http://dx.doi.org/10.1016/j.ccr.2013.01.022] [PMID: 23453623]

[131] Li H, Wang J, Xu H, *et al.* Decreased fructose-1,6-bisphosphatase-2 expression promotes glycolysis and growth in gastric cancer cells. Mol Cancer 2013; 12(1): 110.
[http://dx.doi.org/10.1186/1476-4598-12-110] [PMID: 24063558]

[132] Maekawa M, Taniguchi T, Ishikawa J, Sugimura H, Sugano K, Kanno T. Promoter hypermethylation in cancer silences LDHB, eliminating lactate dehydrogenase isoenzymes 1-4. Clin Chem 2003; 49(9): 1518-20.
[http://dx.doi.org/10.1373/49.9.1518] [PMID: 12928234]

[133] Leiblich A, Cross SS, Catto JW, *et al.* Lactate dehydrogenase-B is silenced by promoter hypermethylation in human prostate cancer. Oncogene 2006; 25(20): 2953-60.
[http://dx.doi.org/10.1038/sj.onc.1209262] [PMID: 16547507]

[134] Desai S, Ding M, Wang B, *et al.* Tissue-specific isoform switch and DNA hypomethylation of the pyruvate kinase PKM gene in human cancers. Oncotarget 2014; 5(18): 8202-10.
[http://dx.doi.org/10.18632/oncotarget.1159] [PMID: 24077665]

[135] Kang YH, Lee HS, Kim WH. Promoter methylation and silencing of PTEN in gastric carcinoma. Lab Invest 2002; 82(3): 285-91.
[http://dx.doi.org/10.1038/labinvest.3780422] [PMID: 11896207]

[136] Salvesen HB, MacDonald N, Ryan A, *et al.* PTEN methylation is associated with advanced stage and microsatellite instability in endometrial carcinoma. Int J Cancer 2001; 91(1): 22-6.
[http://dx.doi.org/10.1002/1097-0215(20010101)91:1<22::AID-IJC1002>3.0.CO;2-S]   [PMID: 11149415]

[137] Soria JC, Lee HY, Lee JI, *et al.* Lack of PTEN expression in non-small cell lung cancer could be

related to promoter methylation. Clin Cancer Res 2002; 8(5): 1178-84.
[PMID: 12006535]

[138]   García JM, Silva J, Peña C, *et al.* Promoter methylation of the PTEN gene is a common molecular change in breast cancer. Genes Chromosomes Cancer 2004; 41(2): 117-24.
[http://dx.doi.org/10.1002/gcc.20062] [PMID: 15287024]

[139]   Alvarez-Nuñez F, Bussaglia E, Mauricio D, *et al.* Thyroid Neoplasia Study Group. PTEN promoter methylation in sporadic thyroid carcinomas. Thyroid 2006; 16(1): 17-23.
[http://dx.doi.org/10.1089/thy.2006.16.17] [PMID: 16487009]

[140]   Lahtz C, Stranzenbach R, Fiedler E, Helmbold P, Dammann RH. Methylation of PTEN as a prognostic factor in malignant melanoma of the skin. J Invest Dermatol 2010; 130(2): 620-2.
[http://dx.doi.org/10.1038/jid.2009.226] [PMID: 19798057]

[141]   Trojan J, Brieger A, Raedle J, Esteller M, Zeuzem S. 5′-CpG island methylation of the LKB1/STK11 promoter and allelic loss at chromosome 19p13.3 in sporadic colorectal cancer. Gut 2000; 47(2): 272-6.
[http://dx.doi.org/10.1136/gut.47.2.272] [PMID: 10896921]

[142]   Esteller M, Avizienyte E, Corn PG, *et al.* Epigenetic inactivation of LKB1 in primary tumors associated with the Peutz-Jeghers syndrome. Oncogene 2000; 19(1): 164-8.
[http://dx.doi.org/10.1038/sj.onc.1203227] [PMID: 10644993]

[143]   Vanharanta S, Shu W, Brenet F, *et al.* Epigenetic expansion of VHL-HIF signal output drives multiorgan metastasis in renal cancer. Nat Med 2013; 19(1): 50-6.
[http://dx.doi.org/10.1038/nm.3029] [PMID: 23223005]

[144]   Herman JG, Latif F, Weng Y, *et al.* Silencing of the VHL tumor-suppressor gene by DNA methylation in renal carcinoma. Proc Natl Acad Sci USA 1994; 91(21): 9700-4.
[http://dx.doi.org/10.1073/pnas.91.21.9700] [PMID: 7937876]

[145]   Schmitt AM, Schmid S, Rudolph T, *et al.* VHL inactivation is an important pathway for the development of malignant sporadic pancreatic endocrine tumors. Endocr Relat Cancer 2009; 16(4): 1219-27.
[http://dx.doi.org/10.1677/ERC-08-0297] [PMID: 19690016]

[146]   Hatzimichael E, Dasoula A, Shah R, *et al.* The prolyl-hydroxylase EGLN3 and not EGLN1 is inactivated by methylation in plasma cell neoplasia. Eur J Haematol 2010; 84(1): 47-51.
[http://dx.doi.org/10.1111/j.1600-0609.2009.01344.x] [PMID: 19737309]

[147]   Rawluszko AA, Bujnicka KE, Horbacka K, Krokowicz P, Jagodzinski PP. Expression and DNA methylation levels of prolyl hydroxylases PHD1, PHD2, PHD3 and asparaginyl hydroxylase FIH in colorectal cancer. BMC Cancer 2013; 13: 526.
[http://dx.doi.org/10.1186/1471-2407-13-526] [PMID: 24195777]

[148]   Place TL, Fitzgerald MP, Venkataraman S, *et al.* Aberrant promoter CpG methylation is a mechanism for impaired PHD3 expression in a diverse set of malignant cells. PLoS One 2011; 6(1): e14617.
[http://dx.doi.org/10.1371/journal.pone.0014617] [PMID: 21297970]

[149]   Agirre X, Novo FJ, Calasanz MJ, *et al.* TP53 is frequently altered by methylation, mutation, and/or deletion in acute lymphoblastic leukaemia. Mol Carcinog 2003; 38(4): 201-8.

[http://dx.doi.org/10.1002/mc.10159] [PMID: 14639659]

[150] Kang JH, Kim SJ, Noh DY, *et al.* Methylation in the p53 promoter is a supplementary route to breast carcinogenesis: correlation between CpG methylation in the p53 promoter and the mutation of the p53 gene in the progression from ductal carcinoma *in situ* to invasive ductal carcinoma. Lab Invest 2001; 81(4): 573-9.
[http://dx.doi.org/10.1038/labinvest.3780266] [PMID: 11304577]

[151] Jesionek-Kupnicka D, Szybka M, Malachowska B, *et al.* TP53 promoter methylation in primary glioblastoma: relationship with TP53 mRNA and protein expression and mutation status. DNA Cell Biol 2014; 33(4): 217-26.
[http://dx.doi.org/10.1089/dna.2013.2201] [PMID: 24506545]

[152] Roth M, Chen WY. Sorting out functions of sirtuins in cancer. Oncogene 2014; 33(13): 1609-20.
[http://dx.doi.org/10.1038/onc.2013.120] [PMID: 23604120]

[153] Rodgers JT, Lerin C, Haas W, Gygi SP, Spiegelman BM, Puigserver P. Nutrient control of glucose homeostasis through a complex of PGC-1alpha and SIRT1. Nature 2005; 434(7029): 113-8.
[http://dx.doi.org/10.1038/nature03354] [PMID: 15744310]

[154] Brunet A, Sweeney LB, Sturgill JF, *et al.* Stress-dependent regulation of FOXO transcription factors by the SIRT1 deacetylase. Science 2004; 303(5666): 2011-5.
[http://dx.doi.org/10.1126/science.1094637] [PMID: 14976264]

[155] Lim JH, Lee YM, Chun YS, Chen J, Kim JE, Park JW. Sirtuin 1 modulates cellular responses to hypoxia by deacetylating hypoxia-inducible factor 1alpha. Mol Cell 2010; 38(6): 864-78.
[http://dx.doi.org/10.1016/j.molcel.2010.05.023] [PMID: 20620956]

[156] Xiao C, Kim HS, Lahusen T, *et al.* SIRT6 deficiency results in severe hypoglycemia by enhancing both basal and insulin-stimulated glucose uptake in mice. J Biol Chem 2010; 285(47): 36776-84.
[http://dx.doi.org/10.1074/jbc.M110.168039] [PMID: 20847051]

[157] Zhong L, D'Urso A, Toiber D, *et al.* The histone deacetylase Sirt6 regulates glucose homeostasis *via* Hif1alpha. Cell 2010; 140(2): 280-93.
[http://dx.doi.org/10.1016/j.cell.2009.12.041] [PMID: 20141841]

[158] Zhong L, Mostoslavsky R. SIRT6: a master epigenetic gatekeeper of glucose metabolism. Transcription 2010; 1(1): 17-21.
[http://dx.doi.org/10.4161/trns.1.1.12143] [PMID: 21327158]

[159] Sebastián C, Zwaans BM, Silberman DM, *et al.* The histone deacetylase SIRT6 is a tumor suppressor that controls cancer metabolism. Cell 2012; 151(6): 1185-99.
[http://dx.doi.org/10.1016/j.cell.2012.10.047] [PMID: 23217706]

[160] Zhang ZG, Qin CY. Sirt6 suppresses hepatocellular carcinoma cell growth *via* inhibiting the extracellular signal-regulated kinase signaling pathway. Mol Med Rep 2014; 9(3): 882-8.
[PMID: 24366394]

[161] Shin JY, He M, Liu YF, Paredes S, Villanova L, Brown K, *et al.* SIRT7 Represses Myc Activity to Suppress ER Stress and Prevent Fatty Liver Disease (vol 5, pg 654, 2013). Cell Reports 2013; 5(5): 1479.
[http://dx.doi.org/10.1016/j.celrep.2013.11.036]

[162] Barber MF, Michishita-Kioi E, Xi Y, *et al.* SIRT7 links H3K18 deacetylation to maintenance of oncogenic transformation. Nature 2012; 487(7405): 114-8.
[PMID: 22722849]

[163] Liu PY, Xu N, Malyukova A, *et al.* The histone deacetylase SIRT2 stabilizes Myc oncoproteins. Cell Death Differ 2013; 20(3): 503-14.
[http://dx.doi.org/10.1038/cdd.2012.147] [PMID: 23175188]

[164] Yamasaki T, Seki N, Yoshino H, *et al.* Tumor-suppressive microRNA-1291 directly regulates glucose transporter 1 in renal cell carcinoma. Cancer Sci 2013; 104(11): 1411-9.
[http://dx.doi.org/10.1111/cas.12240] [PMID: 23889809]

[165] Fei X, Qi M, Wu B, Song Y, Wang Y, Li T. MicroRNA-195-5p suppresses glucose uptake and proliferation of human bladder cancer T24 cells by regulating GLUT3 expression. FEBS Lett 2012; 586(4): 392-7.
[http://dx.doi.org/10.1016/j.febslet.2012.01.006] [PMID: 22265971]

[166] Dai DW, Lu Q, Wang LX, *et al.* Decreased miR-106a inhibits glioma cell glucose uptake and proliferation by targeting SLC2A3 in GBM. BMC Cancer 2013; 13: 478.
[http://dx.doi.org/10.1186/1471-2407-13-478] [PMID: 24124917]

[167] Horie T, Ono K, Nishi H, *et al.* MicroRNA-133 regulates the expression of GLUT4 by targeting KLF15 and is involved in metabolic control in cardiac myocytes. Biochem Biophys Res Commun 2009; 389(2): 315-20.
[http://dx.doi.org/10.1016/j.bbrc.2009.08.136] [PMID: 19720047]

[168] Takahiro H, Ono K, Warraga Y, Nishi H, Nagao K, Kinoshita M, *et al.* MicroRNA-133 regulates the expression of CPT-1b and GLUT4 by targeting SRF and KLF15 and is involved in metabolic control in cardiac myocytes. Circulation 2007; 116(16): 163.
[PMID: 17592079]

[169] Chen YH, Heneidi S, Lee JM, *et al.* miRNA-93 inhibits GLUT4 and is overexpressed in adipose tissue of polycystic ovary syndrome patients and women with insulin resistance. Diabetes 2013; 62(7): 2278-86.
[http://dx.doi.org/10.2337/db12-0963] [PMID: 23493574]

[170] Peschiaroli A, Giacobbe A, Formosa A, *et al.* miR-143 regulates hexokinase 2 expression in cancer cells. Oncogene 2013; 32(6): 797-802.
[http://dx.doi.org/10.1038/onc.2012.100] [PMID: 22469988]

[171] Fang R, Xiao T, Fang Z, *et al.* MicroRNA-143 (miR-143) regulates cancer glycolysis *via* targeting hexokinase 2 gene. J Biol Chem 2012; 287(27): 23227-35.
[http://dx.doi.org/10.1074/jbc.M112.373084] [PMID: 22593586]

[172] Jiang S, Zhang LF, Zhang HW, *et al.* A novel miR-155/miR-143 cascade controls glycolysis by regulating hexokinase 2 in breast cancer cells. EMBO J 2012; 31(8): 1985-98.
[http://dx.doi.org/10.1038/emboj.2012.45] [PMID: 22354042]

[173] Gregersen LH, Jacobsen A, Frankel LB, Wen J, Krogh A, Lund AH. MicroRNA-143 down-regulates Hexokinase 2 in colon cancer cells. BMC Cancer 2012; 12: 232.
[http://dx.doi.org/10.1186/1471-2407-12-232] [PMID: 22691140]

[174] Zhao S, Liu H, Liu Y, *et al.* miR-143 inhibits glycolysis and depletes stemness of glioblastoma stem-like cells. Cancer Lett 2013; 333(2): 253-60.
[http://dx.doi.org/10.1016/j.canlet.2013.01.039] [PMID: 23376635]

[175] Yoshino H, Enokida H, Itesako T, *et al.* Tumor-suppressive microRNA-143/145 cluster targets hexokinase-2 in renal cell carcinoma. Cancer Sci 2013; 104(12): 1567-74.
[http://dx.doi.org/10.1111/cas.12280] [PMID: 24033605]

[176] Kim HR, Roe JS, Lee JE, Cho EJ, Youn HD. p53 regulates glucose metabolism by miR-34a. Biochem Biophys Res Commun 2013; 437(2): 225-31.
[http://dx.doi.org/10.1016/j.bbrc.2013.06.043] [PMID: 23796712]

[177] Ahmad A, Aboukameel A, Kong D, *et al.* Phosphoglucose isomerase/autocrine motility factor mediates epithelial-mesenchymal transition regulated by miR-200 in breast cancer cells. Cancer Res 2011; 71(9): 3400-9.
[http://dx.doi.org/10.1158/0008-5472.CAN-10-0965] [PMID: 21389093]

[178] Castoldi M, Vujic Spasic M, Altamura S, *et al.* The liver-specific microRNA miR-122 controls systemic iron homeostasis in mice. J Clin Invest 2011; 121(4): 1386-96.
[http://dx.doi.org/10.1172/JCI44883] [PMID: 21364282]

[179] Calin GA, Cimmino A, Fabbri M, *et al.* MiR-15a and miR-16-1 cluster functions in human leukemia. Proc Natl Acad Sci USA 2008; 105(13): 5166-71.
[http://dx.doi.org/10.1073/pnas.0800121105] [PMID: 18362358]

[180] Kefas B, Comeau L, Erdle N, Montgomery E, Amos S, Purow B. Pyruvate kinase M2 is a target of the tumor-suppressive microRNA-326 and regulates the survival of glioma cells. Neuro-oncol 2010; 12(11): 1102-12.
[http://dx.doi.org/10.1093/neuonc/noq080] [PMID: 20667897]

[181] Wong TS, Liu XB, Chung-Wai Ho A, Po-Wing Yuen A, Wai-Man Ng R, Ignace Wei W. Identification of pyruvate kinase type M2 as potential oncoprotein in squamous cell carcinoma of tongue through microRNA profiling. Int J Cancer 2008; 123(2): 251-7.
[http://dx.doi.org/10.1002/ijc.23583] [PMID: 18464261]

[182] Kinoshita T, Nohata N, Yoshino H, *et al.* Tumor suppressive microRNA-375 regulates lactate dehydrogenase B in maxillary sinus squamous cell carcinoma. Int J Oncol 2012; 40(1): 185-93.
[PMID: 21922130]

[183] Isozaki Y, Hoshino I, Nohata N, *et al.* Identification of novel molecular targets regulated by tumor suppressive miR-375 induced by histone acetylation in esophageal squamous cell carcinoma. Int J Oncol 2012; 41(3): 985-94.
[PMID: 22752059]

[184] Rathore MG, Saumet A, Rossi JF, *et al.* The NF-κB member p65 controls glutamine metabolism through miR-23a. Int J Biochem Cell Biol 2012; 44(9): 1448-56.
[http://dx.doi.org/10.1016/j.biocel.2012.05.011] [PMID: 22634383]

[185] Gao P, Tchernyshyov I, Chang TC, *et al.* c-Myc suppression of miR-23a/b enhances mitochondrial glutaminase expression and glutamine metabolism. Nature 2009; 458(7239): 762-5.
[http://dx.doi.org/10.1038/nature07823] [PMID: 19219026]

[186] Chan SY, Zhang YY, Hemann C, Mahoney CE, Zweier JL, Loscalzo J. MicroRNA-210 controls mitochondrial metabolism during hypoxia by repressing the iron-sulfur cluster assembly proteins ISCU1/2. Cell Metab 2009; 10(4): 273-84.
[http://dx.doi.org/10.1016/j.cmet.2009.08.015] [PMID: 19808020]

[187] Yu QQ, Wu H, Huang X, *et al.* MiR-1 targets PIK3CA and inhibits tumorigenic properties of A549 cells. Biomed Pharmacother 2014; 68(2): 155-61.
[http://dx.doi.org/10.1016/j.biopha.2014.01.005] [PMID: 24486107]

[188] Hu R, Pan W, Fedulov AV, *et al.* MicroRNA-10a controls airway smooth muscle cell proliferation *via* direct targeting of the PI3 kinase pathway. FASEB J 2014; 28(5): 2347-57.
[http://dx.doi.org/10.1096/fj.13-247247] [PMID: 24522205]

[189] Lang Q, Ling C. MiR-124 suppresses cell proliferation in hepatocellular carcinoma by targeting PIK3CA. Biochem Biophys Res Commun 2012; 426(2): 247-52.
[http://dx.doi.org/10.1016/j.bbrc.2012.08.075] [PMID: 22940133]

[190] Ke XF, Fang J, Wu XN, Yu CH. MicroRNA-203 accelerates apoptosis in LPS-stimulated alveolar epithelial cells by targeting PIK3CA. Biochem Biophys Res Commun 2014; 450(4): 1297-303.
[http://dx.doi.org/10.1016/j.bbrc.2014.06.125] [PMID: 24996183]

[191] Wang Y, Tang Q, Li M, Jiang S, Wang X. MicroRNA-375 inhibits colorectal cancer growth by targeting PIK3CA. Biochem Biophys Res Commun 2014; 444(2): 199-204.
[http://dx.doi.org/10.1016/j.bbrc.2014.01.028] [PMID: 24440701]

[192] Fang YX, Xue JL, Shen Q, Chen JZ, Tian L. MicroRNA-7 inhibits tumor growth and metastasis by targeting the phosphoinositide 3-kinase/Akt pathway in hepatocellular carcinoma (vol 55, pg 1852, 2012). Hepatology 2014; 59(3): 1216.
[http://dx.doi.org/10.1002/hep.27001]

[193] Huang X, Shen Y, Liu M, *et al.* Quantitative proteomics reveals that miR-155 regulates the PI3K-AKT pathway in diffuse large B-cell lymphoma. Am J Pathol 2012; 181(1): 26-33.
[http://dx.doi.org/10.1016/j.ajpath.2012.03.013] [PMID: 22609116]

[194] Guo C, Sah JF, Beard L, Willson JK, Markowitz SD, Guda K. The noncoding RNA, miR-126, suppresses the growth of neoplastic cells by targeting phosphatidylinositol 3-kinase signaling and is frequently lost in colon cancers. Genes Chromosomes Cancer 2008; 47(11): 939-46.
[http://dx.doi.org/10.1002/gcc.20596] [PMID: 18663744]

[195] Meng F, Henson R, Wehbe-Janek H, Ghoshal K, Jacob ST, Patel T. MicroRNA-21 regulates expression of the PTEN tumor suppressor gene in human hepatocellular cancer. Gastroenterology 2007; 133(2): 647-58.
[http://dx.doi.org/10.1053/j.gastro.2007.05.022] [PMID: 17681183]

[196] Zhang JG, Wang JJ, Zhao F, Liu Q, Jiang K, Yang GH. MicroRNA-21 (miR-21) represses tumor suppressor PTEN and promotes growth and invasion in non-small cell lung cancer (NSCLC). Clin Chim Acta 2010; 411(11-12): 846-52.
[http://dx.doi.org/10.1016/j.cca.2010.02.074] [PMID: 20223231]

[197] Xiong B, Cheng Y, Ma L, Zhang C. MiR-21 regulates biological behavior through the PTEN/PI-3 K/Akt signaling pathway in human colorectal cancer cells. Int J Oncol 2013; 42(1): 219-28.

[PMID: 23174819]

[198] Yang SM, Huang C, Li XF, Yu MZ, He Y, Li J. miR-21 confers cisplatin resistance in gastric cancer cells by regulating PTEN. Toxicology 2013; 306: 162-8.
[http://dx.doi.org/10.1016/j.tox.2013.02.014] [PMID: 23466500]

[199] Park JK, Lee EJ, Esau C, Schmittgen TD. Antisense inhibition of microRNA-21 or -221 arrests cell cycle, induces apoptosis, and sensitizes the effects of gemcitabine in pancreatic adenocarcinoma. Pancreas 2009; 38(7): e190-9.
[http://dx.doi.org/10.1097/MPA.0b013e3181ba82e1] [PMID: 19730150]

[200] Dey N, Das F, Ghosh-Choudhury N, *et al.* microRNA-21 governs TORC1 activation in renal cancer cell proliferation and invasion. PLoS One 2012; 7(6): e37366.
[http://dx.doi.org/10.1371/journal.pone.0037366] [PMID: 22685542]

[201] Zaman MS, Thamminana S, Shahryari V, *et al.* Inhibition of PTEN gene expression by oncogenic miR-23b-3p in renal cancer. PLoS One 2012; 7(11): e50203.
[http://dx.doi.org/10.1371/journal.pone.0050203] [PMID: 23189187]

[202] Huse JT, Brennan C, Hambardzumyan D, *et al.* The PTEN-regulating microRNA miR-26a is amplified in high-grade glioma and facilitates gliomagenesis *in vivo*. Genes Dev 2009; 23(11): 1327-37.
[http://dx.doi.org/10.1101/gad.1777409] [PMID: 19487573]

[203] Wu W, Yang J, Feng X, *et al.* MicroRNA-32 (miR-32) regulates phosphatase and tensin homologue (PTEN) expression and promotes growth, migration, and invasion in colorectal carcinoma cells. Mol Cancer 2013; 12: 30.
[http://dx.doi.org/10.1186/1476-4598-12-30] [PMID: 23617834]

[204] Tay Y, Tan SM, Karreth FA, Lieberman J, Pandolfi PP. Characterization of dual PTEN and p53-targeting microRNAs identifies microRNA-638/Dnm2 as a two-hit oncogenic locus. Cell Reports 2014; 8(3): 714-22.
[http://dx.doi.org/10.1016/j.celrep.2014.06.064] [PMID: 25088422]

[205] Poliseno L, Salmena L, Riccardi L, *et al.* Identification of the miR-106b~25 microRNA cluster as a proto-oncogenic PTEN-targeting intron that cooperates with its host gene MCM7 in transformation. Sci Signal 2010; 3(117): ra29.
[http://dx.doi.org/10.1126/scisignal.2000594] [PMID: 20388916]

[206] Beezhold K, Liu J, Kan H, *et al.* miR-190-mediated downregulation of PHLPP contributes to arsenic-induced Akt activation and carcinogenesis. Toxicol Sci 2011; 123(2): 411-20.
[http://dx.doi.org/10.1093/toxsci/kfr188] [PMID: 21750348]

[207] Quintavalle C, Garofalo M, Zanca C, *et al.* miR-221/222 overexpession in human glioblastoma increases invasiveness by targeting the protein phosphate PTPμ. Oncogene 2012; 31(7): 858-68.
[http://dx.doi.org/10.1038/onc.2011.280] [PMID: 21743492]

[208] Hamano R, Miyata H, Yamasaki M, *et al.* Overexpression of miR-200c induces chemoresistance in esophageal cancers mediated through activation of the Akt signaling pathway. Clin Cancer Res 2011; 17(9): 3029-38.
[http://dx.doi.org/10.1158/1078-0432.CCR-10-2532] [PMID: 21248297]

[209] Godlewski J, Nowicki MO, Bronisz A, *et al.* MicroRNA-451 regulates LKB1/AMPK signaling and allows adaptation to metabolic stress in glioma cells. Mol Cell 2010; 37(5): 620-32.
[http://dx.doi.org/10.1016/j.molcel.2010.02.018] [PMID: 20227367]

[210] Mavrakis KJ, Wolfe AL, Oricchio E, *et al.* Genome-wide RNA-mediated interference screen identifies miR-19 targets in Notch-induced T-cell acute lymphoblastic leukaemia. Nat Cell Biol 2010; 12(4): 372-9.
[http://dx.doi.org/10.1038/ncb2037] [PMID: 20190740]

[211] Sampson VB, Rong NH, Han J, *et al.* MicroRNA let-7a down-regulates MYC and reverts MYC-induced growth in Burkitt lymphoma cells. Cancer Res 2007; 67(20): 9762-70.
[http://dx.doi.org/10.1158/0008-5472.CAN-07-2462] [PMID: 17942906]

[212] Lal A, Navarro F, Maher CA, *et al.* miR-24 Inhibits cell proliferation by targeting E2F2, MYC, and other cell-cycle genes *via* binding to "seedless" 3'UTR microRNA recognition elements. Mol Cell 2009; 35(5): 610-25.
[http://dx.doi.org/10.1016/j.molcel.2009.08.020] [PMID: 19748357]

[213] Christoffersen NR, Shalgi R, Frankel LB, *et al.* p53-independent upregulation of miR-34a during oncogene-induced senescence represses MYC. Cell Death Differ 2010; 17(2): 236-45.
[http://dx.doi.org/10.1038/cdd.2009.109] [PMID: 19696787]

[214] Sachdeva M, Zhu S, Wu F, *et al.* p53 represses c-Myc through induction of the tumor suppressor miR-145. Proc Natl Acad Sci USA 2009; 106(9): 3207-12.
[http://dx.doi.org/10.1073/pnas.0808042106] [PMID: 19202062]

[215] Zhen Y, Liu Z, Yang H, *et al.* Tumor suppressor PDCD4 modulates miR-184-mediated direct suppression of C-MYC and BCL2 blocking cell growth and survival in nasopharyngeal carcinoma. Cell Death Dis 2013; 4: e872.
[http://dx.doi.org/10.1038/cddis.2013.376] [PMID: 24157866]

[216] Bhatia S, Kaul D, Varma N. Potential tumor suppressive function of miR-196b in B-cell lineage acute lymphoblastic leukemia. Mol Cell Biochem 2010; 340(1-2): 97-106.
[http://dx.doi.org/10.1007/s11010-010-0406-9] [PMID: 20549547]

[217] Miao LJ, Huang SF, Sun ZT, *et al.* MiR-449c targets c-Myc and inhibits NSCLC cell progression. FEBS Lett 2013; 587(9): 1359-65.
[http://dx.doi.org/10.1016/j.febslet.2013.03.006] [PMID: 23507140]

[218] Lei Z, Li B, Yang Z, *et al.* Regulation of HIF-1alpha and VEGF by miR-20b tunes tumor cells to adapt to the alteration of oxygen concentration. PLoS One 2009; 4(10): e7629.
[http://dx.doi.org/10.1371/journal.pone.0007629] [PMID: 19893619]

[219] Fornari F, Milazzo M, Chieco P, *et al.* MiR-199a-3p regulates mTOR and c-Met to influence the doxorubicin sensitivity of human hepatocarcinoma cells. Cancer Res 2010; 70(12): 5184-93.
[http://dx.doi.org/10.1158/0008-5472.CAN-10-0145] [PMID: 20501828]

[220] Taguchi A, Yanagisawa K, Tanaka M, *et al.* Identification of hypoxia-inducible factor-1 alpha as a novel target for miR-17-92 microRNA cluster. Cancer Res 2008; 68(14): 5540-5.
[http://dx.doi.org/10.1158/0008-5472.CAN-07-6460] [PMID: 18632605]

[221] Ghosh G, Subramanian IV, Adhikari N, *et al.* Hypoxia-induced microRNA-424 expression in human

endothelial cells regulates HIF-α isoforms and promotes angiogenesis. J Clin Invest 2010; 120(11): 4141-54.
[http://dx.doi.org/10.1172/JCI42980] [PMID: 20972335]

[222] Kelly TJ, Souza AL, Clish CB, Puigserver P. A Hypoxia-induced positive feedback loop promotes hypoxia-inducible factor 1 alpha stability through miR-210 suppression of glycerol-3-phosphate dehydrogenase 1-like. Mol Cell Biol 2012; 32(4): 898.
[http://dx.doi.org/10.1128/MCB.06639-11]

[223] Suh SS, Yoo JY, Nuovo GJ, *et al.* MicroRNAs/TP53 feedback circuitry in glioblastoma multiforme. Proc Natl Acad Sci USA 2012; 109(14): 5316-21.
[http://dx.doi.org/10.1073/pnas.1202465109] [PMID: 22431589]

[224] Kumar M, Lu Z, Takwi AA, *et al.* Negative regulation of the tumor suppressor p53 gene by microRNAs. Oncogene 2011; 30(7): 843-53.
[http://dx.doi.org/10.1038/onc.2010.457] [PMID: 20935678]

[225] Herrera-Merchan A, Cerrato C, Luengo G, *et al.* miR-33-mediated downregulation of p53 controls hematopoietic stem cell self-renewal. Cell Cycle 2010; 9(16): 3277-85.
[http://dx.doi.org/10.4161/cc.9.16.12598] [PMID: 20703086]

[226] Le MT, Teh C, Shyh-Chang N, *et al.* MicroRNA-125b is a novel negative regulator of p53. Genes Dev 2009; 23(7): 862-76.
[http://dx.doi.org/10.1101/gad.1767609] [PMID: 19293287]

[227] Swarbrick A, Woods SL, Shaw A, *et al.* miR-380-5p represses p53 to control cellular survival and is associated with poor outcome in MYCN-amplified neuroblastoma. Nat Med 2010; 16(10): 1134-40.
[http://dx.doi.org/10.1038/nm.2227] [PMID: 20871609]

[228] Hu W, Chan CS, Wu R, *et al.* Negative regulation of tumor suppressor p53 by microRNA miR-504. Mol Cell 2010; 38(5): 689-99.
[http://dx.doi.org/10.1016/j.molcel.2010.05.027] [PMID: 20542001]

[229] Tian S, Huang S, Wu S, Guo W, Li J, He X. MicroRNA-1285 inhibits the expression of p53 by directly targeting its 3′ untranslated region. Biochem Biophys Res Commun 2010; 396(2): 435-9.
[http://dx.doi.org/10.1016/j.bbrc.2010.04.112] [PMID: 20417621]

[230] Pichiorri F, Suh SS, Rocci A, *et al.* Downregulation of p53-inducible microRNAs 192, 194, and 215 impairs the p53/MDM2 autoregulatory loop in multiple myeloma development. Cancer Cell 2010; 18(4): 367-81.
[http://dx.doi.org/10.1016/j.ccr.2010.09.005] [PMID: 20951946]

[231] Xiao J, Lin H, Luo X, Luo X, Wang Z. miR-605 joins p53 network to form a p53:miR-605:Mdm2 positive feedback loop in response to stress. EMBO J 2011; 30(3): 524-32.
[http://dx.doi.org/10.1038/emboj.2010.347] [PMID: 21217645]

[232] Yamakuchi M, Ferlito M, Lowenstein CJ. miR-34a repression of SIRT1 regulates apoptosis. Proc Natl Acad Sci USA 2008; 105(36): 13421-6.
[http://dx.doi.org/10.1073/pnas.0801613105] [PMID: 18755897]

[233] Buurman R, Gürlevik E, Schäffer V, *et al.* Histone deacetylases activate hepatocyte growth factor signaling by repressing microRNA-449 in hepatocellular carcinoma cells. Gastroenterology 2012;

143(3): 811-20.e1, 15.
[http://dx.doi.org/10.1053/j.gastro.2012.05.033] [PMID: 22641068]

[234] Zaidi N, Swinnen JV, Smans K. ATP-citrate lyase: A key player in cancer metabolism. Cancer Res 2012; 72(15): 3709-14.
[http://dx.doi.org/10.1158/0008-5472.CAN-11-4112] [PMID: 22787121]

[235] Hatzivassiliou G, Zhao F, Bauer DE, *et al.* ATP citrate lyase inhibition can suppress tumor cell growth. Cancer Cell 2005; 8(4): 311-21.
[http://dx.doi.org/10.1016/j.ccr.2005.09.008] [PMID: 16226706]

[236] Wellen KE, Hatzivassiliou G, Sachdeva UM, Bui TV, Cross JR, Thompson CB. ATP-citrate lyase links cellular metabolism to histone acetylation. Science 2009; 324(5930): 1076-80.
[http://dx.doi.org/10.1126/science.1164097] [PMID: 19461003]

[237] Migita T, Narita T, Nomura K, *et al.* ATP citrate lyase: Activation and therapeutic implications in non-small cell lung cancer. Cancer Res 2008; 68(20): 8547-54.
[http://dx.doi.org/10.1158/0008-5472.CAN-08-1235] [PMID: 18922930]

[238] Lee JV, Carrer A, Shah S, *et al.* Akt-dependent metabolic reprogramming regulates tumor cell histone acetylation. Cell Metab 2014; 20(2): 306-19.
[http://dx.doi.org/10.1016/j.cmet.2014.06.004] [PMID: 24998913]

[239] Knoepfler PS, Zhang XY, Cheng PF, Gafken PR, McMahon SB, Eisenman RN. Myc influences global chromatin structure. EMBO J 2006; 25(12): 2723-34.
[http://dx.doi.org/10.1038/sj.emboj.7601152] [PMID: 16724113]

[240] Edmunds LR, Sharma L, Kang A, *et al.* c-Myc programs fatty acid metabolism and dictates acetyl-CoA abundance and fate. J Biol Chem 2014; 289(36): 25382-92.
[http://dx.doi.org/10.1074/jbc.M114.580662] [PMID: 25053415]

[241] Chiang PK, Gordon RK, Tal J, *et al.* S-Adenosylmethionine and methylation. FASEB J 1996; 10(4): 471-80.
[PMID: 8647346]

[242] James SJ, Pogribny IP, Pogribna M, Miller BJ, Jernigan S, Melnyk S. Mechanisms of DNA damage, DNA hypomethylation, and tumor progression in the folate/methyl-deficient rat model of hepatocarcinogenesis. J Nutr 2003; 133(11) (Suppl. 1): 3740S-7S.
[PMID: 14608108]

[243] Kim YI. Folate and DNA methylation: A mechanistic link between folate deficiency and colorectal cancer? Cancer Epidemiol Biomarkers Prev 2004; 13(4): 511-9.
[PMID: 15066913]

[244] Stern LL, Mason JB, Selhub J, Choi SW. Genomic DNA hypomethylation, a characteristic of most cancers, is present in peripheral leukocytes of individuals who are homozygous for the C677T polymorphism in the methylenetetrahydrofolate reductase gene. Cancer Epidemiol Biomarkers Prev 2000; 9(8): 849-53.
[PMID: 10952104]

[245] Chen RZ, Pettersson U, Beard C, Jackson-Grusby L, Jaenisch R. DNA hypomethylation leads to elevated mutation rates. Nature 1998; 395(6697): 89-93.

[http://dx.doi.org/10.1038/25779] [PMID: 9738504]

[246] Eden A, Gaudet F, Waghmare A, Jaenisch R. Chromosomal instability and tumors promoted by DNA hypomethylation. Science 2003; 300(5618): 455.
[http://dx.doi.org/10.1126/science.1083557] [PMID: 12702868]

[247] Mudd SH, Cerone R, Schiaffino MC, *et al.* Glycine N-methyltransferase deficiency: A novel inborn error causing persistent isolated hypermethioninaemia. J Inherit Metab Dis 2001; 24(4): 448-64.
[http://dx.doi.org/10.1023/A:1010577512912] [PMID: 11596649]

[248] Martínez-Chantar ML, Vázquez-Chantada M, Ariz U, *et al.* Loss of the glycine N-methyltransferase gene leads to steatosis and hepatocellular carcinoma in mice. Hepatology 2008; 47(4): 1191-9.
[http://dx.doi.org/10.1002/hep.22159] [PMID: 18318442]

[249] Fuchs BC, Bode BP. Amino acid transporters ASCT2 and LAT1 in cancer: partners in crime? Semin Cancer Biol 2005; 15(4): 254-66.
[http://dx.doi.org/10.1016/j.semcancer.2005.04.005] [PMID: 15916903]

[250] Haase C, Bergmann R, Fuechtner F, Hoepping A, Pietzsch J. L-type amino acid transporters LAT1 and LAT4 in cancer: uptake of 3-O-methyl-6-18F-fluoro-L-dopa in human adenocarcinoma and squamous cell carcinoma in vitro and in vivo. J Nucl Med 2007; 48(12): 2063-71.
[http://dx.doi.org/10.2967/jnumed.107.043620] [PMID: 18056335]

[251] Possemato R, Marks KM, Shaul YD, *et al.* Functional genomics reveal that the serine synthesis pathway is essential in breast cancer. Nature 2011; 476(7360): 346-50.
[http://dx.doi.org/10.1038/nature10350] [PMID: 21760589]

[252] Locasale JW, Grassian AR, Melman T, *et al.* Phosphoglycerate dehydrogenase diverts glycolytic flux and contributes to oncogenesis. Nat Genet 2011; 43(9): 869-74.
[http://dx.doi.org/10.1038/ng.890] [PMID: 21804546]

[253] Wu Y, Siadaty MS, Berens ME, Hampton GM, Theodorescu D. Overlapping gene expression profiles of cell migration and tumor invasion in human bladder cancer identify metallothionein 1E and nicotinamide N-methyltransferase as novel regulators of cell migration. Oncogene 2008; 27(52): 6679-89.
[http://dx.doi.org/10.1038/onc.2008.264] [PMID: 18724390]

[254] Tang SW, Yang TC, Lin WC, *et al.* Nicotinamide N-methyltransferase induces cellular invasion through activating matrix metalloproteinase-2 expression in clear cell renal cell carcinoma cells. Carcinogenesis 2011; 32(2): 138-45.
[http://dx.doi.org/10.1093/carcin/bgq225] [PMID: 21045016]

[255] Ulanovskaya OA, Zuhl AM, Cravatt BF. NNMT promotes epigenetic remodeling in cancer by creating a metabolic methylation sink. Nat Chem Biol 2013; 9(5): 300-6.
[http://dx.doi.org/10.1038/nchembio.1204] [PMID: 23455543]

[256] Shyh-Chang N, Locasale JW, Lyssiotis CA, *et al.* Influence of threonine metabolism on S-adenosylmethionine and histone methylation. Science 2013; 339(6116): 222-6.
[http://dx.doi.org/10.1126/science.1226603] [PMID: 23118012]

[257] Shiraki N, Shiraki Y, Tsuyama T, *et al.* Methionine metabolism regulates maintenance and differentiation of human pluripotent stem cells. Cell Metab 2014; 19(5): 780-94.

[http://dx.doi.org/10.1016/j.cmet.2014.03.017] [PMID: 24746804]

[258]　Yan H, Parsons DW, Jin G, *et al.* IDH1 and IDH2 mutations in gliomas. N Engl J Med 2009; 360(8): 765-73.
[http://dx.doi.org/10.1056/NEJMoa0808710] [PMID: 19228619]

[259]　Paschka P, Schlenk RF, Gaidzik VI, *et al.* IDH1 and IDH2 mutations are frequent genetic alterations in acute myeloid leukemia and confer adverse prognosis in cytogenetically normal acute myeloid leukemia with NPM1 mutation without FLT3 internal tandem duplication. J Clin Oncol 2010; 28(22): 3636-43.
[http://dx.doi.org/10.1200/JCO.2010.28.3762] [PMID: 20567020]

[260]　Hurley JH, Dean AM, Koshland DE Jr, Stroud RM. Catalytic mechanism of NADP(+)-dependent isocitrate dehydrogenase: implications from the structures of magnesium-isocitrate and NADP+ complexes. Biochemistry 1991; 30(35): 8671-8.
[http://dx.doi.org/10.1021/bi00099a026] [PMID: 1888729]

[261]　Dang L, White DW, Gross S, *et al.* Cancer-associated IDH1 mutations produce 2-hydroxyglutarate. Nature 2010; 465(7300): 966.
[http://dx.doi.org/10.1038/nature09132] [PMID: 20559394]

[262]　Balss J, Meyer J, Mueller W, Korshunov A, Hartmann C, von Deimling A. Analysis of the IDH1 codon 132 mutation in brain tumors. Acta Neuropathol 2008; 116(6): 597-602.
[http://dx.doi.org/10.1007/s00401-008-0455-2] [PMID: 18985363]

[263]　Cairns RA, Iqbal J, Lemonnier F, *et al.* IDH2 mutations are frequent in angioimmunoblastic T-cell lymphoma. Blood 2012; 119(8): 1901-3.
[http://dx.doi.org/10.1182/blood-2011-11-391748] [PMID: 22215888]

[264]　Patel KP, Ravandi F, Ma D, *et al.* Acute myeloid leukemia with IDH1 or IDH2 mutation: frequency and clinicopathologic features. Am J Clin Pathol 2011; 135(1): 35-45.
[http://dx.doi.org/10.1309/AJCPD7NR2RMNQDVF] [PMID: 21173122]

[265]　Ward PS, Patel J, Wise DR, *et al.* The common feature of leukemia-associated IDH1 and IDH2 mutations is a neomorphic enzyme activity converting alpha-ketoglutarate to 2-hydroxyglutarate. Cancer Cell 2010; 17(3): 225-34.
[http://dx.doi.org/10.1016/j.ccr.2010.01.020] [PMID: 20171147]

[266]　Sasaki M, Knobbe CB, Munger JC, *et al.* IDH1(R132H) mutation increases murine haematopoietic progenitors and alters epigenetics. Nature 2012; 488(7413): 656-9.
[http://dx.doi.org/10.1038/nature11323] [PMID: 22763442]

[267]　Lu C, Ward PS, Kapoor GS, *et al.* IDH mutation impairs histone demethylation and results in a block to cell differentiation. Nature 2012; 483(7390): 474-8.
[http://dx.doi.org/10.1038/nature10860] [PMID: 22343901]

[268]　Losman JA, Looper RE, Koivunen P, *et al.* (R)-2-hydroxyglutarate is sufficient to promote leukemogenesis and its effects are reversible. Science 2013; 339(6127): 1621-5.
[http://dx.doi.org/10.1126/science.1231677] [PMID: 23393090]

[269]　Popovici-Muller J, Saunders JO, Salituro FG, *et al.* Discovery of the first potent inhibitors of mutant IDH1 that lower tumor 2-HG *in vivo.* ACS Med Chem Lett 2012; 3(10): 850-5.

[http://dx.doi.org/10.1021/ml300225h] [PMID: 24900389]

[270] Terunuma A, Putluri N, Mishra P, *et al.* MYC-driven accumulation of 2-hydroxyglutarate is associated with breast cancer prognosis. J Clin Invest 2014; 124(1): 398-412.
[http://dx.doi.org/10.1172/JCI71180] [PMID: 24316975]

[271] Figueroa ME, Abdel-Wahab O, Lu C, *et al.* Leukemic IDH1 and IDH2 mutations result in a hypermethylation phenotype, disrupt TET2 function, and impair hematopoietic differentiation. Cancer Cell 2010; 18(6): 553-67.
[http://dx.doi.org/10.1016/j.ccr.2010.11.015] [PMID: 21130701]

[272] Xu W, Yang H, Liu Y, *et al.* Oncometabolite 2-hydroxyglutarate is a competitive inhibitor of α-ketoglutarate-dependent dioxygenases. Cancer Cell 2011; 19(1): 17-30.
[http://dx.doi.org/10.1016/j.ccr.2010.12.014] [PMID: 21251613]

[273] Christensen BC, Smith AA, Zheng S, Koestler DC, Houseman EA, Marsit CJ, *et al.* DNA methylation, isocitrate dehydrogenase mutation, and survival in glioma. J Natl Cancer Inst 2011; 103(2): 143-53.
[http://dx.doi.org/10.1093/jnci/djq497] [PMID: 21163902]

[274] Turcan S, Rohle D, Goenka A, *et al.* IDH1 mutation is sufficient to establish the glioma hypermethylator phenotype. Nature 2012; 483(7390): 479-83.
[http://dx.doi.org/10.1038/nature10866] [PMID: 22343889]

[275] Chowdhury R, Yeoh KK, Tian YM, *et al.* The oncometabolite 2-hydroxyglutarate inhibits histone lysine demethylases. EMBO Rep 2011; 12(5): 463-9.
[http://dx.doi.org/10.1038/embor.2011.43] [PMID: 21460794]

[276] Klose RJ, Kallin EM, Zhang Y. JmjC-domain-containing proteins and histone demethylation. Nat Rev Genet 2006; 7(9): 715-27.
[http://dx.doi.org/10.1038/nrg1945] [PMID: 16983801]

[277] Lee KH, Park JW, Sung HS, Choi YJ, Kim WH, Lee HS, *et al.* PHF2 histone demethylase acts as a tumor suppressor in association with p53 in cancer. Oncogene 2015; 34(22): 2897-909.
[http://dx.doi.org/10.1038/onc.2014.219] [PMID: 25043306]

[278] Niu X, Zhang T, Liao L, *et al.* The von Hippel-Lindau tumor suppressor protein regulates gene expression and tumor growth through histone demethylase JARID1C. Oncogene 2012; 31(6): 776-86.
[http://dx.doi.org/10.1038/onc.2011.266] [PMID: 21725364]

[279] Ene CI, Edwards L, Riddick G, *et al.* Histone demethylase Jumonji D3 (JMJD3) as a tumor suppressor by regulating p53 protein nuclear stabilization. PLoS One 2012; 7(12): e51407.
[http://dx.doi.org/10.1371/journal.pone.0051407] [PMID: 23236496]

[280] Liu Y, Zheng P, Liu Y, *et al.* An epigenetic role for PRL-3 as a regulator of H3K9 methylation in colorectal cancer. Gut 2013; 62(4): 571-81.
[http://dx.doi.org/10.1136/gutjnl-2011-301059] [PMID: 22345654]

[281] Frescas D, Guardavaccaro D, Bassermann F, Koyama-Nasu R, Pagano M. JHDM1B/FBXL10 is a nucleolar protein that represses transcription of ribosomal RNA genes. Nature 2007; 450(7167): 309-13.
[http://dx.doi.org/10.1038/nature06255] [PMID: 17994099]

[282] Venneti S, Felicella MM, Coyne T, *et al.* Histone 3 lysine 9 trimethylation is differentially associated

with isocitrate dehydrogenase mutations in oligodendrogliomas and high-grade astrocytomas. J Neuropathol Exp Neurol 2013; 72(4): 298-306.
[http://dx.doi.org/10.1097/NEN.0b013e3182898113] [PMID: 23481705]

[283]   Pollard PJ, Wortham NC, Tomlinson IP. The TCA cycle and tumorigenesis: the examples of fumarate hydratase and succinate dehydrogenase. Ann Med 2003; 35(8): 632-9.
[http://dx.doi.org/10.1080/07853890310018458] [PMID: 14708972]

[284]   Janeway KA, Kim SY, Lodish M, *et al.* NIH Pediatric and Wild-Type GIST Clinic. Defects in succinate dehydrogenase in gastrointestinal stromal tumors lacking KIT and PDGFRA mutations. Proc Natl Acad Sci USA 2011; 108(1): 314-8.
[http://dx.doi.org/10.1073/pnas.1009199108] [PMID: 21173220]

[285]   Ricketts CJ, Shuch B, Vocke CD, *et al.* Succinate dehydrogenase kidney cancer: an aggressive example of the Warburg effect in cancer. J Urol 2012; 188(6): 2063-71.
[http://dx.doi.org/10.1016/j.juro.2012.08.030] [PMID: 23083876]

[286]   Hensen EF, Bayley JP. Recent advances in the genetics of SDH-related paraganglioma and pheochromocytoma. Fam Cancer 2011; 10(2): 355-63.
[http://dx.doi.org/10.1007/s10689-010-9402-1] [PMID: 21082267]

[287]   Kantorovich V, King KS, Pacak K. SDH-related pheochromocytoma and paraganglioma. Best Pract Res Clin Endocrinol Metab 2010; 24(3): 415-24.
[http://dx.doi.org/10.1016/j.beem.2010.04.001] [PMID: 20833333]

[288]   Hao HX, Khalimonchuk O, Schraders M, *et al.* SDH5, a gene required for flavination of succinate dehydrogenase, is mutated in paraganglioma. Science 2009; 325(5944): 1139-42.
[http://dx.doi.org/10.1126/science.1175689] [PMID: 19628817]

[289]   Toro JR, Nickerson ML, Wei MH, *et al.* Mutations in the fumarate hydratase gene cause hereditary leiomyomatosis and renal cell cancer in families in North America. Am J Hum Genet 2003; 73(1): 95-106.
[http://dx.doi.org/10.1086/376435] [PMID: 12772087]

[290]   Xiao M, Yang H, Xu W, *et al.* Inhibition of α-KG-dependent histone and DNA demethylases by fumarate and succinate that are accumulated in mutations of FH and SDH tumor suppressors. Genes Dev 2012; 26(12): 1326-38.
[http://dx.doi.org/10.1101/gad.191056.112] [PMID: 22677546]

[291]   Letouzé E, Martinelli C, Loriot C, *et al.* SDH mutations establish a hypermethylator phenotype in paraganglioma. Cancer Cell 2013; 23(6): 739-52.
[http://dx.doi.org/10.1016/j.ccr.2013.04.018] [PMID: 23707781]

[292]   Killian JK, Kim SY, Miettinen M, *et al.* Succinate dehydrogenase mutation underlies global epigenomic divergence in gastrointestinal stromal tumor. Cancer Discov 2013; 3(6): 648-57.
[http://dx.doi.org/10.1158/2159-8290.CD-13-0092] [PMID: 23550148]

[293]   Rodríguez-Paredes M, Esteller M. A combined epigenetic therapy equals the efficacy of conventional chemotherapy in refractory advanced non-small cell lung cancer. Cancer Discov 2011; 1(7): 557-9.
[http://dx.doi.org/10.1158/2159-8290.CD-11-0271] [PMID: 22586680]

[294]   Borodovsky A, Salmasi V, Turcan S, *et al.* 5-azacytidine reduces methylation, promotes differentiation

and induces tumor regression in a patient-derived IDH1 mutant glioma xenograft. Oncotarget 2013; 4(10): 1737-47.
[http://dx.doi.org/10.18632/oncotarget.1408] [PMID: 24077805]

[295]   Turcan S, Fabius AW, Borodovsky A, *et al.* Efficient induction of differentiation and growth inhibition in IDH1 mutant glioma cells by the DNMT Inhibitor Decitabine. Oncotarget 2013; 4(10): 1729-36.
[http://dx.doi.org/10.18632/oncotarget.1412] [PMID: 24077826]

[296]   Alcarraz-Vizán G, Boren J, Lee WN, Cascante M. Histone deacetylase inhibition results in a common metabolic profile associated with HT29 differentiation. Metabolomics 2010; 6(2): 229-37.
[http://dx.doi.org/10.1007/s11306-009-0192-0] [PMID: 20445757]

[297]   Wardell SE, Ilkayeva OR, Wieman HL, *et al.* Glucose metabolism as a target of histone deacetylase inhibitors. Mol Endocrinol 2009; 23(3): 388-401.
[http://dx.doi.org/10.1210/me.2008-0179] [PMID: 19106193]

[298]   Amoêdo ND, Rodrigues MF, Pezzuto P, *et al.* Energy metabolism in H460 lung cancer cells: effects of histone deacetylase inhibitors. PLoS One 2011; 6(7): e22264.
[http://dx.doi.org/10.1371/journal.pone.0022264] [PMID: 21789245]

[299]   Rodrigues MF, Carvalho É, Pezzuto P, Rumjanek FD, Amoêdo ND. Reciprocal modulation of histone deacetylase inhibitors sodium butyrate and trichostatin A on the energy metabolism of breast cancer cells. J Cell Biochem 2015; 116(5): 797-808.
[http://dx.doi.org/10.1002/jcb.25036] [PMID: 25510910]

[300]   Bader AG, Brown D, Winkler M. The promise of microRNA replacement therapy. Cancer Res 2010; 70(18): 7027-30.
[http://dx.doi.org/10.1158/0008-5472.CAN-10-2010] [PMID: 20807816]

[301]   Ebert MS, Sharp PA. MicroRNA sponges: progress and possibilities. RNA 2010; 16(11): 2043-50.
[http://dx.doi.org/10.1261/rna.2414110] [PMID: 20855538]

[302]   Li Z, Rana TM. Therapeutic targeting of microRNAs: current status and future challenges. Nat Rev Drug Discov 2014; 13(8): 622-38.
[http://dx.doi.org/10.1038/nrd4359] [PMID: 25011539]

[303]   Pereira DM, Rodrigues PM, Borralho PM, Rodrigues CM. Delivering the promise of miRNA cancer therapeutics. Drug Discov Today 2013; 18(5-6): 282-9.
[http://dx.doi.org/10.1016/j.drudis.2012.10.002] [PMID: 23064097]

[304]   Rohle D, Popovici-Muller J, Palaskas N, *et al.* An inhibitor of mutant IDH1 delays growth and promotes differentiation of glioma cells. Science 2013; 340(6132): 626-30.
[http://dx.doi.org/10.1126/science.1236062] [PMID: 23558169]

[305]   Davis MI, Gross S, Shen M, *et al.* Biochemical, cellular, and biophysical characterization of a potent inhibitor of mutant isocitrate dehydrogenase IDH1. J Biol Chem 2014; 289(20): 13717-25.
[http://dx.doi.org/10.1074/jbc.M113.511030] [PMID: 24668804]

[306]   Wang F, Travins J, DeLaBarre B, *et al.* Targeted inhibition of mutant IDH2 in leukemia cells induces cellular differentiation. Science 2013; 340(6132): 622-6.
[http://dx.doi.org/10.1126/science.1234769] [PMID: 23558173]

[307] Kernytsky A, Wang F, Hansen E, *et al.* IDH2 mutation-induced histone and DNA hypermethylation is progressively reversed by small-molecule inhibition. Blood 2015; 125(2): 296-303.
[http://dx.doi.org/10.1182/blood-2013-10-533604] [PMID: 25398940]

[308] Burdge GC, Lillycrop KA. Nutrition, epigenetics, and developmental plasticity: implications for understanding human disease. Annu Rev Nutr 2010; 30: 315-39.
[http://dx.doi.org/10.1146/annurev.nutr.012809.104751] [PMID: 20415585]

CHAPTER 7

Apoptosis Targeting Therapeutics in Clinical Trials

N.S. Hari Narayana Moorthy[1,2,*], C. Karthikeyan[2], Piyush Trivedi[2]

[1] *Departamento de Química e Bioquímica, Faculdade de Ciências, Universidade do Porto, s/n, Rua do Campo Alegre, 4169-007 Porto, Portugal*

[2] *School of Pharmaceutical Sciences, Rajiv Gandhi Proudyogiki Vishwavidyalaya, Airport Bypass Road, Gandhi Nagar, Bhopal (MP)-462033, India*

Abstract: Apoptosis (called as programmed cell death) is vital for maintaining homeostatic balance between cell survival/cell deaths in metazoan cells. Apoptosis is regulated through extrinsic (or receptor mediated) and intrinsic (or mitochondria mediated) pathways. The pro-apoptotic proteins (*e.g.* Bax, Bak, Bad, Bcl-Xs, Bid, Bik, Bim and Hrk) and the anti-apoptotic proteins (*e.g.* Bcl-2, Bcl-XL, Bcl-W, Bfl-1 and Mcl-1) are crucial to control the apoptotic pathways. Dysfunctions of apoptosis pathways are implicated in cancer as defects in these pathways not only promote tumorigenesis but also confer resistance to cancer cells to most conventional chemotherapies as well as radiotherapy. The apoptosis occurs by imbalanced pro-apoptotic and anti-apoptotic protein levels, impaired or reduced death receptor signalling and caspase function. Hence, targeting apoptosis pathways is considered as an attractive strategy for therapeutic intervention in cancer. The past decade recorded tremendous advances in this area especially small molecular intervention of apoptosis pathways for cancer treatment which resulted in several compounds under clinical development. This chapter reviews the current progressions in the development of bioactive molecules targeting apoptotic pathways with special emphasis on small molecular anticancer drugs under clinical trials. Some excellent examples are; nutlins, MI-888, MI-219 and SM-164 which target MDM2, ABT-263, AT-406 and GX15-070MS which target Bcl-2 family of proteins, birinapant, GDC-0917, HGS-1029 and LCL-161 which target IAPs (inhibitors of apoptotic proteins). The content of this chapter will be enlightening the readers in academic and research to update their knowledge on the anticancer drugs especially target proteins responsible for apoptosis.

* **Corresponding author N.S. Hari Narayana Moorthy:** Departamento de Química e Bioquímica, Faculdade de Ciências, Universidade do Porto, s/n, Rua do Campo Alegre, 4169-007 Porto, Portugal; Tel: +917552678883; Fax: +917552742002; E-mails: hari.moorthy@fc.up.pt, hari.nmoorthy@gmail.com

Atta-ur-Rahman (Ed.)

Keywords: Apoptosis, BCL family proteins, Cancer, Caspase, Clinical trials, IAP, MDM2, Nutlins, p53, Pro-apoptotic protein.

CANCER

Cancer is a life threatening, multifaceted disease that involves disruption of the normal balance of cellular life and death through dysregulation of cellular homeostasis and the prevailing mechanisms responsible for cell growth and replication. Mechanisms responsible for cancer development include dysregulated response to growth signals, angiogenesis, uncontrolled replication, tissue invasion and metastasis, and evasion of apoptosis. Statistically, cancers accounted for 8.2 million deaths and 14 million new cases in 2012 and the number of cancer related deaths is expected to rise to 22 million within the next two decades [1 - 3].

Anticancer drug discovery is a challenging task owing to high attrition rate mainly attributed to lack of efficacy, non-selectivity, toxicity and incompatible pharmacokinetic profiles of anticancer agents which are under clinical development. Hence, discovery of "safe and effective" anticancer drugs remains a priority area for researchers working on cancer worldwide. The effectiveness of drugs used for the cancer therapy is dependent on the type of targets which it modulates. Biochemical pathways necessary for growth and survival of cancer cells are attractive targets for anticancer drug discovery. The former comprises mainly of signal transduction pathways regulating growth and proliferation of cancer cells while the latter comprises of pathways which enhances survival of cancer cells by imparting ability to repair and evade cell death (apoptosis). Targeting apoptosis pathways for anticancer drug discovery is relatively a new avenue compared to the much established therapeutic strategies targeting pathways regulating growth and proliferation of cancer cells. Nevertheless, the increased understanding of molecular mechanisms that regulate apoptosis together with convincing proof-of-principle evidence obtained in several animal models confirming the validity of apoptosis targeted drug discovery for cancer led to the development of several apoptosis-based therapeutics for cancer therapy. This chapter reviews the advancements in the discovery and development of small-molecules attacking apoptotic pathways with special emphasis on the bioactive molecules under clinical trials.

APOPTOSIS

Apoptosis (programmed cell death) is essential for maintaining homeostatic balance between cell survival/cell deaths in metazoan cells. The role of apoptosis in the physiological and the pathological conditions remains to be an intensely investigated area in biological research [4]. Apoptosis is triggered by imbalance in the pro-apoptotic and anti-apoptotic protein levels resulting from impaired or reduced death receptor signalling and caspase functions. Apoptosis is accompanied by a series of biochemical changes including caspases activation, DNA and protein breakdown, membrane changes and recognition by phagocytic cells [5, 6]. Dysfunction of apoptosis pathways are implicated in cancer as defects in these pathways not only promote tumorigenesis but also confer resistance to cancer cells to most conventional chemotherapies as well as radiotherapy. Hence, targeting the apoptosis pathways is considered as an attractive strategy for therapeutic intervention in cancer [7].

MECHANISMS OF APOPTOSIS

Understanding the mechanism of apoptosis formation is vital to comprehending the pathogenic circumstances developed from disordered apoptosis (Fig. **1**) [5]. Apoptosis is triggered either through mitochondria (intrinsic) or death receptor mediated pathways (extrinsic). A myriad of stress signals caused by therapeutics (chemo and radiotherapies) activate the intrinsic pathways of the apoptosis. Subsequently, the signal is relayed to the mitochondria upon the stress, leading to the mitochondrial outer membranes permeabilization (MOMP). This allows the apoptotic proteins including cytochrome c and second mitochondrial-derived activator of caspases (SMAC) to be released into the cytosol from mitochondria. The cytochrome c causes the formation of a multiprotein complex (apoptosome)-cytochrome c, apoptotic protease activating factor 1 (APAF1) and procaspase-9, initially. This causes activation of the caspase-9 activity and downstream caspase cascade from procaspase-9. Further, the release of SMAC stimulates caspase activation by neutralizing IAPs, which regulates apoptosis through inhibition of caspases [5, 6].

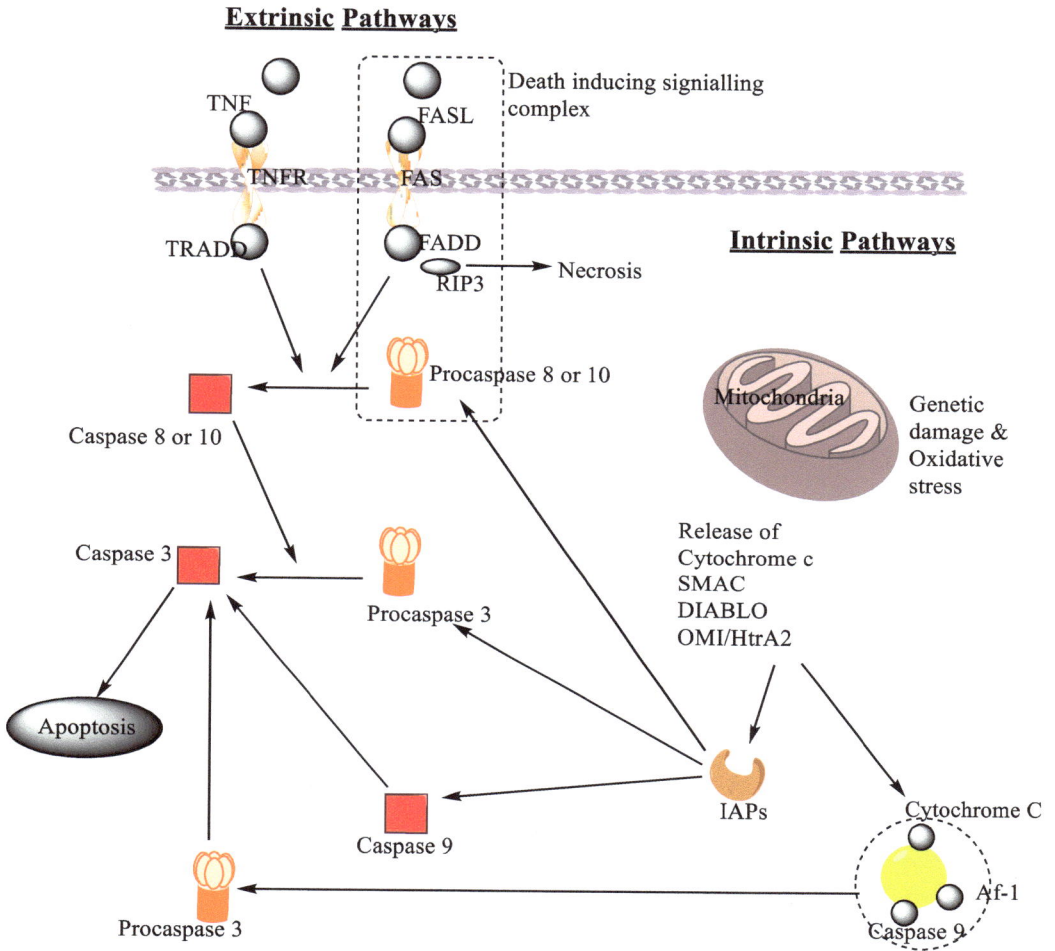

Fig. (1). Mechanism of apoptosis formation [5 - 10].

The extrinsic pathway for the apoptosis regulation is activated through the interactions between the death ligands belong to the tumor necrosis factor (TNF) family *e.g.*, TNFα, TRAIL (TNF-related apoptosis inducing ligand) and the Fas ligand (also known as DR2, CD95 or APO-1) and their cell surface receptors of the TNF receptor (TNFR) superfamily (*e.g.*, TNFR1 and 2, death receptor 4 and 5 and Fas). Similar to the intrinsic pathway, a multiprotein (Fas-FADD and other procaspases) complex is formed at the plasma membrane upon the interactions and this complex makes a signalling platform to activate the initiator caspase-8 (cleaves other non-caspase substrates, such as Bid) and subsequent executioner caspases.

The caspases are grouped as cytokine processing caspases in inflammatory processes (caspase 1 (*e.g.* caspase-1, -4, -5, -13, and -14)) and the caspases play central role in apoptosis (*e.g.* caspase-2, -3, -6, -7,-8, -9 and -10). Those caspases, that are involved in the apoptosis development are further classified into (1) caspases that initiate the apoptotic pathway (initiator caspases (*e.g.* caspase-2, -8, -9 and -10)) and (2) caspases (effector caspases (caspase-3, -6 and -7)), that cleave the cellular components during apoptosis.

The intrinsic and the extrinsic pathways collectively execute the apoptosis is called execution phase and a series of caspases are activated in this phase. The caspase-9 and caspase-8 are the upstream caspase in the intrinsic and extrinsic pathways respectively. These pathways unite at caspase-3, subsequently, the inhibitor of the caspase-activated deoxyribonuclease is cleaved, which results in nuclear apoptosis [5 - 9].

The pro-apoptotic proteins (*e.g.* Bax, Bad, Bcl-Xs, Bid, Bik, Bim and Hrk) and the anti-apoptotic proteins (*e.g.* Bcl-2, Bcl-XL, Bcl-W, Bfl-1 and Mcl-1) are necessary to control the apoptotic pathways. The anti-apoptotic proteins are classified into three major classes such as anti-apoptotic B cell lymphoma 2 (BCL-2) proteins, inhibitor of apoptosis proteins (IAPs) and murine double-minute 2 (MDM2). The BCL family of proteins comprised of pro-apoptotic and anti-apoptotic proteins, which regulate the apoptosis through the intrinsic pathway (act at mitochondrial level) and causes upstream of irreversible cellular damage [10].

TARGETING P53

The p53 is a tumor suppressor protein plays an important role (central role) in the apoptosis regulation, the evasion of antigrowth signals and many other cellular processes including progression of cancer, through both transcription dependent and independent mechanisms. It is also called as tumor protein 53 (or TP53), known as tumor suppressor proteins encoded from TP53 (a tumor suppressor gene) in the chromosome 17 (17p13.1). The name 53 aroused from its molecular weights (53 kDa). Since its discovery in 1979, this protein has become the most intensively investigated proteins in oncology research. Targeting p53-based strategies for cancer treatment are classified as the following categories; 1) gene therapy, 2) immunotherapy and 3) drug therapy [3, 5, 11 - 14].

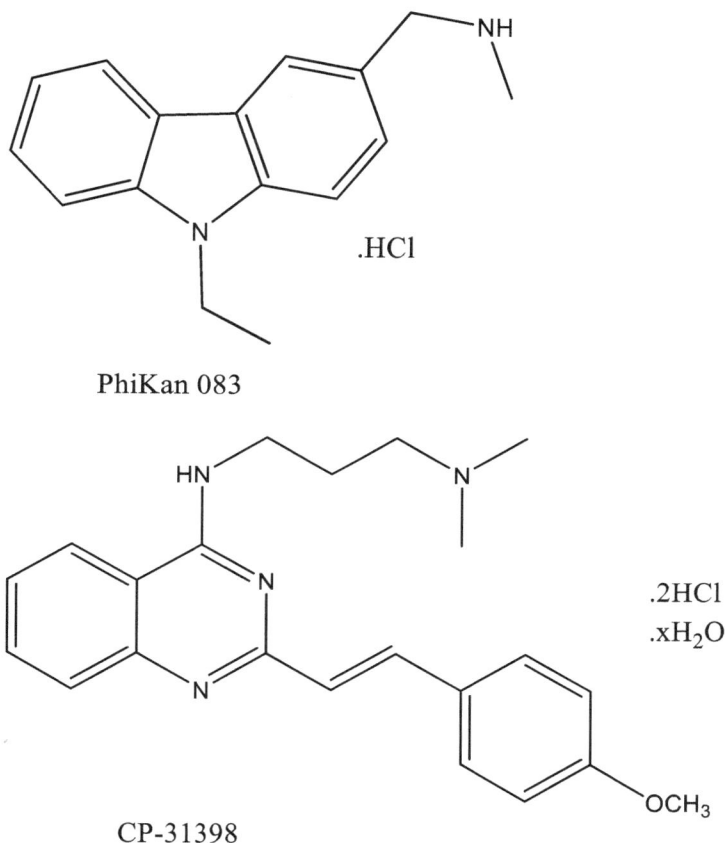

PhiKan 083

CP-31398

Fig. (2). Structure of p53 stabilizing molecules.

p53-based Gene Therapy

The p53-based gene therapy was explored in 1996, using wild-type p53 gene having retroviral vector and was injected into tumor cells of non-small cell lung carcinoma (NSCLC) [15].

p53-based Immunotherapy

p53 vaccines are in clinical research as immunotherapy. A clinical trial conducted by Kuball *et al.* using vaccine made of a recombinant replication-defective adenoviral vector with human wild-type p53 on six patients possess advanced-stage cancer [16].

p53-based Drug Therapy

The drugs that target p53 by different mechanisms including restoration of mutated p53 back to their wild-type functions. Phikan083 (Fig. **2**) is a carbazole derivative interacts with p53 and restore mutant p53. CP-31398 (Fig. **2**) intercalates with DNA causes alteration and destabilization of the DNA-p53 core domain complex, which restores the unstable p53 mutants [17, 18].

ANTI-APOPTOTIC PROTEINS

Targeting the MDM2-p53 Complex

The MDM2 (or its homolog MDMX) is an oncoprotein that inhibits the function of tumor suppressor p53 in almost 50% of the cancer cells through various mechanisms. MDM2 inhibits the function of p53 (transactivation), assists transfer of p53 out of the nucleus, p53 distant to target DNA for transcription and promotes degradation of p53 by the E3 ubiquitin ligase activity. Overexpression of MDM2 in the cells neutralizes the p53 tumor suppressor functions in cell differentiation and can potentiate the tumorigenesis in mice. The inhibitory function occurs by direct binding of MDM2 to p53 create protein-protein interaction complex (MDM2-p53 or MDMX-p53). The inhibition of the MDM2-p53 or MDMX-p53 complex formation, activate p53 in tumor cells and retain its wild-type p53 [19 - 23].

Nutlins

Vassilev and co-workers (2004) (Hoffman-La Roche Inc., Nutley, New Jersey) discovered *cis*-imidazoline analogues for the inhibition of MDM2-p53 complex formation (Fig. **3**). These are first class of MDM2 inhibitors, designated as nutlins and its active enantiomers are randomly named nutlin 1, 2 and 3 [3, 19, 24].

Nutlins mimic p53 by occupying the p53 binding pocket in MDM2, which stabilize and activate the p53 functions in cancer cells [25]. The results of biochemical binding assay on the recombinant MDM2 protein revealed that nutlin-3 is a most potent MDM2 inhibitor (IC_{50}= 90 nM). It has significant cell growth inhibitory activity (IC_{50}= ~1 μM) in p53 wild type cells (SJSA-1, HCT116, and RKO) and decreased activity (IC_{50}= 10 μM) in mutated p53 containing tumor cells (MDA-MB-435 and SW480) [19, 24]. Nutlins also have inhibitory effect on the vascular endothelial growth factor (VEGF), stromal derived factor-1/CXCL12 and osteprotegerin expression and/or release by primary fibroblasts and endothelial cells. Nutlins achieve the therapeutic effects by a direct cytotoxic effect on leukemic cells and an indirect non-cell autonomous effect on tumor stromal and vascular cells. This indirect effect is also used for the treatment of haematological malignancies having p53 mutations [26].

The preclinical studies reported on nutlins suggest that nutlins have different antitumor activity on diverse tumor cell lines carrying dysfunctional wild-type p53. Alongwith doxorubicin, nutlin has synergic antitumor action on wild-type p53 present in chronic B-cell lymphocytic leukemia cells. The antiprostate cancer activity of the nutlin occurred through cell cycle arrest and apoptosis while preserving wild-type p53 and androgen receptor signalling [27, 28]. Currently, nutlin-3 is undergoing phase I study for the treatment of retinoblastoma [29]. Nutlin-3 was also found to be effective in Hodgkin lymphoma and in Ewing's sarcoma cells and has the ability to restore the function of mutated p53 to wild-type p53 [27, 28].

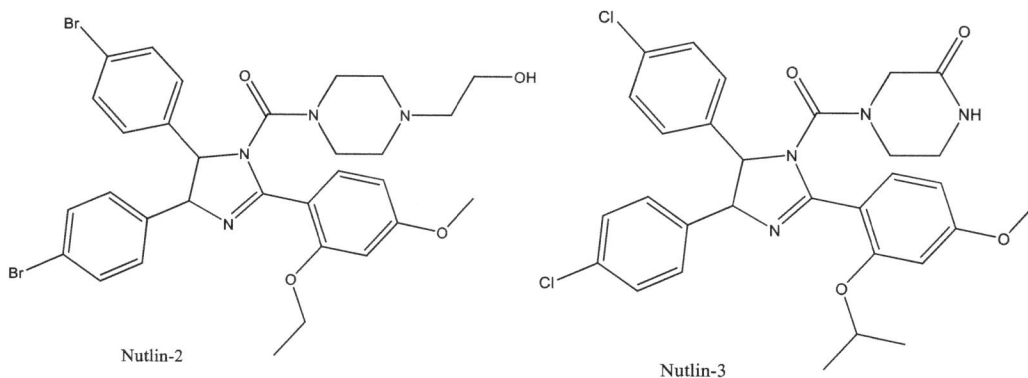

Nutlin-2

Nutlin-3

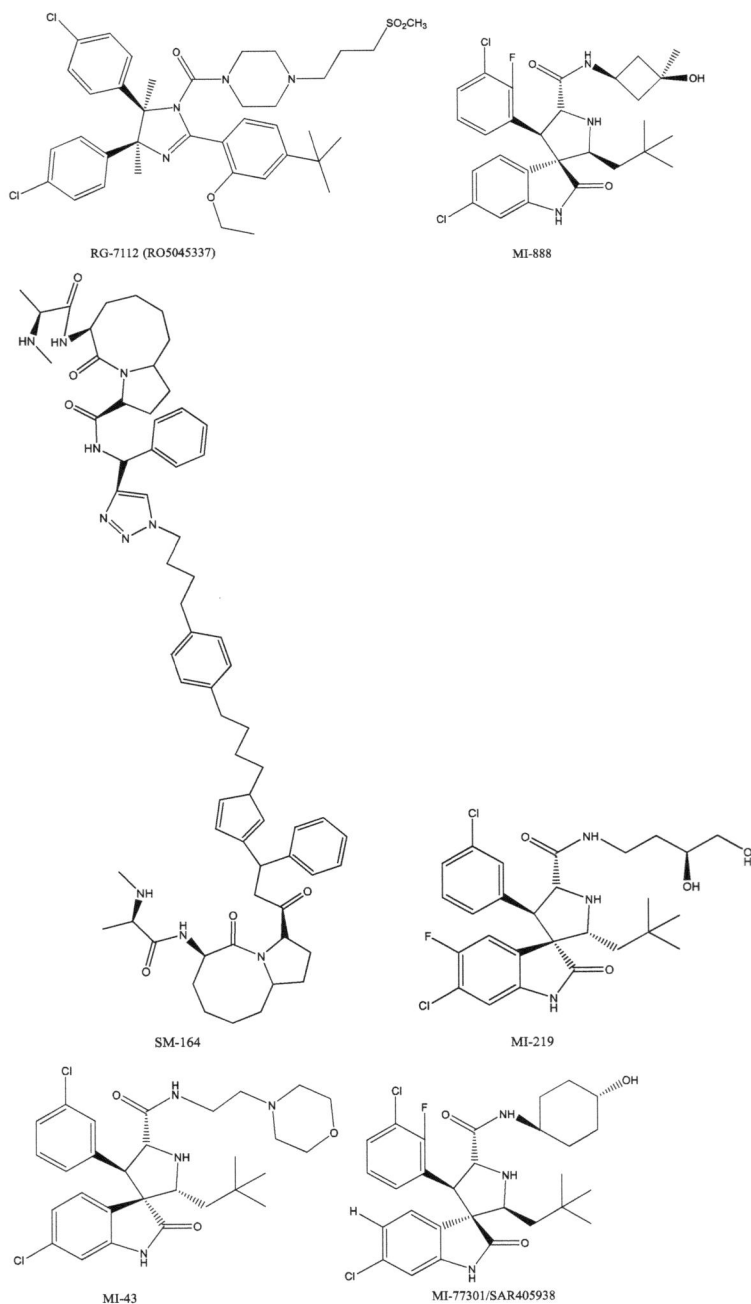

RG-7112 (RO5045337)

MI-888

SM-164

MI-219

MI-43

MI-77301/SAR405938

Fig. (3). Structure of MDM2 and MDMX inhibitors.

RG7112

RG7112 (RO5045337) is the first MDM2 inhibitor to enter clinical trials for a wide range of cancers such as sarcoma, myelogenous leukemia, neoplasms and hematologic neoplasms (ClinicalTrials.gov Identifiers: NCT00559533, NCT00623870, NCT01677780, NCT01164033, NCT01605526, NCT01143740, and NCT01635296) [30]. RG7112 was designed through structure based modification of nutlin-2 and 3 (Fig. **3**). (1) The imidazole ring of the nutlin was substituted with a dimethyl group to reduce or prevent oxidation, (2) The molecular weight was also reduced by the replacement of isopropyl ether in nutlin-3 with ethyl ether in RG7112, while retaining the activity, (3) the metabolic stability of the molecules is enhanced by replacing methyl phenyl ether moiety with *t*-butyl group and (4) a polar group (methyl sulfonyl) was introduced in the urea functionality in RG7112 to improve the MDM2 binding and the pharmacokinetic (PK) properties [19, 31, 32]. The binding affinity of this molecule (RG7112) on MDM2 is enhanced (K_d= 10.7 nM) compared to nutlins. This compound also showed three fold greater growth inhibitory activity than nutlin-3 against cancer cells. Experimental studies in two human osteosarcomas (SJSA-1 and MHMn) and one human prostate tumor (LNCaP) cells in mouse xenograft models revealed that an oral dose at 100 mg/kg daily of RG7112 achieved partial tumor regression [32].

MK-8242 and MI-888

MK-8242 (called as SCH 900242) is in phase I clinical trials for advanced solid tumors or acute myelogenous leukemia as single agent (ClinicalTrials.gov Identifier: NCT01463696 and NCT01451437) [19, 33]. Zhao *et al.* identified the **MI-888** (K_i = 0.44 nM), a MDM2 inhibitor, capable of attaining widespread and durable tumor regression in both SJSA-1 osteosarcoma and RS4;11 acute lymphoblastic leukemia tumor xenograft models. *In vivo* studies on **MI-888** revealed that the molecule showed good *in vivo* efficacy and excellent pharmacokinetic profile [34].

MI-219

The researchers in Wang laboratory at the University of Michigan have developed a spiro-oxindole derivative (MI-219) by structure based *de novo* design, which mimic the key p53 binding residues. This drug binds to MDM2 protein with high affinity, however it has a very high specificity over MDMX and other proteins [6, 35]. MI-219 alone or in combination with MDM2 knockdown, an X-linked inhibitor of apoptosis protein (XIAP) antagonists or etoposide has significant efficacy on a panel of lung cancer cell lines. In WT p53-containing lung cancer cells, MI-219 induces the G1 or G2 arrest in a p53-dependent manner lead to inhibition of growth and has less effect on immortalized cells bearing WT p53. In the combination therapy (with a SMAC mimetic compound (SM-164)), MI-219 increased XIAP expression and SM-164 blocked the XIAP, but SM-164 did not significantly enhance the cytotoxic potency of MI-219 [36 - 38]. MI-219 exerts *in vitro* and *in vivo* antitumor activities through mechanism-based activities. These studies revealed that this drug is not suitable for clinical development because of its high doses (300 mg/kg) and the requirement of an intense schedule (twice daily) to achieve strong antitumor activity *in vivo* [39]. MI-43, an analogue of MI-219, sensitizes the lung cancer cells to etoposide-induced apoptosis. Similar to MI-219, MI-43 kills lung cancer cells harbouring WT p53 selectively [37]. However, the molecule exhibited poor growth inhibition (IC_{50}= 30 µM) in cancer cell lines and also poor oral bioavailability, hence this drug is not further developed in clinical trials [38].

SAR405838 (MI-77301)

The scientists from Wang laboratory, University of Michigan also discovered SAR405838 (MI-77301), analogue of MI-888 with much improved potency and efficacy over MI-219 and is presently undergoing phase I trials (Sanofi S.A in 2012; ClinicalTrials.gov Identifier: NCT01636479). Structurally, SAR405838 differs from MI-219 by its stereochemistry in the quaternary carbon atom, different halogen substitution patterns in both phenyl rings and a conformationally constrained cyclohexanol group. The binding interaction of SAR405838 with MDM2 provided K_i of 0.88 nmol/L, which activates WT p53 *in vitro*. Further, the studies in xenograft tumor tissue of leukemia and solid tumors revealed that SAR405838 causes p53-dependent cell-cycle arrest and/or apoptosis. As MI-888, the SAR405838 also has either durable tumor regression or complete tumor growth inhibition in mouse xenograft models of SJSA-1 osteosarcoma, RS4; acute leukemia, LNCaP prostate cancer and HCT-116 colon cancer at tolerable doses. Interestingly, a single oral dose treatment was found adequate for the entire tumor regression in the SJSA-1 model [19, 39].

CGM097

CGM097 (Novartis), an oral MDM2 inhibitor has progressed into the first human clinical study (phase I study) as single agent for adult patients with selected advanced tumors in 2013 (ClinicalTrials.gov Identifier: NCT01760525) and is characterized by p53 WT status [40]. In oral dose, CGM097 inhibits the interaction between HDM2 protein and the transcriptional activation domain of the tumor suppressor protein p53. Further, the inhibition of the proteosome-mediated enzymatic degradation of p53 leads to the restoration of p53 signalling and apoptosis [41]. The binding kinetics of this complex (CGM097-MDM2) has high association rate constant (K_{on} = 37 x 106 $M^{-1}.s^{-1}$) and a moderate dissociation rate constant (K_{off} = 0.071 s^{-1}). However, CGM097 possessed an 8-fold greater affinity towards MDM2 over nutlin-3 due to its longer residence time [42].

Other MDM2 Inhibitors

DS-3032b developed recently by Daiichi Sankyo Inc, is another MDM2 inhibitor to enter phase I clinical trials (ClinicalTrials.gov Identifier: NCT01877382) [19]. NSC319726 inhibits growth of fibroblasts expression in the p53R175 mutation (IC_{50} = 8 nM) and act as a mutant p53R175 reactivator. This drug is devoid of any inhibitory effects on p53 wild-type cells. MI-773 is an orally available spiro-oxindole exhibits potential antineoplastic activity through inhibiting HDM2 (human double minute 2) [43].

RO5503781 (RG7388, Roche) is a novel class of orally bioavailable MDM2 inhibitor to enter the phase I clinical trials. This drug is being tested as a single agent for advanced malignancies or in combination with cytarabine for AML (ClinicalTrials.gov Identifier: NCT01773408 and NCT01462175) [19, 24]. SJ-172550, a MDMX inhibitor, regulates p53 as MDM2 and directly regulates p53 transcription. Further it is a low micromolar active MDMX inhibitor, binds to the p53 binding pocket of MDMX lead to liberation of p53 to induce apoptosis [44].

Targeting the IAPs

IAPs are 70-80 amino acid segment which plays a key role in the regulation of programmed cell death pathways. IAPs are present at aberrantly high levels in multiple human malignancies hence it acts as favourable targets for the investigation of small-molecular cancer therapeutics. The IAP family made up of eight human proteins and are categorized by the presence of baculovirus IAP repeat (BIR) consist of neuronal IAP (NIAP/BIRC1), cellular IAP1 (cIAP1/BIRC2), cellular IAP2 (cIAP2/BIRC3), X chromosome-linked IAP (XIAP/BIRC4), survivin, BIR-containing ubiquitin-conjugating enzyme (BRUCE/Apollon/BIRC6), livin/melanoma IAP (MLIAP/BIRC7), and IAP-like protein 2 (ILP-2/BIRC8). These protein families contain some structurally and functionally similar proteins responsible for regulation of apoptosis, cytokinine and signal transduction. Targeting IAP-family proteins such as XIAP, cIAP1, Survivin, or Apollon induce apoptosis in tumor cell lines or those cells sensitize to anticancer drugs. IAP proteins such as XIAP, cIAP1, cIAP2 and ML-IAP also contain the Really Interesting New Gene (RING) domain that exhibits E3 ubiquitin ligase activity. Depending on the chain type (*e.g.,* K5-, K11-, K48- or K63-linked chains), ubiquitination can lead to proteasomal degradation of substrates or can alter their signalling properties [5, 7, 25, 45 - 47].

XIAP is reported to be the most important and potent target in all the IAPs for apoptosis development. This protein inhibits both intrinsic as well as extrinsic pathways of apoptosis through action on upstream caspase-9 and the downstream caspases-3 and -7. XIAP interacts to caspase-3, -7, and -9 through its BIR2 or BIR3 domains and inhibits their activities [5, 7, 48].

The binding interactions between the death receptor ligands such as TRAIL, triggers recruitment of adaptor molecules (FADD) and caspase-8 in the extrinsic pathway lead to the activation of caspase-8. Then the link between the extrinsic and the intrinsic pathways is created through caspase-8–mediated cleavage of Bid into tBid. The second mitochondrial activator of caspases (SMAC) is freed into the cytosol, trigger apoptosis by promoting caspase activation. Also the caspases are activated indirectly *via* SMAC-mediated neutralization of IAP proteins. Among the IAP proteins, particularly XIAP, block caspase activation by binding to caspases -3, -7, and -9 through the BIR domains and which affect the intrinsic and the extrinsic apoptosis pathways through negative regulation. The small molecular antagonistics of IAP neutralize the action of IAP and induce apoptosis (Fig. **4**) [5, 7, 45, 49].

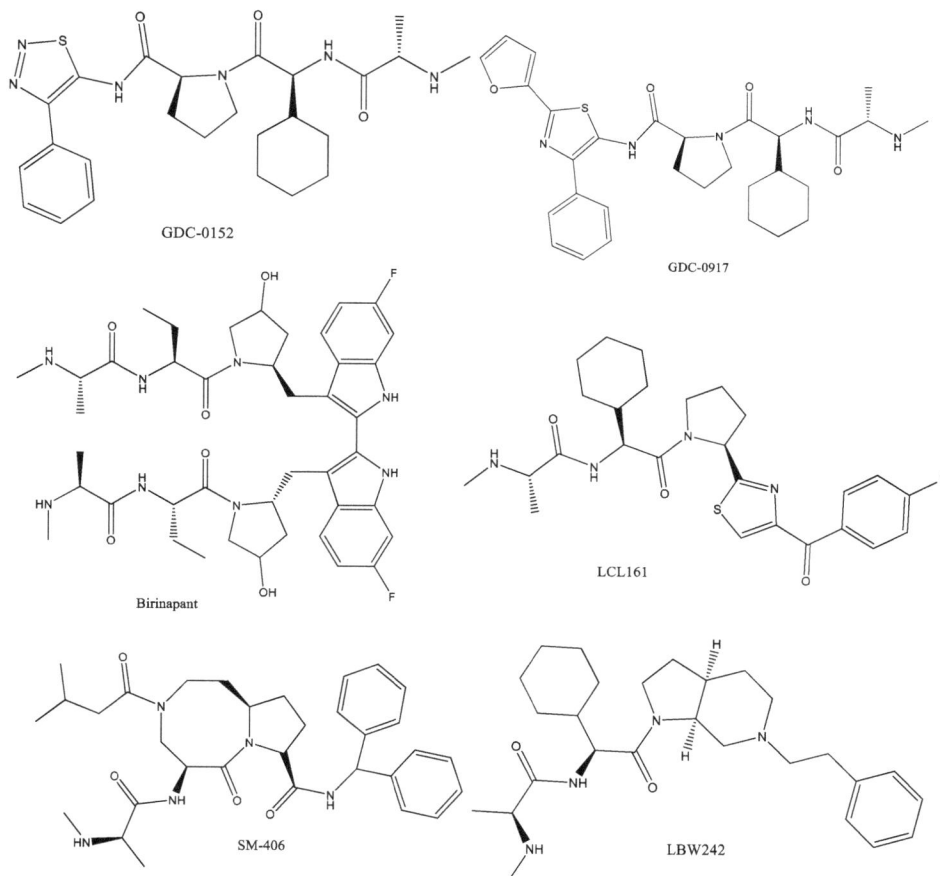

Fig. (4). Structure of IAP antagonists.

OGX-011

OGX-011, an IAP antagonist presently under clinical studies for prostate cancer significantly enhances the apoptotic response and efficacy of chemotherapy, radiation and androgen withdrawal through inhibition of the expression of CLU gene. This drug has been administrated prior to radical prostoctomy and the well tolerated doses has entered into phase II trials [7, 50].

GDC-0152 and GDC-0917 (CUDC-427) (Genentech)

GDC-0152 (S)-1-(S)-2-cyclohexyl-2-([S]-2-methylamino propanamido)acetyl is a potent pan-selective antagonist of IAPs from Genentech and is a first SMAC mimetic compound to enter clinical trials in June 2007. This drug interacts with the BIR3 domain of XIAP, the BIR domain of ML-IAP and the BIR3 domains of cIAP1 and cIAP2 with the Ki values of 28, 14, 17 and 43 nM, respectively. GDC-0152 induces caspase-3/7 activation and apoptosis in tumor cells and also inhibits tumor growth in MDA-MB-231 cells xenografted models. The preclinical pharmacokinetic investigations on the drug administrated through single dose intravenous injection (1 mg/kg) provided high plasma clearance (> 80% of hepatic blood flow) in nude mice, Sprague-Dawley rats and cynomolgus monkeys and a plasma clearance (52% of hepatic blood flow) in beagle dogs. At high doses (100 mg/kg in mice; 20 mg/kg in rats, dogs, and monkeys), significant plasma clearance (saturated) in mouse and rat were observed, while it is less or absent in the monkey and the dog [51, 52]. The human clinical trials on the GDC-0152 showed that it has linear pharmacokinetics on the dose range from 0.049 to 1.48 mg/kg. The allometry and *in vitro/ in vivo* studies gave significant human clearance (9.6 ml/min/kg allometry and 10 ml/min/kg *in vitro- in vivo* extrapolation) in patients (9 ml/min/kg) [51].

More recently, another SMAC mimetic from Genentech, GDC-0917, (S)-1-((S--2-cyclohexyl-2-((S)-2-(methylamino)propanamido)acetyl)-N-(2-(oxazol-2-yl)- 4-phenylthiazol-5-yl)pyrrolidine-2-carboxamide, a potent second-generation IAP antagonist has entered phase I clinical trials as an oral agent. SMAC mimetic (GDC-0917) binds to the SMAC binding groove on IAPs, including XIAP and the cellular IAPs 1 and 2. It inhibits IAP and also promotes the induction of apoptosis through apoptotic signalling pathways. GDC-0917 provides considerable (low to moderate) clearance in the mouse (12.0 ml/min/kg), rat (27.0 ml/min/kg), dog (15.3 ml/min/kg) and significantly high clearance in monkey (67.6 ml/min/kg) [53].

GDC-0917 decreases the cell viability in MDA-MB-231 cancer cells significantly, but showed negligible action on normal human mammary epithelial cells. In contrast to GDC-0152, the GDC-0917 is orally bioavailable. The preclinical toxicology studies using daily dosing in clinic allowed more flexible dosing of drugs. The pharmacokinetic profile of GDC-0917 showed that the drug is mostly eliminated through liver and limited amount *via* kidney. The renal clearance in dog and monkey is estimated to be consistent [51].

Birinapant (TL32711) (TetraLogic Pharmaceuticals): Birinapant, a second generation bivalent SMAC mimetic discovered by TetraLogic pharmaceuticals, induces IAPs and caspase dependent but TNF-α independent apoptosis. Birinapant interacts with the BIR3 domains of cIAP1, cIAP2, XIAP and the BIR domain of ML-IAP *in vitro* and induces autoubiquitylation and proteasomal degradation of cIAP1 and cIAP2 in intact cells, leading to the formation of a RIPK1:caspase-8 complex, caspase-8 activation causes induced tumor cell death. Favourably, this drug (birinapant) also interacts with the TRAF2-associated cIAP1 and cIAP2, subsequently inhibits the TNF-induced NF-kappaB activation. Birinapant in alone or with TNF or TRAIL inhibits TNF-mediated NF-kappaB activity, which induces cell death in a variety of cancer cell lines. The activity of both chemotherapeutic drugs are potentiated in both TNF-dependent and independent manners. Birinapant binds effectively in cIAP1/2 and XIAP in isogenic SUM149- and SUM190-derived cells at nM range and which causes different XIAP expression (SUM149 wtXIAP and SUM190 shXIAP) [6, 54 - 58].

Birinapant was advanced into clinical trials for the treatment of solid tumors and hematological malignancies [59]. The tolerability of this drug is improved with reduced potency to cIAP2 and improved affinity for XIAP BIR3 and also with diminished inhibitory ability to XIAP-dependent signalling pathways. Birinapant does not show any dose-limiting toxicities by intravenous injection reported in phase I study [55]. A phase II study was also performed with the combination of birinapant with irinotecan over irinotecan alone in R/R colorectal cancer patients [57]. Clinical studies are also undergoing for advanced ovarian, fallopian tube and peritoneal cancer [60]. A clinical trial testing of birinapant in combination with the demethylating agent (5-azacytidine) showed synergistic antileukemic effects [61].

GT13402, another SMAC mimetic as Birinapant, has high and low (K_d > 1 μM) binding interaction with cIAP1/2 and XIAP respectively. Furthermore, Birinapant is also shown to cause modest increase in TNF-α production in SUM190 cells not in SUM149 cells [62]. Phase I trials was reported for the IAP antagonists (LCL161, HGS1029 and TL32711) showed well toleration on different cancer cells. These compounds alone or with several combination protocols with IAP antagonists or chemotherapeutics including chemotherapeutic drugs such as taxol, daunorubicin, cytarabine and gemcitabine showed better activity [25, 63 - 65].

AEG40826/HGS1029 (Aegera/Human Genome Sciences)

HGS1029 is a bivalent SMAC mimetic was discovered and licensed by Aegera Therapeutics and Human Genome Sciences respectively for its clinical development, showing a good tolerability profile on transient lymphopaenia (with grade 2) and neutrophilia. The drug also exhibited better pharmacokinetic profiles in advanced solid tumors with the administration of dose-limiting toxicity of HGS1029 on weekly 3 times, repeated every 4 weeks [65 - 67].

LCL161 (Novartis)

LCL161, an orally bioavailable SMAC mimetic (from Novartis), displays antiproliferative activities in tumors as a single agent and synergic effect with paclitaxel in preclinical models. The molecule also entered phase I clinical trials at a weekly dosing schedule (up to 1800 mg weekly dosing) and is well tolerated in patients with advanced cancers with no dose-limiting toxicity. At higher or equal dose (>320 mg of LCL161), the cIAP1 concentrations are reduced steadily which was observed in skin punch biopsies (8 h after the first dose) and in a tumor biopsy (after 24 h). Additionally, a randomized, phase II trial to test weekly dosing of paclitaxel with or without LCL161 in triple negative breast cancer before surgery [64, 67 - 70]. The first-in-human dose-escalation study for the safety, pharmacokinetics and pharmacodynamics of LCL161 in patients with advanced solid tumors has been performed. For this study, 53 patients received at least one dose of LCL161 (dose range, 10 to 3,000 mg) and at 1,800 mg dose, the patients were well tolerated. Further, 1,800 mg of LCL161 as single dose in tablet dosage form is the recommended dose for additional studies [71]. In hepato-cellular carcinoma (HCC) cells, LCL161 induces BCL-2 expression and responsible for anticancer therapy [26].

SM-406/AT-406/Debio 1143 (University of Michigan/Ascenta/DebioPharm)

AT-406 (SM-406/Debio 1143) is a monovalent SMAC mimetic, discovered and licensed for clinical development by University of Michigan [72] and Ascenta Therapeutics/DebioPharm respectively. It is an orally bioavailable compound that interacts with XIAP, cIAP1 and cIAP2 proteins with a binding affinity (K_i) of 66.4, 1.9, and 5.1 nM, respectively. Preclinical studies on the selected cancer cell lines and xenograft tumor models have shown that AT-406 exerts mechanism-based antitumor activity [6, 72]. AT-406 is in two phase I trials including advanced solid tumors and lymphomas, as a single agent and also with other drugs (daunorubicin and cytarabine) [67].

AT-406 was also found to significantly enhance the radiosensitization of HCC193 (TNF-α also contributed sensitization in this sensitive cell) and H460 cells *in vitro* in clinical studies. cIAP1 was depleted in HCC193 cells with lower concentrations of AT-406 than in H460 cells [73]. An appropriate daily dosing (once in a day) on 5 consecutive days in every 3 weeks showed significant pharmacokinetic disposition. However, beyond this dose (>80 mg), no dose relationship was observed between PD and antitumor activity, however all doses induced the degradation of cIAP-1 in PBMCs [74].

SM-164

SM-164 is a bivalent SMAC mimetic which binds to cIAP1 and cIAP2 at low nM range of affinities as AT-406. In cancer cells, especially MDA-MB-231 and other cancer cell lines, SM-164 induces activation of caspases and strong apoptosis as a single agent at <1 nM concentrations. Comparatively, SM-164 is 100–1000 times more potent than its monovalent counterpart (AT-406). Furthermore, intravenous injection of SM-164 in MDA-MB-231 xenograft tumor tissues in mice induces robust apoptosis with a single dose and achieves tumor regression [67, 75, 76].

LBW242

LBW242 is a potent SMAC mimetic discovered by Novartis. LBW242 binds to XIAP and cIAP1 with IC_{50} values of 200 nM and 5 nM, respectively in biotinylated SMAC peptide of the recombinant IAP proteins. As a single agent, it has antitumor activity in human cancer cell lines, including breast cancer cell line (MDA-MB-231). Additionally, it modestly inhibits tumor growth in a model (mouse) of multiple myeloma with oral administration [77 - 79].

Other IAP Antagonists

Several peptidic and non-peptidic molecules including cyclopeptidic SMAC mimetics, 2 and 3 have been demonstrated as IAP antagonists [5, 80]. These molecules have been shown to interact with XIAP and cIAP-1/2 and re-establish the caspases-9 and 3/-7 activities inhibited by XIAP [5, 80].

Targeting the BCL Family of Proteins

The BCL-2 family of proteins inhibit the anti-apoptotic proteins or silencing of the upregulated anti-apoptotic proteins or genes belongs to this family. The apoptosis triggering protein (p53) activates the process in a transcription-independent manner through transporting mono-ubiquitinated p53 to the mitochondria. Subsequently this complex interacts with BCL2 family proteins leading to the activation of Bak or release of Bax from the complexes. This causes the mitochondrial membrane permeabilization, cytochrome-c release and caspase cascade activation [28, 81, 82].

Therapeutic targeting of the pro-survival proteins (BCL family) is one of the promising new targets for anticancer drug development approach that is presently in phase 1/2 clinical trials. The concept of BH3 mimetics is that it mimics the pro-apoptotic BH3-only members through binding and antagonizing the prosurvival members. Designing mimetics of the Noxa BH3 domain, which is a specific antagonistic Mcl-1 ligand, capable of interacting directly with Mcl-1 and efficiently neutralizing its anti-apoptotic activity, which is extremely important to evaluate the clinical significant of patients with CLL [83].

Oblimersen sodium, a BCL-2 antisense has entered clinical trial. This category of the drugs is classified into those affect gene or protein expression (sodium butyrate, depsipetide, fenretinide and flavipirodol) and acting themselves (gossypol, ABT-737, ABT-263, GX15-070, BH3I-1 and HA14-1) (Fig. 5) [5, 84].

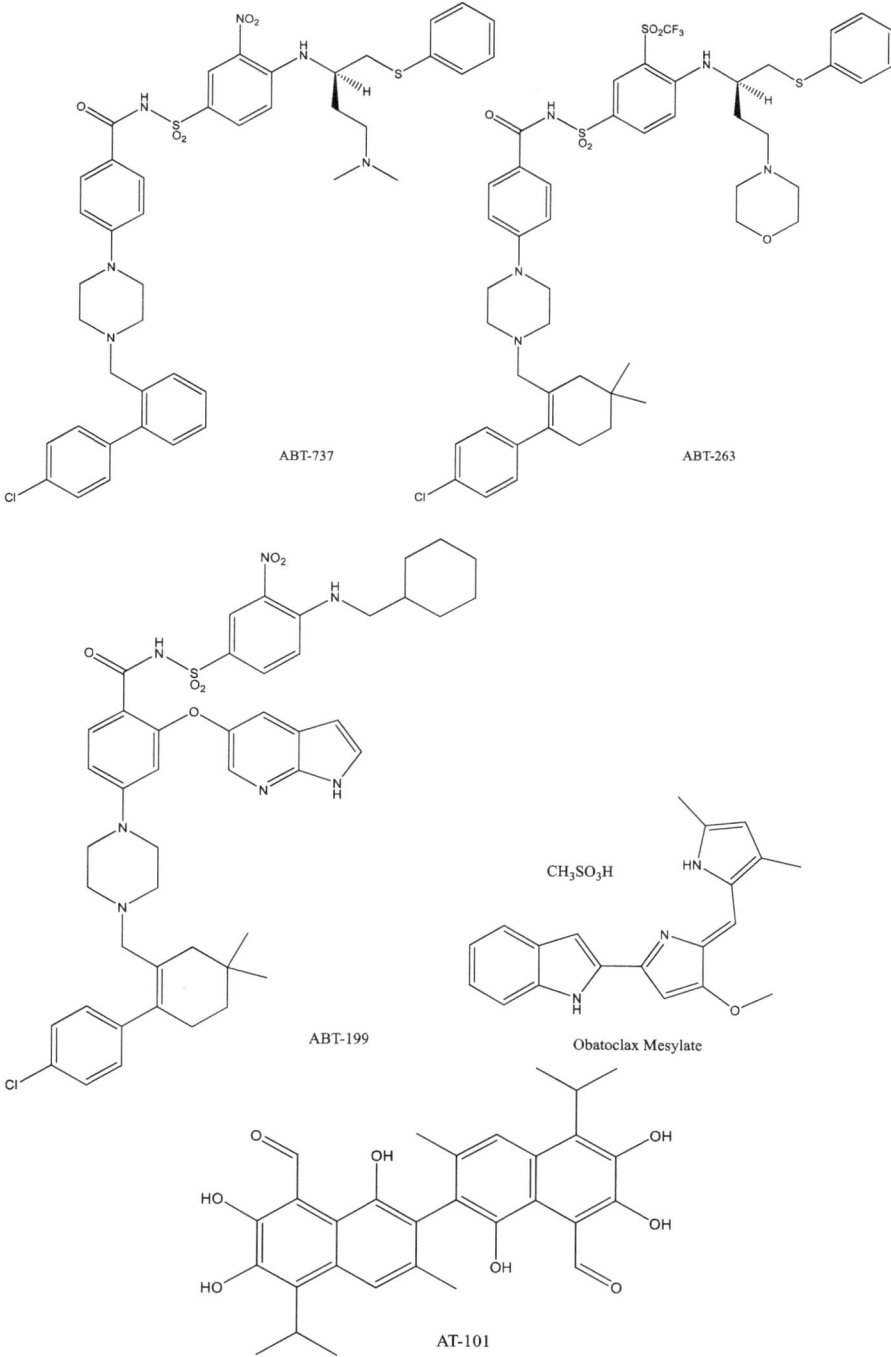

Fig. (5). Structure of drugs targeting BCL family proteins.

ABT-737 and ABT-263 (navitoclax)

ABT-737 is the first small-molecule mimetic discovered to act on the pro-apoptotic BH3 binding domain. It has significant action on multiple BCL family proteins as a single agent and also with other drugs. ABT-737 has equal binding efficiency to BCL-XL, BCL-2, and BCL-w (K_i< 1 nM) but exhibits lower affinity to BFL-1 and Mcl-1 *in vitro*. The molecule was also found to overrule BCL protein mediated apoptosis resistance [85 - 87]. The *in vitro* results on pro-survival BCL proteins (6 proteins) in p53 wild-type or p53-mutant human T-leukemic cells proved that BCL-2 is a better ABT-737 target than BCL-xL and BCL-w. ABT-737 is not effective in displacing BH3-only proteins or Bax from BCL-2 than BCL-xL or BCL-w. ABT-737 exhibited impressive activity profile as a single-agent against leukemias, lymphomas and small-cell lung cancer (SCLC), however it is prone to development of resistance [88].

ABT-263, a structural analogue of ABT-737 is a second-generation Bad-like BH3 mimetic (K_i's of <1 nM/L for BCL-2, BCL-xL and BCL-w) in phase I clinical trials. This molecule was developed to overcome the inefficiencies of ABT-737 [6, 89]. ABT-263 showed 20% to 50% bioavailability according to the type of formulation in preclinical studies. ABT-263 disrupts BCL-2/BCL-xL interactions with Bim protein (a pro-death proteins), which initiates the apoptosis within 2 hr of the post-treatment. The molecule also activates Bax translocation, cytochrome c release and subsequent apoptosis in human tumor cells. Regression of tumors in xenograft models of SCLC and acute lymphoblastic leukemia was observed with oral administration of ABT-263. ABT-263 is currently developed both as a single agent and in combination regimens for the treatment of SCLC and B-cell malignancies [87].

Yamaguchi and co-workers demonstrated that 2-deoxyglucose (2DG) can be used to potentiate ABT-737/263 induced apoptosis in both *in vitro* and *in vivo* on ABT-737/263 resistant cancer cells [90]. ABT-263 has been shown to exhibit synergic action with bortezomib in induction of cancer cell death because of the net neutralization of BCL-XL/BCL-2 (by ABT-263) and Mcl-1 (by bortezomib). ABT-263 also induces a rapid reduction in circulating platelets count in dogs as ABT-737 [87]. Preclinically, both ABT-737 and ABT-263 have been shown to exhibit potent cytotoxicity against a variety of hematologic malignancies. ABT-263 was also shown to induce functional defects in residual circulating platelets, leading to a transient thrombocytopathy undermining its hemostatic function.

HA 14-1, a suggested BCL-2 inhibitor structurally unrelated to ABT-737 and ABT-263, has also been demonstrated to promote apoptosis in tumor cells through its dual actions on the mitochondria and ER initiating ER stress and depleting calcium stores [83, 91].

ABT-199 (GDC-0199/venetoclax, AbbVie)

ABT-199 was developed through structure-guided reverse engineering of ABT-263. ABT-199 showed greater activity in patients with either R/RCLL or R/R non-Hodgkin lymphoma in phase I trials with no significant effects on platelets counts [6, 92]. GDC-0199/ABT-199 inhibits BCL-2 by displacing the sequestered pro-apoptotic proteins which are freely available to promote the release of cytochrome c and the activation of caspases, leading to apoptosis [92 - 94]. ABT-199 monotherapy showed antitumor activity across a range of ABT-199 cohort doses for several NHL subtypes, most notably in Mcl and WM [95].

A phase II study is undergoing to ascertain the pharmacological and safety issues of ABT-199 (GDC-0199) in CLL subjects with relapse or refractory to β-cell receptor signalling pathway inhibitor therapy [96]. A phase II study on ABT-199/GDC-0199 in patients with acute myelogenous leukemia (AML) showed 15.5% overall response rate (ORR) with variation in response. Among the studied patients, complete response observed on all patients but four patients showed incomplete blood count recovery [97].

ABT-263, ABT-737 and ABT-199 were found to accelerate the death of virus infected (with IAV and other viruses) non-cancerous mammalian cells by caspase-9-mediated mitochondria. Further, the administration of these drugs to the infected animals caused premature cell death and affected the innate immune responses to viral infections leading to lower survival rates. Hence, ABT-263, ABT-737 and ABT-199 are hazardous for virus infected cancer patients [98].

ABT-263 and ABT-199 have also demonstrated efficacy in early clinical trials. S1 induces NOXA-dependent sensitization to ABT-737 in a human promyelocytic leukemia cell line (NB4). Furthermore, S1 sensitized CLL cells to ABT-737 (*ex vivo*) and overcame resistance to ABT-737 induced by co-culturing CLL cells with stroma. The deoxyglucose-ABT-263/737 combination is a safe and effective alternative to the genotoxin-based chemotherapies [90].

Obatoclax Mesylate (GX15-070) (Gemin X/Teva)

Obatoclax (GX15-070), a synthetic indole bipyrrole derivative of putative BH3 mimetics, has been shown to interact with BCL-2, BCL-xL and Mcl-1 in low affinity (micromolar range) [99, 100]. It is a promiscuous BCL family inhibitor that binds to BCL-2, BCL-XL, BCL-w, BCLB, BFL-1 and MCL-1 in *in vitro*, albeit with very low affinities than those of ABT-263 to BCL-2, BCL-XL and BCL-w [101, 102]. Phase I trials in leukemia and lymphoma showed that this drug has transient neurotoxicity as single-agent and antitumor activity was reported in several hematologic malignancies, including AML, myelodysplastic syndrome and Hodgkin's and non-Hodgkin's lymphoma. Phase II combination trials are ongoing for hematological malignancies and advanced solid tumors [24, 103 - 105].

Phase 2 study of obatoclax in relapsed or refractory CHL were administrated at least 1 dose of obatoclax and 80 cycles were administrated totally (with the median 4 cycles per patient (range 1-24)). Plasma concentrations of obatoclax evaluated at 3, 23 and 25 hr after the first cycle of therapy in 11 patients showed the median concentrations were 6.25 ± 1.04 ng/mL, 4.96 ± 1.15 ng/mL, and 2.65 ± 0.44 ng/mL, respectively [106, 107]. The phase II studies showed that there is no clinically relevant safety differences between the 20 mg/day (3 hr 63 d; n = 7) and 60 mg/day (24 hr 63 d; n = 5) arms. Obatoclax 20 mg/day was the MTD (3 hr 63 d) in older patients with AML [105].

Dose-finding studies were designed to evaluate the initial safety and pharmacokinetics of intravenously injected obatoclax (once weekly) in patients with solid tumors or lymphoma. Obatoclax was infused initially for 1 hr duration and 3 hr infusion duration in the second study. Patients were continued their treatment as long as obatoclax was well tolerated and there was no evidence of disease progression observed. The BCL-2 anti-apoptotic protein BCL-XL is highly expressed in CNS neurons, suggesting that CNS symptoms may be due to target effects. Another BCL family antagonist, ABT-737 has been shown to alter the recovery of synaptic responses *in vitro* after repetitive synaptic activity, but ABT-737 is too large to transfer the blood-brain barrier. Thus, it is possible that the CNS effects of obatoclax may be due to the target effects [108, 109].

The combination of obatoclax with ABT-737 induced apoptosis in OCI-AML3 leukemic cells. Obatoclax with cytosine arabinoside induced aopotosis in leukemic and in primary AML cell lines. The results on these studies suggest that obatoclax potentiates the effect of other drugs (established drugs) in AML. Clinical trials conducted on obatoclax with other conventional chemotherapeutics have been completed in solid tumors and hematologic malignancies (*e.g.*, NCT00612612, NCT00521144 at clinicaltrials.gov) [105, 110, 111].

AT-101 R-(−)-gossypol (Ascenta)

AT-101, denoted as (-)-gossypol is a polyphenolic compound derived from cotton seeds and roots, possessed pan-BCL-2 inhibitory activity. It mimics the BH3 domain of the cellular BCL-2 protein which affects the prosurvival BCL-2 protein functions and has affinity towards BCL-2, BCL-XL and Mcl-1 at submicromolar concentrations. In tumor cells, AT-101 expressed high levels of BCL-XL and/or BCL-2 than in normal cells (*e.g.* fibroblasts, keratinocytes), leading to apoptosis. Among the two enantiomers of the racemic (±)-gossypol, the (-)-gossypol (called as AT-101) interacts with BCL-XL, BCL-2 and Mcl-1, which induces apoptosis better than (+)-gossypol [112, 113].

AT-101 exerts significant cytotoxicity on drug resistant cell lines and multiple myeloma cell lines through apoptosis initiation. The apoptotic effect was activated through mitochondrial pathway (in multiple myeloma cell lines) by increasing the Bax to BCL-2 ratio, mitochondrial membrane depolarization and caspase activation [113]. Phase I/ II trials of AT-101 in CLL have indicated only limited single-agent therapeutic efficacy. Several gossypol derivatives (acting predominantly through BH3 mimicry) including apogossypolone (ApoG2) were reported to induce apoptosis in CLL cells and are under clinical trials. AT-101 and its derivative ApoG2 are more stable and less toxic than other gossypol-derived compound (TW37) [114 - 116]. Early phase II trials with either monotherapy or combination with conventional chemotherapeutics in prostate and lung cancers have failed to deliver significant clinical activity. Furthermore, several phase II combination trials are undergoing for head and neck squamous cell carcinoma and advanced laryngeal cancer [6].

AT-101 alone or with radiation induces apoptosis in leukemic, Jurkat T and U937 cell lines. This process occurred through the activated SAPK/JNK pathway, which is needed for apoptosis induction and further BCL-XL inhibits activation of SAPK/JNK. The concentration necessary for activation of apoptosis by AT-101 is 1.9 and 2.4 µM (ED$_{50}$) in Jurkat T and U937 cells, respectively. The agonistic action of AT-101 on SAPK/JNK is blocked by the kinase inhibitor SP600125. Combinations of AT-101 and cytotoxic drugs demonstrated to have synergistic antitumor effects *in vitro* and *in vivo* SCLC models [112].

OTHER APOPTOSIS INDUCERS [44]

Apoptolidin A is a 20-membered macrolide produced by *Nocardiopsis* species. Apoptolidin (A-D) induces apoptosis selectively in rat glia cells. All apoptolidins were inhibiting growth of H292 cancer cells (lung carcinoma) in the submicromolar range. Ara-G is an inducer of apoptosis possessed multiple functions as inhibitor of DNA synthesis, antineoplastic and antimetabolite. Cellular kinases convert this drug into the active 5′-triphosphate, Ara-GTP, which can inserted into DNA leads to inhibition of DNA synthesis and apoptosis. BAM7, a selective activator of BAX, binds directly to the BAX trigger site, a distinct BH3 binding site that regulates BAX activation, inducing BAX oligomerization, which enables the release of apoptogenic factors resulting in cell death.

β-cyclodextrin complex of Violacein, an indole derivative, was found to induce apoptosis and cytotoxicity in HL60 leukemic cells. It activates caspases-8, transcription of NF-kappaB target genes and p38-MAPK resembling TNF-α signal transduction for the cytotoxic activity.

Zerumbone is a TRAIL-induced apoptosis potentiator, which plays an active role in the upregulation of DR4 and DR5 expression and downregulation of cFLIP. It is a sesquiterpine, isolated from *Zingiber zerumbet* Smith. Tirapazamine induces apoptosis by inducing breaks in single and double stranded DNA as well as chromosomal breaks. It sensitizes cells to ionizining radiations and anticancer drugs. Taurolidine is used with TRAIL to characterize synergizing effect of other apoptosis related signalling proteins. It also used as a study tool to understand various mechanisms of apoptosis and necrosis.

Ridaifen-B (RID-B), a tamoxifen analog, augments apoptosis inducing effect of TAM in estrogen receptor-negative cells. RID-B was found to induce mitochondria involved apoptosis and activate caspases-3, 8 and 9 in Jurkat cells. The mechanism by which RID-B exerts apoptosis is under investigation. RID-B shows significant cytotoxicity on number of cancer cell lines.

Penta-O-galloyl-β-D-glucose hydrate (PGG) induces apoptosis (caspase dependent) in DU145 and LNCaP cells. PRIMA-1 is a selective reactivator of p53 in mutant tumor cells and it restores sequence specific DNA binding and transactivational activity to mutant p53 proteins. Nitidine chloride is a natural product capable of activating caspase dependent pathway for apoptosis induction. Muristerone, a native phytosteroid induces apoptosis in cell transfected with wild-type Bax and ecdysone-inducible gene expression system. LLP-3, cell permeable survivin inhibitor of survivin-ran complex induces apoptosis in tumor slice cultures. Gambogic acid is a caspase activator and inducer of apoptosis. It irreversibly arrest G2/M phase in the cell cycle. DIM-3-pPhtBu causes apoptotic cell death in KB cells by activation of ER stress. DBeQ potently inhibits cellular proliferation and induces caspase 3/7 activity and apoptosis. CIL-102 acts as an apoptosis inducer and tubulin polymerization inhibitor. CD437 and DMXAA are potent inducers of apoptosis [44].

This chapter concludes that apoptosis and related pathways have now become one of the most important targets for anticancer drug discovery. Our increased understanding of defective pathways regulating apoptosis in cancer has revealed numerous druggable targets for cancer drug discovery. This in turn has resulted in the discovery of many novel agents that specifically targets components (MDM2, IAP and BCL family proteins) of apoptosis pathways in cancer cells with clinical effectiveness either as single agents or in combination with conventional chemo-therapeutic agents and radiation therapy. Concerted efforts towards development of apoptosis-based therapeutics for cancer would help to improve the clinical outcome for wide range of cancers alongwith with existing chemotherapeutic agents.

CONFLICT OF INTEREST

The authors confirm that they have no conflict of interest to declare for this publication.

ACKNOWLEDGEMENTS

N.S.H.N.M. gratefully acknowledges the Fundação para a Ciência e Tecnologia (FCT), Portugal for a Postdoctoral Grant (SFRH/BPD/44469/2008). Authors (N.S.H.N. Moorthy and C. Karthikeyan) have designed and prepared this chapter. All authors contributed have analysed the contents on this chapter and further proof reading. Authors are thankful to all authors of the articles/clinical studies used for this chapter preparation.

REFERENCES

[1]   Available at: http://www.iarc.fr/en/publications/books/wcr/wcr-order.php

[2]   Available at: http://www.who.int/mediacentre/factsheets/fs297/en/

[3]   Costa OD. Nutlins: A novel therapeutic strategy for inhibiting the MDM2-p53 interaction in cancer? TSMJ 2005; 6: 74-7.

[4]   Kerr JF, Wyllie AH, Currie AR. Apoptosis: a basic biological phenomenon with wide-ranging implications in tissue kinetics. Br J Cancer 1972; 26(4): 239-57.
        [http://dx.doi.org/10.1038/bjc.1972.33] [PMID: 4561027]

[5]   Wong RS. Apoptosis in cancer: from pathogenesis to treatment. J Exp Clin Cancer Res 2011; 30: 87.
        [http://dx.doi.org/10.1186/1756-9966-30-87] [PMID: 21943236]

[6]   Bai L, Wang S. Targeting apoptosis pathways for new cancer therapeutics Annu Rev Med 2014; 65: 20.1-20.17..
        [http://dx.doi.org/10.1146/annurev-med-010713-141310]

[7]   Hassan M, Watari H, Almaaty AA, Ohba Y, Sakuragi N. Apoptosis and molecular targeting therapy in cancer. BioMed Res Int 2014; 2014: (Article ID 150845)

[8]   Ghobrial IM, Witzig TE, Adjei AA. Targeting apoptosis pathways in cancer therapy. CA Cancer J Clin 2005; 55(3): 178-94.
        [http://dx.doi.org/10.3322/canjclin.55.3.178] [PMID: 15890640]

[9]   Fink SL, Cookson BT. Apoptosis, pyroptosis, and necrosis: mechanistic description of dead and dying eukaryotic cells. Infect Immun 2005; 73(4): 1907-16.
[http://dx.doi.org/10.1128/IAI.73.4.1907-1916.2005] [PMID: 15784530]

[10]   Gross A, McDonnell JM, Korsmeyer SJ. BCL-2 family members and the mitochondria in apoptosis. Genes Dev 1999; 13(15): 1899-911.
[http://dx.doi.org/10.1101/gad.13.15.1899] [PMID: 10444588]

[11]   Suzuki K, Matusubara H. Recent advances in p53 research and cancer treatment. J Biomed Biotech 2011; 2011: 978312.

[12]   Chène P. p53 as a drug target in cancer therapy. Expert Opin Ther Patents 2001; 11(6): 923-35.

[13]   Levine AJ, Momand J, Finlay CA. The p53 tumour suppressor gene. Nature 1991; 351(6326): 453-6.
[http://dx.doi.org/10.1038/351453a0] [PMID: 2046748]

[14]   Bai L, Zhu WG. p53: structure, function and therapeutic applications. J Cancer Mol 2006; 2(4): 141-53.

[15]   Roth JA, Nguyen D, Lawrence DD, *et al.* Retrovirus-mediated wild-type p53 gene transfer to tumors of patients with lung cancer. Nat Med 1996; 2(9): 985-91.
[http://dx.doi.org/10.1038/nm0996-985] [PMID: 8782455]

[16]   Kuball J, Schuler M, Antunes Ferreira E, *et al.* Generating p53-specific cytotoxic T lymphocytes by recombinant adenoviral vector-based vaccination in mice, but not man. Gene Ther 2002; 9(13): 833-43.
[PMID: 12080377]

[17]   Boeckler FM, Joerger AC, Jaggi G, Rutherford TJ, Veprintsev DB, Fersht AR. Targeted rescue of a destabilized mutant of p53 by an *in silico* screened drug. Proc Natl Acad Sci USA 2008; 105(30): 10360-5.
[http://dx.doi.org/10.1073/pnas.0805326105] [PMID: 18650397]

[18]   Rippin TM, Bykov VJ, Freund SM, Selivanova G, Wiman KG, Fersht AR. Characterization of the p53-rescue drug CP-31398 *in vitro* and in living cells. Oncogene 2002; 21(14): 2119-29.
[http://dx.doi.org/10.1038/sj.onc.1205362] [PMID: 11948395]

[19]   Zhao Y, Bernard D, Wang S. Small molecule inhibitors of MDM2-p53 and MDMX-p53 interaction as new cancer therapeutics. Biodiscovery 2013; 8: 4.
[http://dx.doi.org/10.7750/BioDiscovery.2013.8.4]

[20]   Freedman DA, Wu L, Levine AJ. Functions of the MDM2 oncoprotein. Cell Mol Life Sci 1999; 55(1): 96-107.
[http://dx.doi.org/10.1007/s000180050273] [PMID: 10065155]

[21]   Wu X, Bayle JH, Olson D, Levine AJ. The p53-mdm-2 autoregulatory feedback loop. Genes Dev 1993; 7(7A): 1126-32.
[http://dx.doi.org/10.1101/gad.7.7a.1126] [PMID: 8319905]

[22]   Juven-Gershon T, Oren M. MDM2: the ups and downs. Mol Med 1999; 5(2): 71-83.
[PMID: 10203572]

[23]   Ganguli G, Abecassis J, Wasylyk B. MDM2 induces hyperplasia and premalignant lesions when

expressed in the basal layer of the epidermis. EMBO J 2000; 19(19): 5135-47.
[http://dx.doi.org/10.1093/emboj/19.19.5135] [PMID: 11013216]

[24]   Vassilev LT, Vu BT, Graves B, *et al. In vivo* activation of the p53 pathway by small-molecule antagonists of MDM2. Science 2004; 303(5659): 844-8.
[http://dx.doi.org/10.1126/science.1092472] [PMID: 14704432]

[25]   Fulda S. Molecular pathways: targeting inhibitor of apoptosis proteins in cancer--from molecular mechanism to therapeutic application. Clin Cancer Res 2014; 20(2): 289-95.
[http://dx.doi.org/10.1158/1078-0432.CCR-13-0227] [PMID: 24270683]

[26]   Tian A, Wilson GS, Lie S, *et al.* Synergistic effects of IAP inhibitor LCL161 and paclitaxel on hepatocellular carcinoma cells. Cancer Lett 2014; 351(2): 232-41.
[http://dx.doi.org/10.1016/j.canlet.2014.06.006] [PMID: 24976294]

[27]   Drakos E, Thomaides A, Medeiros LJ, *et al.* Inhibition of p53-murine double minute 2 interaction by nutlin-3A stabilizes p53 and induces cell cycle arrest and apoptosis in Hodgkin lymphoma. Clin Cancer Res 2007; 13(11): 3380-7.
[http://dx.doi.org/10.1158/1078-0432.CCR-06-2581] [PMID: 17545546]

[28]   Puszynski K, Gandolfi A, d'Onofrio A. The pharmacodynamics of the p53-MDM2 targeting drug Nutlin: the role of gene-switching noise. PLOS Comput Biol 2014; 10(12): e1003991.
[http://dx.doi.org/10.1371/journal.pcbi.1003991] [PMID: 25504419]

[29]   Secchiero P, Bosco R, Celeghini C, Zauli G. Recent advances in the therapeutic perspectives of Nutlin-3. Curr Pharm Des 2011; 17(6): 569-77.
[http://dx.doi.org/10.2174/138161211795222586] [PMID: 21391907]

[30]   Ray-Coquard I, Blay JY, Italiano A, *et al.* Effect of the MDM2 antagonist RG7112 on the P53 pathway in patients with MDM2-amplified, well-differentiated or dedifferentiated liposarcoma: an exploratory proof-of-mechanism study. Lancet Oncol 2012; 13(11): 1133-40.
[http://dx.doi.org/10.1016/S1470-2045(12)70474-6] [PMID: 23084521]

[31]   Vu B, Wovkulich P, Pizzolato G, *et al.* Discovery of RG7112: A small-molecule MDM2 inhibitor in clinical development. ACS Med Chem Lett 2013; 4(5): 466-9.
[http://dx.doi.org/10.1021/ml4000657] [PMID: 24900694]

[32]   Tovar C, Graves B, Packman K, *et al.* MDM2 small-molecule antagonist RG7112 activates p53 signaling and regresses human tumors in preclinical cancer models. Cancer Res 2013; 73(8): 2587-97.
[http://dx.doi.org/10.1158/0008-5472.CAN-12-2807] [PMID: 23400593]

[33]   Perez-Moreno P, Brambilla E, Thomas R, Soria JC. Squamous cell carcinoma of the lung: molecular subtypes and therapeutic opportunities. Clin Cancer Res 2012; 18(9): 2443-51.
[http://dx.doi.org/10.1158/1078-0432.CCR-11-2370] [PMID: 22407829]

[34]   Zhao Y, Yu S, Sun W, *et al.* A potent small-molecule inhibitor of the MDM2-p53 interaction (MI-888) achieved complete and durable tumor regression in mice. J Med Chem 2013; 56(13): 5553-61.
[http://dx.doi.org/10.1021/jm4005708] [PMID: 23786219]

[35]   Shangary S, Qin D, McEachern D, *et al.* Temporal activation of p53 by a specific MDM2 inhibitor is selectively toxic to tumors and leads to complete tumor growth inhibition. Proc Natl Acad Sci USA 2008; 105(10): 3933-8.

[http://dx.doi.org/10.1073/pnas.0708917105] [PMID: 18316739]

[36]   Gu L, Zhu N, Zhang H, Durden DL, Feng Y, Zhou M. Regulation of XIAP translation and induction by MDM2 following irradiation. Cancer Cell 2009; 15(5): 363-75.
[http://dx.doi.org/10.1016/j.ccr.2009.03.002] [PMID: 19411066]

[37]   Sun SH, Zheng M, Ding K, Wang S, Sun Y. A small molecule that disrupts MDM2-p53 binding activates p53, induces apoptosis and sensitizes lung cancer cells to chemotherapy. Cancer Biol Ther 2008; 7(6): 845-52.
[http://dx.doi.org/10.4161/cbt.7.6.5841] [PMID: 18340116]

[38]   Zheng M, Yang J, Xu X, Sebolt JT, Wang S, Sun Y. Efficacy of MDM2 inhibitor MI-219 against lung cancer cells alone or in combination with MDM2 knockdown, a XIAP inhibitor or etoposide. Anticancer Res 2010; 30(9): 3321-31.
[PMID: 20944104]

[39]   Wang S, Sun W, Zhao Y, *et al.* SAR405838: an optimized inhibitor of MDM2-p53 interaction that induces complete and durable tumor regression. Cancer Res 2014; 74(20): 5855-65.
[http://dx.doi.org/10.1158/0008-5472.CAN-14-0799] [PMID: 25145672]

[40]   A phase I dose escalation study of CGM097 in adult patients with selected advanced solid tumors (CCGM097X2101). https://clinicaltrials.gov/ct2/show/NCT01760525, [20/03/2015]

[41]   p53/HDM2 interaction inhibitor CGM097. http://www.cancer.gov/drug-dictionary?cdrid=744999, [20/03/2015]

[42]   Valat T, Masuya K, Baysang F, *et al.* Abstract 1798: Mechanistic study of NVP-CGM097: a potent, selective and species specific inhibitor of p53-MDM2. Cancer Res 2014; 74: 1798.
[http://dx.doi.org/10.1158/1538-7445.AM2014-1798]

[43]   NVP-CGM097(CGM-097) is a potent and selective MDM2 inhibitor; an orally bioavailable HDM2 antagonist with potential antineoplastic activity. http://www.medchem-express.com/ NVP-CGM097.html, [20/03/2015]

[44]   http://www.sigmaaldrich.com/life-science/cell-biology/cell-biology-products.html?TablePage=956032 3., [20/03/2015]

[45]   Fulda S, Vucic D. Targeting IAP proteins for therapeutic intervention in cancer. Nat Rev Drug Discov 2012; 11(2): 109-24.
[http://dx.doi.org/10.1038/nrd3627] [PMID: 22293567]

[46]   Fulda S. Regulation of cell migration, invasion and metastasis by IAP proteins and their antagonists. Oncogene 2014; 33(6): 671-6.
[http://dx.doi.org/10.1038/onc.2013.63] [PMID: 23474760]

[47]   Vucic D, Dixit VM, Wertz IE. Ubiquitylation in apoptosis: a post-translational modification at the edge of life and death. Nat Rev Mol Cell Biol 2011; 12(7): 439-52.
[http://dx.doi.org/10.1038/nrm3143] [PMID: 21697901]

[48]   Dai Y, Lawrence TS, Xu L. Overcoming cancer therapy resistance by targeting inhibitors of apoptosis proteins and nuclear factor-kappa B. Am J Transl Res 2009; 1(1): 1-15.
[PMID: 19966933]

[49] Fulda S, Debatin KM. Extrinsic *versus* intrinsic apoptosis pathways in anticancer chemotherapy. Oncogene 2006; 25(34): 4798-811.
[http://dx.doi.org/10.1038/sj.onc.1209608] [PMID: 16892092]

[50] John M, Hinke A, Stauch M, *et al.* FAKT Study Group. Weekly paclitaxel plus trastuzumab in metastatic breast cancer pretreated with anthracyclines-a phase II multipractice study. BMC Cancer 2012; 12: 165.
[http://dx.doi.org/10.1186/1471-2407-12-165] [PMID: 22559145]

[51] Wong H, Gould SE, Budha N, *et al.* Learning and confirming with preclinical studies: modeling and simulation in the discovery of GDC-0917, an inhibitor of apoptosis proteins antagonist. Drug Metab Dispos 2013; 41(12): 2104-13.
[http://dx.doi.org/10.1124/dmd.113.053926] [PMID: 24041744]

[52] Flygare JA, Beresini M, Budha N, *et al.* Discovery of a potent small-molecule antagonist of inhibitor of apoptosis (IAP) proteins and clinical candidate for the treatment of cancer (GDC-0152). J Med Chem 2012; 55(9): 4101-13.
[http://dx.doi.org/10.1021/jm300060k] [PMID: 22413863]

[53] https://www.tititudorancea.net/z/smac_mimetic_gdc_0917.htm, [10/03/2015]

[54] Allensworth JL, Sauer SJ, Lyerly HK, Morse MA, Devi GR. SMAC mimetic Birinapant induces apoptosis and enhances TRAIL potency in inflammatory breast cancer cells in an IAP-dependent and TNF-α-independent mechanism. Breast Cancer Res Treat 2013; 137(2): 359-71.
[http://dx.doi.org/10.1007/s10549-012-2352-6] [PMID: 23225169]

[55] Amaravadi RK, Schilder RJ, Dy GK, *et al.* Phase 1 study of the SMAC mimetic TL32711 in adult subjects with advanced solid tumors and lymphoma to evaluate safety, pharmacokinetics, pharmacodynamics, and antitumor activity. 102nd Proc Annu Meet Am Assoc Cancer Res. Apr. 2–6; Orlando, FL. 2011.

[56] Amaravadi RK, Senzer NN, Martin L, *et al.* A phase I study of birinapant (TL32711) combined with multiple chemotherapies evaluating tolerability and clinical activity for solid tumor patients. J Clin Oncol 2013; 31. [Suppl.].

[57] Senzer N, LoRusso P, Martin L, *et al.* Phase II clinical activity and tolerability of the SMAC mimetic birinapant (TL32711) plus irinotecan in irinotecan-relapsed/refractory metastatic colorectal cancer. J Clin Oncol 2013; 31. [Suppl.].

[58] Benetatos CA, Mitsuuchi Y, Burns JM, *et al.* Birinapant (TL32711), a bivalent SMAC mimetic, targets TRAF2-associated cIAPs, abrogates TNF-induced NF-κB activation, and is active in patient-derived xenograft models. Mol Cancer Ther 2014; 13(4): 867-79.
[http://dx.doi.org/10.1158/1535-7163.MCT-13-0798] [PMID: 24563541]

[59] Condon SM, Mitsuuchi Y, Deng Y, *et al.* Birinapant, a SMAC-mimetic with improved tolerability for the treatment of solid tumors and hematological malignancies. J Med Chem 2014; 57(9): 3666-77.
[http://dx.doi.org/10.1021/jm500176w] [PMID: 24684347]

[60] Birinapant for advanced ovarian, fallopian tube, and peritoneal cancer. https://clinicaltrials.gov/ct2/show/NCT01681368, [10/03/2015]

[61] Steinhart L, Belz K, Fulda S. SMAC mimetic and demethylating agents synergistically trigger cell

death in acute myeloid leukemia cells and overcome apoptosis resistance by inducing necroptosis. Cell Death Dis 2013; 4: e802.
[http://dx.doi.org/10.1038/cddis.2013.320] [PMID: 24030154]

[62]   Allensworth JL, Sauer SJ, Lyerly HK, Morse MA, Devi GR. SMAC mimetic birinapant induces apoptosis and enhances TRAIL potency in inflammatory breast cancer cells in an IAP-dependent and TNF-α-independent mechanism. Breast Cancer Res Treat 2013; 137(2): 359-71.
[http://dx.doi.org/10.1007/s10549-012-2352-6] [PMID: 23225169]

[63]   Frey NV, Luger S, Mangan J, *et al.* A phase I study using single agent birinapant in patients with relapsed myelodysplastic syndrome and acute myelogenous leukemia. 56th ASH Annual Meeting and Exposition. Dec 6-9, 2014; San Francisco, CA. 2014.

[64]   Infante JR, Dees EC, Burris HA, *et al.* A phase I study of LCL-161, an oral inhibitor, in patients with advanced cancer. Proceedings of the 2010 Annual Meeting of the American Association for Cancer Research. Washington, DC. 2010.

[65]   Sikic BI, Eckhardt SG, Gallant G, *et al.* Safety, pharmocokinetics (PK), and pharmacodynamics (PD) of HGS1029, an inhibitor of apoptosis protein (IAP), in patients (Pts.) with advanced solid tumors: Results of a phase I study. J Clin Oncol 2012; 29. [suppl].

[66]   A study of HGS1029 (AEG40826-2HCl) in subjects with advanced solid tumors.https://clinicaltrials.gov/ct2/show/NCT00708006, [13/03/2015]

[67]   Wang S, Bai L, Lu J, Liu L, Yang CY, Sun H. Targeting inhibitors of apoptosis proteins (IAPs) for new breast cancer therapeutics. J Mammary Gland Biol Neoplasia 2012; 17(3-4): 217-28.
[http://dx.doi.org/10.1007/s10911-012-9265-1] [PMID: 23054134]

[68]   Sharma SK, Straub C, Zawel L. Development of peptidomimetics targeting IAPs. Int J Pept Res Ther 2006; 12(1): 21-32.
[http://dx.doi.org/10.1007/s10989-005-9003-2] [PMID: 19617919]

[69]   Dienstmann R, Vidal L, Dees EC, *et al.* A phase Ib study of LCL161, an oral inhibitor of apoptosis (IAP) antagonist, in combination with weekly paclitaxel in patients with advanced solid tumors Cancer Res 2012; 72((Suppl. 24)): P6–11-06.

[70]   Houghton PJ, Kang MH, Reynolds CP, *et al.* Initial testing (stage 1) of LCL161, a SMAC mimetic, by the Pediatric Preclinical Testing Program. Pediatr Blood Cancer 2012; 58(4): 636-9.
[http://dx.doi.org/10.1002/pbc.23167] [PMID: 21681929]

[71]   Infante JR, Dees EC, Olszanski AJ, *et al.* Phase I dose-escalation study of LCL161, an oral inhibitor of apoptosis proteins inhibitor, in patients with advanced solid tumors. J Clin Oncol 2014; 32(28): 3103-10.
[http://dx.doi.org/10.1200/JCO.2013.52.3993] [PMID: 25113756]

[72]   Cai Q, Sun H, Peng Y, *et al.* A potent and orally active antagonist (SM-406/AT-406) of multiple inhibitor of apoptosis proteins (IAPs) in clinical development for cancer treatment. J Med Chem 2011; 54(8): 2714-26.
[http://dx.doi.org/10.1021/jm101505d] [PMID: 21443232]

[73]   Liu1 N, Tao Z, Le Blanc JM, *et al.* Debio 1143, an antagonist of multiple inhibitor-of-apoptosis proteins, activates apoptosis and enhances radiosensitization of non-small cell lung cancer cells *in*

vitro. Am J Cancer Res 2014; 4(6): 943-51.

[74]   Hurwitz HI, Smith DC, Pitot HC, *et al.* Safety, pharmacokinetics, and pharmacodynamic properties of oral DEBIO1143 (AT-406) in patients with advanced cancer: results of a first-in-man study. Cancer Chemother Pharmacol 2015; 75(4): 851-9.
        [http://dx.doi.org/10.1007/s00280-015-2709-8] [PMID: 25716544]

[75]   Varfolomeev E, Blankenship JW, Wayson SM, *et al.* IAP antagonists induce autoubiquitination of c-IAPs, NF-kappaB activation, and TNF alpha-dependent apoptosis. Cell 2007; 131(4): 669-81.
        [http://dx.doi.org/10.1016/j.cell.2007.10.030] [PMID: 18022362]

[76]   Vince JE, Wong WW, Khan N, *et al.* IAP antagonists target cIAP1 to induce TNF alpha-dependent apoptosis. Cell 2007; 131(4): 682-93.
        [http://dx.doi.org/10.1016/j.cell.2007.10.037] [PMID: 18022363]

[77]   Chauhan D, Neri P, Velankar M, *et al.* Targeting mitochondrial factor SMAC/DIABLO as therapy for multiple myeloma (MM). Blood 2007; 109(3): 1220-7.
        [http://dx.doi.org/10.1182/blood-2006-04-015149] [PMID: 17032924]

[78]   Gaither A, Porter D, Yao Y, *et al.* A SMAC mimetic rescue screen reveals roles for inhibitor of apoptosis proteins in tumor necrosis factor-alpha signaling. Cancer Res 2007; 67(24): 11493-8.
        [http://dx.doi.org/10.1158/0008-5472.CAN-07-5173] [PMID: 18089776]

[79]   Li L, Thomas RM, Suzuki H, De Brabander JK, Wang X, Harran PG. A small molecule SMAC mimic potentiates TRAIL- and TNFalpha-mediated cell death. Science 2004; 305(5689): 1471-4.
        [http://dx.doi.org/10.1126/science.1098231] [PMID: 15353805]

[80]   Sun H, Liu L, Lu J, *et al.* Cyclopeptide SMAC mimetics as antagonists of IAP proteins. Bioorg Med Chem Lett 2010; 20(10): 3043-6.
        [http://dx.doi.org/10.1016/j.bmcl.2010.03.114] [PMID: 20443226]

[81]   Tian XJ, Liu F, Zhang XP, Li J, Wang W. A two-step mechanism for cell fate decision by coordination of nuclear and mitochondrial p53 activities. PLoS One 2012; 7(6): e38164.
        [http://dx.doi.org/10.1371/journal.pone.0038164] [PMID: 22679490]

[82]   Chipuk JE, Kuwana T, Bouchier-Hayes L, *et al.* Direct activation of Bax by p53 mediates mitochondrial membrane permeabilization and apoptosis. Science 2004; 303(5660): 1010-4.
        [http://dx.doi.org/10.1126/science.1092734] [PMID: 14963330]

[83]   Schoenwaelder SM, Jackson SP. Bcl-xL-inhibitory BH3 mimetics (ABT-737 or ABT-263) and the modulation of cytosolic calcium flux and platelet function. Blood 2012; 119(5): 1320-1.
        [http://dx.doi.org/10.1182/blood-2011-10-387399] [PMID: 22308285]

[84]   Kang MH, Reynolds CP. Bcl-2 inhibitors: targeting mitochondrial apoptotic pathways in cancer therapy. Clin Cancer Res 2009; 15(4): 1126-32.
        [http://dx.doi.org/10.1158/1078-0432.CCR-08-0144] [PMID: 19228717]

[85]   Chen S, Dai Y, Harada H, Dent P, Grant S. Mcl-1 down-regulation potentiates ABT-737 lethality by cooperatively inducing Bak activation and Bax translocation. Cancer Res 2007; 67(2): 782-91.
        [http://dx.doi.org/10.1158/0008-5472.CAN-06-3964] [PMID: 17234790]

[86]   Oltersdorf T, Elmore SW, Shoemaker AR, *et al.* An inhibitor of Bcl-2 family proteins induces regression of solid tumours. Nature 2005; 435(7042): 677-81.

[http://dx.doi.org/10.1038/nature03579] [PMID: 15902208]

[87]   Tse C, Shoemaker AR, Adickes J, *et al*. ABT-263: a potent and orally bioavailable Bcl-2 family inhibitor. Cancer Res 2008; 68(9): 3421-8.
[http://dx.doi.org/10.1158/0008-5472.CAN-07-5836] [PMID: 18451170]

[88]   Rooswinkel RW, van de Kooij B, Verheij M, Borst J. Bcl-2 is a better ABT-737 target than Bcl-xL or Bcl-w and only Noxa overcomes resistance mediated by Mcl-1, Bfl-1, or Bcl-B. Cell Death Dis 2012; 3: e366.
[http://dx.doi.org/10.1038/cddis.2012.109] [PMID: 22875003]

[89]   Soderquist R, Pletnev AA, Danilov AV, Eastman A. The putative BH3 mimetic S1 sensitizes leukemia to ABT-737 by increasing reactive oxygen species, inducing endoplasmic reticulum stress, and upregulating the BH3-only protein NOXA. Apoptosis 2014; 19(1): 201-9.
[http://dx.doi.org/10.1007/s10495-013-0910-y] [PMID: 24072590]

[90]   Yamaguchi R, Janssen E, Perkins G, Ellisman M, Kitada S, Reed JC. Efficient elimination of cancer cells by deoxyglucose-ABT-263/737 combination therapy. PLoS One 2011; 6(9): e24102.
[http://dx.doi.org/10.1371/journal.pone.0024102] [PMID: 21949692]

[91]   Vogler M, Hamali HA, Sun XM, *et al*. BCL2/BCL-X(L) inhibition induces apoptosis, disrupts cellular calcium homeostasis, and prevents platelet activation. Blood 2011; 117(26): 7145-54.
[http://dx.doi.org/10.1182/blood-2011-03-344812] [PMID: 21562047]

[92]   Souers AJ, Leverson JD, Boghaert ER, *et al*. ABT-199, a potent and selective BCL-2 inhibitor, achieves antitumor activity while sparing platelets. Nat Med 2013; 19(2): 202-8.
[http://dx.doi.org/10.1038/nm.3048] [PMID: 23291630]

[93]   Touzeau C, Dousset C, Le Gouill S, *et al*. The Bcl-2 specific BH3 mimetic ABT-199: a promising targeted therapy for t(11;14) multiple myeloma. Leukemia 2014; 28(1): 210-2.
[http://dx.doi.org/10.1038/leu.2013.216] [PMID: 23860449]

[94]   Selective BCL-2 inhibitor (GDC-0199/ABT-199) BCL-http://www.biooncology.com/pipeline-molecules/bcl-2, 2015

[95]   Davids MS, Seymour JF, Gerecitano JF, *et al*. Phase I study of ABT-199 (GDC-0199) in patients with relapsed/refractory (R/R) non-Hodgkin lymphoma (NHL): Responses observed in diffuse large B-cell (DLBCL) and follicular lymphoma (FL) at higher cohort doses J Clin Oncol 2014; 32: 5s. (suppl; abstract 8522)

[96]   A phase 2 open-label study of the efficacy and safety of ABT-199 (GDC-0199) in chronic lymphocytic leukemia (CLL) subjects with relapse or refractory to B-cell receptor signaling pathway inhibitor therapy. https://clinicaltrials.gov/ct2/show/NCT02141282, [13/03/2015]

[97]   AbbVie presents results from phase 2 study of investigational compound venetoclax (ABT-199/GD-0199) in acute myelogenous leukemia at the 56th American Society of Hematology Annual Meeting. http://www.prnewswire.com/news-releases/abbvie-presents-results-fr, [13/03/2015]

[98]   Kakkola L, Denisova OV, Tynell J, *et al*. Anticancer compound ABT-263 accelerates apoptosis in virus-infected cells and imbalances cytokine production and lowers survival rates of infected mice. Cell Death Dis 2013; 4: e742.
[http://dx.doi.org/10.1038/cddis.2013.267] [PMID: 23887633]

[99]   Lessene G, Czabotar PE, Colman PM. BCL-2 family antagonists for cancer therapy. Nat Rev Drug Discov 2008; 7(12): 989-1000.
[http://dx.doi.org/10.1038/nrd2658] [PMID: 19043450]

[100]   Khaw SL, Huang DC, Roberts AW. Overcoming blocks in apoptosis with BH3-mimetic therapy in haematological malignancies. Pathology 2011; 43(6): 525-35.
[http://dx.doi.org/10.1097/PAT.0b013e32834b1b34] [PMID: 21881535]

[101]   Zhai D, Jin C, Satterthwait AC, Reed JC. Comparison of chemical inhibitors of antiapoptotic Bcl--family proteins. Cell Death Differ 2006; 13(8): 1419-21.
[http://dx.doi.org/10.1038/sj.cdd.4401937] [PMID: 16645636]

[102]   Nguyen M, Marcellus RC, Roulston A, *et al.* Small molecule obatoclax (GX15-070) antagonizes MCL-1 and overcomes MCL-1-mediated resistance to apoptosis. Proc Natl Acad Sci USA 2007; 104(49): 19512-7.
[http://dx.doi.org/10.1073/pnas.0709443104] [PMID: 18040043]

[103]   Schimmer AD, O'Brien S, Kantarjian H, *et al.* A phase I study of the pan Bcl-2 family inhibitor obatoclax mesylate in patients with advanced hematologic malignancies. Clin Cancer Res 2008; 14(24): 8295-301.
[http://dx.doi.org/10.1158/1078-0432.CCR-08-0999] [PMID: 19088047]

[104]   Hwang JJ, Kuruvilla J, Mendelson D, *et al.* Phase I dose finding studies of obatoclax (GX15-070), a small molecule pan-BCL-2 family antagonist, in patients with advanced solid tumors or lymphoma. Clin Cancer Res 2010; 16(15): 4038-45.
[http://dx.doi.org/10.1158/1078-0432.CCR-10-0822] [PMID: 20538761]

[105]   Schimmer AD, Raza A, Carter TH, *et al.* A multicenter phase I/II study of obatoclax mesylate administered as a 3- or 24-hr infusion in older patients with previously untreated acute myeloid leukemia. PLoS One 2014; 9(10): e108694.
[http://dx.doi.org/10.1371/journal.pone.0108694] [PMID: 25285531]

[106]   Parikh SA, Kantarjian H, Schimmer A, *et al.* Phase II study of obatoclax mesylate (GX15-070), a small-molecule BCL-2 family antagonist, for patients with myelofibrosis. Clin Lymphoma Myeloma Leuk 2010; 10(4): 285-9.
[http://dx.doi.org/10.3816/CLML.2010.n.059] [PMID: 20709666]

[107]   Oki Y, Copeland A, Hagemeister F, *et al.* Experience with obatoclax mesylate (GX15-070), a small molecule pan-Bcl-2 family antagonist in patients with relapsed or refractory classical Hodgkin lymphoma. Blood 2012; 119(9): 2171-2.
[http://dx.doi.org/10.1182/blood-2011-11-391037] [PMID: 22383790]

[108]   Hickman JA, Hardwick JM, Kaczmarek LK, Jonas EA. Bcl-xL inhibitor ABT-737 reveals a dual role for Bcl-xL in synaptic transmission. J Neurophysiol 2008; 99(3): 1515-22.
[http://dx.doi.org/10.1152/jn.00598.2007] [PMID: 18160428]

[109]   Hwang JJ, Kuruvilla J, Mendelson D, *et al.* Phase I dose finding studies of obatoclax (GX15-070), a small molecule pan-BCL-2 family antagonist, in patients with advanced solid tumors or lymphoma. Clin Cancer Res 2010; 16(15): 4038-45.
[http://dx.doi.org/10.1158/1078-0432.CCR-10-0822] [PMID: 20538761]

[110] Rahmani M, Aust MM, Attkisson E, Williams DC Jr, Ferreira-Gonzalez A, Grant S. Inhibition of Bcl-2 antiapoptotic members by obatoclax potently enhances sorafenib-induced apoptosis in human myeloid leukemia cells through a Bim-dependent process. Blood 2012; 119(25): 6089-98.
[http://dx.doi.org/10.1182/blood-2011-09-378141] [PMID: 22446485]

[111] Parikh SA, Kantarjian H, Schimmer A, *et al.* Phase II study of obatoclax mesylate (GX15-070), a small-molecule BCL-2 family antagonist, for patients with myelofibrosis. Clin Lymphoma Myeloma Leuk 2010; 10(4): 285-9.
[http://dx.doi.org/10.3816/CLML.2010.n.059] [PMID: 20709666]

[112] Leal TA, Schelman WR, Traynor AM, *et al.* A phase I study of r-(-)-gossypol (AT-101, NSC 726190) in combination with cisplatin (P) and etoposide (E) in patients with advanced solid tumors and extensive-stage small cell lung cancer (ES-SCLC). J Clin Oncol. 28(15 suppl): e13030-289. ASCO Annual Meeting Abstracts

[113] Kline MP, Rajkumar SV, Timm MM, *et al.* R-(-)-gossypol (AT-101) activates programmed cell death in multiple myeloma cells. Exp Hematol 2008; 36(5): 568-76.
[http://dx.doi.org/10.1016/j.exphem.2008.01.003] [PMID: 18346839]

[114] Billard C. Apoptosis inducers in chronic lymphocytic leukemia. Oncotarget 2014; 5(2): 309-25.
[http://dx.doi.org/10.18632/oncotarget.1480] [PMID: 24525395]

[115] Billard C. Development of Noxa-like BH3 mimetics for apoptosis-based therapeutic strategy in chronic lymphocytic leukemia. Mol Cancer Res 2012; 10(6): 673-6.
[http://dx.doi.org/10.1158/1541-7786.MCR-12-0015] [PMID: 22466256]

[116] Balakrishnan K, Aggarwal S, Wierda W, Gandhi V. Bax and Bak are required for apogossypolone, a BH3 mimetic, induced apoptosis in chronic lymphocytic leukemia Leuk Lymphoma 2012; 54: 1097-100.
[http://dx.doi.org/10.1158/1541-7786.MCR-12-0015] [PMID: 22466256]

SUBJECT INDEX

A

Acetylation 390, 402, 403, 409, 410, 412

Acetyl CoA 278, 279, 281, 303, 306, 410, 411, 415

Acetyl-coenzyme A 387

Acetyl group 391, 411

Activation of AMPK 396, 401, 408

Activity 13, 272, 273, 304, 309
  anticancer 272, 273, 304
  significant 13, 309

Acute myeloid leukemia (AML) 286, 293, 301, 349, 351, 390, 416, 419, 465, 475, 476, 477

Adenocarcinomas 41, 292, 293, 295

Adoptive cell-therapy 326

Advanced lung cancer 14

Advanced melanoma 221, 227, 231, 234, 236, 237, 241, 242, 243, 244, 245

Advanced NSCLC 14, 15, 31, 33, 63, 65, 302

Advanced solid tumors 295, 296, 299, 300, 304, 463, 470, 471, 476

Aerobic glycolysis 272, 277, 282, 283, 284, 286, 310, 311, 388, 394, 406

Aerobic respiration 277, 278, 280, 299, 305, 311

Afatinib 3, 9, 18, 45, 51, 64, 79, 142, 145, 185

Agios pharmaceuticals 294, 295, 296

Aipha-ketoglutarate 286, 313, 395, 416, 417, 418, 420, 421, 422

Alkylating agents 219, 220, 222, 336

American joint committee on cancer (AJCC) 218

Amino acids 4, 40, 54, 391, 394, 413, 415

Amphiregulin 4, 20, 81, 188

AMPK activity in cancer cells 396

Anderson cancer center 289, 290, 291, 292, 293, 297

Anthracycline 13, 290, 335

Anti-apoptotic proteins 454, 458, 460, 472

Anticancer 273, 288, 299, 301, 305, 308, 309

Anticancer drug discovery 455, 479

Anticancer drugs 303, 454, 466, 479

Anti-EGFR agents 26, 29, 34, 48, 53, 62, 66, 68, 76, 77, 142, 147, 164, 181, 187

Anti-EGFR inhibitors 9, 10, 56, 59, 69, 74, 75, 158, 159, 175, 176, 181, 183, 185, 186

Anti-EGFR therapeutics 3, 9, 80, 142, 164, 186

Anti-EGFR therapy 19, 20, 43, 54, 57, 61, 63, 64, 68, 73, 146, 150, 159, 166, 175
  resistance mechanisms to 5, 164

Antigen-presenting cells (APCs) 234, 236

Antigens 230, 234, 350, 351, 353, 354, 356, 358, 359
  cancer-testis 230, 232

Anti-idiotype vaccines 325, 326

Antitumor activity 348, 461, 471, 472, 476

Apoptosis 10, 285, 454, 455, 456, 457, 458, 464, 465, 466, 467, 468, 474, 475, 477, 478, 479
  formation 456, 457

H

I